Rob & Smith's
Operative Surgery

Surgery of the Colon, Rectum and Anus

Fifth Edition

General Editors

David C. Carter MD, FRCS(Ed), FRCS(Glas)
Regius Professor of Clinical Surgery, Royal Infirmary,
Edinburgh, UK

R. C. G. Russell MS, FRCS
Consultant Surgeon, Middlesex Hospital and Royal National
Throat, Nose and Ear Hospital, London, UK

Consulting Editor

Hugh Dudley CBE, ChM, FRCS(Ed), FRACS, FRCS
Emeritus Professor, St Mary's Hospital, London, UK

Art Editor

Gillian Lee FMAA, HonFIMI, AMI, RMIP
15 Little Plucketts Way, Buckhurst Hill, Essex, UK

Other volumes available in the series

Rob & Smith's
Operative Surgery

Surgery of the Colon, Rectum and Anus

Edited by

L. P. Fielding MB, FRCS, FACS

Chief of Surgery, St Mary's Hospital, Waterbury, Connecticut, Clinical Professor of Surgery, Yale University School of Medicine, New Haven, Connecticut, USA and Visiting Clinical Scientist, St Mary's Hospital, London, UK

S. M. Goldberg MD, FACS, FRACS

Clinical Professor of Surgery and Director, Division of Colon and Rectal Surgery, University of Minnesota Medical School, Minneapolis, Minnesota, USA

Fifth Edition

Butterworth–Heinemann Ltd
Linacre House, Jordan Hill, Oxford OX2 8DP, UK

ℛ A member of the Reed Elsevier group

OXFORD   LONDON   BOSTON
MUNICH   NEW DELHI   SINGAPORE   SYDNEY
TOKYO   TORONTO   WELLINGTON

First published 1993

First edition 1957
Second edition 1969
Third edition 1977
Fourth edition 1983

British Library Cataloguing in Publication Data
Rob & Smith's Operative Surgery. –
Surgery of the Colon, Rectum and Anus. –
5Rev.ed
  I. Fielding, L. P.
  II. Goldberg, Stanley M.
  617.4

  ISBN 0-7506-1255-X

Library of Congress Cataloging-in-Publication Data
(Revised for vol. 2)
Rob & Smith's operative surgery. – 5th ed.
   Includes bibliographical references and index.
   Contents: [1] Genitourinary – [2] Surgery of the colon, rectum, and anus.
   1. Surgery, Operative. I. Rob, Charles.
II. Smith of Marlow, Rodney Smith, Baron, 1914–
III. Dudley, Hugh A. F. (Hugh Arnold Freeman)
IV. Carter, David C. (David Craig) V. Russell,
R. C. G. V. Title: Rob and Smith's operative
surgery. [DNLM: 1. Surgery, Operative.
WO 500/R6282]
RD32R63 1993   617'.91   92-22884
ISBN 0-7506-1255-X

Composition by Genesis Typesetting, Laser Quay, Rochester, Kent
Printed and bound in Hong Kong

Contributors

J. Alexander-Williams MD, FRCS, FACS
Professor of Gastrointestinal Surgery, The General Hospital, Birmingham B4 6NH, UK

T. G. Allen-Mersh MD, FRCS
Consultant Surgeon, Westminster Hospital, London SW1P 2AP, UK

D. N. Armstrong MD, FRCSEd
Department of Surgery, Yale University School of Medicine, New Haven, Connecticut 06511, USA

R. W. Bailey MD
Division Head, General Surgery, Greater Baltimore Medical Center, Baltimore, Maryland 21202, USA

L. W. Baker FRCSEd, FRCS, MSc, FNU
Professor Emeritus, Department of Surgery, University of Natal, Durban 4052, South Africa

G. H. Ballantyne MD, FACS, FASCRS
Associate Professor of Surgery, Department of Surgery, Yale University School of Medicine, New Haven, Connecticut 06511, USA

D. C. C. Bartolo MS, FRCS, FRCSEd
Consultant Surgeon, Department of Surgery, University of Edinburgh, Royal Infirmary, Edinburgh EH3 9YW, UK

J. U. Bascom MD, PhD, FACS
Consulting and Attending Surgeon, Sacred Heart General Hospital, 655 E 11th Avenue, Eugene, Oregon 97401, USA

R. W. Beart Jr MD
Professor of Surgery, Mayo Clinic, 13400 East Shea Boulevard, Scottsdale, Arizona 85259, USA

D. E. Beck MD, FACS, FASCRS
Staff Colorectal Surgeon, Department of Colon and Rectal Surgery, Oschner Clinic, New Orleans, Louisiana, USA

A. Berger MD
Consultant Surgeon, Hôpital Laennec, 42 rue de Sèvres, F-75007 Paris, France

O. Bernell MD
General Surgeon, Department of Surgery, Huddinge University Hospital, S-14186 Huddinge, Sweden

E. L. Bokey MS, FRACS
University of Sydney, Department of Colon and Rectal Surgery, Concord Hospital, Concord, New South Wales, Australia

J. C. Bonello MD
Associate Professor of Surgery and Head, Department of Surgery, University of Illinois College of Medicine at Urbana-Champaign, and Program Director, Colon and Rectal Residency Program, Carle Clinic Association, Urbana, Illinois 61801, USA

B. Bordelon MD
Department of Surgery, University of Utah School of Medicine, 50 North Medical Drive, Salt Lake City, Utah 84132, USA

H. Brevinge MD
Department of Surgery, Sahlgrenska Hospital, 413 45 Göteborg, Sweden

M. P. Bubrick MD
Associate Professor, Department of Surgery, University of Minnesota and Chief of Surgery, Hennepin County Medical Center, Minneapolis, Minnesota 55415, USA

G. Buess MD, FRCSEd
Minimal Invasive Surgery, Department of Surgery, Eberhard-Karl University, Schnarrenberg Hospital, D7400 Tübingen, Germany

P. H. Chapuis DS, FRACS
University of Sydney, Department of Colon and Rectal Surgery, Concord Hospital, Concord, New South Wales, Australia

A. M. Cohen MD
Chief, Colorectal Service, Department of Surgery, Memorial Sloan-Kettering Cancer Center, 1275 York Avenue, New York, NY 10021, USA

Z. Cohen MD, FRCS(C), FACS
Professor of Surgery, University of Toronto, 600 University Avenue, STE 451, Toronto, Ontario, Canada

D. E. Cutait MD, FACS, FRCS(Hon)
Associate Professor of Surgery, Medical School of the University of São Paulo and Clinical Director, Hospital Sírio-Libanês, São Paulo 01427, Brazil, South America

R. Cutait MD, TCBC
Associate Professor of Surgery, Medical School of the University of São Paulo, São Paulo 01427, Brazil, South America

T. I. Davidson ChM, MRCP, FRCS
Lecturer in Surgery, Westminster Hospital, London SW1P 2AP, UK

H. B. Devlin MA, MD, MCh, FRCS, FRCSI, FACS
Lecturer in Clinical Surgery, University of Newcastle upon Tyne and Consultant Surgeon, North Tees General Hospital, Stockton-on-Tees, Cleveland TS19 8PE, UK

S. A. Dolk MD
Department of Surgery, Karolinska Institute, Danderyd Hospital, S-182 88 Danderyd, Sweden

R. R. Dozois MD, MS, FACS
Professor of Surgery, Mayo Clinic, 2000 1st Street SW, Rochester, Minnesota 55905, USA

T. E. Eisenstat MD, FACS, FASCRS
Clinical Professor of Surgery, University of Medicine and Dentistry, Robert Wood Johnson Medical School, New Brunswick, New Jersey 07060, USA

G. R. Ekelund MD, PhD
Associate Professor and Chairman, Department of Surgery, Malmö General Hospital, University of Lund, S-214 01 Malmö, Sweden

M. T. El Riwini MB, BCh
Faculty of Medicine, University of Alexandria, Egypt

J.-L. Faucheron MD
Chief Resident, Department of Surgery, Hôpital Saint-Antoine, 184 rue du Fg Saint-Antoine, 75012 Paris, France

V. W. Fazio FRACS, FACS
Chairman, Department of Colorectal Surgery, Cleveland Clinic Foundation, 9500 Euclid Avenue, Cleveland, Ohio 44106, USA

L. P. Fielding MB, FRCS, FACS
Chief of Surgery, St Mary's Hospital, Waterbury, Connecticut 06706, Clinical Professor of Surgery, Yale University School of Medicine, Connecticut, USA and Visiting Clinical Scientist, St Mary's Hospital, London, UK

F. J. Figliolini MD, TCBC, FACS
Rua Ministro Rocha Azevedo, 1409-10 Andar, Sao Paulo 01410, Brazil, South America

E. W. Fonkalsrud MD
Professor and Chief of Pediatric Surgery, UCLA School of Medicine, Los Angeles, California 90024, USA

J. B. J. Fozard MS, FRCS
Consultant Surgeon, Royal Bournemouth Hospital, Bournemouth, Dorset BH7 7DW, UK

P. Frileux MD
Professor of Surgery, Hôpital Laennec, 42 rue de Sèvres, F-75007 Paris, France

H. S. Goh BSc, FRCS
Senior Consultant and Head, Department of Colorectal Surgery, Singapore General Hospital, Outram Road, Singapore 0316

S. M. Goldberg MD, FACS, FRACS
Clinical Professor of Surgery and Director, Division of Colon and Rectal Surgery, University of Minnesota Medical School, Minneapolis, Minnesota 55402, USA

P. H. Gordon MD, FRCSC, FACS
Professor of Surgery, McGill University and Director, Colon and Rectal Surgery, Sir Mortimer B. Davis Jewish General Hospital, Montreal, Quebec H3T 1E2, Canada

R. H. Grace FRCS
Consultant Surgeon, The Royal Hospital, Cleveland Road, Wolverhampton, West Midlands WV2 1BT, UK

J. D. Hardcastle MA, MChir, FRCS, FRCP
Department of Surgery, University Hospital, Queen's Medical Centre, Nottingham NG7 2UH, UK

P. R. Hawley MS, FRCS
Senior Consultant Surgeon, St Mark's Hospital for Diseases of the Rectum and Colon and Consultant Surgeon, King Edward VII Hospital, London, UK

R. J. Heald MA, MChir, FRCS, FRCSEd
Consultant Surgeon, Colorectal Research Unit, Basingstoke District Hospital, Basingstoke, Hampshire, UK

G. Hellers MD, PhD
Chairman, Department of Surgery, Huddinge University Hospital, S-14186 Huddinge, Sweden

M. M. Henry MB, FRCS
Consultant Surgeon, Central Middlesex Hospital, Honorary Consultant Surgeon, St Mark's Hospital for Diseases of the Rectum and Colon, and Senior Lecturer, Academic Surgical Unit, St Mary's Hospital, London, UK

K. Hojo MD
Chief of Proctology, National Cancer Centre, Tokyo and Professor of Surgery, Tokyo Medical University, 5-1-1 Tsukiji, Tokyo, Japan

B. F. Holmstrom MD
Department of Surgery, Karolinska Institute, Danderyd Hospital, S-182 88 Danderyd, Sweden

C. N. Hudson MChir, FRCS, FRCOG, FRACOG
Director, Clinical Academic Department of Obstetrics and Gynaecology, Medical College of St Bartholomew's Hospital, West Smithfield, London EC1A 7BE, UK

L. Hultén MD, PhD
Professor of Surgery, Surgical Department II, Sahlgrenska Hospital, University of Göteborg, S-413 45 Göteborg, Sweden

J. G. Hunter MD
Department of Surgery, Emory University Hospital, Atlanta, Georgia, USA

R. D. Hurst MD
Assistant Professor of Surgery, Yale University School of Medicine, 333 Cedar Street, New Haven, Connecticut, USA

T. T. Irvin PhD, ChM, FRCSEd
Consultant Surgeon, Royal Devon and Exeter Hospital, Barrack Road, Exeter, Devon EX2 5DW, UK

M. Irving MD, ChM, FRCS
Professor of Surgery and Consultant Surgeon, Hope Hospital, University of Manchester School of Medicine, Salford M6 8HD, UK

B. T. Jackson MS, FRCS
Consultant Surgeon, St Thomas' Hospital, London SE1 7EH, UK

D. G. Jagelman MS, FRCS, FACS
Chairman, Division of Surgery and Chairman, Department of Colorectal Surgery, Cleveland Clinic Florida, 300 Cypress Creek Road, Fort Lauderdale, Florida 33309, USA

H. Jiborn MD, PhD
Associate Professor, Department of Surgery, Malmö General Hospital, University of Lund, S-214 01 Malmö, Sweden

M. R. B. Keighley MS, FRCS
Barling Professor of Surgery, Department of Surgery, Queen Elizabeth Hospital, Birmingham B15 2TH, UK

K. A. Kelly MD, FACS, FRCSEd
Professor and Chair, Department of Surgery, Mayo Clinic and Mayo Medical School, Rochester, Minnesota, USA

H. L. Kennedy MD, FACS
Assistant Clinical Professor of Surgery, University of California, 1020 29th Street, Suite 350, Sacramento, California 95816, USA

J. Kewenter MD, PhD
Department of Surgery, Sahlgrenska Hospital, 413 45 Göteborg, Sweden

E. S. Kiff MD, FRCS
Consultant Surgeon, University Hospital of South Manchester, Manchester M20 9BX, UK

M. Killingback FRCS, FRCSEd, FRACS
Sydney Adventist Hospital, Sydney, Australia

Patrick F. Leahy MCh, FRCSI
Consultant Surgeon, Blackrock Clinic, Dublin, Eire

H. Lee MD
Mayo Clinic, Scottsdale, Arizona, USA

M. M. Lirici MD
Department of Surgery, La Sapienza University Medical School, Policlinico Umberto I, Rome 00161, Italy

H. W. Loose FRCR
Consultant Radiologist, Freeman Hospital, Newcastle-upon-Tyne, UK

A. C. Lowry MD, FACS
Clinical Assistant Professor of Surgery, Division of Colon and Rectal Surgery, University of Minnesota Medical School, Minneapolis, Minnesota 55435, USA

F. M. Luvuno FRCSEd, FRCS(Glas)
Senior Consultant Surgeon, King Edward VIII Hospital and Senior Lecturer, Department of Surgery, University of Natal, PO Box 17039, Congella 4013, South Africa

R. D. Madoff MD
Clinical Assistant Professor of Surgery, Division of Colon and Rectal Surgery, University of Minnesota Medical School, Minneapolis, Minnesota 55402, USA

C. V. Mann MA, MCh, FRCS
Consulting Surgeon, The Royal London Hospital and St Mark's Hospital for Diseases of the Rectum and Colon, London, UK

D. T. Martin MD, FACS
Assistant Professor, University of New Mexico School of Medicine, Albuquerque, New Mexico, USA

A. McLeish MD, FRACS
Senior Colorectal Surgeon, Austin Hospital, Heidelberg, Victoria, Australia 3084

I. M. Modlin MD, PhD, FACS, FRCSEd, FCS
Professor of Surgery, Yale University School of Medicine, 333 Cedar Street, New Haven, Connecticut, USA

J. J. Murray MD
Staff Surgeon, Department of Colon and Rectal Surgery, Lahey Clinic Medical Center, Burlington, Massachusetts 01805, USA

T. Muto MD, DMSc
Professor of Surgery, University of Tokyo, 7-3-1 Hongo, Bunkyo-ku, Tokyo 113, Japan

G. L. Newstead FRACS, FRCS, FACS
Senior Lecturer in Surgery, University of New South Wales and Associate Director, Division of Surgery, Prince of Wales Hospital, Randwick, NSW 2031, Australia

R. J. Nicholls MChir, FRCS
Consultant Surgeon, St Mark's Hospital for Diseases of the Rectum and Colon, City Road, London EC1V 2PS, UK

B. Nordlinger MD
Professor of Surgery, Centre de Chirurgie Digestive, Hôpital Saint-Antoine, 184 rue du Fg Saint-Antoine, 75012 Paris, France

J. M. A. Northover MS, FRCS
Consultant Surgeon, St Mark's Hospital for Diseases of the Rectum and Colon, City Road, London EC1V 2PS, UK

M. J. Notaras FRCS, FRCSEd, FACS
Consultant Surgeon, Barnet General Hospital and Honorary Senior Lecturer and Consultant Surgeon, University College Hospital, London, UK

J. R. Oakley FRACS
Staff Surgeon and Head, Section of Enterostomal Therapy, Department of Colorectal Surgery, Cleveland Clinic Foundation, 9500 Euclid Avenue, Cleveland, Ohio 44106, USA

S. O'Dwyer MD, FRCS
Consultant Surgeon, The General and Queen Elizabeth Hospitals, Birmingham, UK

G. C. Oliver MD
Associate Clinical Professor of Surgery, Robert Wood Johnson Medical School and Muhlenberg Hospital, Plainfield, New Jersey 07060, USA

D. P. Otchy MD, FACS
Assistant Chief, General Surgery Service, Brooke Army Medical Center and Assistant Professor of Surgery, Uniformed Services University of the Health Sciences, San Antonio, Texas 78234-6200, USA

R. F. Parc MD
Professor of Surgery, Hôpital Saint-Antoine, 184 rue du Fg Saint-Antoine, 75012 Paris, France

T. G. Parks MCh, FRCSEd, FRCS(Glas), FRCSI
Professor of Surgical Science, The Queen's University of Belfast, Belfast, UK

J. H. Pemberton MD
Associate Professor of Surgery, Colon and Rectal Surgery, Mayo Clinic, 200 First Street SW, Rochester, Minnesota 55905, USA

R. K. S. Phillips MS, FRCS
Consultant Surgeon, St Mark's Hospital for Diseases of the Rectum and Colon and Homerton Hospital, London and Honorary Lecturer, St Bartholomew's Hospital Medical School, London, UK

D. Rosenthal MD, FACS
Surgical Consultant, Brooke Army Medical Center and Clinical Professor of Surgery, Uniformed Services Univesity of the Health Sciences, San Antonio, Texas 78234-6200, USA

T. M. Ross MD, FRCS(C), FACS
Assistant Professor of Surgery, Women's College Hospital, University of Toronto, 60 Grosvenor Suite 317, Toronto, Ontario, Canada

D. A. Rothenberger MD
Clinical Professor of Surgery and Chief, Division of Colon and Rectal Surgery, University of Minnesota Medical School, Minneapolis, Minnesota 55102, USA

R. J. Rubin MD
Clinical Professor of Surgery, Robert Wood Johnson Medical School and Muhlenberg Hospital, Plainfield, New Jersey 07060, USA

J. M. Sackier MB, FRCS
Associate Professor of Surgery, University of California, San Diego, California 92103-9981, USA

E. P. Salvati MD, FACS
Clinical Professor of Surgery, University of Medicine and Dentistry, Robert Wood Johnson Medical School, New Brunswick, New Jersey 07060, USA

D. J. Schoetz Jr MD
Chairman, Department of Colon and Rectal Surgery, Lahey Clinic Medical Center, Burlington, Massachusetts 01805, USA

P. F. Schofield MD, FRCS
Consultant Surgeon, Withington and Christie Hospitals and Honorary Reader in Surgery, University Hospital of South Manchester, Manchester M20 9BX, UK

S. I. Schwartz MD
Department of Surgery, University of Rochester, Medical Center, 601 Elmwood Avenue, Rochester, New York 14642, USA

W. Silen MD
Johnson and Johnson Professor of Surgery, Harvard Medical School, 330 Brookline Avenue, Boston, Massachusetts 02215, USA

H. S. Stern MD, FRCS(C), FACS
Associate Professor of Surgery, Mount Sinai Hospital, University of Toronto, 600 University Avenue No. 1225, Toronto, Ontario, Canada

T. Takahashi MD
Chief, Surgical Department, Tokyo Metropolitan Komagome Hospital, 3-18-22 Honkomagome, Bunkyo-ku, Tokyo, Japan

J. P. S. Thomson DM, MS, FRCS
Consultant Surgeon and Clinical Director, St Mark's Hospital for Diseases of the Rectum and Colon, City Road, London EC1V 2PS, UK

S. R. Thomson ChM, FRCS
Senior Lecturer, Department of Surgery, University of Natal, Natal, South Africa

A. G. Thorson MD, FACS
Associate Professor of Surgery and Program Director, Section of Colon and Rectal Surgery, Creighton University School of Medicine and Clinical Assistant Professor of Surgery, University of Nebraska College of Medicine, Omaha, Nebraska 68102, USA

J. Utsunomiya MD
Second Department of Surgery, Hyogo College of Medicine, 1-1 Mukogawa-cho, Nishinomiya, Hyogo 663, Japan

M. C. Veidenheimer MD
Staff Surgeon, Department of Colon and Rectal Surgery, Lahey Clinic Medical Center, Burlington, Massachusetts 01805, USA

A. M. Vernava III MD
Assistant Professor of Surgery, St Louis Medical University, St Louis, Missouri, USA

S. D. Wexner MD, FACS, FASCRS, FACG
Staff Colorectal Surgeon, Residency Program Director, Department of Colorectal Surgery and Director of Anorectal Physiology Laboratory, Cleveland Clinic Florida, Fort Lauderdale, Florida, USA

R. L. Whelan MD
Assistant Professor of Surgery and Director, Section of Colon and Rectal Surgery, Columbia Presbyterian Medical Center, Columbia University College of Physicians and Surgeons, New York, USA

C. B. Williams FRCP
Consultant Physician, St Marks Hospital for Diseases of the Rectum and Colon, St Bartholomew's Hospital and King Edward VII Hospital for Officers, and Honorary Consultant Physician, The Hospital for Sick Children, London, UK

J. G. Williams MCh, FRCS
Lecturer in Surgery, University of Birmingham, Queen Elizabeth Hospital, Birmingham, UK

N. S. Williams MS, FRCS
Professor of Surgery and Director, Surgical Unit, The Royal London Hospital, London E1 1BB, UK

P. Wind MD
Assistant Professor, Centre de Chirurgie Digestive, Hôpital Saint-Antoine, 184 rue du Fg Saint-Antoine, 75012 Paris, France

W. D. Wong MD
Clinical Assistant Professor of Surgery, Division of Colon and Rectal Surgery, University of Minnesota Medical School, Minneapolis, Minnesota 55102, USA

K. A. Zucker MD, FACS
Professor of Surgery, University of New Mexico School of Medicine, Albuquerque, New Mexico 87131, USA

Contributing Medical Artists

Antoine Barnaud
11 Rue Jacques Dulud,
92200 Neuilly sur Seine, France

Angela Christie MMAA
14 West End Avenue, Pinner,
Middlesex HA5 1BJ, UK

Peter Cox RDD, MMAA, AIMI
2 Frome Villas, Frenchay,
Bristol BS16 1LT, UK

Patrick Elliott BA(Hons), ATC, MMAA, AIMBI
46 Stone Delf,
Sheffield S10 3QX, UK

Jenny Halstead MMAA
The Red House, 85 Christchurch Road, Reading,
Berkshire RG2 7BD, UK

Diane Kinton BA(Hons)
Gillian Lee Illustrations,
15 Little Plucketts Way, Buckhurst Hill,
Essex IG9 5QU, UK

The late Robert Lane MMAA
Studio 19A, Edith Grove,
London SW10, UK

Gillian Lee FMAA, HonFIMI, AMI, RMIP
Gillian Lee Illustrations,
15 Little Plucketts Way, Buckhurst Hill,
Essex IG9 5QU, UK

Gillian Oliver MMAA, AIMI
15 Bramble Road, Hatfield,
Hertfordshire AL10 9RZ, UK

Marks Creative Consultants
31 Waddon Road, Croydon,
Surrey CR0 4LH, UK

Richard Neave FMAA, AIMI
Unit of Art in Medicine,
Department of Cell and Structural Biology,
University of Manchester, Manchester M13 9PT, UK

Paul Richardson BA(Hons)
54 Wellington Road,
Orpington BR5 4AQ, Kent

Denise Smith BA(Hons), MMAA
Unit of Art in Medicine,
Department of Cell and Structural Biology,
University of Manchester, Manchester M13 9PT, UK

The Editors gratefully acknowledge the support of United States Surgical Corporation (Connecticut, USA) in the production of this volume and for making available stapling instruments to the medical illustrators.

Contents

Endoscopy and laparoscopic techniques

Stomas

Preface

This fifth edition of *Surgery of the Colon, Rectum and Anus* is, we believe, a substantial improvement over the last edition of this text published 10 years ago. The 88 chapters are arranged in ten sections with each section having its own introductory comment to place the segment of the book into general perspective. Some sections are new, others are expanded, and we have also taken the opportunity of consolidating certain areas of the text where there is more unanimity of opinion concerning technique or where the usage of certain operations now seems to be outmoded. Despite these changes which signify a great expansion of this subject in recent years, the overall purpose of the text has not changed. We have asked each author to place great emphasis on the special details of technique ('tricks-of-the-trade') which make the difference between success and failure.

We have taken a new look at the section on general principles, recognizing that applied surgical anatomy is fundamental and crucial to surgical outcome. The prevention of sepsis, positioning of patients for effective surgery, and the greatly expanded techniques of achieving bowel continuity are discussed in considerable detail. We have attempted to extend the horizons of colorectal and general surgeons by the inclusion of a section on radiological techniques indicating the multidisciplinary nature of the team now required. In addition, the rise of AIDS-related colorectal problems require us to pay particular attention to surgical technique so that all members of the operative team might be protected from infection.

Although endoscopy is well established, minimal access surgery using television-guided laparoscopic-assisted surgery is in its infancy, and we fully expect the details of technique to change and to be developed in the near future. However, this youthful section signifies our predictions for the future. The fashioning of stomas continues to be a challenging subject which requires meticulous technique, but the methods themselves have become standardized in recent years. The inclusion of a short section on small intestinal surgery is justified on the grounds that colorectal surgeons are not limited by the ileocaecal valve, but are more willing to accept an anatomical demarcation nearer the ligament of Treitz. The descriptions of intra-abdominal colonic surgery, as well as pelvic and rectal surgery, form the bedrock of this discipline. We have chosen to have a substantial section on pouch procedures and the alternative techniques currently available. We have taken a similar approach to the substantial number of alternative procedures for the surgical management of rectal prolapse. The multiplicity of methods in these two sections speaks to the continued developmental aspects of pouch procedures and the relatively mixed results being obtained for the various rectal prolapse operations.

The clinical management and laboratory investigation of patients with incontinence has received much attention in recent years. We fully support an expansion in the numbers of clinical laboratories investigating these patients and an increase in the numbers of operative procedures for the treatment of faecal incontinence. The final section on anorectal conditions is, we believe, comprehensive and clear and addresses the operative problems associated with these common conditions which cause so much morbidity.

All in all an attempt has been made to combine the old with the new; greater emphasis has been laid on the overall management of patients, the indications and contraindications for surgery, and in the more controversial areas the results that can be expected from a particular operative treatment are outlined.

By undertaking this more comprehensive approach to surgical methods and technique, we hope to provide the reader not only with descriptions of the surgical procedures, but also with some of that most elusive essential for success – technical and clinical judgement.

We hope that this text will help foster the concept that clinical results can be significantly improved by heightening technical expertise in this challenging and expanding field of surgery.

L. Peter Fielding
Stanley M. Goldberg

General principles: introductory comment

S. I. Schwartz MD
Department of Surgery, University of Rochester, Rochester, New York, USA

Determination of elements that constitute 'general principles' is the domain of the editors; it is a critical responsibility. As the first segment to which the reader is exposed, the 'general principles' section serves as the standard for the entire text and provides an appropriate and meaningful basis for the subject matter of the work.

Considerations of applied anatomy, preoperative assessment and preparation, positioning of patients for operations, anastomotic techniques, management of anastomotic leaks and consequent sepsis, and the role of diagnostic and interventional radiology, transcend all disorders of concern for the surgeon caring for a patient with a colorectal or anal disorder and are thus pertinent to the entire book.

The three chapters on anatomy are designated as 'applied' anatomy and bring into focus those anatomical features that are critical for the success of the procedures. Separate presentations of intra-abdominal, pelvic/perineal, and anal regions stress the features specifically applicable in these distinct areas. A knowledge of the visceral anatomy, vascular supply, and relationships with important adjacent structures contributes to the safe and expeditious removal and anastomosis of segments of the intraperitoneal colon. Dissection of the rectum depends on an appreciation of the fascial connections that must be divided by the surgeon, and consideration needs also to be given to other pelvic organs such as the uterus, ovaries and ureter. The more in-depth emphasis of the applied anatomy including the muscular support so vital for continence, and definition of the anorectal spaces that harbour the complex abscesses that develop in these areas, is critical for the successful management of clinical problems. The addenda of cross-sectional tomographic imaging and intrarectal ultrasonography contribute to this thorough presentation of anatomy. As William Hunter wrote: 'Who are the men in the profession that would persuade students that a little anatomy is enough for a physician, and a little more too much for a surgeon? God help them!'

The section on rectal biopsy presents the necessary directions for providing the specimen required to define the pathology of the lesion and to dictate therapy.

Successful colorectal surgery is relatively unique; the intellectually prepared surgeon must operate on a bacteriologically prepared patient. Unlike the upper regions of the gastrointestinal tract, the colon and rectum are colonized with potential pathogens, and the prevention of sepsis during the preoperative and postoperative periods is integral to overall general principles.

Patient positioning, an often neglected issue in the description of operative technique, is given attention.

Most operative procedures on the colon and rectum incorporate exploration, excision and reconstruction of continuity of the bowel. Knowledge of anatomy and pathology is essential for appropriate exploration and excision. Reconstruction of continuity focuses on creating the anastomosis which, in the modern surgical world, incorporates a choice of sutures, staples and biodegradable rings. Each has advantages, disadvantages and specific applications, but all achieve equivalent results. The oldest of these techniques – suturing – is presented with step-by-step clarity and many variations are described. This technique is appropriately emphasized because it remains the most adaptable and is therefore relied on in tenuous and compromised circumstances. The stapling technique has been refined to expeditiously create an anastomosis equivalent to the sutured anastomosis; the newly rejuvenated anastomosis button (best known in the past as the 'Murphy button') is described in its current biodegradable form.

As surgical techniques to anastomose the colon and rectum by sutures, staples or rings have matured to the point of anticipated success, the dreaded complication of anastomotic leak has become a less frequent occurrence. It has not, and never will, completely disappear, however. The only surgeon who does not require complete expertise in the management of complications is the surgeon who does not operate. The diagnosis and management of anastomotic leakage and subsequent sepsis are therefore an integral part of general principles of colon and rectal surgery and, for the affected patient, the most critical consideration. In modern colorectal surgery the interventional radiologist has become a powerful ally in the management of anastomotic leaks, sepsis and colonic bleeding. The capabilities of diagnostic procedures and the results of radiologically directed intervention must be understood.

The final chapter in this section discusses the principles of operating on the immunocompromised patient and includes the management of affected patients and the prevention of infection in personnel involved in the care of such patients. This subject is becoming increasingly important and will be needed by surgeons well into the 21st century.

Applied surgical anatomy: intra-abdominal contents

J. B. J. Fozard MS, FRCS
Consultant Surgeon, Royal Bournemouth Hospital, Bournemouth, Dorset, UK

J. H. Pemberton MD
Associate Professor of Surgery, Mayo Clinic, Rochester, Minnesota, USA

The disposition of the colon within the peritoneal cavity is extremely variable, depending on individual build and the length and presence or absence of mesenteric attachments. This description of the anatomy of the intra-abdominal contents will be restricted and related to the colon encountered under 'normal' circumstances.

1 The distinguishing feature of the large intestine is the condensation of longitudinal muscle into three strips or taenia coli giving rise to its haustral appearance. The taenia coli arise at the base of the appendix on the caecum and fuse at the rectosigmoid junction to give a uniform longitudinal muscle coat to the rectum. The course of the large intestine is well demonstrated by double-contrast barium enema. Of note, the hepatic flexure lies lower than the splenic flexure, which is high on the left.

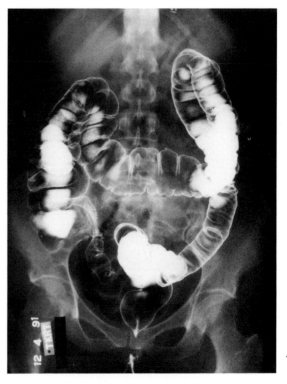

1

2 The ascending and descending colons are usually retroperitoneal structures. Both the sigmoid and transverse colons have mesenteries. If access to the abdomen is limited, the transverse colon is identified by the attached greater omentum and the sigmoid colon by the more obvious appendices epiploicae.

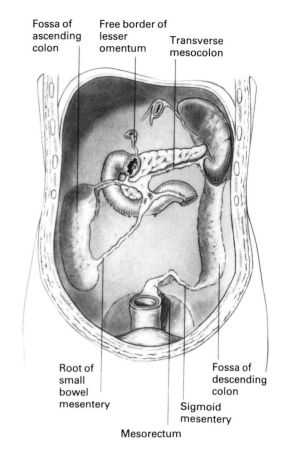

Fossa of ascending colon

Free border of lesser omentum

Transverse mesocolon

Root of small bowel mesentery

Mesorectum

Sigmoid mesentery

Fossa of descending colon

2

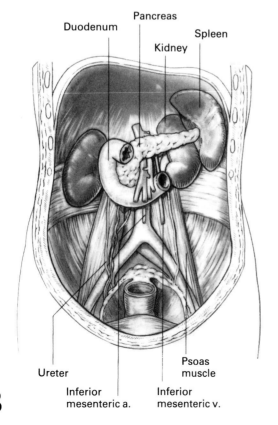

Duodenum

Pancreas

Kidney

Spleen

Ureter

Inferior mesenteric a.

Inferior mesenteric v.

Psoas muscle

3

Right colon

3 The right colon comprises the caecum (that portion below the ileocaecal valve) and the ascending colon to the hepatic flexure. It is largely a retroperitoneal structure and bound down to the right posterior abdominal wall and associated structures, although in 10% of individuals the caecum and ascending colon are mobile. The peritoneal reflection from the right colon onto the posterior abdominal wall is marked by the line of Toldt. Incision of the peritoneum along this line is a preliminary step in mobilization.

4a, b Of note, the right colon is related posteriorly to the right ureter, gonadal vessels, duodenum and kidney.

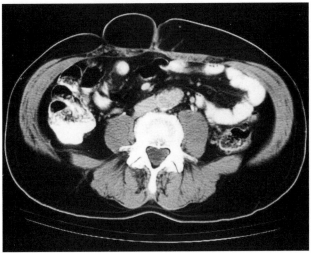

4a

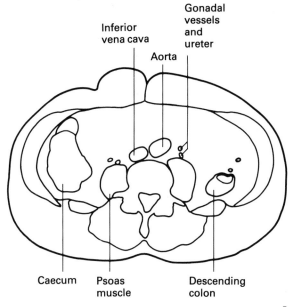

Inferior vena cava

Gonadal vessels and ureter

Aorta

Caecum   Psoas muscle   Descending colon

4b

5a, b With the peritoneum divided along the line of Toldt, the right colon is mobilized medially to the root of the small intestinal mesentery, exposing the posterior structures (*see Illustration 2*). The right ureter and gonadal vessels run caudally on the surface of the psoas muscle. More cranially, the hepatic flexure may be free or adherent to the gallbladder. When mobilized, the hepatic flexure mesentery crosses over between the second and third part of the duodenum, with the C loop and head of the pancreas exposed.

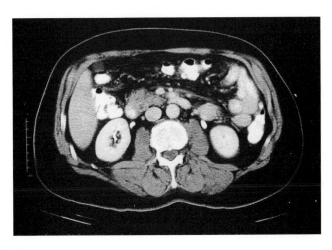

5a

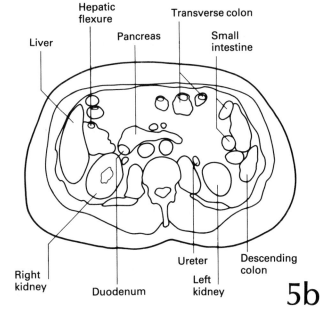

Hepatic flexure

Liver

Pancreas

Transverse colon

Small intestine

Right kidney

Duodenum

Ureter

Left kidney

Descending colon

5b

Transverse colon

6 The transverse colon extends between the hepatic and splenic flexures, forming a loop of varying dependency. It is attached to the greater curvature of the stomach by the gastrocolic omentum. The greater omentum is attached to the transverse colon on its superior surface, and posterosuperiorly the colon is suspended from the posterior abdominal wall by the transverse mesocolon. The key to mobilization of the transverse colon, to identify its posterior relations, is to open the lesser sac.

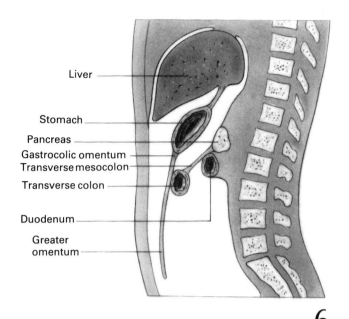

Liver

Stomach

Pancreas

Gastrocolic omentum

Transverse mesocolon

Transverse colon

Duodenum

Greater omentum

6

7, 8 Access to the lesser sac may be gained to the left of the midline by two routes: either by separating the greater omentum from the transverse colon along the bloodless plane of Pauchet or by dividing the gastrocolic omentum outside the gastroepiploic arcade.

The body of the pancreas lies within the lesser sac, just superior to the transverse mesocolon. To the right,

the lesser sac is obliterated, but an avascular plane can usually be developed between the first part of the duodenum, pancreas and remaining transverse mesocolon. On the posterior abdominal wall, the transverse mesocolon crosses from the superior mesenteric vessels, superior to the duodenojejunal flexure and ends just beyond this point where the descending colon is again a retroperitoneal structure (*see Illustration 2*).

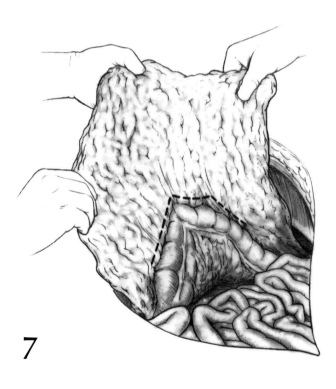

7

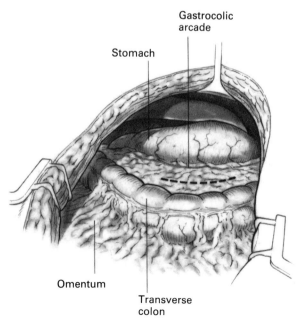

Gastrocolic arcade

Stomach

Omentum

Transverse colon

8

Splenic flexure

9 The splenic flexure lies at a higher level than the hepatic flexure, generally tucked well up under the left costal margin and closely related to the spleen. The splenic flexure is attached to the diaphragm postero-laterally by the phrenocolic ligament, which appears as a band of thickened peritoneum running below the lower pole of the spleen. The splenic flexure may be free of the spleen or attached by adhesions to the splenic capsule. Before mobilization these adhesions should be freed with cautery to avoid a capsular tear. Working with fingers simultaneously, laterally from the lesser sac and medially under the phrenocolic ligament, the attachments of the splenic flexure are defined. Although there are no named vessels in this attachment, it is often wise to divide between clamps.

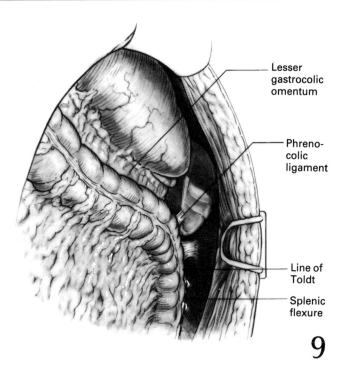

Lesser gastrocolic omentum

Phreno-colic ligament

Line of Toldt

Splenic flexure

9

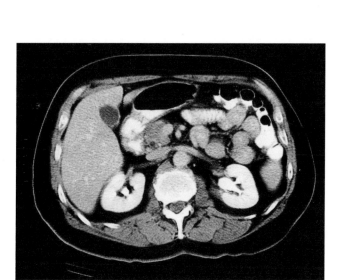

10a

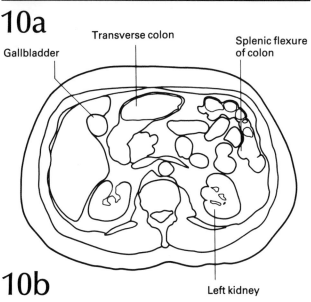

Gallbladder

Transverse colon

Splenic flexure of colon

Left kidney

10b

10a, b The major relationships of the splenic flexure are to the left kidney, adrenal gland, tail of the pancreas and spleen. As the splenic flexure is mobilized caudally and medially, its thin mesentery peels off Gerota's fascia. Of some importance, the inferior mesenteric vein drains cranially at the base of this mesentery just lateral to the duodenojejunal flexure and joins the splenic vein after passing posterior to the pancreas.

Descending colon

The descending colon from the splenic flexure to the medial border of the psoas major muscle inferiorly is plastered to the posterior abdominal wall. Laterally, the line of mobilization is again marked on the peritoneal reflection by the line of Toldt (*see Illustration 9*). The descending colon is related posteriorly to the muscles and nerves of the posterior abdominal wall, and on mobilization medially, the mesentery can be separated from the ureter and gonadal vessels which lie on the medial aspect of the psoas major muscle (*see Illustrations 4 and 5*).

Sigmoid colon

11a, b In the region of the pelvic brim, the colon angles anteriorly and acquires a mesentery. This marks the junction of the descending with the sigmoid colon, which becomes the rectum at the sacral promontory. The sigmoid colon is very variable in length, position and fixity. A long meso-sigmoid colon with a short base predisposes to volvulus (as described in the chapter on pp. 420–435). Commonly, the sigmoid colon loops down into the pelvis with its apex lying anterior to the rectum. Adhesions to the lateral wall of the iliac fossa are usually present. If these are divided and the sigmoid colon is stretched to the right, the intersigmoid fossa and line of Toldt are readily appreciated. Incision of the peritoneal reflection along this line allows mobilization of the sigmoid colon, and the intersigmoid fossa acts as a guide to the position of the left ureter. The ureter descends on the psoas muscle along with the gonadal vessels and crosses into the pelvis at the bifurcation of the common iliac artery.

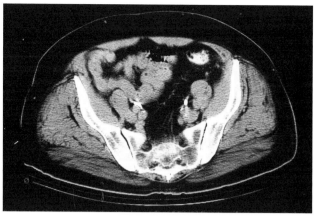

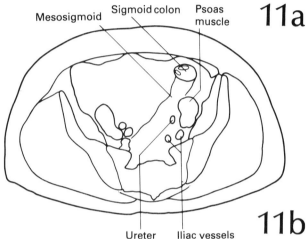

Mesosigmoid   Sigmoid colon   Psoas muscle   **11a**

Ureter   Iliac vessels   **11b**

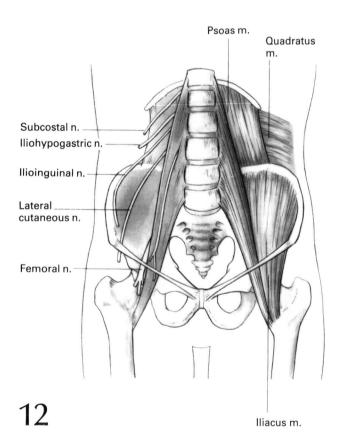

Psoas m.

Quadratus m.

Subcostal n.

Iliohypogastric n.

Ilioinguinal n.

Lateral cutaneous n.

Femoral n.

12

Iliacus m.

Muscles and nerves of the posterior abdominal wall

12 Extended radical *en bloc* resections for cancer may incorporate part of the posterior abdominal wall to achieve clear resection margins. This particularly applies to caecal, ascending and descending colonic carcinoma, which may invade the muscles (psoas, quadratus lumborum, transverse abdominis and iliac). Of more importance from a functional point of view are the nerves of the posterior abdominal wall running in close proximity. The genitofemoral nerve runs inferiorly on the psoas muscle and supplies the cremaster muscle and skin overlying the femoral triangle and scrotum or labia. The lateral cutaneous nerve of the thigh passes obliquely across the iliac muscle. The ilioinguinal and iliohypogastric nerves supply the lower lateral portion of the anterolateral abdominal wall, and damage may lead to muscular weakness and possible hernia. The femoral nerve runs between the psoas and iliacus muscles below the iliac crest and enters the thigh lateral to the femoral sheath. It may be damaged during extended resection of the caecum, resulting in paralysis of the quadriceps femoris muscle and sensory loss on the anterior and lateral aspects of the thigh.

Vasculature

Knowledge of the blood supply to the colon and ileum is essential, because an adequate blood supply must be maintained to an anastomosis or pouch after resection. In addition, lymphatic drainage mirrors arterial supply, which is important in cancer surgery and the potential for ischaemic colitis is increased in areas of the colon in which there are diminished mesenteric arterial communications.

13–15 Although there are many variations to the theme, the right colon generally lies within the superior mesenteric territory, deriving its supply from the ileocolic, right colic and middle colic arteries. The left colon is supplied from the inferior mesenteric artery via the left colic artery and between two and six sigmoidal branches. The long anastomosis of Riolan completes the marginal artery between superior and inferior mesenteric territories. Following ligation or occlusion of the inferior mesenteric artery, blood supply to the left colon depends on the integrity of the arc of Riolan. For this reason, ischaemic colitis tends to occur in the splenic flexure. Conversely, after low anterior resection the splenic flexure may be mobilized to provide the colon with an adequate blood supply for anastomosis. As an alternative, avoidance of a high tie on the inferior mesenteric artery has been shown not to jeopardize prognosis and has the added benefit of preserving the blood supply via the ascending left colic artery.

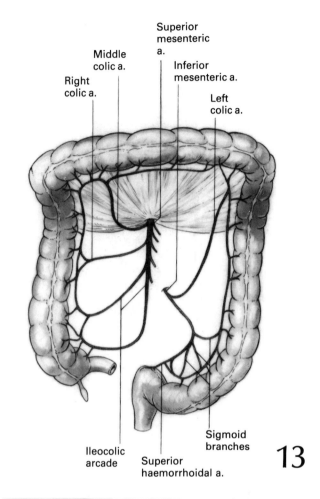

13

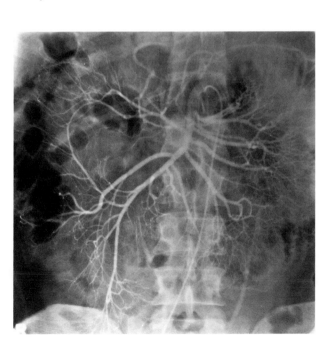

14

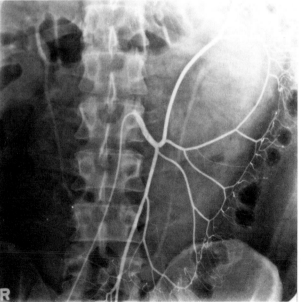

15

The ileocolic artery is constant and bifurcates into a colic and ileal branch. An ileocolic arcade is present in 78% of patients and a recurrent ileal artery in 39%. Sacrifice of the ileocolic artery may produce terminal ileum of dubious viability, unsuitable for anastomosis or pouch construction. This anatomy should also be taken into account before dividing vessels to achieve adequate length for ileal pouch–anal anastomosis. The right colic artery may arise as a single trunk with the middle colic artery and very occasionally from the ileocolic artery. It is occasionally absent (2%).

The term 'middle colic artery' is a relative misnomer. It arises at the lower border or behind the pancreas and tends to run towards the hepatic flexure. It is absent in 3% of patients and may arise occasionally from the coeliac axis. Accessory middle colic arteries are present in 8% of patients. The splenic branch of the middle colic artery forms part of the arc of Riolan.

The inferior mesenteric artery has its origin 3–4 cm above the aortic bifurcation and may be just inferior to the third part of the duodenum (*see Illustration 15*). The left colic artery arises 2.5–3 cm from the origin of the inferior mesenteric artery and ascends towards the splenic flexure. The sigmoidal arteries vary in size and number. The first may arise from either the left colic or inferior mesenteric artery. The inferior mesenteric artery continues as the superior rectal artery.

In relation to ligation of the inferior mesenteric artery and its immediate branches, it is important to recognize that the left ureter may be intimately associated with this vessel and must be protected.

The venous anatomy mirrors the arterial anatomy except for the inferior mesenteric vein which runs in the base of the descending colon 'mesentery', lateral to the duodenojejunal flexure to anastomose with the splenic vein posterior to the pancreas. High ligation of the inferior mesenteric vein may be helpful in gaining length for a left-sided colorectal anastomosis.

Further reading

Siddharth P, Ravo B. Colorectal neurovasculature and anal sphincter. *Surg Clin North Am* 1988; 68: 1185–200.

Smith L, Friend WG, Medwell SJ. The superior mesenteric artery. The critical factor in the pouch pull-through procedure. *Dis Colon Rectum* 1984; 27: 741–4.

Applied surgical anatomy: pelvic contents

J. B. J. Fozard MS, FRCS
Consultant Surgeon, Royal Bournemouth Hospital, Bournemouth, Dorset, UK

J. H. Pemberton MD
Associate Professor of Surgery, Mayo Clinic, Rochester, Minnesota, USA

This chapter details surgical anatomy of the pelvic contents, with specific relevance to the colon and rectal surgeon. Detail is restricted to the anatomical relationships, tissue planes and spaces that enable a safe operation on the rectum and anus and avoid damage to vital structures.

Rectum

1 The rectum varies in length with age, sex and body habitus. In some anatomical descriptions it is suggested that the rectum starts opposite the body of vertebra S3. This landmark, however, has no relevance to the surgeon, who should use the sacral promontory as the appropriate reference point for the commencement of the rectum.

Proctoscopically, the rectosigmoid junction is visualized 14–16 cm from the anal verge, but functionally the sigmoid colon properly terminates at the confluence of the taenia coli. Although the confluence occurs at a variable distance from the sacral promontory, it is this anatomical feature that determines adequacy of distal resection for diverticular disease.

The rectum extends into the pelvis following the sacral curve, and at the level of the pelvic floor (anorectal ring) angles acutely backwards making the junction with the anal canal. The anal canal is 4 cm in length, with its axis in line with the umbilicus, and terminates at the anal verge.

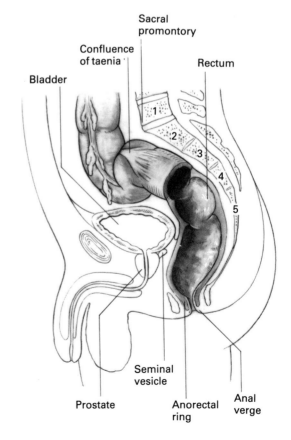

1

2a, b The rectum has three lateral curves: upper and lower convex to the right and middle convex to the left, represented on its intraluminal aspect as the valves of Houston. Of significance for biopsy or polypectomy purposes, the middle valve of Houston is taken to mark the anterior peritoneal reflection. Straightening of the curves during mobilization of the rectum 'lengthens' the rectum by 5 cm. The rectal wall is made up of four layers: mucosa, submucosa, inner circular and outer longitudinal muscles. Over its upper third, the rectum is closely invested with peritoneum on its anterior and lateral surfaces and with the mesorectum posteriorly. As the rectum descends into the pelvis, the peritoneum fans out to cover only its anterior surface, with a layer of fat of variable thickness interposed. The anterior peritoneal reflection is variable in health and disease, occurring usually at 7–9 cm above the anal verge in men and 5–7.5 cm in women. The peritoneum is reflected directly onto the bladder in men and onto the vagina and uterus in women, with the potential space of the pouch of Douglas in between. Digital transanal palpation of the pouch of Douglas may reveal peritoneal tumour seeding, pelvic abscess, or other abnormal pathology.

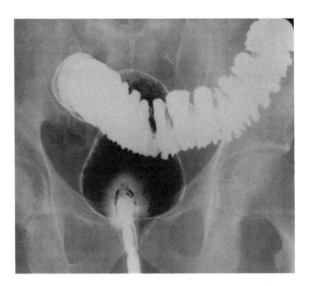

2a

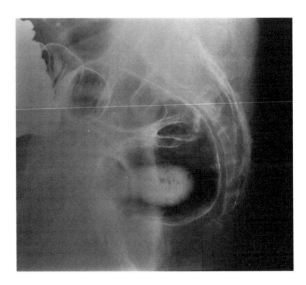

2b

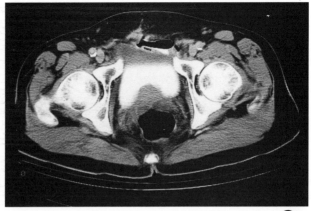

3a

3a–c The gross relations of the rectum are thus, posteriorly, the sacrum, coccyx, levator ani muscles, median sacral vessels and the roots of the sacral nerve plexus. Anteriorly in men the rectum is related to the bladder, prostate and seminal vesicles. The ureters are crossed by the vas deferens running vertically down the anterolateral wall of the pelvis. Exposure of the ureter in men may be achieved by incising the peritoneum from the common iliac artery bifurcation down the pelvic side wall, thus opening the lateral retroperitoneal space.

In women, the rectum is related to the uterus and vagina. Laterally, below the peritoneal reflection, the rectum is separated from the side wall of the pelvis by the ureter and iliac vessels.

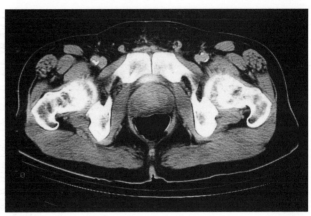

3b

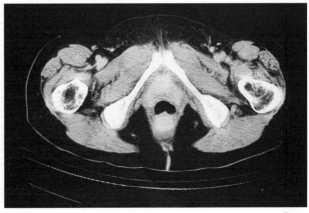

3c

Fascial relationships of the rectum

4 Knowledge of the fascial relationships of the rectum is intrinsic to successful mobilization of the rectum. With the sigmoid colon mobilized and the sigmoid mesentery stretched, a window between the inferior mesenteric artery and posterior abdominal wall structures below the aortic bifurcation can be developed (as described in the chapter on pp. 3–10).

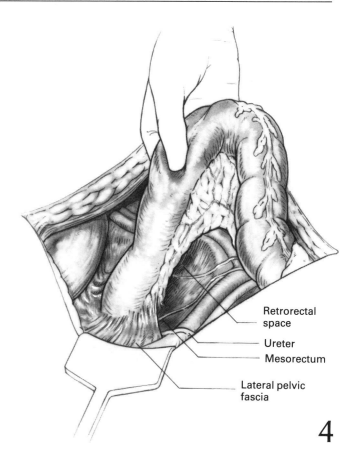

Retrorectal space

Ureter

Mesorectum

Lateral pelvic fascia

4

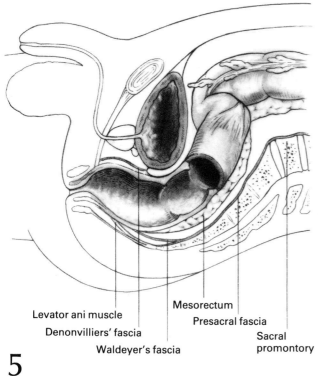

Levator ani muscle

Denonvilliers' fascia

Waldeyer's fascia

Mesorectum

Presacral fascia

Sacral promontory

5

5 Advancing the dissection over the sacral promontory, a tissue plane of loose areolar tissue is found between the mesorectum anteriorly, invested by the fascia propria of the rectum, and the presacral fascia posteriorly, protecting the median sacral vessels, nerve roots, presacral nerve and bony sacrum. This posterior plane is crucial to posterior mobilization because an inadvertent breach of the presacral fascia may lead to difficult venous bleeding and possible pelvic nerve damage.

6 By developing the posterior plane, lifting the rectum upwards and forwards, at the S4 level a dense fascial layer is encountered. The rectosacral or Waldeyer's fascia extends forwards to attach to the fascia propria of the rectum just above the anorectal ring. This must be incised sharply to complete mobilization down onto the levator ani muscles.

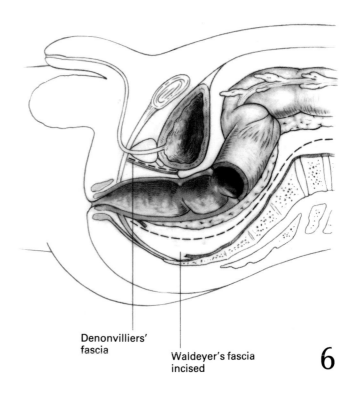

Denonvilliers' fascia

Waldeyer's fascia incised

6

Seminal vesicles

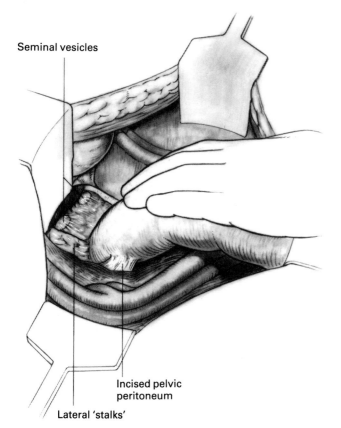

Incised pelvic peritoneum

Lateral 'stalks'

7

7 Incising the anterior peritoneal reflection, a layer of fascia known as Denonvilliers' fascia extends caudally to the urogenital diaphragm, separating extraperitoneal rectum from the anterior structures: seminal vesicles, periprostatic plexus and prostate in the male, or vagina in the female. With posterior and anterior dissection completed, two wings of the lateral pelvic fascia connecting the rectum to the pelvic side wall anterolaterally remain. This loose fatty tissue, possibly containing accessory branches of the middle haemorrhoidal artery, is divided and, with strong traction of the rectum, it is possible to define the lateral ligaments or rectal stalks which lie at the level just above the levator ani muscles. The lateral ligaments are definite structures but many surgeons mistakenly apply this term to describe the rather tenuous, more superficial, lateral pelvic fascia.

Female pelvic organs

8 Because of proximity to the rectum, the female organs are not uncommonly involved in disease processes. In particular, with a rectal carcinoma invading anteriorly or severe endometriosis involving the rectum, an *en bloc* resection will be required. The uterus is supported in the pelvis, anterior to the rectum, by five ligaments. The broad ligaments are reflections of peritoneum over the uterus and pelvic organs to the lateral pelvic walls. Running anterolaterally, the round ligaments extend from the fundus of the uterus to pass throught the deep inguinal ring. Connective tissue – the uterovesical ligament – attaches the bladder to the lower uterine segment. Posteriorly, the uterosacral ligaments are bands of fascia extending from the cervix around the rectum to the sacrum. The cardinal ligaments extend from the uterus to the lateral pelvic wall, and contain the uterine artery as it crosses over the ureter.

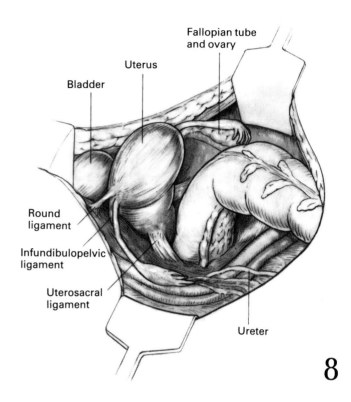

9 Initial division of the round ligament followed by incision of the broad ligament opens up the loose areolar tissue of the lateral retroperitoneal space and is the key to safe exposure of the ureter and pelvic vessels. The ureter crosses the bifurcation of the common iliac artery and descends into the pelvis, medial to the internal iliac vessels and just lateral to the uterosacral ligaments. Encased in the cardinal ligaments, the ureter is crossed by the uterine artery, and anteriorly it enters the upper outer angle of the trigone of the bladder.

The ovaries are attached by the ovarian ligament and lie in close relation to the fimbriae of the fallopian tube. The ovarian artery and vein descend into the pelvis in the infundibulopelvic ligament. Within the ovarian ligament is a utero–ovarian arterial anastomosis, which can give rise to significant bleeding.

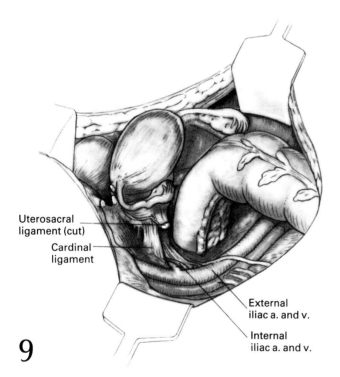

Anal canal

The terminal portion of the intestinal tract extends over a distance of about 4 cm from the anorectal ring to the hairy skin of the anal verge. The lining of the anal canal has important anatomical features, and the musculature of the anorectal region is essential for continence. Posteriorly, the anal canal is related to the coccyx, laterally to the ischiorectal fossa and its contents, and anteriorly to the urethra in men and to the perineal body and vagina in women.

Anal canal lining

10 The important anatomical landmark in the anal canal is the dentate or pectinate line. This line of anal valves lies 2 cm from the anal verge and corresponds to the junction of the middle and lower thirds of the internal anal sphincter which is relevant to the operation of internal sphincterotomy (as described in the chapter on pp. 871–879). Extending cranially from the dentate line, the mucosa is pleated into the 12–14 columns of Morgagni, and at the base of these columns above each anal valve lie the anal crypts. Opening into the crypts are a variable number of anal glands (4–10) which traverse the submucosa, two-thirds entering the internal sphincter and half terminating in the intersphincteric plane. Commonly, perianal fistulae are cryptoglandular in origin, and the internal opening can thus be expected to be probed at the corresponding anal crypt.

Cranial to the dentate line in the region of the columns of Morgagni, the mucosa consists of several layers of cuboidal cells (anal transitional zone) giving way over a distance of 0.5–1 cm to a single layer of cuboidal columnar cells characteristic of rectal mucosa. A corresponding colour change is seen from the deep purple of the transitional zone to pink of rectal mucosa in the region of the anorectal ring.

Caudal to the dentate line, the anal canal is lined by anoderm, a modified squamous epithelium devoid of hair, and glands over a distance of 1.5 cm. At the anal verge, the lining acquires the characteristics of normal skin including apocrine glands. For this reason, hidradenitis suppurativa (described in the chapter on pp. 806–813) does not extend into the anal canal and may be excised without anal stenosis.

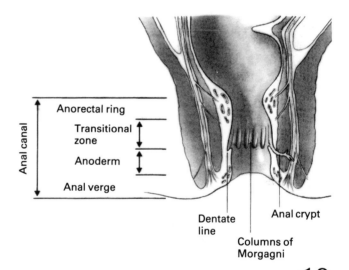

Anal canal

Anorectal ring

Transitional zone

Anoderm

Anal verge

Dentate line

Anal crypt

Columns of Morgagni

10

Anal canal musculature

Internal anal sphincter

11 This is the caudal continuation of the circular smooth muscle of the rectum, which becomes thickened and rounded to end 1.5 cm caudal to the dentate line and slightly cranial to the subcutaneous aspect of the external anal sphincter. With a Pratt speculum inserted through the anus stretching the internal sphincter, the tip of the finger may be rolled over the rim of the internal sphincter to palpate the intersphincteric groove.

Conjoined longitudinal muscle

The longitudinal muscle coat of the rectum, with some fibres from the pubococcygeus muscle, descends as a thin band between the internal and external anal sphincter. Some fibres traverse the internal sphincter, Treitz's muscle, or the muscularis submucosae ani, to form a supporting network around the haemorrhoidal venous plexus. Inferiorly, fibres run through the internal and external anal sphincters with dermal terminations, the so-called corrugator cutis ani (*see Illustration 11*).

External anal sphincter

This is an elliptical, continuous sleeve of striated muscle, enveloping the anal canal and internal anal sphincter and extending slightly beyond, to terminate in a subcutaneous position (*see Illustration 11*). Superiorly, it is continuous with the puborectalis and levator ani muscles. The whole muscle is a single unit, without subcutaneous, superficial, or deep divisions as previously described. Posteriorly, the external anal sphincter is attached to the skin superficially, and at a slightly deeper level to the coccyx, by the anococcygeal ligament. The deeper portion of the external sphincter has no posterior attachment and becomes continuous with the

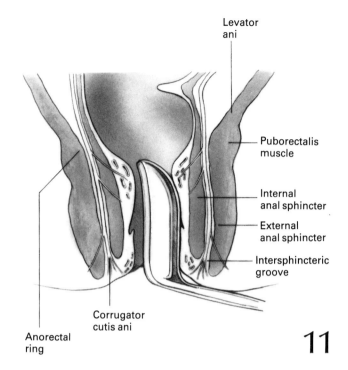

Levator ani

Puborectalis muscle

Internal anal sphincter

External anal sphincter

Intersphincteric groove

Corrugator cutis ani

Anorectal ring

11

puborectalis muscle at the level of the anorectal ring. Anteriorly, the external anal sphincter is attached to the skin superficially, then to the transverse perineal muscles, and most deeply fuses with the puborectalis muscle.

Perineal body

This is the central portion of the perineum, where external sphincter, bulbospongiosus and superficial and deep transverse perineal muscles meet. This tendinous intersection separates the anus from the vagina in women and is believed to support the perineum. Obstetric injury to the sphincter mechanism inevitably involves a repair of this structure.

Pelvic floor

12 The greater part of the pelvic floor is formed by the paired levator ani muscles. These have a funnel configuration with the outlet at the puborectalis sling. Each consists of two constituent muscles. The iliococcygeus muscle originates from the ischial spine and the obturator fascia and inserts into the sacrum (S4, S5), and coccyx and fuse medially as the anococcygeal raphe. The pubococcygeus muscle originates from the obturator fascia and pubic symphysis and inserts into the sacrum and coccyx. Fibres decussate medially with the contralateral side, fusing with the perineal body, prostate and vagina, and forming part of the conjoint longitudinal muscle of the anal canal; posteriorly, the fibres fuse in the midline as the anococcygeal raphe.

The puborectalis muscle is regarded separately. It originates from the pubic symphysis and superior fascia of the urogenital diaphragm and slings around the posterior aspect of the rectum, marking the anorectal ring. Awareness of this landmark during fistula and abscess surgery is of crucial importance for preservation of continence.

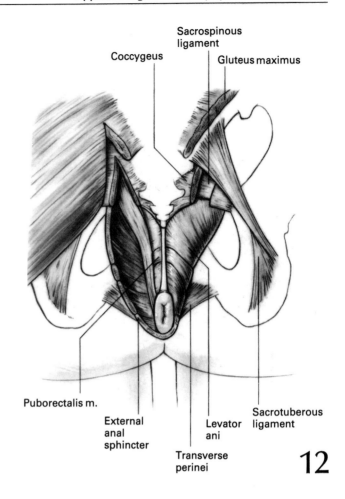

12

13 Other paired muscles make up the remainder of the pelvic floor. Posteriorly, the coccygeus muscles originate from the ischial spines and insert medially into S5 and the coccyx. Fibres blend with the sacrospinous ligament as a single unit. Dividing the pelvic floor into rectal and urogenital parts, the superficial transverse perineal muscles originate from the pelvic floor laterally, and insert into the central perineal raphe and external anal sphincter medially. The deep transverse perineal muscles originate from the ischium and in men merge medially with the urethral sphincter. During abdominoperineal resection of the rectum, recognition of the transverse perineal muscles guides the initial anterior dissection so that injury to the male urethra is avoided.

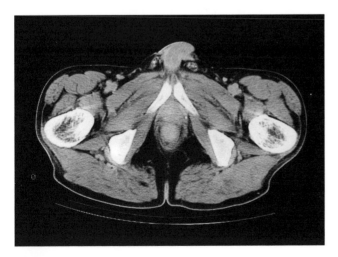

13

Perianal and pararectal spaces

Knowledge of the anatomy of the anorectal spaces and their potential communications and extensions is essential for effective treatment of the common problem of anorectal sepsis.

Ischiorectal fossa

14, 15 A more correct anatomical description would be the ischioanal space. The apex of this space is at the origin of the levator ani muscles from the obturator fascia, and the floor inferiorly is the skin of the perineum. The space is bounded anteriorly by the transverse muscles of the perineum, posteriorly by the sacrotuberous ligaments and gluteus maximus muscles, medially by the external anal sphincter and levator ani muscles, and laterally by the obturator internus muscle and obturator fascia. Running within the lateral wall and coursing from the ischial spine is Alcock's canal, containing the internal pudendal vessels and pudendal nerve. The space itself contains coarsely lobulated fat, the inferior haemorrhoidal vessels and nerves, and the scrotal or labial vessels. An ischioanal abscess may very occasionally extend anteriorly above the urogenital diaphragm.

Perianal space

The perianal space surrounds the anal verge and is bounded by the corrugator cutis ani. It contains the most caudal rim of the external anal sphincter, branches of the inferior haemorrhoidal vessels and the external haemorrhoidal plexus. Trauma to this plexus results in exquisitely painful perianal haematoma. Important communications for perianal abscess are laterally with the fat of the buttock and caudally the intersphincteric space.

Intersphincteric space

The intersphincteric space is a potential space between the internal and external anal sphincters and is continuous with the perianal space. The intersphincteric space is a common site for abscesses of cryptoglandular origin and fistula extension.

Postanal spaces

The ischioanal spaces communicate posteriorly through the superficial and deep postanal spaces. The superficial space runs between the skin and the anococcygeal ligament. Of more significance, the deep postanal space runs between the anococcygeal ligament and the anococcygeal raphe of the levator ani muscles. This posterior communication is responsible for the so-called 'horseshoe' abscess, and failure effectively to recognize and drain the deep postanal space results in persistent sepsis.

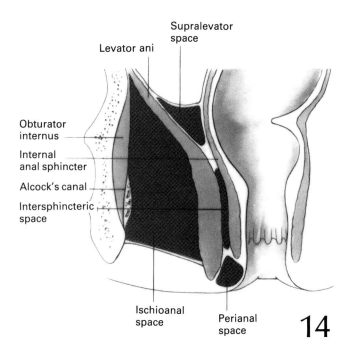

14

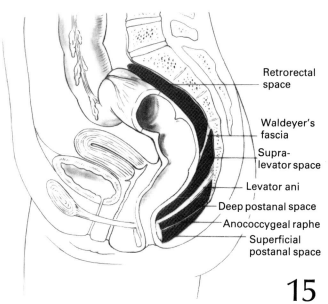

15

Retrorectal and supralevator spaces

Above the pelvic floor are two surgically important and distinct potential spaces. The retrorectal space begins cranial to Waldeyer's fascia and extends upwards between the fascia propria, enveloping the mesorectum and rectum anteriorly, the presacral fascia posteriorly, and the pelvic fascia and peritoneum laterally and superiorly. It is this space that is opened initially during posterior mobilization of the rectum. At a deeper level, between Waldeyer's fascia and the levator ani muscles, is the supralevator space, bounded laterally by the obturator fascia.

Pelvic vasculature

16a, b At the body of L4, the aorta bifurcates into the right and left common iliac arteries. These diverge as they descend towards the pelvis and bifurcate at the sacroiliac joint into external and internal iliac arteries. Branches of the internal iliac artery, arising from the pelvic wall, are responsible for blood supply to the pelvic viscera, walls, perineum and gluteal region. Internal iliac artery and vein ligation may be considered before sacrumectomy for advanced rectal carcinoma.

The blood supply to the rectum and anal canal comes mainly from the superior, middle and inferior rectal arteries. The superior rectal artery is the continuation of the inferior mesenteric artery after giving off the sigmoid branches. This artery lies at the base of the sigmoid mesocolon, where it bifurcates and is in very close relation to the presacral nerves posteriorly, just proximal to the sacral promontory, before descending into the mesorectum. This is one of the key regions for potential autonomic nerve damage during rectal mobilization.

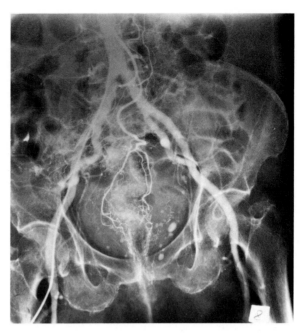

16a

The mesorectum is triangular, with its base on the posterior rectal wall, thinning to end at the pelvic floor. Running within the mesorectum are the superior rectal artery and vein branches and tributaries, and proximal draining lymphatics. The surgical importance of the mesorectum lies in its complete excision during low anterior resection for carcinoma, which is believed to lessen the risk of local tumour recurrence (as described in the chapter on pp. 456–471). Within the mesorectum, the superior rectal artery bifurcates in a variable fashion with an average of five branches reaching the haemorrhoidal zone. Contrary to historical dogma, there is no direct positional relationship to the primary haemorrhoidal groups.

The branching arrangement of the superior rectal vessels, forming a V shape within the triangular mesorectum, facilitates mobilization close to the rectal wall, as few vessels penetrate in the midline posteriorly. This approach may be used to protect the nerves during proctectomy for benign disease.

The inferior rectal arteries arise from the internal pudendal artery, which is a branch of the internal iliac artery. The middle rectal artery arises from the internal iliac artery and traverses deep to the levator fascia to reach the rectal wall. It may be encountered during anterior mobilization of the rectum, close to the seminal vesicles and prostate or upper part of the vagina. One-quarter of patients possess an accessory middle rectal artery traversing the lateral stalks. Very occasionally, the superior rectal artery is small, and under these circumstances caution is advised, as the middle

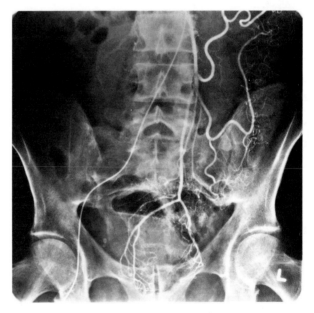

16b

rectal artery may be substantial. The superior and inferior rectal arteries are major contributors to a rich intramural anastomotic network, such that the rectal viability is preserved after division of the superior rectal artery.

Venous drainage of the rectum and anal canal mirrors the arterial supply. Middle and inferior rectal veins drain systemically, and the superior rectal vein drains into the portal system via the splenic vein.

Anal cushions

17 These are constant and normal structures above the dentate line in the anal canal. Three primary positions – left lateral, right anterior and right posterior – with intermediate minor groups are described. The cushions consist of dilated submucosal haemorrhoidal venous plexuses fed by direct arteriovenous communications, which account for bright red 'anal canal' bleeding. Treitz's muscle, with contributions from the internal anal sphincter and conjoint longitudinal muscle, forms a supporting scaffold. The sliding anal canal theory for haemorrhoids rests on stretching and disruption of this support. Rubber band 'ligation' or injection sclerotherapy is correctly applied *above* the haemorrhoidal venous plexus and effectively 'refixes' the anal cushions.

Lymphatic drainage

18 The microscopic distribution of lymphatics within the wall of the rectum or colon is important with reference to the ability of a tumour to become invasive with metastatic potential. Some lymphatics are present in the lowest part of the lamina propria, intimately associated with the muscularis mucosae, but they are plentiful in the submucosa and muscularis propria. For practical purposes, the muscularis mucosae is taken as the dividing line, with tumours superficial to this plane being described as 'adenomas' with varying degrees of 'dysplasia'. Once the muscularis mucosae has been reached, the neoplasm is defined as a 'carcinoma' with metastatic potential.

Lymphatic drainage of the rectum and anus tends to be segmental, mirroring the arterial supply (*see Illustration 16*). Lymph from the proximal two-thirds of the rectum drains with the superior rectal artery to the inferior mesenteric nodes. The lower one-third of the rectum drains both proximally via superior rectal lymphatics and laterally via middle rectal lymphatics to the internal iliac nodes. In women, lymphatic spread may occur to the posterior vaginal wall, uterus, broad ligaments, ovaries and pouch of Douglas. In general, retrograde spread only occurs after extensive involvement of perirectal tissues, proximal and perineural lymphatics, and with venous infiltration. This information is pertinent when assessing the advisability of a more radical resection, in particular ileal lymphadenectomy, hysterectomy and bilateral oophorectomy.

From the anal canal above the dentate line, lymphatics drain both proximally by the superior rectal nodes to the inferior mesenteric nodes, and laterally via middle rectal and inferior rectal vessels to the internal iliac nodes. Generally, below the dentate line primary drainage is to the inguinal lymph nodes. In the presence of obstruction, lymph from the lower anal canal may also take the superior rectal and inferior rectal routes.

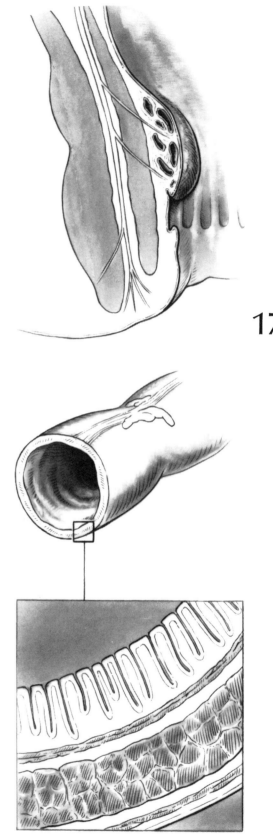

17

18

Innervation

19 During rectal mobilization, pelvic autonomic neurological damage may occur. It is of paramount importance to avoid bladder dysfunction, impotence and retrograde ejaculation, but this will depend in part on the pathological process and type of surgery being performed.

The lower rectum, bladder and sexual organs receive their sympathetic supply via the presacral nerves. These are formed from the aortic plexus and lumbar splanchnic nerves. The presacral nerves descend over the bifurcation of the aorta and sacral promontory, closely related anteriorly to the superior rectal artery. During the initial phase of rectal mobilization, the presacral nerves are liable to be tented up with the superior rectal artery, and attention must be given to their preservation at this point. Below the sacral promontory, the presacral nerves run bilaterally around the pelvic wall, protected initially by the presacral fascia (and the 'potential' retrorectal space), to reach their respective pelvic plexus.

The parasympathetic outflow to the pelvis arises from the anterior roots of S3 and S4. The nervi erigentes pass laterally, forwards and upwards to join the presacral nerve at the pelvic plexus, providing visceral branches to the bladder, ureters, seminal vesicles, prostate, rectum, membranous urethra and corpora cavernosa. The pelvic plexus is located anteriorly on the pelvic side wall at the level of the lower third of the rectum and lateral to the rectal stalks. In men, its midpoint is related to the tip of the seminal vesicle, and in women, the anterior part lies lateral to the upper third of the vagina, with its upper fibres extending into the cardinal ligament. Excessive traction on the rectum, particularly laterally, before division of the rectal stalks may damage the pelvic plexus. Where pelvic lymphadenectomy is considered, preservation of the S4 root may preserve a degree of urinary function.

The periprostatic plexus is an important subdivision of the pelvic plexus, supplying fibres to the prostate, seminal vesicles, corpora cavernosa, vas deferens, urethra, ejaculatory ducts and bulbourethral glands. Erection of the penis is mediated by both parasympathetic (arteriolar vasodilatation) and sympathetic (inhibition of vasoconstriction) inflow. Sympathetic activity is

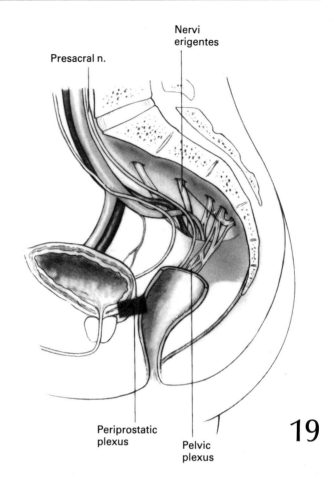

responsible for emission and parasympathetic activity for ejaculation. Fibres from the periprostatic plexus are protected by Denonvilliers' fascia and therefore sexual function may be protected by dissection below Denonvilliers' fascia.

Further reading

Mundy AR. An anatomical explanation for bladder dysfunction following rectal and uterine surgery. *Br J Urol* 1982; 54: 501–4.

Pemberton JH. Anatomy and physiology of the anus and rectum. In: Condon RE, ed. *Shackleford's Surgery of the Alimentary Tract.* Volume IV. Philadelphia: WB Saunders, 1991: 242–74.

Thomson WHF. The nature of haemorrhoids. *Br J Surg* 1975; 62: 542–52.

Applied surgical anatomy: perineal and anal canal

David J. Schoetz Jr MD
Chairman, Department of Colon and Rectal Surgery, Lahey Clinic Medical Center, Burlington, Massachusetts, USA

Topographical anatomy

1 Inspection of the anal region shows that the anal orifice itself lacks hair and other skin appendages. The perianal skin is corrugated symmetrically around the anus. Palpation at the anal verge permits discrimination between the internal (smooth muscle) and external (skeletal muscle) sphincters at the lateral border of the haemorrhoids; this is the intersphincteric groove, an important landmark for operative surgery. Bony prominences that form the boundaries of the perianal region include the coccyx posteriorly and the ischium bilaterally. The perineal body separates the posterior from the anterior perineal triangles anteriorly.

Anal canal

Frontal view

2 The anal canal measures 3–4 cm from the anorectal junction superiorly to the anal verge and is lined by smooth squamous epithelium in its lower half. Approximately 2 cm inside the anal verge is the junction between rectal mucosa and anoderm. This junction assumes a 'saw-toothed' appearance and is the dentate line. Pleated rectal mucosa above the dentate line forms the columns of Morgagni, numbering from six to 14. At the lower end of the columns are the anal papillae. Between the columns, just above the dentate line, are the anal crypts into which the anal glands discharge. Obstruction of the crypts is believed to be responsible for most pararectal abscesses and fistulae. The rectal epithelium is composed of mucin-secreting columnar cells, while that of the anal canal is composed of squamous cells. The transitional zone between these two structures is gradual, measuring 6–12 mm and characterized by a cuboidal epithelium. This zone is also referred to as the cloacogenic zone and is the source of some neoplasms of the anal canal.

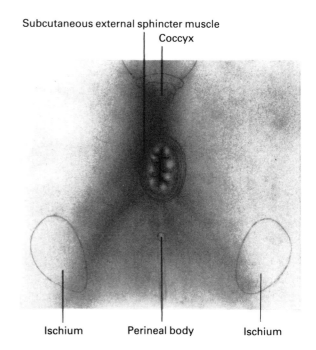

Subcutaneous external sphincter muscle
Coccyx

Ischium Perineal body Ischium

1

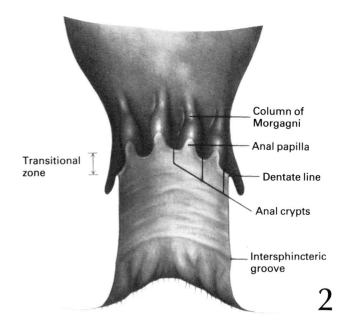

Transitional zone

Column of Morgagni

Anal papilla

Dentate line

Anal crypts

Intersphincteric groove

2

Longitudinal section

3 Circular muscle fibres of the colon and rectum enlarge in the distal end to form the internal sphincter. This involuntary sphincter, responsible for maintenance of resting tone of the anal canal, extends from above the dentate line superiorly to within 1 cm of the anal verge. Voluntary skeletal muscle makes up the external sphincter complex. The puborectalis muscle, merged with the levator ani muscle, is the deepest muscle and is crucial for maintenance of anal continence. The deep, superficial and subcutaneous portions of the external sphincter are continuous with each other. The subcutaneous portion of the external sphincter is distal to the internal sphincter.

Between the external and internal sphincters is the longitudinal muscle, a continuation of the longitudinal muscle of the colon and rectum. Fibres from the longitudinal muscle pierce the internal sphincter and penetrate through and insert into the submucosa of the distal rectal mucosa. These mucosal suspensory ligaments are believed to anchor the mucosa, preventing prolapse. The remainder of the longitudinal muscle inserts into the dermis of the perianal skin by small ramifications called the corrugator cutis ani muscle. Anal glands, lined by stratified columnar epithelium, open directly into the anal crypts. Half of these glands cross into the intersphincteric plane and are the source of most pararectal abscesses.

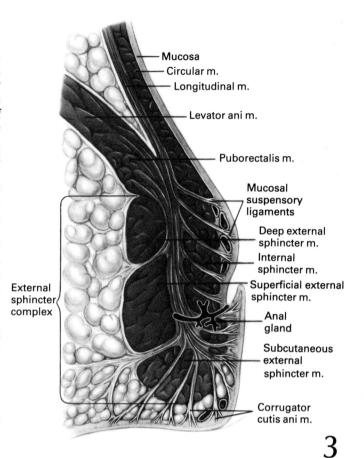

3

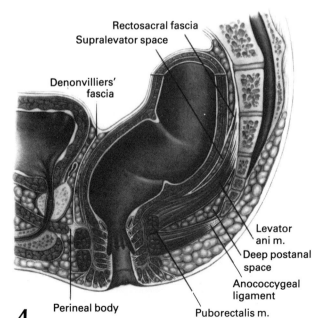

4

Lateral view

4 Fascial attachments of the rectum below the peritoneal reflection include Denonvilliers' fascia anteriorly and the rectosacral fascia (Waldeyer's) posteriorly. Denonvilliers' fascia extends from the anterior peritoneal reflection to the urogenital diaphragm. Laterally, this fascia blends with the anterior fascia of the lateral ligaments. Posteriorly, the rectosacral fascia originates from the presacral fascia and extends downward and anteriorly to insert in the posterior aspect of the rectum above the puborectalis muscle. Inferior to the rectosacral fascia is the supralevator space. Posteriorly, the external sphincter is anchored to the coccyx by the anococcygeal ligament. The puborectalis muscle has no posterior attachment. The potential space between the levator ani muscle and the anococcygeal ligament is the deep postanal space, the origin of most horseshoe abscesses and fistulae. Anteriorly, the deep portion of the external sphincter merges with the transverse perineal muscles and inserts into the central tendon of the perineum, the perineal body.

Levator ani muscle

5a–d Viewed from above (*Illustration 5a*, male; *Illustration 5b*, female), the levator ani muscle arises laterally from the tendinous arch that adheres firmly to the pelvic bones. The iliococcygeus muscle is the most lateral portion of the muscle, with its medial insertion in the anococcygeal raphe and lower sacrum. The pubococcygeus muscle arises from the back of the pubic symphysis and attaches posteriorly at the anococcygeal raphe and coccyx. The puborectalis muscle is the most medial portion of the levator muscle; it arises from the posterior symphysis and forms a sling around the anorectal junction, attaching to the opposite symphysis. Lack of a posterior attachment permits the muscle to pull forward, closing off the anorectal junction and preserving continence. Inferior views of these structures are shown in *Illustrations 5c* (male) and *5d* (female).

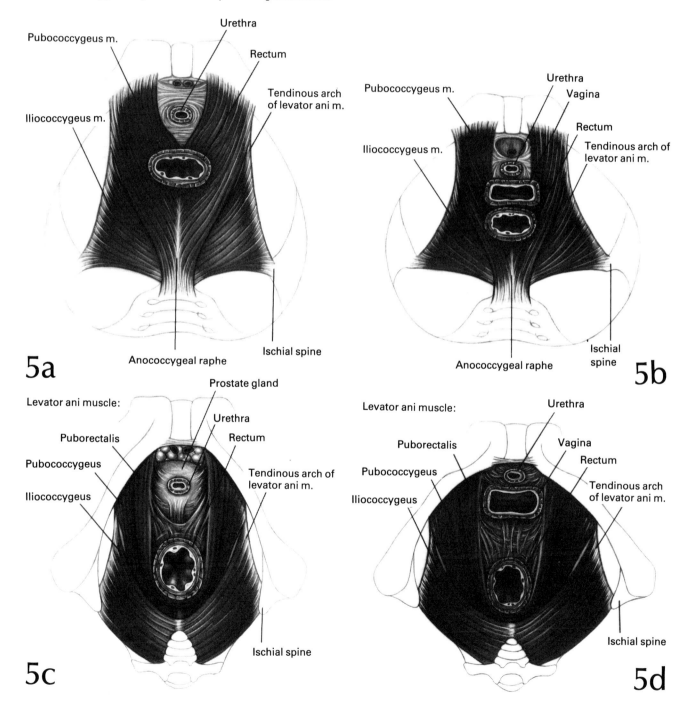

Perineum

Inferior view

6a, b The superficial transverse perineal muscles, which insert centrally into the perineal body, separate the perineum into anterior and posterior triangles (*Illustration 6a*, male; *Illustration 6b*, female).

The arterial and venous supplies are paired. The internal pudendal artery and vein originate from the internal iliac artery and vein and pass through Alcock's canal at the superolateral border of the ischiorectal fossa. The internal pudendal artery and vein give rise to the inferior rectal artery and vein, which supply the distal rectum and anal canal as well as the external sphincter muscles. The perineal artery and vein cross into the anterior triangle to supply the urogenital structures.

The internal pudendal nerve, also in Alcock's canal, gives rise to the inferior rectal nerve that traverses the ischiorectal fossa and supplies the external sphincter with motor innervation and the anal canal and perianal region with sensory innervation. In addition, motor innervation of the levator muscle is derived from the deep perineal nerve below and branches of the fourth sacral nerve above.

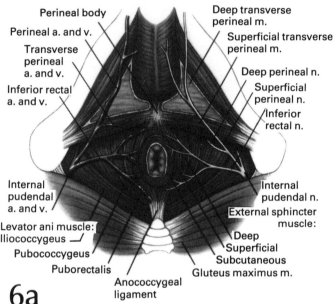

6a

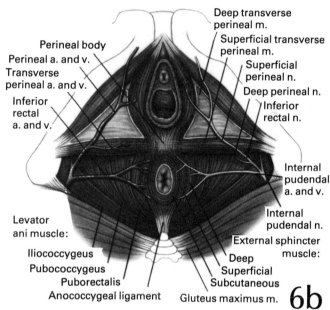

6b

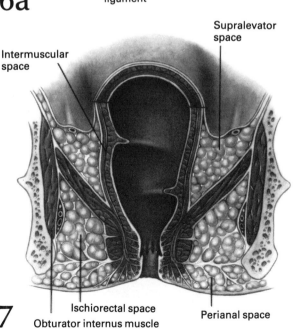

7

Anorectal spaces

Frontal view

7 The perianal space is in the area of the anal verge. Laterally it is continuous with the subcutaneous fat of the buttocks, and medially it extends up to the dentate line.

The ischiorectal space is a pyramid-shaped area bounded superiorly by the levator ani, laterally by the obturator internus muscle and the obturator fascia overlying the ischium, medially by the levator and external sphincter, anteriorly by the superficial and deep perineal muscles, posteriorly by the gluteus maximus, and inferiorly by the perineal skin.

The supralevator space is situated on either side of the rectum and is bounded superiorly by the peritoneum, laterally by the pelvic wall, medially by the rectum, and inferiorly by the levator muscles.

The intermuscular space (intersphincteric space) lies between the internal and external sphincter muscles and extends superiorly within the rectal wall.

Anorectal abscesses

Frontal view

8 Abscesses corresponding to the described anorectal spaces are shown: A, perianal abscess; B, ischiorectal abscess; C, intermuscular abscess; and D, supralevator abscess.

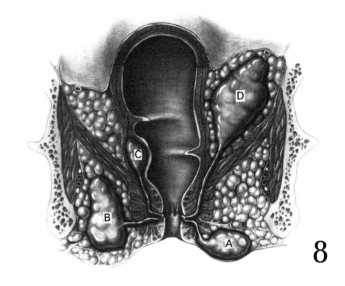

8

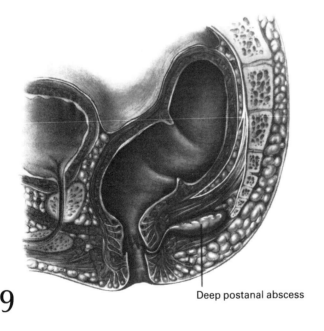

9

Deep postanal abscess

Abscess in deep postanal space

9 An abscess in the deep postanal space is located posterior to the rectum in the area superior to the anococcygeal ligament and inferior to the levator muscle. Pus may dissect into one or both ischiorectal fossae, resulting in a horseshoe abscess. External inflammatory signs are frequently lacking. Drainage is accomplished by an extrasphincteric incision between the posterior aspect of the sphincter and the coccyx.

Arterial supply of rectum and anus

Frontal view

10 The superior rectal artery is the termination of the inferior mesenteric artery, descending within the mesentery of the sigmoid. Bifurcation occurs at the level of the third sacral segment. A single branch supplies the left (L) side of the distal rectum, whereas the right side splits into anterior (RA) and posterior (RP) branches.

The middle rectal artery arises from the anterior branch of the internal iliac artery, coursing superior to the levator muscle and traversing the lateral ligaments to supply the lower rectum and upper anal canal.

The course of the inferior rectal artery has already been described (*see Illustration 6*).

The middle sacral artery arises posteriorly above the bifurcation of the aorta and descends over the lower lumbar vertebrae, sacrum and coccyx to the level of the anococcygeal raphe. Surgical injury to this vessel can occur during mobilization of the distal rectum.

Multiple anastomoses among these arteries provide a rich collateral circulation to the rectum and anus.

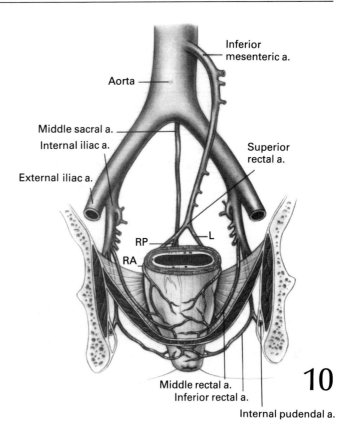

Venous drainage of rectum and anus

Frontal view

11 Veins in this region accompany the corresponding arteries. The superior rectal vein drains the rectum and upper anal canal into the inferior mesenteric vein, which drains into the portal vein by way of the splenic vein. The middle rectal veins drain the same area into the systemic venous system by way of the internal iliac veins. The inferior rectal veins drain the anal canal by way of the internal pudendal into the internal iliac veins.

Potential portosystemic communications exist within the submucosal plexus of veins in the lower rectum and anal canal. The external rectal (haemorrhoidal) plexus drains into the systemic venous system by the inferior rectal veins, whereas the internal rectal (haemorrhoidal) plexus drains into the portal venous system by the superior rectal vein.

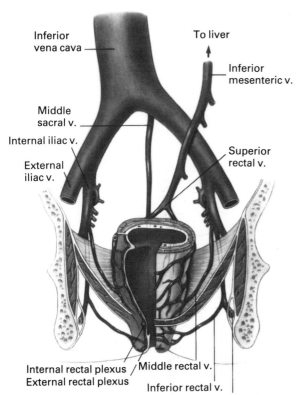

Presacral venous anatomy

12a, b

(Illustration 12a, frontal view; Illustration 12b, lateral view.) Two separate venous systems exist within the presacral space. On the anterior surface of the sacrum is the presacral venous plexus, a network of veins that drain by way of the lateral sacral vein and the middle sacral vein into the inferior vena cava. These veins also communicate with the basivertebral venous system, which penetrates directly to the sacral foramina to join the internal vertebral venous system within the substance of the sacrum. Adventitia of the basivertebral veins blends with the sacral periosteum, making control by suture ligature extremely difficult, if not impossible, when the veins are disrupted during rectal mobilization. The vertebral venous system is a complex network of valveless venous sinuses around the dura of the spinal cord that communicates with the vertebral vein superiorly. Numerous branches from the vertebral venous system communicate with the inferior vena cava to form a large pool of blood that accounts for life-threatening haemorrhage during rectal excision when the veins are injured.

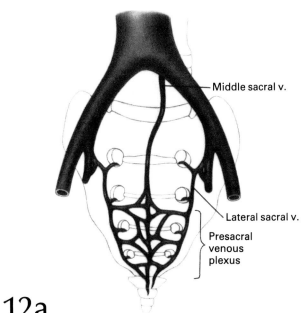

Middle sacral v.

Lateral sacral v.

Presacral venous plexus

12a

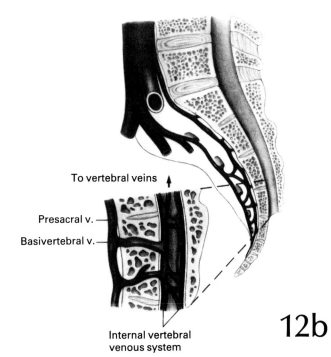

To vertebral veins

Presacral v.

Basivertebral v.

Internal vertebral venous system

12b

Lymphatic drainage of the rectum and anus

13 Lymphatic vessels follow the arterial supply. Rich intramural lymphatic vessels found in the submucosa penetrate into the pararectal tissues and follow the arteries. Lymphatic drainage from the intraperitoneal rectum is exclusively upward along the course of the superior rectal artery to the inferior mesenteric nodes and to the preaortic nodes. Lateral spread from the lower rectum is along the course of the middle rectal arteries to the internal iliac nodes and posteriorly to the sacral nodes. Extension farther upward through the common iliac nodes leads to the preaortic nodes.

Downward spread follows the inferior rectal artery to the pararectal nodes within the ischial rectal fossa and to the internal iliac nodes. In addition, the anal canal drains by way of the subdermal lymphatic system to the inguinal nodes in the groin. As a result, tumours of the distal rectum and anal canal may spread to the inguinal nodes and to the lateral pelvic nodes.

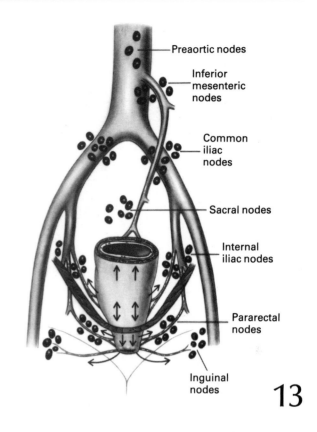

Preaortic nodes

Inferior mesenteric nodes

Common iliac nodes

Sacral nodes

Internal iliac nodes

Pararectal nodes

Inguinal nodes

13

Autonomic and somatic nerves

14 Motor innervation to the external sphincter arises from the second, third and fourth sacral nerves by way of the internal pudendal nerve to the inferior rectal nerves. Levator ani muscles are supplied by nerve fibres from the fourth sacral nerve on the superior aspect and, on the inferior aspect, by the inferior rectal and perineal nerves.

Sensory innervation below the dentate line is supplied by afferent fibres of the inferior rectal nerves.

Sympathetic innervation arises from the sympathetic ganglia of the first, second and third lumbar nerves with sympathetic fibres to the preaortic plexus. Fibres travel inferiorly to the inferior mesenteric plexus, some fibres following the inferior mesenteric artery and its branches to supply the colon and rectum. The remainder of the sympathetic fibres unite below the bifurcation of the aorta in the hypogastric plexus. Two main hypogastric nerves carry sympathetic innervation to the pelvic plexus on either side of the rectum.

Parasympathetic innervation arises from the second, third and fourth sacral nerves and gives rise to the nervi erigentes, which unite with the sympathetic nerves in the pelvic plexus. From the pelvic plexus, combined sympathetic and parasympathetic nerves are distributed to the pelvic organs, including the rectum and the genitourinary system.

Sympathetic chain   Spinal cord

L1

Preaortic plexus

Inferior mesenteric plexus

Hypogastric plexus

Hypogastric n.

Pelvic plexus

To pelvic organs

To pelvic organs

Inferior rectal n.

Perineal n.

L1
L2
L3
L4
L5
S1
S2
S3
S4
S5

Nervi erigentes

Internal pudendal n.

14

—— Sympathetic
······· Parasympathetic
– – – Somatic

Pelvic nerves

Frontal view

15 Injury to the autonomic nerves may occur at several points, as illustrated, during rectal mobilization:

1. High ligation of the inferior mesenteric artery flush with the aorta may injure sympathetic nerves to the rectum and the internal sphincter.
2. Dissection below the aortic bifurcation may injure the hypogastric plexus and result in sympathetic denervation of the sexual apparatus (ejaculatory dysfunction) or urinary sphincter (urinary frequency).
3. Failure to stay in the presacral plane may injure the hypogastric nerves and result in sympathetic denervation.
4. Nervi erigentes are short and enter the pelvic plexus in the posterolateral pelvis. Consequently, isolated parasympathetic denervation is rare.
5. Mixed parasympathetic and sympathetic nerves may be injured during division of the lateral ligaments when dissection is on the lateral pelvic side wall. More often, these nerves are injured as they progress anteriorly toward the seminal vesicles and prostate gland. Injury to these nerves results in parasympathetic denervation of the sexual organs (erectile impotence) and bladder (flaccid neurogenic bladder).

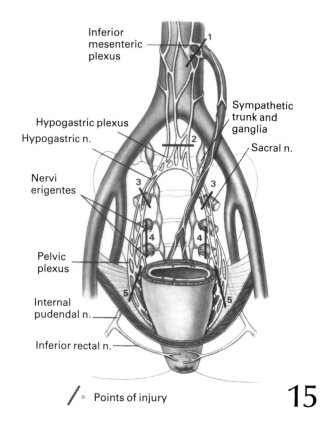

/ = Points of injury

15

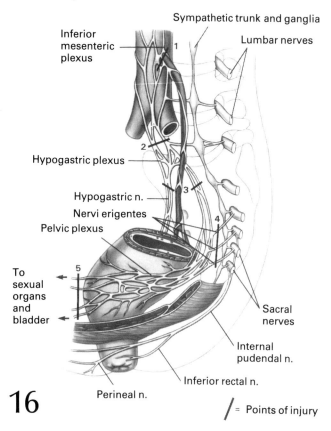

16

/ = Points of injury

Lateral view

16 The possibility of injuring fibres from the pelvic plexus can be better appreciated in this lateral view.

Cross-sectional imaging

17 With the increasing application of computed tomography, cross-sectional anatomy of the perineum is routinely observed. In this example from a normal male pelvis, the bony prominences of the pubis (Pu), the coccyx (C) and the ischium bilaterally (I) frame the perineal structures. The anococcygeal ligament (AL) is seen attaching the anorectal junction (A) to the coccyx posteriorly. The inferior border of the puborectalis muscle (P) is seen forming a sling around the anorectal junction. The proximity of the prostate (Pr) to the anterior rectum is readily identified. The ischiorectal spaces (IS) on either side are accentuated by their fat content, contrasting them with the surrounding structures. The gluteus muscles (G) make up the posterior boundary of the ischiorectal space.

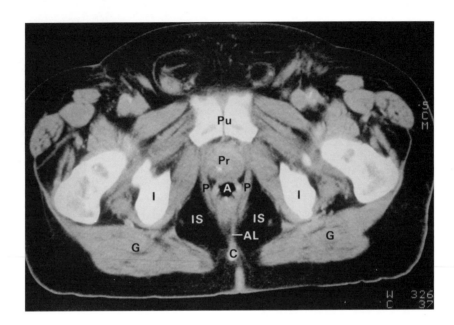

17

Intrarectal ultrasonography

18 The development of intrarectal ultrasonography has permitted more accurate diagnosis of conditions that affect the prostate as well as the rectum. A transducer is inserted transanally, and a balloon is inflated with degassed water in which the transducer rotates. Alternating light and dark bands correspond to the layers of the rectum. The inner dark circle represents the balloon; 1, the first white band represents the mucosa; 2, a black band represents the muscularis mucosa; 3, a white band represents the submucosa; 4, a black band represents the muscularis propria; and 5, a white band represents the interface between the muscularis propria and the perirectal fat.

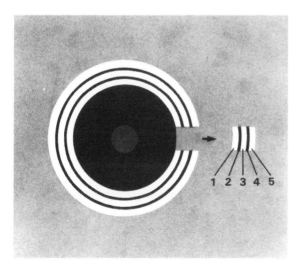

18

19 This study demonstrates an anterior rectal tumour (T) with an intact interface between the muscularis and perirectal fat immediately behind the prostate (Pr).

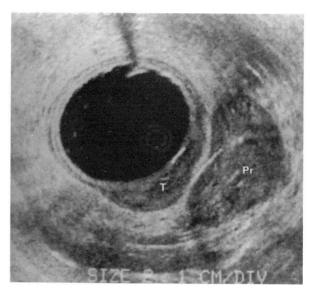

19

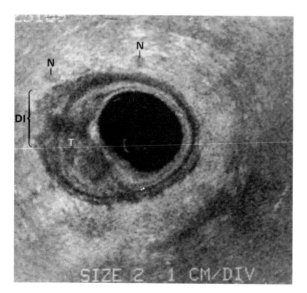

20

20 This study demonstrates a posterior rectal tumour (T) with destroyed interface (DI) between the muscularis and perirectal fat. Two enlarged lymph nodes (N) are also seen.

Acknowledgements

Illustrations 1–16 and *18* are reprinted with kind permission of the Lahey Clinic Medical Centre.

Illustrations by Gillian Lee and the late Robert Lane

Rectal biopsy

Robin K. S. Phillips MS, FRCS
Consultant Surgeon, St Mark's Hospital For Diseases of the Rectum and Colon and Homerton Hospital, London and Honorary Lecturer, St Bartholomew's Hospital Medical School, London, UK

Biopsy is a diagnostic procedure which, unless carried out correctly, may fail in its purpose. The biopsy may be mucosal, excisional, full-thickness, or taken from an abnormal structure. Each requires special care to achieve the best results.

Operations

MUCOSAL BIOPSY

1, 2 A simple mucosal biopsy is carried out for diseases which are primarily superficial, e.g. ulcerative, Crohn's and ischaemic colitis, amoebic disease, and solitary ulcer syndrome. No anaesthetic is required. The procedure is usually easy but may be difficult when the mucosa is very atrophic as in the chronic inactive phase of ulcerative colitis. A satisfactory result can be obtained with an 'Officer's' heavy biopsy forceps; the piece of mucosa is twisted off by rotating the instrument until the specimen comes away without traction. This reduces the possibility of bleeding from the biopsy site.

Sharp cutting forceps (including suction biopsy apparatus) should not be used unless the edges are sharpened regularly because, when blunt, bleeding may occur.

With flexible instruments there is also the opportunity for 'hot' biopsy. With this technique, the appropriate endoscopic biopsy forceps grasp the lesion, which is tented up. A coagulating diathermy current is then passed until the apex of the tented mucosa turns white, and the biopsy is taken. The technique is appropriate for sampling and destroying small polyps, but larger polyps require snare removal. Diathermy artefacts and the small risk of secondary haemorrhage make the use of the 'hot' procedure inappropriate for routine diagnostic biopsy.

Regardless of the method used, pathologists prefer a specimen that is not fixed 'curled-up' because the glandular structure becomes distorted. The biopsy should be pressed down, mucosa upwards, on a piece of ground glass, thick blotting paper or card before being placed in a fixative solution. It is probably wise to defer a barium enema examination for at least 1 week after a biopsy has been taken because of the small risk of intestinal perforation.

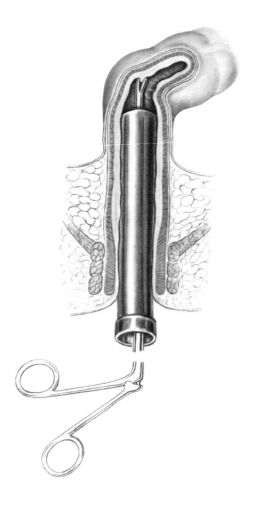

1

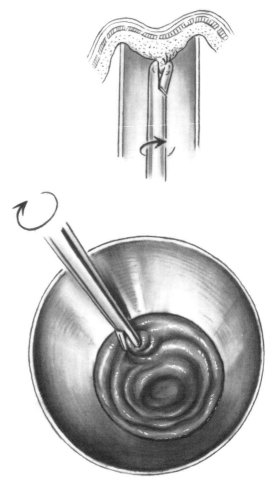

2

EXCISION BIOPSY

3 The forceps or snare is placed over the lesion or around its base and the whole structure is removed. In the case of a pedunculated lesion, the wire loop of the snare is passed over the polyp which is gently shaken until the wire lies around the stalk. The loop is tightened until it grips the stalk and then the instrument is retracted slightly so that minimal traction is exerted on the stalk. The diathermy current is passed using multiple very short bursts at 5-s intervals, tightening the wire slowly until the polyp is removed. *A long continuous current must never be used.*

If the pedicle bleeds, it should be touched with a fulgurating button using a coagulating current, or a swab of 1:1000 topical adrenaline may be applied.

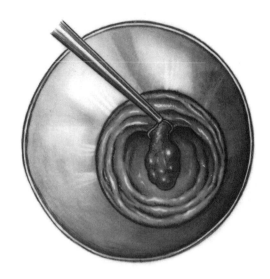

3

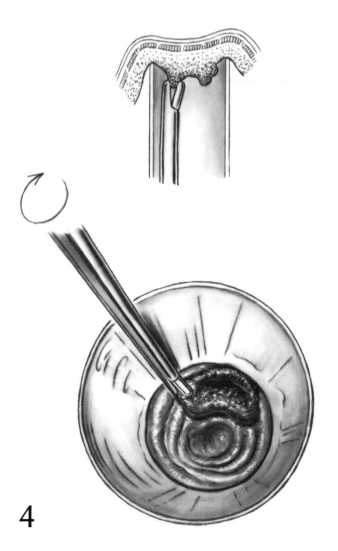

4

BIOPSY OF ABNORMAL STRUCTURES

When an abnormal structure such as a tumour is seen, two decisions must be made – whether it can be removed completely (excision biopsy) and, if not, from which area is a correct diagnosis (diagnostic biopsy) most likely to be obtained. All biopsies are liable to sampling error if only a part of the lesion is sampled. Thus, if a tumour is small or pedunculated, it should usually be removed totally either by twisting or by snaring using electrocoagulation. This can be done without an anaesthetic and the intestine does not normally require any special cleansing.

4 If the lesion is larger and not completely removable, the biopsy should be taken with Officer's forceps, from the edge where the mucosa alters its characteristics, e.g. the rolled everted edge of a malignant ulcer. If the lesion is within reach of the finger it may be reasonable to take the biopsy from the most indurated area. This is particularly necessary for patients with a villous adenoma, which is very soft when benign but becomes indurated when malignant, when it is recurrent, or after previous diathermy treatment.

It is very unwise and dangerous to make a blind 'grab' at a lesion, particularly when it is of uncertain nature, because bleeding and perforation may occur. If a whole polyp is removed, its stalk or base should be identified with a stitch because this is the area where tumour infiltration needs to be sought by the pathologist.

FULL-THICKNESS RECTAL BIOPSY

A full-thickness rectal biopsy may be required on some occasions to diagnose Hirschsprung's disease (aganglionosis) or some similar rare disorders with either hyperganglionosis or hypoganglionosis. In infants a full-thickness biopsy is usually unnecessary because the diagnosis of Hirschsprung's disease may be made: (1) by seeing abnormal nerve fibres in the submucosa of the mucosal biopsy; (2) by special staining techniques; (3) supported physiologically by an absent anorectal inhibitory reflex. In the adult in whom the diagnosis is suspected or if a megacolon is present, however, a full-thickness biopsy should be taken. These patients are usually very constipated and therefore it may be necessary to spend several days clearing the intestine. It is essential that the intestine should be clear before this diagnostic procedure is carried out to avoid dangerous extrarectal sepsis. A general anaesthetic is required.

Position of patient

The patient is placed either in the lithotomy or prone jack-knife position (*see* pp. 47–50) and an Eisenhammer or Parks' speculum is inserted. The biopsy is best taken from the left posterior quadrant. It must be from above the upper limit of the internal sphincter muscle, which is normally an aganglionic area. The anorectal ring is palpated to determine the upper limit of the sphincter complex.

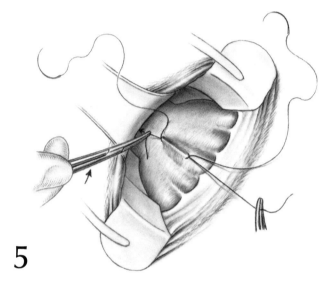

5

Incision

5, 6 Stay sutures of 2/0 absorbable material are placed through the thickness of the rectal wall 2–3 cm apart and tied. If they are correctly placed, incorporating muscle, a characteristic blanching occurs as they are secured. One end of the upper stitch is gripped in an artery forceps which is pushed forwards and upwards by an assistant. The lower stitch is pulled downwards and backwards by the operator. The other end of the upper suture with the needle attached is left in order to oversew the defect in one full-thickness layer when the piece of tissue has been removed. Thus, the purpose of the two stay sutures is to raise and control a full-thickness ridge of rectal wall and to facilitate removal of the tissue. Suction to remove blood may be helpful.

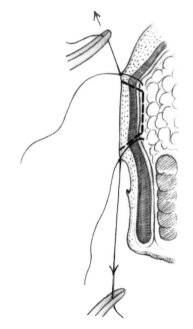

6

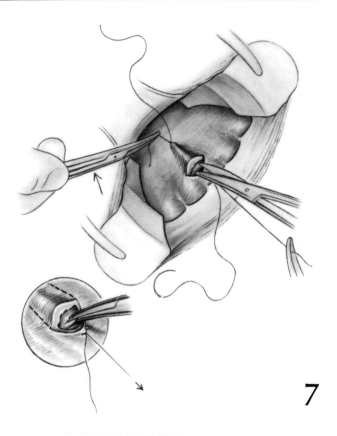

7 A transverse incision is made with scissors or with diathermy set on a coagulating current directly through the full thickness of the intestinal wall, just above the lower stay stitch. As soon as the muscle coat is seen, it should be grasped with Allis' forceps; the muscle layer should not be relinquished, otherwise it will retract and a mucosal biopsy can easily result.

7

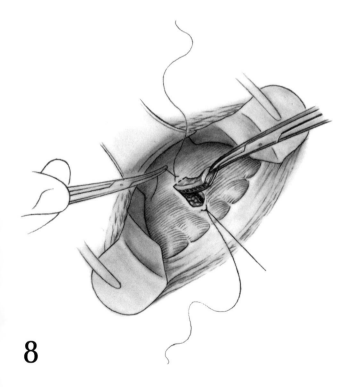

8 Parallel cuts 3 mm apart are made vertically up the rectum (longitudinally) to the upper stay suture and the specimen is removed.

8

Wound closure

9 The defect is closed with interrupted 2/0 absorbable sutures taking all layers of the intestinal wall.

The retractor is closed slightly to see whether bleeding has been controlled. A further full-thickness stitch may be inserted if necessary and a piece of haemostatic gauze placed on the area.

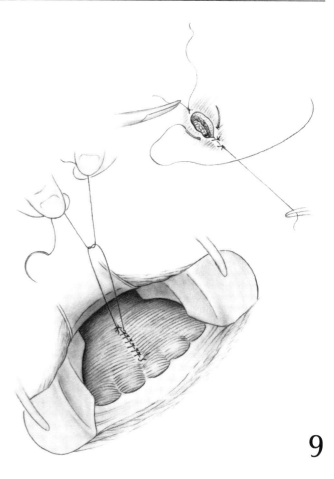

9

Postoperative care and complications

No special treatment is needed after operation, but bulk stool softeners are preferred to oil-containing laxatives. No postrectal abscesses or fistulae have resulted from this procedure, nor has secondary haemorrhage occurred in the author's experience.

Sepsis prevention in colorectal surgery

Steven D. Wexner MD, FACS, FASCRS, FACG
Staff Colorectal Surgeon, Residency Program Director, Department of Colorectal Surgery, and Director of Anorectal Physiology Laboratory, Cleveland Clinic Florida, Fort Lauderdale, Florida, USA

David E. Beck MD, FACS, FASCRS
Staff Colorectal Surgeon, Department of Colon and Rectal Surgery, Oschner Clinic, New Orleans, Louisiana, USA

Operative technique is one of the most important factors that can limit morbidity and mortality rates in colorectal surgery. The measures described in this chapter complement but cannot replace good technique. Each surgeon uses multiple measures to obtain good results. Thus, the large number of factors involved has made it difficult to study the influence of each measure on the incidence of septic complications.

Biology of tissue contamination

Wound infections result from contamination with either skin or bowel flora, while intra-abdominal abscesses result from contamination with bowel contents. An adequate number of bacteria and a suitable environment must be present for an 'infection' to become established. A colony count of at least ten is usually required to produce infection in normal tissue. The presence of devitalized tissue, foreign bodies or haematoma reduces the number of bacteria required, re-emphasizing the importance of good surgical technique.

Skin flora contains predominantly Gram-positive cocci, whereas the intestine contains a mixture of bacteria (*Table 1*).

Patient factors are also important. The presence of a distant infection, such as within the urinary tract, significantly increases the incidence of postoperative sepsis. Patients with diabetes and other immunocompromised patients have well documented higher incidences of infections, probably caused by their reduced ability to suppress bacteria.

Bowel preparation

The major septic risk associated with a colonic resection is from colonic bacterial contamination. Preoperative preparation to 'clean' the bowel has become standard practice in colonic and rectal surgery, and consists of two components: mechanical cleansing and antibiotic preparation. A 'clean' colon reduces the incidence of infectious complications and anastomotic disruption, simplifies colonic surgery, and is certainly more aesthetically pleasing to the surgeon. The ideal mechanical bowel preparation would be safe, cost-effective, rapid, provide good cleansing, and cause minimal patient discomfort and inconvenience. Furthermore, it should be easy to administer, for both inpatient and outpatient usage. Several methods are available, but no method has yet fulfilled all these criteria.

Mechanical preparation options

Dietary restriction

This method is insufficient by itself to cleanse the colon adequately. However, 1–5 days of a clear liquid diet may be used as an adjunctive preparatory measure.

Cathartics

Cathartics stimulate bowel evacuation. Medications commonly used include castor oil, magnesium citrate, senna concentrate or bisacodyl. Regimens that employ these medications usually require 2–3 days to empty the colon of stool and are frequently combined with enemas and dietary restrictions. These agents have been associated with dehydration and electrolyte changes, and frequently cause abdominal cramps and anal irritation. In controlled trials using cathartics, adequate cleansing occurred in only 75% of patients. Some surgeons have reverted to the use of a phosphate soda preparation.

Enemas

Enemas (saline, soap suds, tap water) work by dilution or irritation. They are messy and uncomfortable for patients and the nursing staff, and rarely provide adequate cleansing when used alone. They may be helpful in patients with an obstructing lesion who should not be given any oral bowel preparation.

Oral lavage

Oral lavage methods, which usually require only 2–4 h, have been developed to reduce the time required for mechanical cleansing.

Three solutions have been described. The first is saline (1.5–2 l/h via a small 10-Fr nasogastric tube for 4–5 h), which has been associated with fluid and electrolyte disturbances and weight gain. It should not be used in patients with compromised renal or cardiovascular status and is rarely used in current clinical practice.

Mannitol is an osmotic agent which is not absorbed. It causes clinical dehydration and is metabolized by colonic bacteria, resulting in increased infection rates and combustible gas production. Because of these disadvantages and the risk of bowel gas explosions, mannitol should seldom be used.

Polyethylene glycol electrolyte gastrointestinal lavage (PEG lavage) is an isosmotic solution composed of polyethylene glycol 3350 and an electrolyte solution (sodium, 125 mmol/l; sulphate, 40 mmol/l; chloride, 35 mmol/l; bicarbonate, 20 mmol/l; and potassium,

10 mmol/l). In the USA, this solution is available commercially as Golytely and Colyte. It provides excellent cleansing in 90–100% of patients and is associated with neither fluid nor electrolyte problems. It has a mildly salty taste, is well tolerated by most patients, and clinical trials have demonstrated its superiority over other methods. A new solution, NuLytely, has an improved taste and, in controlled trials, appears to clean as well as other PEG lavage solutions.

Intraoperative lavage methods have been described for patients requiring emergency operations. Proponents of these techniques suggest that their use may allow the safe accomplishment of a primary anastomosis after resection (*see* chapter on pp. 397–415).

The transrectal method involves placing a large Malecot or de Pezzar latex catheter (32–34 Fr) into the rectum via the anus. This allows irrigation of the left colon, which may be accomplished before or during the operation.

Although cumbersome, these latter two methods may adequately cleanse the colon, thus permitting a primary anastomosis in selected cases.

Antibiotic preparation options

Mechanical cleansing of the bowel reduces the amount of stool and bacteria, but does not alter the concentration of bacteria remaining in the colon. Use of appropriate prophylactic antibiotics in several prospective studies has reduced the incidence of infectious complications associated with colonic resections from 40–50% to approximately 5–10%. To be effective, the drugs must cover the spectrum of both Gram-negative and anaerobic bacteria adequately. Furthermore, they must be administered before bacterial contamination to provide adequate intraluminal and tissue levels. Finally, the duration of use must be short to reduce the development of resistant bacterial strains (less than 24–48 h).

Bowel flora

The colon contains a large number of bacteria. The species of bacteria and their mean stool concentrations are listed in *Table 1*. Bacteriological studies have demonstrated that there is a wide variation in the bacterial species between individuals, but that the flora of each person remains relatively stable over time.

Methods

Luminal antibiotics are inexpensive and effective. Overgrowth of resistant bacteria is avoided if these agents are used for less than 24 h. The systemic absorption of these agents is variable and there is controversy about the importance of luminal and tissue concentrations. These medications may cause gastrointestinal discomfort or diarrhoea. Appropriate agents are listed in *Table 2*. Product information should be consulted to confirm dosages.

Systemic (parenteral) antibiotics produce results equal to those produced by luminal medications if the appropriate drugs are used and if they are administered immediately before surgery. Adequate tissue levels must be present at the time of contamination. Appropriate agents and their recommended dosages are described in *Table 3*. Again the dosages should be confirmed before use.

Table 1   Colonic bacteria

Organism	Concentration in stool*
Anaerobic	
Gram-negative bacilli	
Bacteroides fragilis	10^9
Bacteroides spp.	10^8
Gram-positive cocci	10^7
Gram-positive bacilli	
Clostridia spp.	10^7
Aerobic	
Gram-negative bacilli	
Escherichia coli	10^8
Klebsiella spp.	10^6
Gram-positive cocci	
Streptococcus (*Enterococcus*)	
faecalis	10^6
Staphylococcus aureus	10^6

* Log counts/g stool

Table 2   Oral antibiotic agents

Medication	Bacterial cover*	Dosage
Erythromycin	Gram-positive, anaerobic	1 g
Neomycin	Gram-negative	1 g
Metronidazole	Anaerobic	500 mg

* An anti-aerobic agent must be combined with an anti-anaerobic agent. Acceptable combinations include erythromycin and neomycin or metronidazole and neomycin (see text)

Table 3   Parenteral antibiotic agents

Medication	Spectrum of cover	Dosage
Cefotetan	Gram-positive, Gram-negative, anaerobic	1 g (every 12 h)
Cefotaxime	Gram-positive, Gram-negative, anaerobic	1–2 g (every 8 h)
Cefoxitin	Gram-positive, Gram-negative, anaerobic	1–2 g (every 6 h)
Gentamicin	Gram-negative, aerobic	80 mg (every 8 h)
Clindamycin	Aerobic, anaerobic	150 mg (every 6 h)
Metronidazole	Anaerobic	500 mg (every 6 h)

Topical antibiotics can also be used at surgery. These have been found to be equivalent to other methods of prophylactic antibiotic administration in reducing infectious complications.

Combinations of antibiotic methods are difficult to justify because of the additional cost. When single methods have been compared with a combination of methods in prospective trials, there has been no statistical improvement unless the single method has an unusually large infection rate. However, despite the lack of consistent scientific support, the majority of surgeons utilize a combination of methods, usually oral and systemic agents together.

Recommendations

A 1-day preparation provides good cleansing and its short duration makes it cost effective.

Mechanical cleansing (PEG lavage preparation)

A clear liquid diet is started on the day before surgery. In the morning, PEG lavage is started: 240 ml orally every 10 min (1.5 l/h) until diarrhoea becomes clear and free of particulate matter.

Some surgeons also administer metoclopramide, 10 mg by mouth, 1 h before beginning PEG lavage as it may reduce nausea and bloating. Two bisacodyl tablets may also be administered after completing the PEG lavage to evacuate any remaining colonic fluid. Although clinically helpful in selected patients, these adjunctive medications have not demonstrated a significant improvement in controlled trials.

Antibiotics

One or more of the following regimens may be selected.

Oral antibiotics

Three doses of neomycin (1 g orally) and erythromycin (1 g orally) the day before surgery at 13.00, 14.00 and 23.00 hours. Metronidazole (1 g orally) may be substituted for the erythromycin.

Parenteral antibiotics

Any one of the following may be chosen.

1. Intravenous cefotetan, 1 g, on call to the operating room.

2. Intravenous cefoxitin, 1 g, on call to the operating room and every 6 h for three doses after surgery.
3. Intravenous cefotaxime, 2 g, and intravenous metronidazole, 1 g, on call to the operating room.

Topical

A first generation cephalosporin can be used, e.g. cefapirin sodium, 1 g/l of saline. The abdomen and wound should be irrigated at the end of the operation.

Intraoperative limitations of contamination

During surgery the important principles of adequate exposure, haemostasis and the correct operation performed in the proper manner remain extremely important. Bowel preparation as described above reduces but does not eliminate the potential for contamination. Additional measures are thought to be helpful but it has been difficult to document this in well controlled studies.

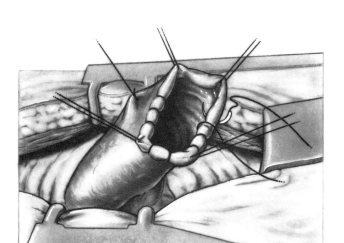

1

1   Traction sutures or atraumatic clamps can be used to keep the open ends of the bowel elevated. This in turn reduces the chances of intestinal contents spilling into the surgical field.

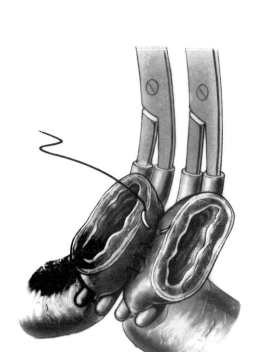

2

2   Atraumatic bowel clamps such as Glassman, Dennis or Satinsky clamps, or ties (umbilical tapes or Penrose drains) prevent retained intestinal contents from spilling into the open ends of the bowel and contaminating the abdominal cavity or wound. Swabbing the ends of the open bowel with povidone-iodine or an antibiotic solution may also aid in reducing infectious complications. Packing loops of bowel away from open ends of bowel and covering exposed loops with laparotomy pads or towels helps limit gross particulate contamination.

3 Sponges and plastic barrier drapes can be placed on the exposed wound edges: these probably help to prevent wound contamination. They have not, however, been proven statistically to reduce the incidence of wound infections.

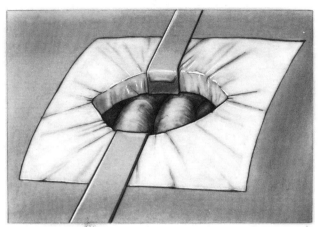

3

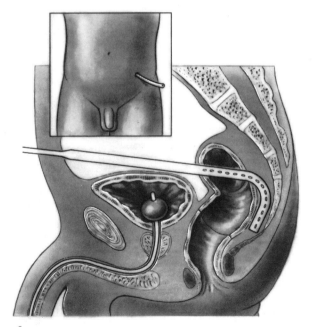

4

Drains

4 Multiple prospective studies have evaluated the use of abdominal drains. It is generally accepted that drains are ineffective in the abdominal cavity. However, the pelvis is different because it forms a rigid non-collapsible space that can store blood or peritoneal fluid. Both of these substances are excellent culture media for bacteria. Therefore, although placement of pelvic drains is reasonable, their use is not mandatory.

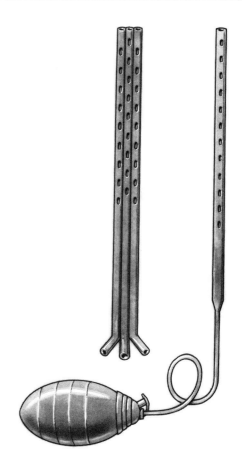

5 When suction drains are used they are generally removed on the second postoperative day. All studies have shown a reduced incidence of infection with closed suction drains when compared with Penrose drains.

Some authors have proposed irrigation of the pelvis to assist in evacuation of retained pelvic secretions and blood. However, a prospective controlled trial demonstrated no difference between suction sump drains with irrigation and those in which suction alone was employed.

5

Wounds

Historically, the incidence of wound infection after colonic resection averaged 30–40%. These high incidences were associated with poor mechanical preparation. However, these studies were often uncontrolled and the antibiotics used would not have been considered effective by today's standards. Recent studies in which appropriate antibiotics were used have shown higher infection rates only in patients in whom inadequate cleansing was present. However, the difference frequently failed to reach statistical significance. Current postoperative wound infection rates are usually in the range below 5–10%.

Despite high residual colonic bacterial concentrations, an adequate bowel preparation generally permits primary skin reapposition. Packing the subcutaneous wound open with gauze is very effective in preventing superficial wound infections. This measure is appropriate in emergency operations on unprepared bowel in which gross faecal contamination is noted.

Further reading

Beck DE, DiPalma JA. A new oral lavage solution versus cathartics and enema method for preoperative colonic cleansing. *Arch Surg* 1991; 126: 552–5.

Condon RE. Intestinal antisepsis: rationale and results. *World J Surg* 1982; 6: 182–7.

Gorbach SL, Nahas L, Lerner PI, Weinstein L. Studies of intestinal microflora. *Gastroenterology* 1967; 53: 845–55.

Hares MM, Alexander-Williams J. The effect of bowel preparation on colonic surgery. *World J Surg* 1982; 6: 175–81.

Saadia R, Schein M. The place of intraoperative antegrade colonic irrigation in emergency left-sided colonic surgery. *Dis Colon Rectum* 1989; 32: 78–81.

Vernava AM III, Dean P. Preoperative and postoperative management. In: Beck DE, Wexner SD, eds. *Fundamentals of Anorectal Surgery.* New York: McGraw-Hill, 1992: 50–6.

Wilson SE, Sokol T. Antimicrobials in elective colon surgery. *Infect Surg* 1985; 10: 609–11.

Patient positioning for colorectal surgery

Theodore M. Ross MD, FRCS(C), FACS
Assistant Professor of Surgery, Women's College Hospital, University of Toronto, Toronto, Ontario, Canada

Hartley S. Stern MD, FRCS(C), FACS
Associate Professor of Surgery, Director of Surgical Oncology Program and General Surgeon, Mount Sinai Hospital, University of Toronto, Toronto, Ontario, Canada

The choice of position for patients on the operating table, although often dominated by an individual surgeon's preference, should be decided by taking account of three important considerations: operative access and visibility; anaesthetic requirements; and potential complications related to positioning. The ideal position provides excellent exposure for the surgeon with minimal risk of nerve damage and respiratory compromise for the patient.

The three most common positions used in colon and rectal surgery are supine, lithotomy, and prone or jack-knife.

Supine position

1 The supine position on the operating table is the most common for colonic operations. Patients lie flat on their backs with their arms at the side (tucked in using a drawsheet) or abducted on an arm board. A padded foot board should be used to prevent foot-drop. Padding should also be provided over the following pressure points: calcaneum, sacrum, coccyx, olecranon process and occiput.

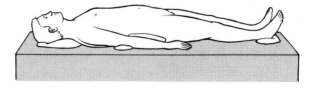

1

Lithotomy (Trendelenburg) position

The lithotomy position may be used for operations on the left colon, rectum, or perineum, but is modified depending on whether the surgeon intends to open the abdomen.

The patient is placed with the coccyx just above the perineal cut-out of the operating table. If the buttocks extend beyond this point, the lumbosacral ligaments may be strained. With the patient in this position, the feet will extend beyond the end of the operating table; therefore a padded table or an assistant is required to support the patient's legs and feet. There are two methods to elevate the legs into the lithotomy position: the ankle-strap and the leg–foot support methods.

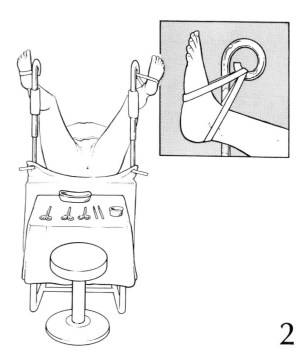

Ankle-strap method

2   One stirrup is placed under the ankle and the other around the sole of the patient's mid-foot. No part of the patient's legs should touch the metal posts. This method is suitable for relatively short operations on the perineum. If longer procedures are contemplated or the surgeon intends to enter the abdomen, then the leg–foot support method is preferable.

2

Leg–foot support method

3   The stirrups, of either the Lloyd-Davies type or the more modern Allen stirrup type, must be well padded to prevent popliteal pressure, which may cause vessel thrombosis. In addition, it is critical to carefully position and adequately pad the knee, leg and foot, to prevent pressure on the common peroneal nerve. The patient's legs may be covered with cotton stockings without creases to provide warmth and reduce shedding of epithelium and bacteria. Alternatively, anti-embolism stockings may be used.

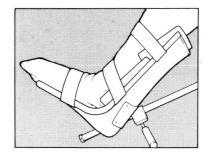

After the legs are placed in stirrups, the operating table pad over the foot segment is removed and this section is lowered. The patient's hands should not extend beyond the break in the table because they may be crushed when the foot section is later raised.

It is essential that the legs be raised and lowered *simultaneously* to prevent straining the lumbosacral muscles and joints. In addition, when the legs are lowered the patient may become hypotensive because of the sudden increase in blood flow to the legs. (This is more likely to occur in the ankle-strap method.) Therefore, the legs must be lowered slowly.

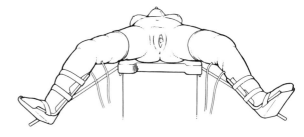

3

Prone or jack-knife position

This position may be used for most anorectal procedures. After induction of anaesthesia, the patient is intubated on a stretcher and then turned onto the operating table. A minimum of four people is required for the patient to be safely turned, with particular attention required for safe delivery of the head and neck.

4 In the jack-knife position, the respiratory system may be compromised because of reduced movement of both chest and diaphragm. Therefore, padded supports (rolls) are placed under the shoulders and hips to allow for satisfactory air movement into the chest. Care must be taken to prevent undue pressure on the breasts in women and the genitalia in men.

The patient's head is turned to the side with a soft foam doughnut protecting the ear. Padding is used under the knees and ankles to prevent plantar flexion of the feet and possible pressure on the toes. The arms, bent at the elbows, are placed on boards. The patient's hips must be positioned over the break point of the operating table. Conversion from the prone to the jack-knife position occurs when the bed is flexed to raise the hips and lower the head and feet.

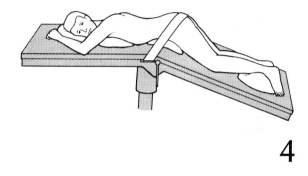

4

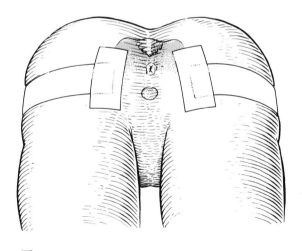

5

5 Adhesive tape may be applied to the buttocks and then fastened to the sides of the operating table for additional peritoneal exposure. The ends of the tape may be covered with a waterproof surface (Steridrape) to prevent the tape from becoming dislodged during the procedure. Patients in the jack-knife position may have pooling of the blood in the upper body and legs, adversely affecting the heart and circulation. Therefore, an increased intravenous fluid infusion rate may be necessary to prevent hypotension.

Choice of position: abdominal operations

For most colonic operations, the supine position is most commonly used because of its simplicity, ease in positioning assistants and lack of major complications.

There is some controversy about proper positioning for operations on the distal left colon and rectum. The extended lithotomy or lithotomy (Trendelenburg) position is the authors' personal preference for these procedures because it allows a wide choice of technical methods (including transanal insertion of a circular stapling device for low anterior resection) without turning or moving the patient once the operation has begun. It is also possible to work separately in the abdomen or in the perineum or synchronously with two teams of surgeons; a third assistant may be placed between the patient's legs, which aids retraction for pelvic dissection. These techniques are usually associated with a shortening of the operative time.

The proper position of the patient, however, in the lithotomy (Trendelenburg) position must be achieved, because a prolonged procedure increases the risk of compression complications, specifically foot drop from common peroneal nerve compression. The most common mechanism of injury to this nerve is by direct compression producing local ischaemia. The neurological injury produces displacement and intussusception of paranodal myelin along the nerve, which results in segmental areas of local compression that amplify the original injury.

Another mechanism of nerve injury is from a stretch force on the sciatic nerve, which may be fixed at the sciatic notch and at the fibular neck. The stretch force may result in rupture of nutrient arteries. The length of surgery, usually greater than 6 h, appears to be a critical factor in these nerve injuries.

As an alternative, a staged approach may be used for an abdominoperineal excision of the rectum. The first stage, in the supine position, is the completion of the abdominal portion of the procedure including closure of the pelvic peritoneum, fashioning the colostomy and abdominal wall closure. The patient is then placed in the lithotomy position or alternatively turned into the prone jack-knife position to complete the proctectomy. The advantages of the delayed use of the lithotomy position are that the time spent in this position is reduced, thus diminishing the risk of common peroneal nerve compression, and easier positioning of the operative assistants during the abdominal phase of the procedure may be possible.

The prone position, as the second stage, allows excellent access by the surgeon and assistant for the proctectomy. One of the authors (H.S.) prefers this position for abdominoperineal resection, particularly for anteriorly placed tumours. In men, it allows for much greater control of troublesome prostatic bed bleeding, and in women it enables *en bloc* excision of the posterior vaginal wall when so indicated.

The major disadvantages of this two-stage positioning approach are the inability to use cooperative synchronous surgery for excision of the rectum, the need to turn the patient during surgery, potential respiratory problems, and a slightly prolonged operative time.

Choice of position: anorectal procedures

Prone jack-knife position

For most anorectal procedures, the prone jack-knife position provides excellent operative exposure and positioning of assistants. Lighting can easily be directed onto the operative site and bleeding drains away from the operative field. This position is ideal for procedures being carried out under local, caudal, or epidural anaesthesia. Its major disadvantage is the need for endotracheal intubation when a general anaesthetic is required. Despite this problem, the jack-knife position provides superb exposure for rectovaginal fistula repair, anal sphincter repair, haemorrhoidectomy and excision of anterior low rectal neoplasms.

Lithotomy position

In this position the surgeon may sit with a low table across the knees. Assistants may be placed on the surgeon's right or left and all types of anaesthesia (local, caudal, epidural, or general) may be used.

This position has the advantage of not necessitating endotracheal intubation with a general anaesthetic. Good lighting may be slightly more difficult to achieve, but in problem cases this can be overcome by a mobile light or head light. Bleeding does not drain away and therefore may obscure the operative field. Despite these problems, the ease of patient positioning and the lack of the need for endotracheal intubation make this position useful for anal fistulotomy, sphincterotomy, treatment of condylomata and excision of a posterior rectal neoplasm. The prone or jack-knife position may be used for these procedures if carried out under local, caudal, or epidural anaesthesia and is preferred for the more complex cases.

Left lateral position

A few surgeons prefer this position for some anorectal procedures with the buttocks over the side of the table. It is less comfortable for the surgeon and requires an assistant to retract the upper buttock, which otherwise overhangs the anal canal and obscures the operative field. This method can be used with all forms of anaesthesia.

Anastomotic suturing techniques

Thomas T. Irvin PhD, ChM, FRCSEd
Consultant Surgeon, Royal Devon and Exeter Hospital (Wonford), Exeter, Devon, UK

History

The basic principles of intestinal suture were established more than 100 years ago by Travers, Lembert, Czerny and Halsted, and have since undergone little modification. However, these pioneers recognized the dangers of intestinal anastomosis. The breakdown or disruption of a suture line in the large intestine may result in peritonitis, faecal fistulation and serious or fatal septic complications. The factors that result in such complications are now well established, and it is apparent that safety in anastomosis of the intestine depends to a large extent on the technical expertise and judgement of the operating surgeon.

The development of stapling instruments for anastomosis of the intestine has added a new dimension to colorectal surgery. There is no difference in the healing properties of stapled or sutured anastomoses, but colorectal surgeons need to be familiar with both methods. Interestingly, it appears that techniques of hand suture have a longer learning curve than stapling methods[1].

Principles and justification

The factors that influence the healing of an anastomosis of the large intestine can be considered under two broad headings: surgeon-related variables and patient-related variables.

Surgeon-related variables

The multicentre Large Bowel Cancer Project co-ordinated from St Mary's Hospital, London[2], established that there was an enormous difference in the incidence of disruption of large bowel anastomoses in the hands of different surgeons, the incidence ranging from 0.5% to more than 30%. Such a wide variation could not be explained by differences in the patients undergoing surgery, and the results of this study imply that there are wide variations in the technical expertise and/or judgement of surgeons performing colonic and colo-rectal anastomoses.

The technical factors which may affect the outcome of anastomosis include: access and exposure, blood supply, suture technique, the use of drains and diversion of the faecal stream.

Access and exposure

Intestinal anastomoses will prove difficult if surgical access and exposure are unsatisfactory. This may result from inadequate anaesthesia, an inappropriate or inadequate incision, and imperfect illumination of the operative field. Poor access may also result from inadequate mobilization of the viscera, a problem which is especially likely to occur in operations involving a low rectal anastomosis.

The surgeon should never have to struggle with an anastomosis because of limited access. When difficulty is encountered, the problem should be carefully assessed and an attempt must be made to improve the exposure. If the difficulty seems insurmountable it is prudent to consider an alternative procedure which avoids an anastomosis or, if possible, to call upon a surgeon with greater experience of such surgery.

Blood supply

A good blood supply is vital to the healing of all wounds, and the preparation for an anastomosis must be meticulous to avoid disturbance of the blood supply to the cut edges of the bowel. The only absolute criterion of an adequate blood supply is the presence of free arterial bleeding from the cut edges of the gut. The absence of a visible or palpable arterial pulse is not necessarily of significance, but blanching or cyanosis of the edges of the bowel and the presence of a dark, venous type of bleeding are signs of an inadequate and thus an unacceptable blood supply.

Blood flow to an anastomosis may be compromised in several ways: undue tension on the suture line resulting from inadequate mobilization of the viscera; devascular-ization of the bowel during mobilization or preparation for the anastomosis; strangulation of the tissues by tightly knotted sutures; and the excessive use of diathermy coagulation to achieve haemostasis in the cut ends of the bowel.

Before starting an anastomosis the surgeon should ensure that the ends of the bowel can easily be apposed: if the bowel ends overlap it can be safely assumed that there will be no tension on the suture line. Haemostasis in the cut edges of the bowel may be achieved either by individual ligation of vessels or by the use of diathermy coagulation. The latter method has the disadvantage that it may result in a greater degree of tissue necrosis at the suture line, but it is certainly a less tedious technique than the ligation of vessels and, in practice, little tissue damage will result if diathermy is limited to controlling only major bleeding points. Minor oozing should be ignored, but significant arterial bleeding should be checked because these vessels retract within the tissues and produce unpleasant haematomas.

Some surgeons place non-crushing occlusion clamps across the bowel to avoid soiling of the operative field during intestinal anastomosis. However, it is important that these clamps are applied lightly and never across the mesentery of the intestine for fear of damaging the blood supply to the anastomosis.

Suture technique

Secure healing of an intestinal anastomosis is dependent on accurate apposition of the serosal or outer surfaces of the bowel, and this is achieved by the use of a suture technique which inverts the cut edges of the gut.

Most surgeons use an open method of intestinal anastomosis. 'Aseptic' or closed techniques of anasto-mosis achieved some popularity in the earlier part of this century because of the belief that the breakdown of anastomoses resulted from the bacterial contamination of the peritoneum which occurred during the construc-tion of the open type of anastomosis. Several ingenious techniques of 'aseptic' anastomosis were devised, but they were not generally accompanied by a reduction in the incidence of anastomotic dehiscence. Some surgeons still use closed types of anastomosis for aesthetic reasons.

One aspect of the technique of intestinal suture which has remained the subject of controversy is the use of either one layer or two layers of sutures in an anastomosis. Probably a majority of surgeons now use a single layer of sutures on the grounds that it may cause less ischaemia, tissue necrosis or narrowing of the lumen than a two-layer method.

1a–d

The two-layer anastomosis (*Illustration 1a*) consists of an inner layer of sutures incorporating the full thickness of the bowel wall and an outer layer of sutures inserted through all layers except the mucosa. This second layer is frequently referrred to as a seromuscular stitch, but it should in fact include the collagenous submucosal layer of the bowel since more superficial sutures have a tendency to cut out. Single-layer techniques of suture are shown in *Illustrations 1b–d*. In *Illustration 1b* the suture is inserted from the mucosal aspect of the bowel through the full thickness of the bowel wall and inversion of the anastomosis results when the suture is tied. The Gambee stitch (*Illustration 1c*) is inserted through all layers of the bowel wall and is passed twice through the mucosa on each side of the anastomosis to secure mucosal inversion. The Gambee suture technique thus results in minimal inversion of the cut edges of the bowel. In *Illustration 1d* the suture is a submucosal stitch inserted from the serosal aspect of the bowel, as in the outer layer of a two-layer anastomosis. Matheson and Irving[3] have reported excellent results with this 'serosubmucosal suture' and other experts in colorectal surgery have now adopted this method.

The author uses a single-layer suture technique for colonic and colorectal anastomoses, and a two-layer method for anastomoses involving the caecum or terminal ileum.

Various absorbable and non-absorbable suture materials have been used for anastomosis of the intestine. Experimental studies have suggested that anastomoses made with absorbable sutures are weaker than those made with non-absorbable materials during the early phase of healing, but the difference is slight and probably has no clinical significance. It is usual for two-layer anastomoses to be made with absorbable sutures for the inner layer and non-absorbable sutures for the outer layer. Single-layer anastomoses are usually fashioned with non-absorbable materials.

Chromic catgut is the most popular absorbable suture material, and there is no convincing evidence that other materials such as polyglycolic acid, polyglactin, or polydioxanone are superior for intestinal suture. However, an increasing number of surgeons are using polyglactin (Vicryl) even in single-layer anastomoses.

Non-absorbable suture materials include silk, polypropylene and various synthetic polyesters. There are theoretical advantages to the use of monofilament non-absorbable suture materials (stainless steel wire, nylon or polypropylene) in that these materials provoke less tissue reaction than braided sutures, but these differences are slight and the monofilament sutures have inferior handling characteristics. The author prefers braided non-absorbable suture materials.

The size or gauge of the suture material used in anastomosis of the intestine is not standard, but 2/0 or 3/0 sutures are in common use in adult surgery. The use of ultrafine suture materials for adults is probably

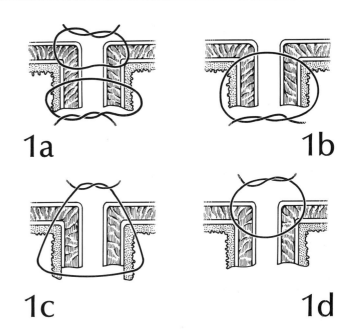

misguided because these sutures may cut through the bowel wall.

Use of drains

The use of peritoneal drains is regarded by some surgeons as a necessary feature of the management of anastomoses, particularly in surgery of the colon and rectum. Many protagonists of the use of drains claim that they safeguard the patient against anastomotic leakage by permitting the development of an enterocutaneous fistula when anastomotic dehiscence occurs rather than a diffusing faecal peritonitis. However, experimental studies have shown that foreign bodies, including drains, placed close to anastomoses actually increase the probability of anastomotic disruption. The value of drains is in removing any blood or serum which may collect in dead space, particularly after low anterior resection of the rectum when such collections may account for a significant incidence of 'late' dehiscence of the suture line.

The author uses small-calibre (Redivac) closed suction drains for the purpose of removing any blood or serum which may collect after operations involving significant dissection or mobilization of the viscera, and in operations complicated by significant faecal contamination. The drains are deliberately not placed in the vicinity of anastomoses and are removed after 48 h.

Faecal diversion

There has been considerable debate concerning the value of a temporary loop colostomy, caecostomy or loop ileostomy to protect anastomoses in the left colon or rectum. These procedures are usually reserved for 'high-risk' anastomoses such as a very low colorectal or coloanal anastomosis or an anastomosis made in the presence of unfavourable local conditions. There is no evidence that proximal faecal diversion prevents anastomotic dehiscence, but it does appear that the septic complications of dehiscence may be less serious when the faecal stream has been diverted.

It is therefore a matter of judgement as to when faecal diversion should be used to protect an anastomosis, and it is apparent from the literature and informal discussion with surgeons that there is considerable variation in the use of such methods. In the case of low colorectal anastomoses, some surgeons use intraoperative leakage tests as a guide to the need for a defunctioning colostomy. In such tests the rectum is distended with air and a colostomy is used if sites of visible leakage of air cannot be repaired. However, other surgeons have suggested that demonstration of an airtight anastomosis is no guarantee of uncomplicated postoperative healing.

In recent years, an intracolonic bypass procedure has been developed as an alternative to faecal diversion by colostomy or ileostomy for the protection of distal left-sided anastomoses in the large intestine[4]. A soft latex tube with a reinforced collar is sutured to the mucosa and submucosa of the bowel wall with absorbable sutures proximal to the anastomosis, thus creating a watertight seal and excluding the anastomosis from contact with the faecal content of the bowel. The device separates spontaneously from the bowel wall and is passed rectally after 2 weeks.

The author uses a loop transverse colostomy to protect the colorectal anastomosis in the following circumstances:

1. When the anastomosis is 6 cm or less from the anal verge.
2. When the anastomosis is close to the site of previous fistulation between the large intestine and the vagina or urinary bladder.
3. When the rectum has suffered irradiation injury.
4. When there are unusual technical difficulties with the anastomosis because of restricted access or obesity.
5. When a very large pelvic dead space exists following operations for extensive malignancies.

This protocol has resulted in complete freedom from life-threatening or fatal complications of anastomotic dehiscence in the author's unit during the past 15 years.

Some surgeons use a loop ileostomy in preference to a colostomy. However, it should be noted that closure of a loop ileostomy is technically more difficult than closure of a loop colostomy and the author would not recommend the use of a defunctioning loop ileostomy unless the surgeon is familiar with the technique of closure of this stoma.

The surgeon should avoid an anastomosis in the presence of established peritoneal sepsis and the bowel should be exteriorized as a colostomy or ileostomy.

Alimentary continuity can be re-established at a later date as an elective procedure.

Postoperative peritoneal sepsis and anastomotic complications may result when significant faecal contamination or soiling of the peritoneum occurs during surgery. In some cases, as in the surgery of advanced tumours of the large intestine, some degree of soiling may be unavoidable, but it should always be regarded as a serious complication. When gross faecal soiling occurs in conjunction with other local factors which may propagate peritoneal infection (residual tumour, extensive retroperitoneal dissection or traumatic injuries to other viscera), it is advisable to avoid an anastomosis and to exteriorize the bowel.

Patient-related variables

Bowel preparation

Faecal loading of the colon has an adverse effect on the healing of colonic or rectal anastomoses. The mechanical state of the bowel may determine the success or failure of anastomoses in the left colon or rectum, and is a major factor in the high incidence of dehiscence which follows primary anastomosis of the left colon in operations for acute obstruction.

In elective colonic surgery, thorough mechanical preparation of the bowel is an integral factor in the safe conduct of colonic and rectal anastomoses, but may be relatively ineffective when there is some degree of colonic obstruction. Dudley et al.[5] described an ingenious method of intraoperative colonic irrigation followed by primary anastomosis in cases complicated by obstruction. This method has found favour with other surgeons but the majority still prefer to avoid an anastomosis and exteriorize the bowel in the presence of gross large bowel obstruction. Alimentary continuity is re-established at a second operation. The author believes that there is a place for both methods. Intraoperative colonic lavage adds significantly to the operating time and may be inappropriate in operations on unfit patients.

Surprisingly, the bacterial content of the colon remains high despite mechanical preparation and it is customary to use antimicrobial agents to reduce the infectivity of the colonic contents. There is no convincing evidence that prophylactic antimicrobial therapy prevents anastomotic dehiscence, but it results in a reduction in the incidence of abdominal wound infection after intestinal surgery and the septic complications of anastomotic dehiscence may be less severe when the bowel is prepared with antibiotics. Most oral antibiotic regimens effective in 'sterilizing' the intestinal contents have the potential disadvantage that they may cause a clostridial pseudomembranous colitis, but the short-term use of systemic antibiotics is less likely to lead to this complication.

Systemic factors

The precise role of systemic abnormalities in the pathogenesis of anastomotic dehiscence has not been clearly defined, but it seems probable that such factors are of much less significance than the presence of local sepsis, colonic obstruction, or surgeon-related variables. The systemic factors which do appear to exert an unfavourable effect on anastomotic healing include advanced malignancy, malnutrition and colorectal operations resulting in excessive blood loss.

Severe malnutrition leads to reduced collagen synthesis and impaired healing of colonic anastomoses, and several factors may account for the relationship between excessive blood loss and the healing of anastomoses. Traumatic or bloody operations on the colon in experimental animals result in peritoneal sepsis and, as a consequence, an increased incidence of anastomotic dehiscence. This factor may partly account for the high incidence of anastomotic dehiscence in patients with advanced malignant disease since this seems to be largely a complication of extensive operations for the removal of fixed tumours. Moreover, major intraoperative blood loss has disproportionately severe effects on the splanchnic circulation, and the resulting intestinal ischaemia may have adverse effects on colonic healing.

Preoperative

Preoperative assessment must take account of the general medical status or fitness of the patient as well as specific consideration of the intestinal disease and the appropriate method of surgical treatment. It should be noted that the majority of fatalities after surgery of the large intestine are due to complications of coexisting medical disease rather than to specific complications of surgery, and the risks are greatly increased in the elderly and in emergency operations. The surgeon is ultimately responsible for the safety of the patient, but the preoperative assessment is a joint exercise involving the anaesthetist and, on occasions, specialist physicians.

Preoperative investigations to determine the extent of the large bowel pathology will not be discussed here. The issues which do require discussion are: selection of the appropriate surgeon for the operation, informed consent, preparation of the large intestine, and perioperative antibiotic therapy.

Selection of surgeon

It is essential that the surgeon and anaesthetist have appropriate skills to treat the patient. This may seem an elementary point but the Confidential Enquiry into Perioperative Deaths[6] showed that surgeons and anaesthetists undertaking the treatment of patients who are seriously ill are sometimes lacking in appropriate skills or experience. It is the responsibility of the consultant in charge of the patient to ensure that the surgeon actually performing the operation has the appropriate experience.

Informed consent

Patients undergoing surgical operations in the UK remain less informed than their counterparts in the USA but this situation is changing. Department of Health guidelines suggest that patients must be informed of any substantial risk associated with the proposed treatment, and that they have the right to refuse certain types of treatment.

It is essential that the surgeon discusses with the patient the possibility of a stoma as part of the operative treatment, carefully explaining the reasons why such an arrangement might become necessary, and whether it is likely to be temporary or permanent. Some patients may not wish to have a stoma under any circumstances and the surgeon must be aware of this before embarking upon the operation.

Preparation of large intestine

Mechanical preparation

2 In the absence of partial or complete obstruction of the bowel, modern methods of mechanical preparation should ensure that the large intestine is virtually empty. These new methods achieve mechanical cleansing of the gut more rapidly than the traditional methods of purging or enema, and they involve the use of whole gut irrigation or powerful stimulant laxatives.

The original technique of whole gut irrigation involved the administration of 4 litres of normal saline by nasogastric tube every hour for a period of 3 h, but patient compliance was rather poor and there was some risk of salt and water absorption resulting in fluid overload in the elderly. The modern technique involves the administration of 3–4 litres of a polyethylene glycol electrolyte solution over a period of 3 h by oral ingestion or by nasogastric tube. The appearance of the colonic lumen through the colonoscope after whole gut irrigation is shown.

The most effective stimulant laxative is Picolax (sodium picosulphate and magnesium citrate). Two sachets are taken on the day before surgery, one in the morning and a second in the afternoon. This is the method used by the author.

Preoperative mechanical preparation should not be attempted if there is evidence of obstruction of the intestine, even if the obstruction is incomplete. The preparation will be ineffectual, unhelpful and potentially dangerous. In such circumstances, the surgeon must consider alternative strategies such as intraoperative colonic irrigation, resection of the obstructed bowel, the use of an intracolonic bypass tube or avoidance of a primary anastomosis.

Antimicrobial preparation

Various antibiotic regimens are used to reduce the infectivity of the gut content and to minimize the effects of faecal spillage during operations on the large intestine. Some surgeons limit the use of antibiotics to the perioperative period, while others also administer antimicrobial agents during preoperative mechanical preparation of the bowel.

The author gives patients oral metronidazole, 200 mg every 8 h, for 48 h before surgery.

Perioperative antibiotic therapy

It has been shown that perioperative use of intravenous broad-spectrum antibiotics results in a significant reduction in the incidence of abdominal wound sepsis in colorectal surgery. Such therapy may also reduce the risks of intra-abdominal septic complications, particularly in cases complicated by significant faecal soiling of

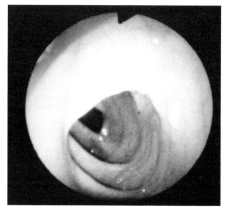

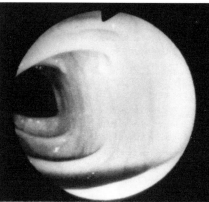

2

the peritoneum, and some surgeons use perioperative intravenous antibiotics in preference to preoperative oral medication. The antibiotics in most common use are second or third generation cephalosporins, and many surgeons combine these drugs with metronidazole because of its activity against *Bacteroides* spp.

The author uses the following regimen: cefuroxime, 1.5 g, is given by intravenous injection with induction of anaesthesia, and two further intravenous doses of 750 mg are given at intervals of 8 h. Metronidazole is not given routinely unless there is evidence of significant sepsis or faecal soiling at operation. In such cases, this drug is given in a dose of 500 mg every 6 h by intravenous infusion, and is continued together with cefuroxime for 3–5 days.

Anaesthesia

Nearly all abdominal operations on the large intestine are carried out under general anaesthesia with full muscle relaxation, although it is possible to carry out resections and anastomoses under spinal anaesthesia. Some significance has been attached to the use of parasympathomimetic drugs such as neostigmine in the reversal of muscle relaxants since the muscarinic effects on the large intestine might result in disruption of an anastomosis. The author is not convinced that such dangers exist in actual practice and has not encountered a case in which such complications ensued.

Operations

Anastomoses may be made end-to-end, end-to-side, side-to-end or side-to-side. In this section the indications for the use of the different types of anastomosis and the techniques of intestinal suture will be described.

END-TO-END ANASTOMOSIS

This method of anastomosis is applicable at any level in the large intestine. The anastomosis can be made either with a two-layer or a single-layer method of suture but the author, in common with many other surgeons, prefers the single-layer method for most colonic and colorectal anastomoses.

Single-layer method

Braided non-absorbable suture materials such as silk or a synthetic polyester are generally preferred, but some surgeons use an absorbable polyglactin (Vicryl) suture.

Methods of suture

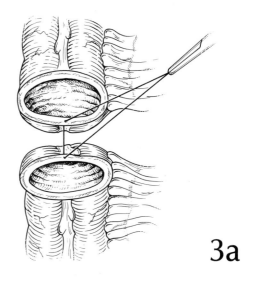

3a

3a–c Various suture techniques are used in single-layer anastomoses, and more than one technique may be used in an individual anastomosis. The suture may be a serosubmucosal stitch (*Illustration 3a*), a full thickness vertical stitch (*Illustration 3b*), or a horizontal mattress suture (*Illustration 3c*). Most anastomoses are made by the open method, but a closed technique of end-to-end anastomosis may be used if the colon is sufficiently mobile for the application of special occlusive clamps. Closed techniques of anastomosis were commonly used some 50 years ago when they were believed to be safer than open methods, but they are seldom used in modern surgical practice although they have considerable aesthetic value.

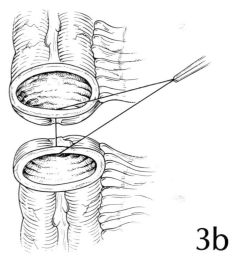

3b

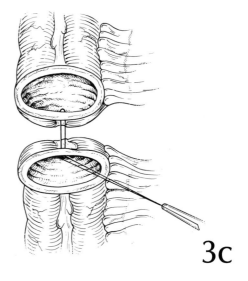

3c

Colonic anastomosis: serosubmucosal suture (open method)

4a–e Stay sutures are inserted at the mesenteric and antimesenteric borders of the intestine and at the midpoint of the posterior aspect of the anastomosis (*Illustration 4a*). The remaining sutures on the posterior aspect of the anastomosis are inserted at intervals not exceeding 5 mm (*Illustration 4b*) and the sutures are held in forceps until the layer is complete. The anterior layer is created in a similar fashion, beginning with a suture at the midpoint of the anastomosis (*Illustration 4c*). The sutures are held in forceps until the layer is completed (*Illustration 4d*), and secure inversion of the mucosa is achieved when they are tied (*Illustration 4e*).

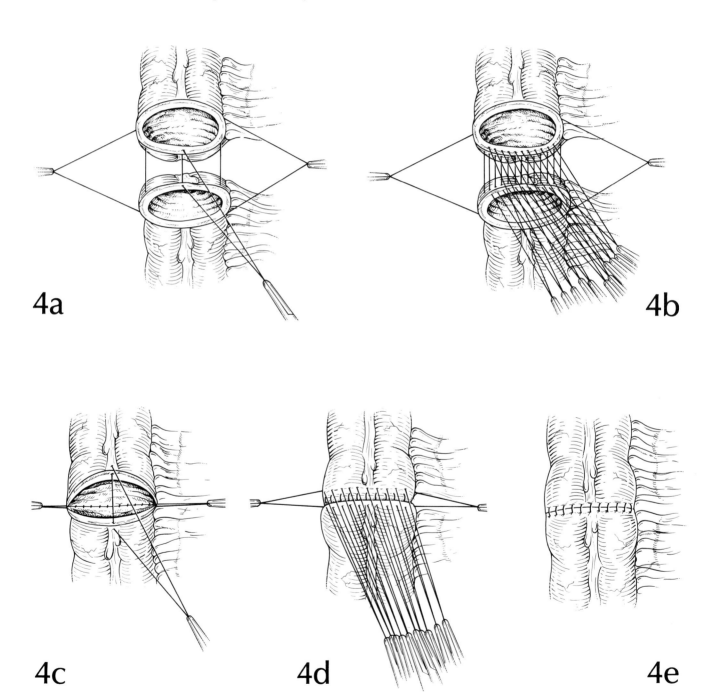

4a

4b

4c

4d

4e

Colonic anastomosis: serosubmucosal suture (closed method)

5a–c This method requires the use of Wangensteen's clamps and is applicable only when both ends of the bowel are sufficiently mobile and the access is sufficiently good to permit the use of these clamps. The technique thus has limited application and is mainly used in ileocolic anastomoses or anastomoses in the proximal colon; it is not suitable for colorectal anastomoses.

The ends of the bowel are held in the occlusive clamps and the posterior layer of serosubmucosal sutures is inserted in a similar fashion to an open anastomosis (*Illustration 5a*). The stitches should be inserted at least 5 mm from the edge of the clamp so that the clamps can be easily rotated, and each stitch must be sufficiently deep to incorporate the submucosal layer of the bowel wall. The sutures are tied after completion of the posterior layer. The clamps are then rotated and are held together with a double collar while the anterior layer of the anastomosis is completed (*Illustration 5b*). The stitches for the anterior layer can be placed closer to the occlusion clamps. The sutures of the completed anterior layer are held taut while the clamps are removed and are then tied, starting with the angle sutures at the mesenteric and antimesenteric borders.

An essential step on completion of the anastomosis is to separate the crushed ends of the bowel by firm pressure between finger and thumb (*Illustration 5c*). The surgeon must be absolutely certain that patency of the lumen has been established.

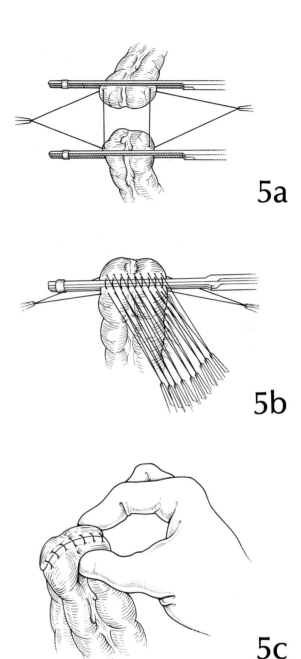

5a

5b

5c

Colorectal anastomosis: single-layer open technique

6a–g In the author's opinion, a single-layer suture technique is infinitely preferable to a two-layer method for colorectal anastomosis. Indeed, a two-layer technique is virtually impossible to use in the construction of very low colorectal anastomoses when access is limited.

A braided suture material such as silk is used, and the anastomosis begins with the insertion of three sutures through all layers of the bowel wall (*Illustration 6a*). The first two sutures are inserted at the mesenteric and antimesenteric borders of the intestine and a third suture is inserted at the midpoint between these sutures. The presence of this central stitch assists greatly in the subsequent insertion of equidistant sutures in the posterior aspect of the anastomosis. The posterior layer is completed with a series of through-and-through sutures incorporating all layers of the bowel wall, and the sutures are held in forceps until the layer is complete (*Illustration 6b*). The interval between each suture should be relatively small; otherwise there is a tendency for eversion of the mucosa to occur when the sutures are tied. Alternative suture methods may be used, such as a mattress technique (*Illustration 6c*) or a submucosal suture (*Illustration 6d*), but these sutures become more difficult in very low anastomoses. The author uses the method shown in *Illustrations 6a* and *6b*. The anterior layer of the anastomosis is made with a similar series of full thickness sutures knotted on the mucosa (*Illustration 6e*). A small gap in the suture line finally remains in the centre of the anterior layer, and this is closed with a submucosal suture inserted parallel to the edge of the suture line (*Illustration 6f*).

An alternative method of construction of the anterior layer is to use a series of vertical submucosal sutures as shown in *Illustration 4d* or horizontal mattress sutures (*Illustration 6g*).

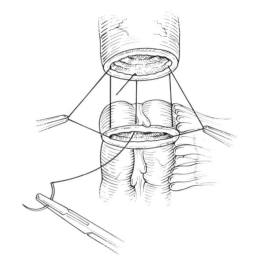

6a

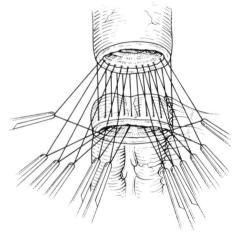

6b

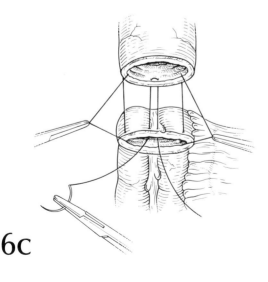

6c

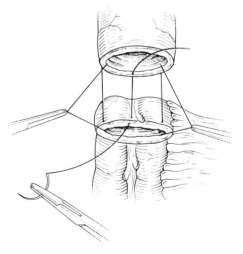

6d

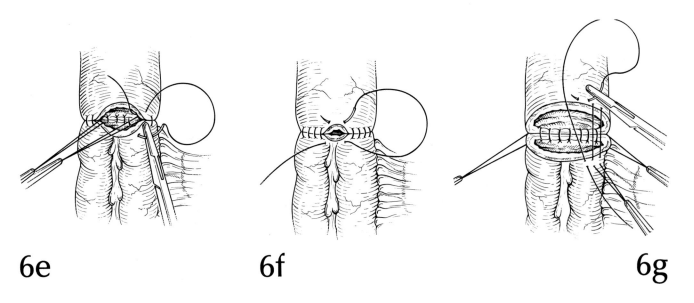

6e

6f

6g

Coloanorectal anastomosis

7a, b An end-to-end, overlapping, or sleeve-type anastomosis may be made between the colon and the upper part of the anal canal. In the Parks operation, the colon is pulled through a short rectal stump (after excision of the rectal mucosa) and anastomosed to the anal canal above the dentate line. A single-layer anastomosis is made with sutures which incorporate the anal mucosa, the internal sphincter muscle and the full thickness of the colonic wall

(*Illustration 7a*). A bivalve anal speculum or retractor is required for this anastomosis, and the author uses a single layer of interrupted silk sutures, although absorbable sutures of chromic catgut or polyglactin may be equally satisfactory. Some surgeons insert a second layer of sutures through the outer edge of the rectal stump and the serosal layer of the colon (points A and A[1] of *Illustration 7b*), but the author finds this unnecessary and unusually difficult.

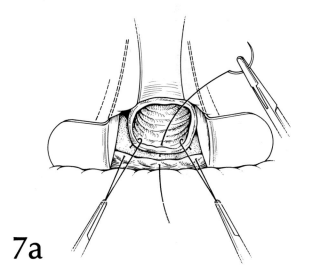

7a

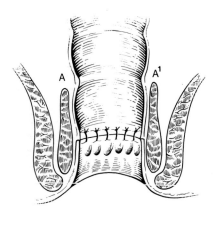

7b

Two-layer method

The author uses chromic catgut and non-absorbable sutures in these anastomoses, but some surgeons use polyglactin for all layers with excellent results.

Insertion of posterior outer layer of sutures

8a–c The divided ends of the bowel are held in crushing clamps and light occlusion clamps are applied across the bowel, care being taken to avoid the mesentery. The two-layer inverting anastomosis commences with the insertion of the outer layer of interrupted submucosal sutures on the posterior aspect of the anastomosis (*Illustrations 8a, b*). Non-absorbable sutures of silk or other braided material are used and they are inserted first at the mesenteric and antimesenteric borders of the intestine. The sutures are tied when this layer is complete and the crushing clamps can then be amputated (*Illustration 8c*), thus opening the bowel lumen.

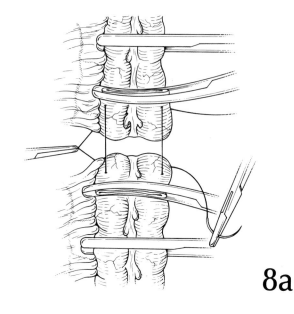

8a

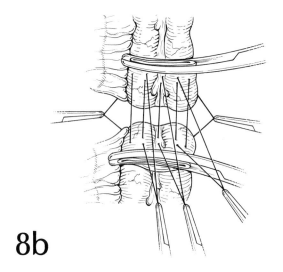

8b

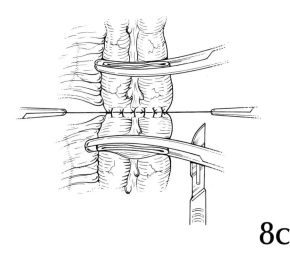

8c

Inner layer of sutures

9a–g A continuous chromic catgut suture which begins at the antimesenteric border is used for the inner layer of the anastomosis. The suture is inserted through all layers of the bowel wall and tied on the serosal aspect (*Illustration 9a*). A forceps is applied to the short end of the suture which will be used again on completion of this layer. A continuous over-and-over suture technique is used for the posterior aspect of the anastomosis, care being taken to include all coats of the bowel wall (*Illustration 9b*). The mesenteric corner of the anastomosis is securely invaginated by the use of the Connell suture technique (*Illustration 9c*) and inversion of the edges of the

bowel is achieved when the suture is pulled taut (*Illustration 9d*). The anterior aspect of the inner layer of the anastomosis may be completed with an over-and-over suture technique, but a continuous Connell technique may be preferred (*Illustration 9e*). The mucosa and edges of the bowel on the antimesenteric aspect are invaginated as the last Connell stitch is pulled tight (*Illustration 9f*), and the suture is tied to its other end (*Illustration 9g*).

Some surgeons prefer to start the inner all-coats catgut layer in the midline posteriorly, using catgut with a needle at each end. This avoids knots at the weakest points – the mesenteric and antimesenteric borders.

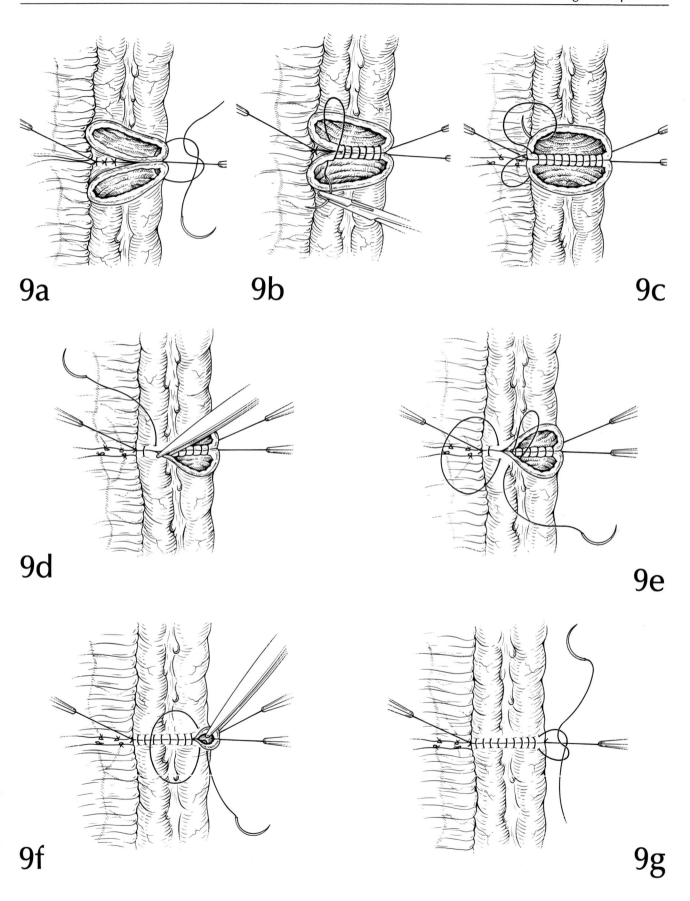

9a

9b

9c

9d

9e

9f

9g

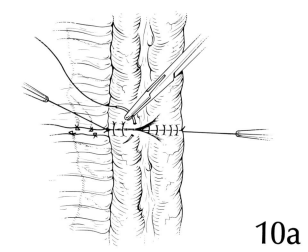

10a

Insertion of anterior outer layer of sutures

10a, b Interrupted non-absorbable submucosal sutures are then inserted on the anterior aspect of the bowel (*Illustration 10a*), and the anastomosis is completed (*Illustration 10b*).

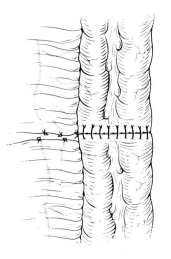

10b

Anastomosis starting with inner layer of sutures

11a–d Some surgeons prefer to begin the two-layer anastomosis with the insertion of the inner layer of catgut (*Illustrations 11a, b*). When this layer is complete, the outer layer of sutures is inserted on the anterior aspect of the anastomosis and the anastomosis is then rotated (*Illustration 11c*) so that the outer layer can be completed on the posterior aspect (*Illustration 11d*). This method is apt to prove unsatisfactory in obese subjects when the mesentery is laden with fat because, after completion of the inner layer, insertion of the outer layer of sutures on the posterior aspect of the anastomosis is difficult to achieve with precision when the mesenteric fat encroaches on the bowel wall.

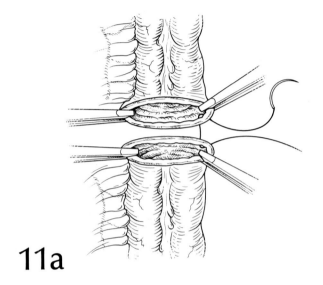

11a

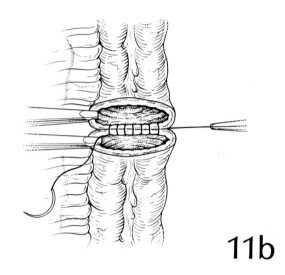

11b

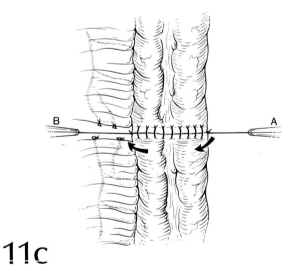

11c

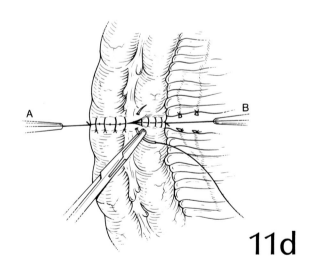

11d

Ileocolic anastomosis: correction for unequal ends of bowel

12a–d An end-to-end anastomosis is possible even when there is considerable disparity in the size of the two ends of bowel. This situation may arise in anastomosis of the ileum to the colon after right hemicolectomy or in operations for small bowel obstruction (*Illustration 12a*). The problem is solved by widening the orifice of the smaller lumen: the outer layer of submucosal sutures is inserted in an oblique fashion away from the cut edge of the bowel on the antimesenteric aspect in the end of the smaller calibre lumen (*Illustration 12b*), and the open end of the bowel is widened by cutting along the antimesenteric border (*Illustrations 12c, d*).

Most problems of disparity can be solved in this way, but some surgeons prefer to use an end-to-side technique of anastomosis in these circumstances.

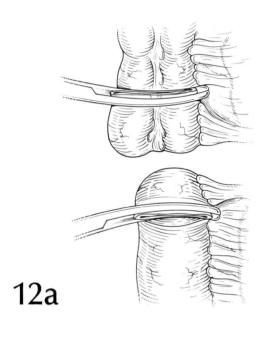

12a

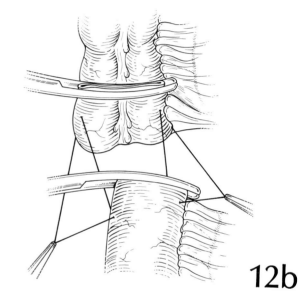

12b

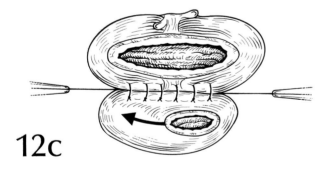

12c

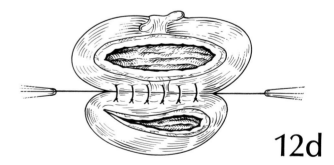

12d

Colorectal anastomosis

It is the author's view that a two-layer suture technique has only limited application in colorectal anastomoses and that it is inappropriate for low colorectal anastomosis.

13a–d A modified suture technique is used in a two-layer anastomosis in the extraperitoneal rectum. In a low colorectal anastomosis, where access may be restricted, it is often simpler to insert the outer layer of submucosal sutures parallel to the cut edge of the rectum as horizontal mattress sutures (*Illustrations 13a, b*). The use of this stitch in the extraperitoneal rectum is desirable also in that it is placed at right angles to the longitudinal muscle fibres, and there is less tendency for it to cut through the muscle tissue than a conventional vertical suture. The sutures are held in forceps until the outer layer is complete (*Illustration 13c*), and inversion of the suture line is achieved when these are tied (*Illustration 13d*).

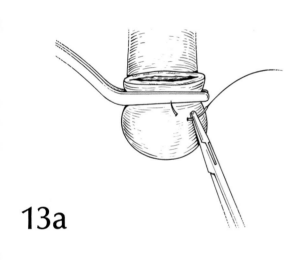

13a

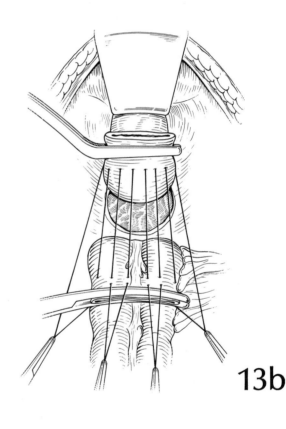

13b

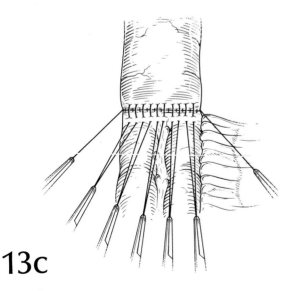

13c

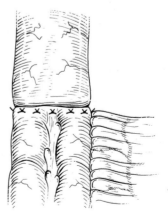

13d

Caecorectal anastomosis

14 An end-to-end anastomosis may be made between the caecum and rectum after subtotal colectomy. A two-layer suture technique is used, but the author prefers a side-to-end reconstruction for this anastomosis, as shown in *Illustrations 17a–d.*

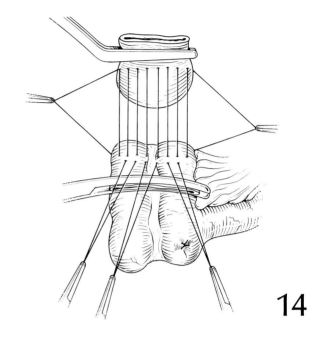

14

END-TO-SIDE AND SIDE-TO-END ANASTOMOSES

These methods are used less frequently than end-to-end anastomoses. The side-to-end method is used by some surgeons for caecorectal, ileorectal and colorectal anastomoses, and it appears to be the most common method for anastomosis of the ileum to the anal canal in the operation of restorative proctocolectomy. The end-to-side technique is favoured by some surgeons for ileocolic anastomosis, particularly when there is a significant disparity in the two ends of bowel.

Technique for closure of end of bowel

15a–h When an end-to-side or side-to-end anastomosis of the small or large intestine is performed, one end of the bowel must be closed. A two-layer inverting suture technique is used. The bowel is held in a crushing clamp, and a chromic catgut suture mounted on a straight needle is inserted through all layers of the bowel wall at the antimesenteric border (*Illustration 15a*). The suture is knotted, and the first layer starts as a continuous horizontal mattress suture (*Illustrations 15b, c*). The crushing clamp is removed as the suture is again knotted at the mesenteric border of the intestine. The suture is then returned towards the antimesenteric end as a continuous over-and-over stitch incorporating all layers of the bowel wall (*Illustrations 15d, e*) and is finally knotted at the antimesenteric end (*Illustration 15f*). Interrupted submucosal sutures of silk or other braided material are then inserted (*Illustration 15g*), and the end of the bowel is securely invaginated (*Illustration 15h*).

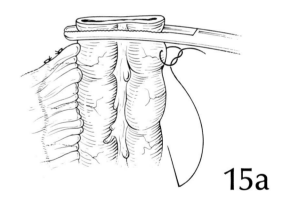

15a

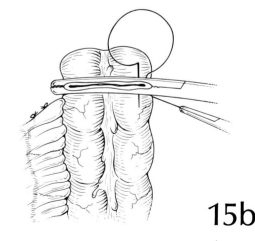

15b

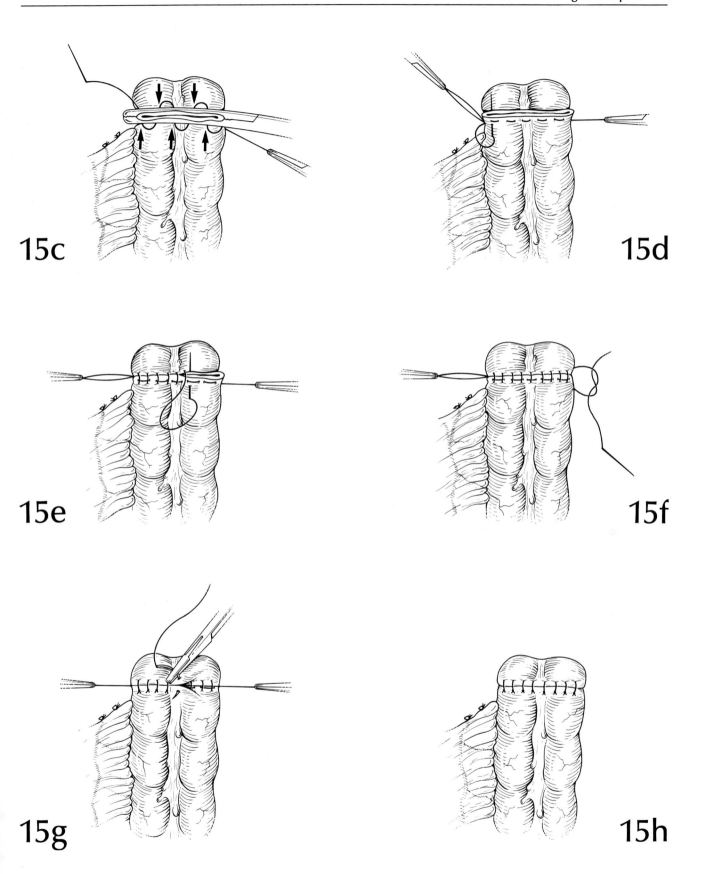

15c

15d

15e

15f

15g

15h

Ileocolic and ileorectal/colorectal anastomoses

16a–d
In an end-to-side reconstruction after the operation of right hemicolectomy, the end of the colon is closed and the end of the ileum is anastomosed to the side of the colon using a standard two-layer inverting technique (*Illustrations 16a–c*).

In side-to-end colorectal anastomosis, the side of the colon is anastomosed to the end of the rectal stump (*Illustration 16d*). The author never uses this method in colorectal anastomosis but finds it useful in anastomosis of the caecum to the rectum and in anastomosis of the ileum to the rectum after the operation of subtotal colectomy if there is marked disparity in the size of the ileum and rectum.

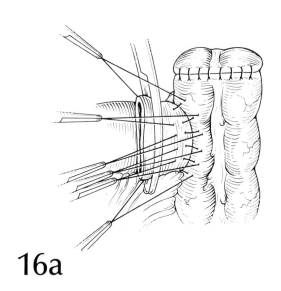

16a

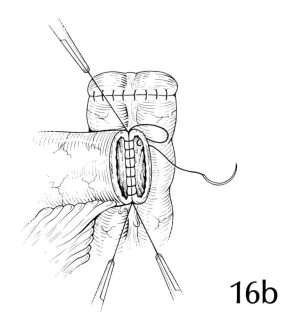

16b

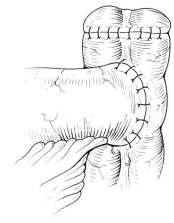

16c

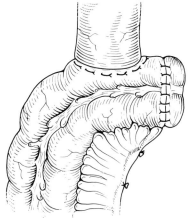

16d

Caecorectal anastomosis

17a–d In the method of anastomosis favoured by the author, the end of the caecum is closed (*Illustration 17a*) using the technique shown in *Illustrations 15a–h* and the side of the caecum is anastomosed to the cut end of the rectum. A two-layer suture technique is used, beginning with the insertion of an outer posterior row of silk submucosal mattress sutures (*Illustration 17b*). The inner layer of the anastomosis is made with a continuous chromic catgut suture incorporating all layers of the bowel wall (*Illustration 17c*) and the anastomosis is completed with an anterior layer of silk submucosal mattress sutures (*Illustration 17d*).

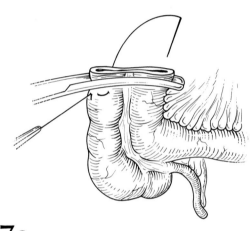

17a

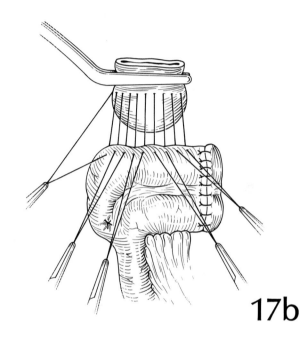

17b

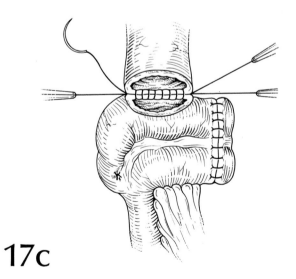

17c

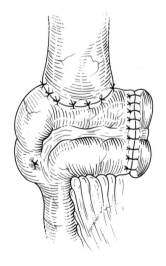

17d

Ileoanal pouch anastomosis

18 The most common method of anastomosis in the operation of restorative proctocolectomy involves suture of the side of the most dependent part of the ileal pouch to the lumen of the anal canal at or above the dentate line. A single-layer suture technique is favoured although some surgeons use a stapled anastomosis. It is customary and advisable to protect the anastomosis with a defunctioning loop ileostomy.

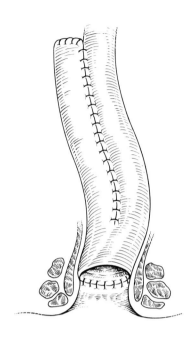

18

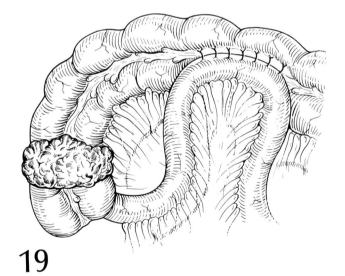

19

SIDE-TO-SIDE ANASTOMOSIS

19 The chief application of side-to-side anastomosis in the large intestine is in the relief of obstructions caused by irremovable neoplasms, particularly in the right colon. The ileum is anastomosed to the transverse colon beyond the site of obstruction using a two-layer suture technique.

A previous generation of surgeons frequently used side-to-side techniques of anastomosis in preference to the end-to-end method, but there is no evidence that the former method is safer and it may result in 'blind loop' problems associated with the closure of the two ends of bowel.

Postoperative care

Peritoneal drains are removed after 48 h, their purpose being to remove any collections of blood or serum during the early postoperative period.

Systemic antibiotics are usually limited to the perioperative period, but may be continued for 3–5 days when there is significant faecal soiling or bacterial contamination during surgery. Intravenous cefuroxime and metronidazole are used by the author.

A period of alimentary motor dysfunction inevitably follows anastomosis of the intestine and may or may not be apparent clinically. Nasogastric tubes are not required routinely but oral intake should be introduced cautiously. Early oral intake may result in abdominal distension and vomiting. In the author's practice, oral intake is restricted until the patient passes flatus, which usually occurs on about the fourth day.

Prolonged intolerance of oral intake, vomiting, fever or protracted ileus may indicate that anastomotic dehiscence has occurred. Gross disruption of an anastomosis is usually accompanied by evidence of peritonitis, fistulation or systemic signs of gross sepsis, but the signs may be less explicit in elderly subjects. A marked leucocytosis accompanying a non-specific general deterioration in the condition of the elderly patient should alert the surgeon to the possibility that anastomotic dehiscence has occurred.

Dehiscence is a complication which begins during the first few days after operation when the integrity and strength of the anastomosis are largely dependent on the sutures. Clinical features of dehiscence seldom arise de novo after the first postoperative week, although this may not be true for stapled anastomoses.

Anastomoses in the left colon or rectum may be examined radiologically on the 12th day using a water-soluble contrast medium such as Gastrografin. In most cases the study is of academic interest only, although small anastomotic leaks which are unassociated with clinical signs may be revealed. Occasionally, the study will confirm the clinical impression that a more serious degree of anastomotic disruption has occurred.

Ultrasonographic examination of the abdomen is helpful in the diagnosis of localized leaks, and perianastomotic abscesses may be drained percutaneously under ultrasonographic guidance. However, most abscesses associated with colorectal anastomoses will discharge spontaneously through the suture line. It may require considerable judgement on the part of the surgeon to determine when further surgery is indicated for the complications of anastomotic dehiscence.

Outcome

In expert hands, major resectional surgery of the large intestine is associated with a mortality rate of less than 5%, and most deaths are due to complications of coexisting medical disease rather than problems with the anastomosis. Fatalities due to disruption of the anastomosis are rarely encountered in the hands of skilled and experienced surgeons.

References

1. Friend PJ, Scott R, Everett WG, Scott IHK. Stapling or suturing for anastomoses of the left side of the large intestine. *Surg Gynecol Obstet* 1990; 171: 373–6.

2. Fielding LP, Stewart-Brown S, Blesovsky L, Kearney G. Anastomotic integrity after operations for large-bowel cancer: a multicentre study *BMJ* 1980; 281: 411–14.

3. Matheson NA, Irving AD. Single layer anastomosis after rectosigmoid resection. *Br J Surg* 1975; 62: 239–42.

4. Ravo B, Ger R. Temporary colostomy – an outmoded procedure? A report on the intracolonic bypass. *Dis Colon Rectum* 1985; 28: 904–7.

5. Dudley HAF, Radcliffe AG, McGeehan D. Intraoperative irrigation of the colon to permit primary anastomosis. *Br J Surg* 1980; 67: 80–1.

6. Buck N, Devlin HB, Lunn JN. *The Report of a Confidential Enquiry into Perioperative Deaths.* London: Nuffield Provincial Hospitals Trust, 1987.

Stapling in colorectal surgery

R. W. Beart Jr MD, FACS
Professor of Surgery, Mayo Clinic, Scottsdale, Arizona, USA

History

Surgeons continue to be interested in identifying the best way to create an intestinal anastomosis. In 1893, Nicholas pointed out that '...the ideal method of uniting intestinal wounds is yet to be devised'. Through the years, surgeons have devised numerous types of suture material; absorbable, non-absorbable, synthetic, non-synthetic, braided and monofilament, to create intestinal anastomoses. Mechanical stapling devices might be traced to the early work of Denans in Marseilles, whose work preceded the more famous Murphy Button by 66 years. In 1826, he invaginated intestinal ends over two silver rings, and then approximated the bowel with a special pair of forceps. Inversion was accomplished, and the entire circumferences of the serosal surfaces were opposed. Stapling devices were developed to overcome inadequacies with traditional suturing methods. Hultl produced a stapling instrument in 1911. It was cumbersome, weighed over 4.5 kg, and took hours to assemble. Petz designed an instrument, similar to Payr's crushing clamp, which placed a row of staples along both edges close to the stomach during gastrectomy. Between 1945 and 1950, a group of Russian engineers in Moscow, including Gudov and Androsov, developed methods to staple blood vessels together, prompted by the difficulties with traditional suture techniques experienced during World War II. Their developments continued up until 1970, and included many gastrointestinal stapling instruments[1].

Since that time, Ravitch and Steichen should be given the greatest credit for the proliferation of these instruments[2]. They initiated numerous publications outlining surgical techniques for the use of staplers to perform pneumonectomy, lobectomy, gastrectomy, end-to-end bowel anastomosis, and transection of multiple vessels. These instruments have now become commonplace and approximately 40% of intestinal anastomoses in the USA are created with these devices. It is appropriate to review the advantages of these instruments as well as the potential disadvantages that have been identified since the early 1970s.

When performing colonic surgery with staplers, there are four fundamental techniques which should be mastered: functional end-to-end anastomosis, end-to-side anastomosis, end-to-end anastomosis, and double/triple stapling methods.

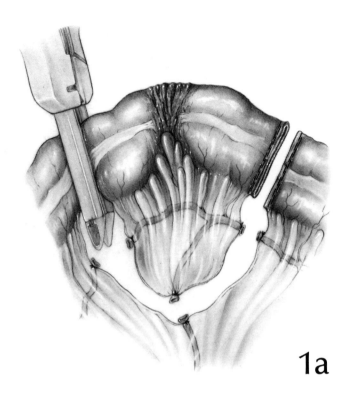

1a

Functional end-to-end anastomosis

1a, b In the functional end-to-end method, the bowel is mobilized completely, making sure that all tension has been relieved. The mesentery is dissected to the point where the bowel is to be transected. This can be achieved with a linear stapler which cuts as it divides and seals both ends of the bowel (*Illustration 1a*).

Alternatively, a clamp can be placed on the section to be removed and a stapling device placed across the end to be preserved (*Illustration 1b*). The stapler should be placed in the antimesenteric to mesenteric direction.

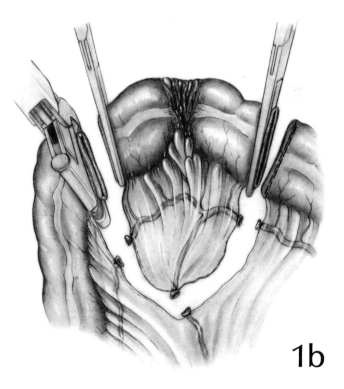

1b

2 The anastomosis is inspected on the inside of the bowel to look for bleeding points which may occasionally need to be ligated. The length of the anastomosis should not be less than 6 cm to provide an adequate lumen. If less than 6 cm, then a second linear staple cartridge should be used in the linear stapler.

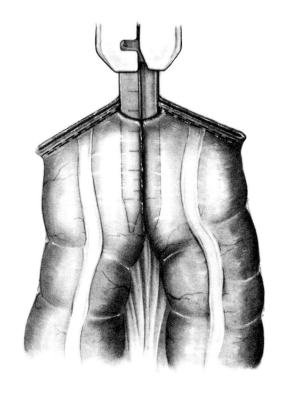

2

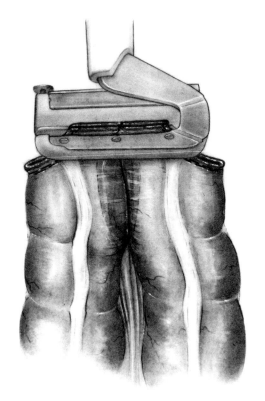

3

3 This leaves a defect at the site where the staplers were inserted, which can be closed with either a mechanical stapler or a traditional hand sewn technique. In either case, the closure should be from staple line to staple line, by distracting the two staple lines to form a triangular anastomotic defect. Two limbs of the triangle are the staple lines and the third limb is the closure of the defect. This creates a functional end-to-end anastomosis, which has been shown to heal well and function as well as an end-to-end anastomosis[3].

End-to-side anastomosis

4 An end-to-side anastomosis can be created as an alternative to the functional end-to-end anastomosis. The bowel is similarly mobilized and divided, but the ends of the remaining bowel are not sutured shut. Instead, a purse-string suture is placed around the end of the distal bowel (e.g. the transverse colon). After sizing the proximal bowel, the appropriate circular staple device is placed through the end of the proximal bowel (e.g. the terminal ileum) without the anvil.

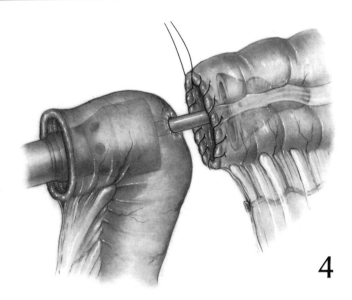

4

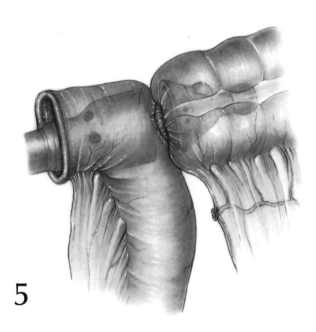

5

5 The circular stapler shaft is then extended through the antimesenteric side of the ileum and the anvil attached. The anvil is then placed into the end of the transverse colon and the purse-string tied around the shaft of the anvil, which is retracted into the stapling instrument.

6 An end-to-side anastomosis is created with a circular stapler, which is then withdrawn. The end of the ileum through which the stapler had been placed must then be closed with a linear stapler.

These two anastomotic techniques are used in similar situations. The functional end-to-end anastomosis requires four staple cartridges and is, therefore, somewhat more expensive than the end-to-side anastomosis. However, the end-to-side anastomosis has a short but real 'blind end', which theoretically may, at a future time, cause problems by the formation of a pulsion diverticulum. In both cases, the mesenteric defect can be closed. Neither anastomotic technique has been shown to be more secure or more rapid than traditional hand-sewn techniques. Therefore it becomes a matter of personal preference as to which technique a surgeon chooses to use.

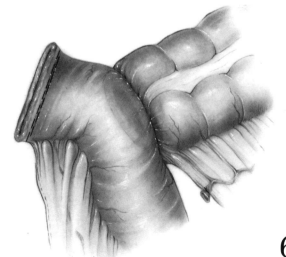

6

End-to-end anastomosis

The end-to-end anastomosis is most commonly created with the circular stapler. Typically, such an anastomosis will be created in the pelvis where the descending or sigmoid colon is being anastomosed to the rectum. With this technique, the patient must be placed in a modified lithotomy position (*see* chapter on pp. 47–50) so that access to the anus is possible. The bowel is mobilized and the mesentery ligated and resected to the point where the bowel is to be divided. Distally, a clamp is placed across the bowel at the proximal margin of transection, and the distal rectum is irrigated with water or cytotoxic agent to minimize the presence of any viable cancer cells.

7 A non-crushing bowel clamp can then be placed across the distal bowel, the bowel can be transected and a purse-string suture placed around the open rectum. Proximally, the bowel is transected and a purse-string suture needs to be placed, which can be done with a purse-string clamp. Automatic purse-string devices can be used both proximally and distally, but are quite expensive and probably offer minimal advantage.

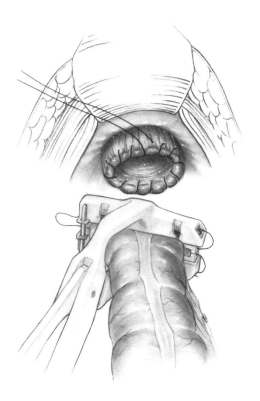

7

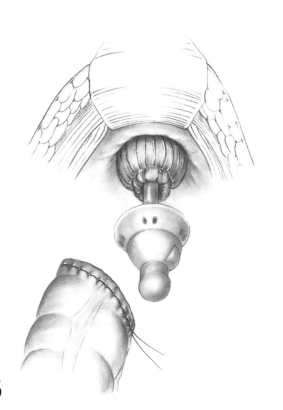

8

8 Once the purse-strings are placed, the circular stapler is inserted through the anus and advanced through the rectum. As it approaches the rectal purse-string, the assistant opens the stapling device, passing the anvil through the purse-string suture. The purse-string is then tightened around the shaft and the instrument is opened completely.

9 The proximal bowel is then placed over the anvil. Placing the bowel over the anvil can be difficult and, before doing this, the edge of the proximal bowel should be grasped with three narrow Allis' clamps, one-third of the circumference apart. The bowel can be dilated with ring forceps and glucagon can be given to relax the bowel. The Allis' forceps are then used to place the lumen over the posterior aspect of the anvil and, using blunt-tipped forceps, the anterior lip of the bowel is brought over the anvil anteriorly. The purse-string can then be tightened around the shaft of the anvil.

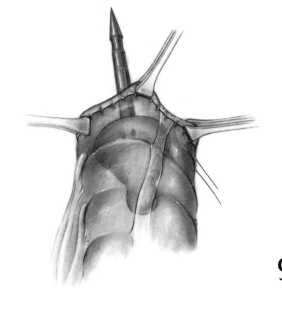

9

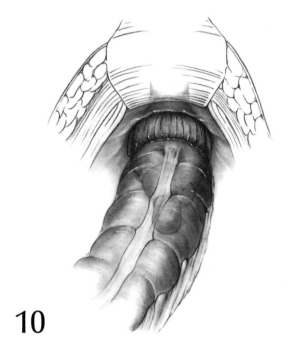

10

10 Under direct vision and making sure the bowel is not rotated, the anvil can then be tightened and the stapler can be fired. The stapler is then opened minimally and, using a rotating motion, is withdrawn from the anus. The operating surgeon, working the abdomen, should make an effort to place traction on the rectum to ease the stapler across the anastomosis because the anastomosis is smaller than the cartridge and removal of the stapler can be somewhat difficult.

At this point, the surgeon must ensure that the anastomosis is not under tension. This is done by making sure that the bowel is laying in the hollow of the sacrum. If there is any 'bow-stringing' across the hollow of the sacrum, the left colon and splenic flexure must be mobilized to remove any evidence of tension. The stapler rings should be inspected. They should be removed from the stapler carefully, maintaining their orientation, and the purse-string sutures should be cut so the rings can be opened fully. Unless the purse-string sutures are cut, small defects in the rings can be hidden. If a defect in the ring is identified, its location in the circumference of the bowel should be noted; this is made possible by having preserved its orientation. If the anastomosis cannot be adequately inspected, the rectum should be insufflated with air through the anus and the leak identified. If this can be repaired with sutures, diversion may be unnecessary. If a leak cannot be identified, or if there is any question about the integrity of the anastomosis, a diverting stoma is appropriate.

Double/triple stapling techniques

11 A double or triple staple technique is used in a similar situation to an end-to-end anastomosis. With these techniques, the bowel is similarly mobilized and the mesentery ligated and divided. The distal bowel is transected with a linear stapler.

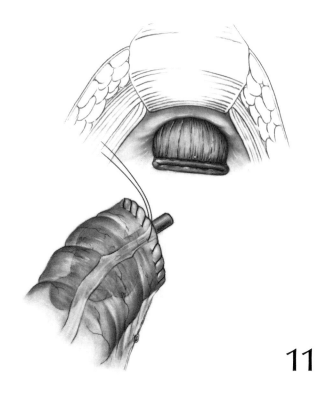

11

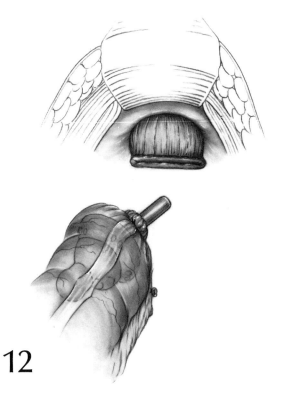

12

12 In the double stapling method, a purse-string suture is then placed in the proximal bowel after its division between clamps, and the detachable anvil inserted proximally with the purse-string suture being tied snugly onto the shaft of the anvil.

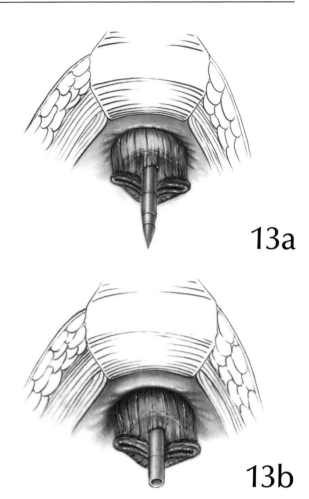

13a, b The circular stapler (without the anvil which has already been placed in the proximal bowel) is then passed through the anus and placed under some pressure against the rectal stump. The shaft of the instrument is then advanced and allowed to perforate the blind stump of the rectum adjacent to the staple line.

13a

13b

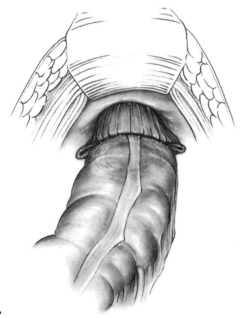

14 The anvil and the stapler are then reunited, making sure that the bowel is not rotated. The stapler is closed, fired and removed. However, it is vital to ensure that neither the vagina nor other pelvic structures are included in the anastomosis, and after the instrument is closed, all sides of the anastomosis must be carefully inspected before firing the apparatus.

It is desirable to ensure that the linear staple lines are not juxtaposed when this technique is used, and the bowel must not be under tension after the anastomosis has been completed.

14

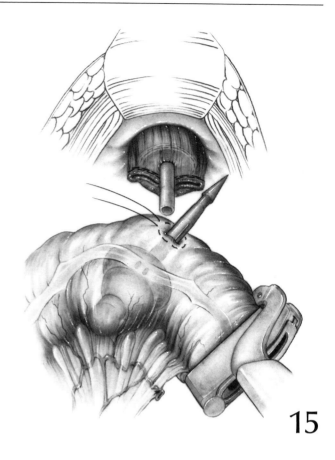

15 In the triple stapling technique, an enterotomy is made in the proximal bowel a few centimetres from its open end. The anvil is introduced, the colotomy closed with a purse-string suture, and the bowel is then transected distally.

15

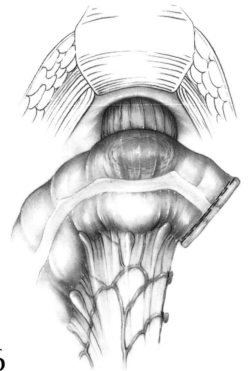

16

16 The anastomosis is completed as for the double stapling method described above.

Stapled pouch procedures

Stapling devices can be used to construct various types of ileoanal pouches with sutures or staples. The latter technique is less time consuming, although more expensive.

Advantages and disadvantages of staplers

Staplers have been proven to be an effective way of anastomosing the bowel. Traditional Halstedian techniques requiring inversion anastomosis have not been found to be necessary with staplers and an everted anastomosis is secure. It has not been shown that staplers save a significant amount of operative time for most anastomoses[3, 4]. For low-lying rectal anastomoses, it has been shown that perhaps as many as 15% of rectums will be preserved in situations where a traditional two-layered anastomosis cannot be performed[2]. Questions have been raised about whether or not metal is a promoter of carcinogenesis or may promote recurrence of cancer[5, 6]. However, the preponderance of recent data suggests that when the rectum is irrigated and margins of normal bowel are resected around cancers, local recurrences do not appear to be increased when compared with hand-sutured techniques[1, 5].

Stricturing has been noted with an increased frequency when the circular stapler is used. It is unclear whether this is a vascular problem or if there are other aetiologies. Most often, the stricture is a very thin web and can be easily dilated; it occurs in 30–40% of patients, but is functionally significant in only about 2%. It is also important to note that these staple lines are not haemostatic, and care must be taken to confirm that there are no bleeding vessels coming through the anastomosis. If this occurs, the bleeding point must be ligated. Staplers are clearly a more costly way to anastomose the bowel, and the prudent surgeon may choose not to staple anastomoses in all situations. However, these techniques are clearly advantageous in specific situations and should be part of the armamentarium of all general surgeons[7, 8].

References

1. Fraser I. An historical perspective on mechanical aids in intestinal anastomosis. *Surg Gynecol Obstet* 1982; 155: 566–74.

2. Ravitch MM, Ong TH, Gazzola L. A new, precise, and rapid technique of intestinal resection and anastomosis with staples. *Surg Gynecol Obstet* 1974; 139: 6–10.

3. Scher KS, Scott-Conner C, Jones CW, Leach M. A comparison of stapled and sutured anastomoses in colonic operations. *Surg Gynecol Obstet* 1982; 155: 489–93.

4. Beart RW, Kelly KA. Randomized prospective evaluation of the EEA stapler for colorectal anastomoses. *Am J Surg* 1981; 141: 143–7.

5. Gertsch P, Baer H, Kraft R, Maddern GJ, Altermatt HJ. Malignant cells are collected on circular staplers. *Dis Colon Rectum* 1992; 35: 238–41.

6. Phillips RKS, Cook HT. Effect of steel wire sutures on the incidence of chemically induced rodent colonic tumours. *Br J Surg* 1986; 73: 671–4.

7. Dziki A, Duncan M, Harmon J *et al.* Advantages of handsewn over stapled bowel anastomosis. *Dis Colon Rectum* 1991; 34: 442–8.

8. Heald RJ, Allen DR. Stapled ileo-anal anastomosis: a technique to avoid mucosal proctectomy in the ileal pouch operation. *Br J Surg* 1986; 73: 571–2.

9. Heald RJ. Towards fewer colostomies – the impact of circular stapling devices on the surgery of rectal cancer in a district hospital. *Br J Surg* 1980; 67: 198–200.

10. Hurst PA, Prout WG, Kelly JM, Bannister JJ, Walker RT. Local recurrence after low anterior resection using the staple gun. *Br J Surg* 1982; 69: 275–6.

Biodegradable anastomotic ring (BAR) technique

Melvin P. Bubrick MD
Associate Professor, Department of Surgery, University of Minnesota and Chief of Surgery, Hennepin County Medical Center, Minneapolis, USA

History

Despite almost two centuries of controversy over the optimum procedure or device for anastomosing two ends of intestine together, most surgeons invariably agree on the requisite qualities for the ideal intestinal anastomosis: adequate blood supply, accurate serosal apposition, absence of tension on the suture line, an uncompromised lumen diameter and a watertight seal[1]. Mechanical devices to anastomose the bowel have been in use since the early 19th century and inverting intraluminal anastomotic devices were described by Denans in 1827, Bonnier in 1885 and Murphy in 1892. The Murphy button was by far the most widely used of these devices, primarily because of its speed and simplicity, although it eventually lost popularity because of some definite shortcomings[2]. These deficiencies included the weight of the device, which made it heavy and cumbersome to use, the presence of necrosis of the inverted bowel ends which was caused by the rings coming together too tightly, and the narrow internal diameter which sometimes made early postoperative bowel obstruction a problem.

Hardy and associates[3] described the Valtrac biodegradable anastomotic ring (BAR) to take advantage of the speed and simplicity of the Murphy button while making it more suitable for contemporary use by remedying its specific shortcomings. The device is made of two interlocking rings of polyglycolic acid polymer which contain barium sulphate. It has the feel of a lightweight plastic material and is designed to fragment after polymer hydrolysis has softened the material, allowing it to pass from the bowel lumen 2–3 weeks after surgery when external mechanical support is no longer needed. The lumen is large enough to prevent obstructive episodes and the two interlocking rings have serrated edges to prevent necrosis of the inverted intestinal ends.

Principles and justification

Indications

Although the BAR has been used successfully in the emergency setting when bowel preparation has not been possible, use of the device necessitates opening both ends of the intestine. The risks of anastomotic leakage in this setting must always be weighed against the overall risk and benefit of performing a temporary stoma and then performing an elective anastomosis at a later time.

The BAR is not suitable for low pelvic anastomoses because a transanal inserting instrument is not yet available. It is best to plan to use the device for small bowel or colonic anastomoses within the abdominal cavity and above the peritoneal reflection.

The device is also not designed for anastomosis of two ends of bowel with widely disparate diameters. Although it is possible to angulate the smaller of the two ends to fit the device, in general, if one end of intestine is greater than 50% larger in diameter than the other, then alternative suturing or stapling methods are preferable. This decision should be made during the operation and is based on both the size and the elasticity of the bowel ends; the smaller of the two ends of intestine can often be dilated to a size that is suitable for the BAR.

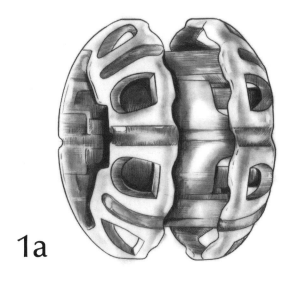

1a

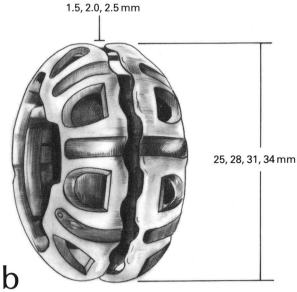

1.5, 2.0, 2.5 mm

25, 28, 31, 34 mm

1b

BAR device sizes

1a, b External diameter and gap size are the two measurements that need to be considered when selecting the appropriate size Valtrac BAR device. The external diameters of the currently available devices are 25, 28, 31 and 34 mm. The 25-, 28- and 31-mm devices have a gap size of either 1.5 mm or 2.0 mm. The 34-mm devices have either a 2.0- or 2.5-mm gap size. The gap size is created when the BAR is in the closed position and determination of the appropriate gap size depends upon the thickness of the walls of the two ends that are being anastomosed together.

Preoperative

Mechanical and antibiotic bowel preparation should be performed for all elective intestinal anastomotic procedures.

Operation

2 The segment of bowel is mobilized and the blood supply is taken in the same fashion as is done for resection and anastomosis using suture or staple techniques. The proximal and distal points of the anastomosis are defined by dividing the mesocolon or mesentery alongside the bowel with small haemostats and devascularizing a zone of 1–2 cm. The intervening mesocolon or mesentery between these two segments is then divided between clamps and ligated.

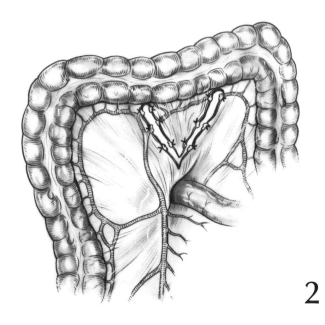

2

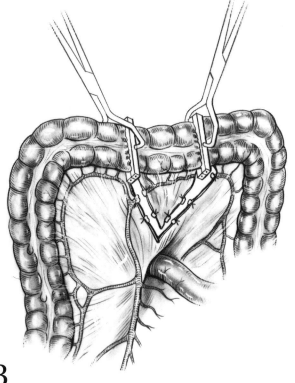

3

3 The two ends of bowel are not divided until after the purse-string suture has been applied through a purse-string clamp. Each purse-string clamp is applied across the previously marked proximal and distal ends of intestine and the instrument is closed. The instrument should not be clamped tightly because this might encourage crossover sutures across the anterior and posterior wall of the bowel.

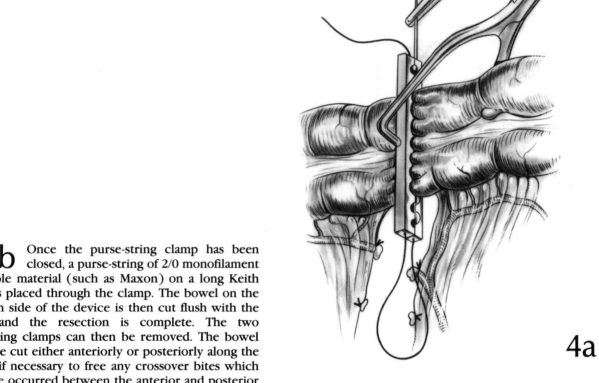

4a, b Once the purse-string clamp has been closed, a purse-string of 2/0 monofilament absorbable material (such as Maxon) on a long Keith needle is placed through the clamp. The bowel on the specimen side of the device is then cut flush with the device and the resection is complete. The two purse-string clamps can then be removed. The bowel should be cut either anteriorly or posteriorly along the mucosa if necessary to free any crossover bites which may have occurred between the anterior and posterior walls.

4a

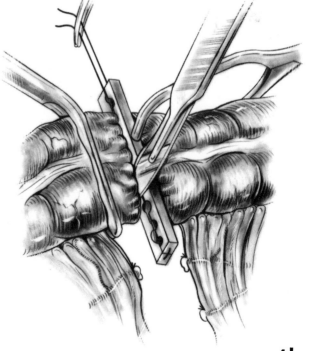

4b

5 Occasionally the bites are placed so far apart that a gaping defect is created between bites. It is best to apply simple 'pulley' sutures in this case. The same type of absorbable suture material is used on a taper needle and bites are taken through the full thickness of the bowel wall to include the purse-string suture. The pulley suture is then tied down loosely enough so that the purse-string suture still pulls freely.

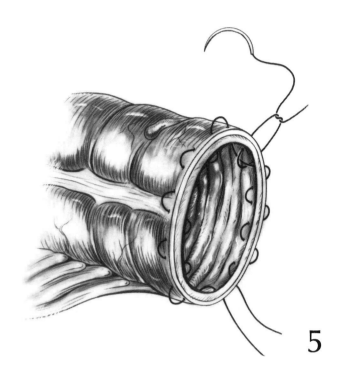

5

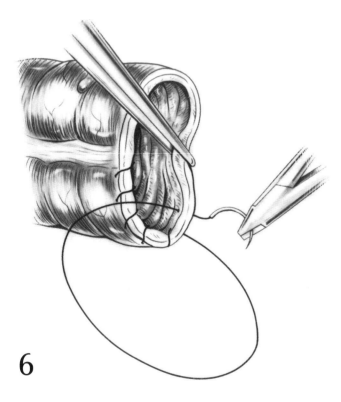

6

6 If a purse-string device is not available, the purse-string suture can be applied manually, taking small 1–2-mm bites out of the full thickness of the bowel wall circumferentially. The use of the purse-string suture device greatly facilitates applying the purse-string and generally saves time.

7 A sizer (used for the circular stapling technique) should then be applied to both proximal and distal ends of the bowel to determine what external diameter size BAR should be used. The BAR size corresponds to the same external diameter size of a circular stapling cartridge. If there is wide disparity in the size of the two ends of bowel, gentle dilatation of the smaller lumen may be tried to make the two approximate each other more closely.

The gap size is then determined. For most colonic anastomoses the 2.0-mm gap size is ideal. If the bowel is unusually thin, as is sometimes the case for the small intestine, a 1.5-mm gap size may be more suitable. Occasionally the two segments will be so large and thick that a device with a 34-mm external diameter and a 2.5-mm gap is needed.

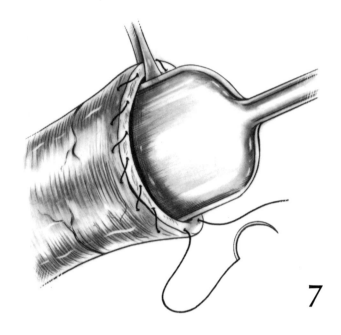

7

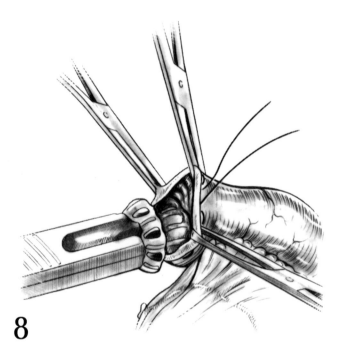

8

8 The BAR is then inserted into the proximal end of the anastomosis with the aid of an inserting handle. The free ends of the bowel are triangulated by grasping them with Allis' forceps and the BAR is gently passed into the lumen. The purse-string suture is tightly secured around the BAR.

9 The inserting device is then removed by gently pushing the release flanges on the handle and pulling the inserting handle from the BAR.

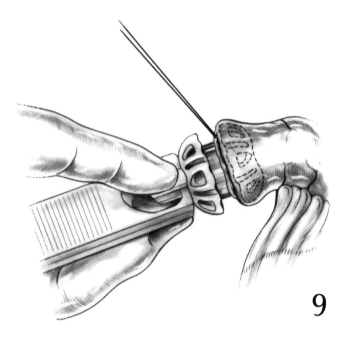

9

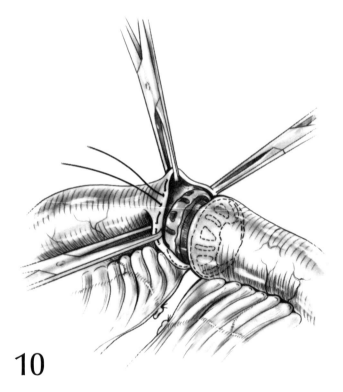

10

10 Using the same triangulation techniques, the distal end of the bowel is then grasped with three Allis' forceps and the second ring of the BAR is advanced into the bowel lumen. The purse-string is again tightened down securely onto the BAR.

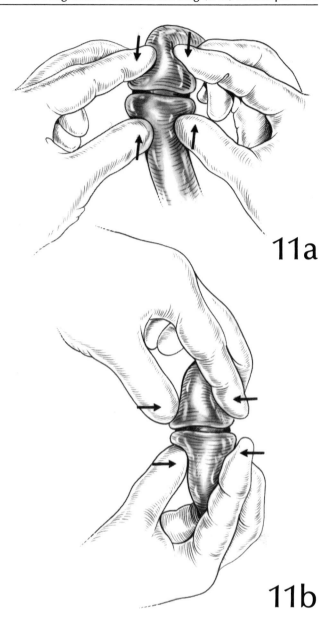

11a, b Direct pressure is applied with the thumb and index finger of each hand and the device is snapped into the closed position until an audible clicking sound is heard. It is safest to apply pressure on the BAR a second time from a different angle to be certain that the door frame locks have been closed. If the device is snapped into place with the operator's fingers at the 3 o'clock and 9 o'clock positions initially, it is then best to apply pressure at the 12 o'clock and 6 o'clock positions to ensure adequate closure.

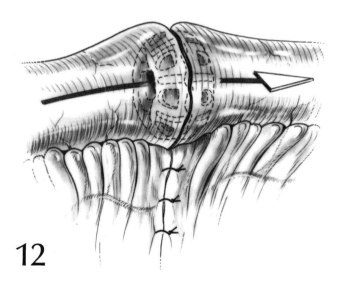

12 The defect in the mesentery or mesocolon is then closed in the usual fashion with interrupted or running sutures.

Postoperative care

Postoperative management of a patient having an anastomosis with the BAR technique is identical to the management of a patient undergoing anastomosis by suturing or stapling techniques. It is best to keep the patient on 'nil by mouth' and on intravenous fluids until peristalsis has returned, as indicated by the presence of bowel sounds, passage of flatus or the first bowel movement. The author prefers to use nasogastric suction during the early period of postoperative ileus for most patients.

The BAR contains barium sulphate which renders it radio-opaque and its position can always be checked with an abdominal film if there is a delay in the return of peristalsis or if the patient is suspected of developing other intra-abdominal complications. When peristalsis returns the patient may be started on a clear liquid diet and advanced to a general diet as tolerated. There are no specific dietary restrictions in the early postoperative period, although it is wise for the patient to avoid constipating foods. The use of a psyllium bulk-forming laxative agent or stool softener may be helpful. The patient is discharged from the hospital when a normal diet is tolerated, which usually occurs between the fifth and eighth postoperative day.

The device softens, fragments and passes into the bowel lumen usually during the third postoperative week. The patient is generally unaware of this occurring. Occasionally a patient will pass the device intact and notice some discomfort associated with the event. Rarely, the device is passed as early as the end of the first postoperative week. Should this occur it is safest to watch the patient closely for 48–72 h, and to continue a liquid diet until it is clear that the anastomotic site did not sustain any trauma during the early passage of the device.

Outcome

In a recent multicentre multinational controlled randomized trial[1] of 782 patients having colorectal anastomoses by either sutured, stapled or BAR techniques, there was no difference in any outcome parameters between the three anastomotic methods. Complications such as wound infection, bleeding and dehiscence, intra-abdominal abscess, bleeding, anastomotic leak, ileus and obstruction were assessed. The overall complication rate in the study for all three anastomotic techniques was the same. When complications occur with the BAR device they should be treated in an identical fashion to those that follow other anastomotic techniques.

References

1. Bubrick MP, Corman ML, Cahil CJ *et al*. Prospective, randomized trial of the biofragmentable anastomosis ring. *Am J Surg* 1991; 161: 136–43.

2. Ravitch MM. Development of intestinal anastomotic devices. *South Med J* 1982; 75: 1520–4.

3. Hardy TG, Pace WG, Maney JW, Katz AR, Kaganov AL. A biofragmentable ring for sutureless bowel anastomoses: an experimental study. *Dis Colon Rectum* 1985; 28: 484–90.

Illustrations by Richard Neave and the late Robert Lane

Surgical management of anastomotic leakage and intra-abdominal sepsis

Miles Irving MD, ChM, FRCS
Professor of Surgery and Consultant Surgeon, Hope Hospital, University of Manchester School of Medicine, Salford, UK

Sarah O'Dwyer MD, FRCS
Consultant Surgeon, The General and Queen Elizabeth Hospitals, Birmingham, UK

Principles and justification

Leakage from anastomosed bowel is almost always the result of bad judgement and/or poor technique at the time of construction. Leakage rates vary widely between surgeons and, although anastomotic leakage occurs even in the best of hands, very low rates can be attained and this must be the goal of all gastrointestinal surgeons.

Anastomotic failure occurs when the bowel is ischaemic, when it is inadequately mobilized (resulting in tension on the anastomosis), and when seromuscular apposition of the divided intestinal ends is inaccurate. Furthermore, the presence of severe malnutrition and intra-abdominal sepsis also compromise anastomotic healing and, therefore, when conditions for anastomotic healing are not ideal the surgeon should not hesitate to exteriorize the intestinal ends and reconstruct the intestine at a later date. It may be appropriate to protect a primary anastomosis by fashioning a proximal diverting stoma which can be closed when the anastomosis has healed. The role of intraluminal devices such as the Coloshield in protecting an anastomosis is unclear, and they have not gained wide acceptance. Should anastomotic leakage occur, prompt institution of the correct management will limit the risk of further major complications and death. The approach to this problem will depend upon the type of leakage and the general condition of the patient.

Anastomotic leaks can be categorized into four principal types:

1. Asymptomatic leaks.
2. Leaks associated with generalized peritonitis.
3. Leaks associated with localized infection or abscess formation.
4. Leaks associated with an enterocutaneous fistula.

Clinical presentation

Leakage associated with generalized peritonitis

Disruption of an anastomosis with leakage of enteric content can occur at any time after surgery but is most usual 2–5 days following the procedure. Bowel contents discharge into the abdominal cavity and the patient becomes tachycardic and shows signs of generalized peritonitis. In a short time peripheral circulatory failure develops, urine output falls and vital signs deteriorate. The degree of abdominal distension depends on the amount of gas leakage and may lead to a tense tympanitic abdomen with radiological evidence of pneumoperitoneum. The diagnosis of an anastomotic leak can be difficult, particularly in immunosuppressed and elderly patients where an intra-abdominal catastrophe can present as progressive postoperative confusion or deterioration in respiratory function. In most cases an experienced surgeon will be able to make a clinical diagnosis of anastomotic leakage, following which resuscitation and urgent laparotomy are required.

Leakage associated with abscess formation

An abscess should be suspected in a patient who fails to progress or where there is evidence of low-grade swinging pyrexia. Where there is a track to the surface erythema of the skin, swelling and tenderness indicate the site for drainage. Assessment of the pelvis by rectal examination may reveal a boggy swelling in the presacral space. A low pelvic abscess can be drained rectally or through the perineum. If such an abscess is associated with leakage from a colonic anastomosis, a defunctioning stoma may be necessary to prevent further pelvic abscess formation.

Leakage associated with an enterocutaneous fistula

In some cases of anastomotic leak, the surrounding inflammatory reaction is so marked that the leakage is confined and a generalized peritonitis does not occur. In these cases the patient develops pain and swelling in the area of leakage, which is associated with a raised temperature and constitutional disturbance. The remaining part of the abdomen remains soft although there may be a degree of intestinal obstruction, but normal bowel function may continue.

Eventually a fistula presents through the wound or drain site with the discharge of pus, gas and enteric content (singly or in combination), usually followed by relief of constitutional and obstructive symptoms.

Preoperative

Asymptomatic leakage

Small leaks from low rectal anastomoses are seen in a proportion of cases in which the integrity of the anastomosis is routinely checked postoperatively by radio-opaque enema. Similar small leaks almost certainly occur in anastomoses higher in the intestinal tract but these are rarely subject to such checks. Providing the leak is not associated with infection, as evidenced by persistent swinging pyrexia and signs of inflammation, and normal bowel function has returned, no intervention is required. The leak will heal spontaneously without complications.

Leakage associated with generalized peritonitis

The patient with generalized peritonitis requires aggressive intravenous fluid resuscitation using both crystalloid and colloid solutions and should be transferred to a high-dependency or intensive therapy unit before surgery if possible.

Measurement of central venous and pulmonary wedge pressures aids in the determination of the degree of circulatory failure and allows optimal fluid resuscitation with minimal cardiac overload. Arterial blood gases and acid–base status should be measured and mechanical ventilation may be necessary to reverse acidosis and to support pulmonary function. Blood cultures should be taken and intravenous antibiotics (such as metronidazole and cefuroxime) should be given immediately the diagnosis has been established. A urinary catheter is inserted at the outset of resuscitation and, wherever possible, surgery should be delayed until urinary flow is established. Pharmacological support (e.g. using dopamine and noradrenaline) may be required to bring about a satisfactory cardiac response and to maintain systemic vascular resistance. However, the presence of faecal peritonitis may prevent complete correction of circulatory failure before reoperation.

Leakage associated with abscess

Supplementary investigations (e.g. ultrasonography, computed tomography (CT) and indium-labelled leucocyte scanning) are useful in defining the anatomy and localizing occult collections of pus. In some cases, when there are strong clinical grounds for suspecting an abscess but radiological investigation has been inconclusive, laparotomy is justifiable.

Operations

Incision

Wherever practicable the previous incision should be reopened and extended as necessary to obtain adequate access. On opening the peritoneal cavity faecal fluid should be sucked out and a sample sent for urgent microbiological assessment.

MANAGEMENT OF LEAKS ASSOCIATED WITH GENERALIZED PERITONITIS

1 The soft fibrinous adhesions binding the abdominal contents together should be separated to release pockets of fluid that lie between the loops of intestine. This is best achieved by gentle digital dissection, gradually separating the tissues and following the bowel down to the site of the anastomosis. Every effort should be made to avoid perforating the intestine during this dissection.

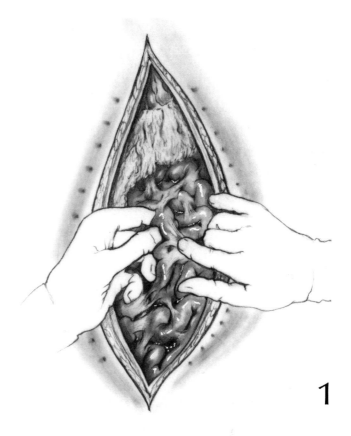

1

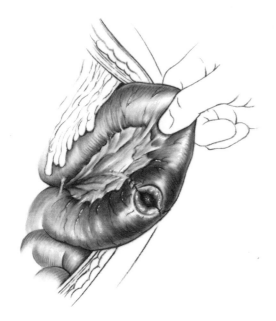

2

2 The leakage usually arises from a hole in one part of the anastomosis: only rarely will the whole anastomosis have come apart (although this may occur on exploration and mobilization). A small defect may be resutured, but this should not be performed in the great majority of patients. Similarly, taking down the anastomosis, resecting the area and then constructing a new anastomosis is dangerous because this second anastomosis, fashioned in the presence of generalized peritonitis, is also likely to leak. Even a loop stoma proximal to the disrupted bowel may be insufficient because there remains a length of 'loaded' bowel between the stoma and the point of leakage.

3 Once the site of leakage has been established the anastomosis is taken down and the ends separated. The abdominal cavity should be irrigated with copious quantities of saline at body temperature. Careful separation of loops of intestine and irrigation of paracolic, subdiaphragmatic and pelvic recesses must be continued until the irrigation fluid is no longer turbid or contains debris. Fibrinous exudates can be left as radical debridement has not been shown to be of value and may lead to blood loss and tissue damage.

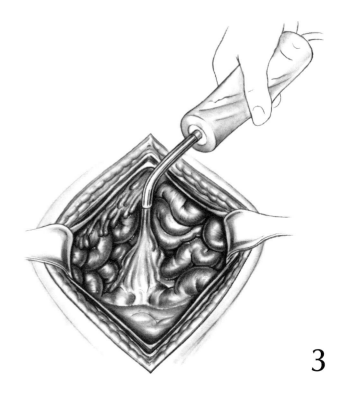

3

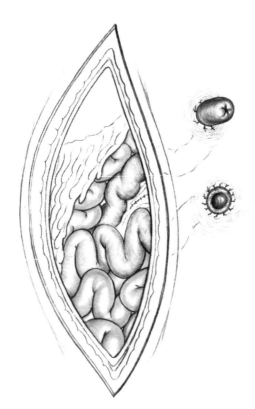

4

4 The intestinal ends must be separated and excised back to healthy tissue. Ideally, both ends should be brought to the surface through stab incisions away from the main wound and fixed with mucocutaneous sutures. It is important for the proximal stoma to be in a site where a bag can be applied successfully and this stoma should be constructed as a formal end ileostomy (*see* pp. 243–269) or colostomy (*see* pp. 274–283). When the inflammatory reaction to generalized or prolonged peritonitis is severe, thickened mesentery and oedema of the intestinal wall may prevent eversion of the mucosa. In order to avoid a flush ileostomy, where possible about 5 cm of ileum should be brought out and tacked to the abdominal wall. Eversion can be performed under local anaesthesia a few days later.

5   Where there is only a short segment of bowel beyond the disrupted anastomosis (such as a rectal stump following an anterior resection), or where separation of the small bowel mesentery is difficult because of oedema, the stump or distal bowel should be closed in the manner of a Hartmann's operation and only the proximal limb brought out to the surface.

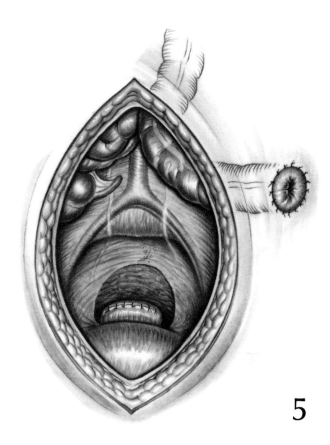

5

Wound closure

6a–c Following stoma formation the peritoneal cavity is washed with 1 litre of saline containing 1 g tetracycline. Sump suction drains are inserted into the right and left paracolic gutters positioned in the hepatorenal and rectovesical pouches, respectively. In the case of moderate peritoneal contamination it may be possible to close the deep layers of the abdominal wall with interrupted sutures of 1 polydioxanone, taking 1-cm bites of muscle and peritoneum on each side as a one-layer 'mass' closure. Tension sutures should not be used in closure of abdominal wounds. The skin and subcutaneous tissues are irrigated with tetracycline in saline lavage and primary closure is performed using monofilament sutures or metal clips. If there has been severe faecal contamination, the superficial layers can be left open and packed with gauze soaked in saline. The gauze pack is changed every 12 h until healthy granulation tissue is seen and the wound is clean. It may then be closed under local anaesthesia, usually some time after the fourth postoperative day.

In some cases of long-standing peritonitis it can be difficult to close the abdominal wall because oedema and inflammation render the intestine difficult to reduce into the abdominal cavity and because the abdominal wall is rigid. In such circumstances the authors recommend the use of relaxing incisions into the muscles of the abdominal wall at the lateral border of the anterior rectus sheath on either side of the midline wound.

In a very small number of cases, where contamination of the abdominal cavity is extremely severe or long-standing, or if there is a large intra-abdominal cavity unsuitable for treatment by tube drains alone, formal laparostomy may be necessary. Following thorough intra-abdominal toilet and siting of suction drains the abdomen or the abscess cavity is packed with saline-soaked gauze. In order to prevent coughing disturbing the packs, patients are ventilated for 24 h after laparostomy. The packs are changed 12–18 h after surgery and then twice daily, allowing absorption of purulent fluid into the packs and thereby preventing occult intracavity abscess formation.

Formation of granulation tissue, epithelialization and contraction of the wound occurs over 2–3 months and occasionally incisional hernia repair is required at a later date.

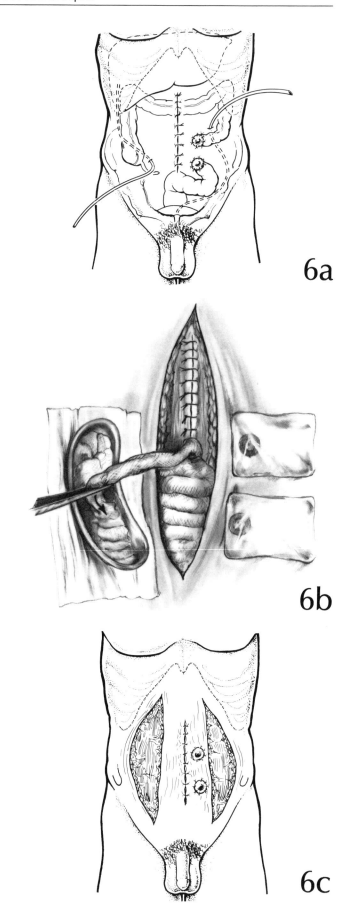

6a

6b

6c

MANAGEMENT OF LEAKS ASSOCIATED WITH ABSCESS FORMATION

7 Whenever a well-localized abscess is detected it should be drained by direct incision or, preferably, ultrasound- or CT-guided drainage. Following anatomical delineation of the abscess a drain is inserted and pus sent for microbiological culture. If preoperative scanning indicates evidence of loculation, further drains can be inserted to facilitate complete emptying of the cavities. If the abscess is chronic and has a thick wall, drains must be left *in situ* until repeat scanning indicates complete collapse of the cavity. Irrigation of the cavity may be necessary to remove any debris which collects as the abscess heals.

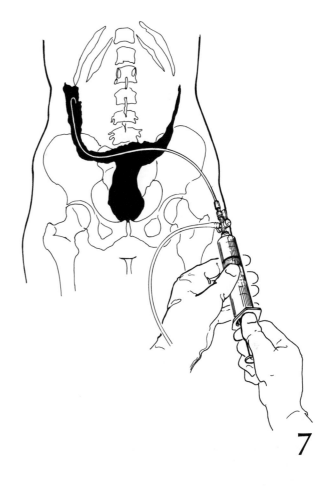

7

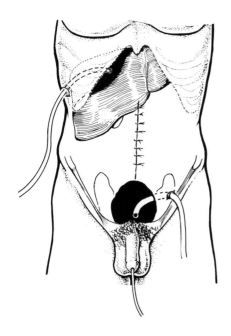

8

8 Abscesses which cannot be safely or adequately drained with the aid of scanning techniques require a formal surgical approach. In the case of an inadequately draining abscess with a track to the surface, this track can be used as a guide to the deeper cavity. In some cases laparotomy may be necessary to achieve satisfactory placement of large tube drains which should be positioned to allow drainage of debris and pus.

MANAGEMENT OF LEAKS ASSOCIATED WITH ENTEROCUTANEOUS FISTULA

With correct management 60–80% of enterocutaneous fistulae will heal with no operative intervention other than to drain abscesses. Five principles of management of such fistulae should be undertaken in the following sequence:

1. Fluid and electrolyte disturbances should be corrected.
2. The skin should be protected by application of stoma appliances.
3. Nutritional support should be started.
4. Focal sepsis should be detected and eliminated.
5. The anatomy of the fistula should be investigated and a decision made for conservative or surgical management.

Correction of fluid and electrolyte disturbances

9 A high output fistula, defined as one with a loss of over 500 ml in 24 h, can lead to rapid dehydration. Continuous replacement of the lost water and electrolytes is necessary until the loss ceases. During this time, application of a dependent drainage device may allow the patient to mobilize and minimizes the need for repetitive emptying of stoma bags.

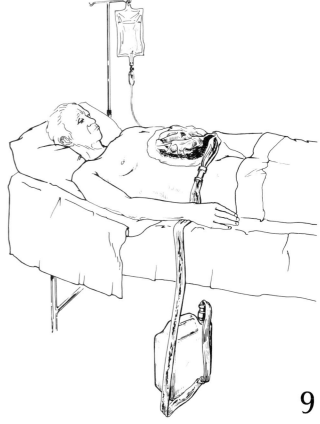

9

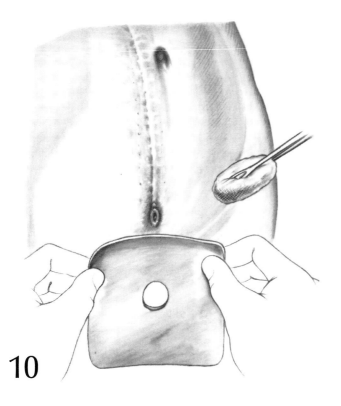

10

Protection of the skin around the fistula

10 The mouth of the fistula should be isolated with protective material such as Karaya or Stomahesive placed over the surrounding skin and a stoma bag fitted over this protective barrier.

11 For confluent fistulae or those arising in large broken-down wounds it is important to prevent pooling of liquid bowel contents, and protection of the skin may necessitate introduction of suction catheters and the application of an extensive appliance on the abdominal wall.

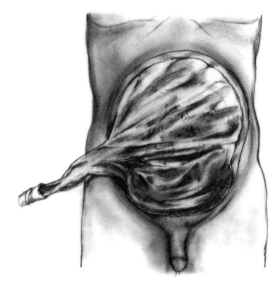

11

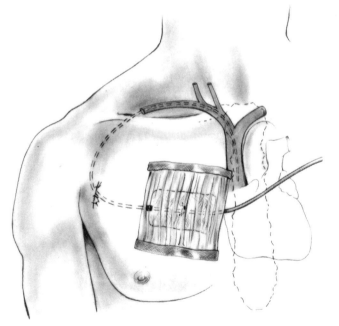

12

Nutritional support

12 Once fluid and electrolyte deficits have been corrected, parenteral nutrition should be commenced through a catheter positioned in a large vein, preferably with the tip in the superior vena cava. Tunnelling the feeding line so that it emerges on the anterior chest wall allows better access for the nursing staff, who should be trained in strict aseptic technique. By using dedicated feeding lines and trained staff exogenous line infection can be almost eliminated. Patients with terminal ileal or large bowel fistulae can usually be converted rapidly to enteral nutrition using a liquid low-residue formula. Peripheral intravenous feeding may be an alternative means of short-term adaptation to enteral feeding.

13 Patients with a high small intestinal fistula, a persistent high-output stoma or significant malnutrition will require parenteral nutrition until the fistula closes or reanastomosis of the bowel takes place. Using compact pumps it is possible to decrease the duration of feeding gradually so that the daily requirements are infused over 12 h during the evening and night. This allows the patient to exercise during the day when the feeding line is closed off using a heparin lock.

Detection and elimination of focal sepsis

The patient should be examined to establish whether sepsis is present, to determine the anatomy of the fistula and to ascertain whether there is obstruction distal to the fistula. Abscesses can be detected by a combination of clinical signs, CT, ultrasonography and isotope scanning and sinography. The anatomy of the fistula can be established by radio-opaque contrast studies and fistulography.

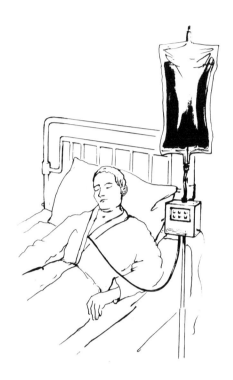

13

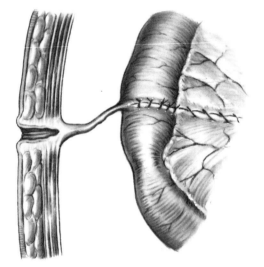

14

Continuing management of the fistula

14 If a fistula has a low output, and is shown on contrast study to be lateral and without distal obstruction then it will close with the management regimen outlined above, provided that there is no residual sepsis. Where there is a persistent track, fistuloscopy and insertion of tissue sealants can be helpful in occluding the track.

15a–d If the bowel is completely disrupted (*Illustration 15a*), there is distal obstruction (*b*), an associated abscess (*c*), or muco-cutaneous continuity (*d*), the fistula will not close spontaneously. In these circumstances surgical operation is necessary and the type of surgery is dictated by the maturation of the fistula and the nutritional state of the patient. If, as a result of good nutritional management, the patient is well nourished (serum albumin >28 g/dl), and if sepsis has been eliminated, it is permissible to resect the fistula and reconstruct the anastomosis. If, however, the patient is anaemic, hypoalbuminaemic or septic, the bowel ends should be exteriorized as previously described. Reanastomosis can take place later when the patient is no longer septic and malnourished.

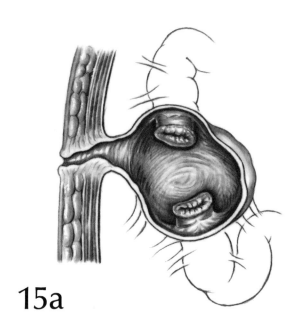

15a

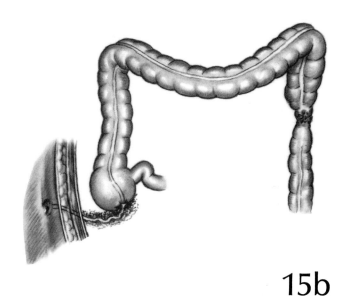

15b

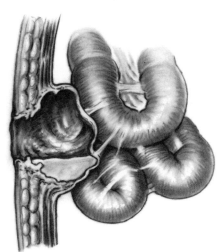

15c

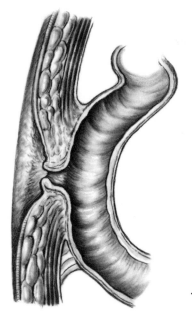

15d

Postoperative care

In the immediate postoperative period the patient may be haemodynamically unstable and is best managed in a high-dependency or intensive care area. Respiratory support may be required but prolonged mechanical ventilation is associated with increased complications and must be avoided wherever possible. Intravenous infusions should be continued until the stoma starts functioning, at which time oral intake can commence.

Postoperative antibiotics should be considered only if there has been gross contamination of the abdominal cavity or if there is recurrent septicaemia. Abscesses should be drained percutaneously following ultrasonographic or CT localization but surgical drainage may occasionally be necessary. Should the patient show evidence of ongoing sepsis a full infection screen is required and, if an infective focus cannot be identified or drained percutaneously, further laparotomy is necessary.

Restoration of intestinal continuity

Reanastomosis of the bowel should not be contemplated until all sepsis has subsided and the patient has regained lost weight. At the earliest this will be 3 months after all wounds have healed, but it may be better to leave the patient even longer, to allow intra-abdominal inflammation to subside and to make restoration technically easier. Early intervention increases the risk of bowel injury during division of adhesions and separation of bowel loops.

Interventional radiology in colorectal surgery

Henry W. Loose FRCR
Consultant Radiologist, Freeman Hospital, Newcastle-upon-Tyne, UK

Principles and justification

The development of new imaging methods, in particular the techniques of computed tomography (CT) and real time ultrasonography, has enabled precise localization of disease foci. The introduction of more refined fluoroscopic and angiographic equipment in parallel with the development of small-diameter catheters, guidewires and drainage tubes has rendered many abnormalities accessible for biopsy and drainage using guided percutaneous techniques.

The colon is readily examined by colonoscopy, but the paracolic tissues and other organs cannot be visualized, and severe haemorrhage may render colonoscopy ineffective. Angiography is often quicker and more precise, and embolization of the bleeding vessel through the arterial catheter may be a simple therapeutic measure, either as a definitive treatment or to enable resuscitation of the patient before surgical resection of the underlying pathological lesion.

Surgical relief of colonic obstruction is traditional and remains the treatment of choice, but a small proportion of patients can be treated using interventional radiological techniques, e.g. percutaneous caecostomy for relief of pseudo-obstruction, barium reduction of intussusception and balloon dilatation of colonic strictures.

Metastases from colonic carcinoma, particularly in the liver parenchyma, have on the whole defied successful therapy. Selective angiographic catheter placement and embolization or injection of cytotoxic agents have been shown to prevent tumour growth and are under active investigation.

Preoperative

Personnel

These techniques should be performed by radiologists who have specialized as full-time 'interventionalists'. It is important that the department offers adequate equipment, trained staff (both radiographic and nursing), as well as sufficient clinical experience to justify the substantial capital expenditure that is involved in maintaining a complete range of disposable equipment.

Anaesthesia

Local anaesthesia with mild sedation (diazepam, 10 mg intravenously) is usually sufficient for most procedures, and may be potentiated with pethidine hydrochloride, 25–50 mg intravenously if required. Some centres prefer oral diazepam in doses appropriate to the age of the patient and an intramuscular narcotic 1 h before the procedure.

Anxious patients benefit from papaverine, 20 mg intramuscularly 30 min before the procedure. In a long procedure or in patients who require dilatation of a tract to a gauge larger than 8.5 Fr, a combination of midazolam hydrochloride, 5–10 mg intravenously with fentanyl citrate, 50–100 µg intravenously, is effective. All patients must be monitored with a visual display of pulse rate, blood pressure and oxygen saturation.

General anaesthesia is seldom required with the exception of children, and is contraindicated because the development of pain is a pertinent indication of ischaemia or overdilatation, which can only be appreciated if the patient is able to communicate with the operator.

Patient preparation

The appropriate puncture site, usually the femoral artery at the groin, should be shaved. Fluid by mouth should be encouraged because the incidence of depression of renal function secondary to the toxic effects of contrast medium rises significantly if fluid is withheld.

Diagnostic angiography causes little discomfort apart from a transient warmth and occasional feeling of micturition if the internal iliac vessels are filled.

Embolization of a solid organ, however, causes ischaemic pain that may require intravenous narcotics for 24–48 h after the procedure. An intravenous infusion should be *in situ* before embolization.

Extensive embolization may also cause a low-grade fever secondary to tissue destruction, nausea and a feeling of lassitude which has been termed 'postembolization syndrome'. These may require supportive therapy.

If angiography is to be performed for localization of the site of haemorrhage, additional personnel are required to monitor the vital signs and to maintain adequate fluid balance, blood volume and the airway, to enable the attention of the operating radiologist to be directed to the procedure.

Informed consent

The procedure should be discussed with the patient and informed consent obtained, preferably by the 'operating' radiologist. The radiologist should not proceed to intervene without full and complete discussion with other appropriate clinicians who are responsible for the care of the patient.

Equipment

Standard disposable catheters (5 Fr or 7 Fr) and wires (0.035 inch) in sterile packs are used. The 'sidewinder' shape facilitates entry into the coeliac and superior and inferior mesenteric vessels from a femoral approach, as the tip enters in a caudal direction after the catheter has been formed in the aortic arch.

Embolic materials

Autologous clotted blood is absorbed within 12 h and therefore is of little practical value. The most practical materials for vessel embolization are the absorbable haemostatic materials, such as surgical gelatin sponge (Gelfoam) cut into small fragments 0.25–1 mm in diameter. These are drawn into a syringe in 50% normal saline and 50% contrast medium and injected under fluoroscopy when the contrast medium is visible, which allows close monitoring of any change in flow pattern. Slow hand injection is required. As soon as the flow in the vessel is slowed, the catheter is withdrawn a few millimetres to ensure that the vessel is not obstructed, and contrast medium is injected to clear the catheter and repeated every 5 min. Further particles may be required if flow continues or a steel coil can be placed behind the surgical gelatin sponge to obstruct residual flow. Gelatin sponge is absorbed within a few days, but the clot will have consolidated at the point of haemorrhage. The coil causes permanent obstruction, but is soon bypassed by collateral flow.

Tumour embolization requires more permanent materials that are not absorbed such as polyvinyl alcohol (Ivalon), a plastic sponge that expands when wet. It is available ready packed and sterile as spheres or sheets which can be cut into fragments of appropriate size (150–590 μm) in the angiography room.

A most effective embolizing agent is absolute alcohol (70%), which is painful on injection but toxic to the endothelium and produces rapid permanent vessel closure. Alcohol can be used in end arteries, e.g. the hepatic or renal vessels, with distal catheter placement but it is inappropriate for embolization of intestine or other sites of dual arterial supply, such as the internal iliac vessel.

Steel coils or detachable balloons are used for occlusion of larger vessels and act in a fashion equivalent to surgical ligation. Coils are essentially short segments of wire (0.038 inch) with a circular memory. Dacron threads are tied around the wire and stimulate clot formation *in vivo*. Detachable balloons are used to close fistulae and the necks of aneurysms, but otherwise have little advantage over the coils and are more cumbersome to use. Liquid plastic polymers are used, but require extra skills and are outside the scope of this text.

If it is not possible to achieve good distal catheter placement, then embolization is unsafe. This can be overcome by the introduction of a coaxial 3-Fr catheter passed with a 0.025-inch steerable guidewire through the lumen of the diagnostic catheter and steered to a more peripheral position. Steel coils (0.025 inch) are available, and gelatin or polyvinyl alcohol sponges are made in a powder form (200 μm) for use through the small coaxial catheter.

An alternative to particulate embolization is the infusion of a vasoconstrictive drug through the arterial catheter, which may be left *in situ* for up to 24 h. Satisfactory persisting vasoconstriction is monitored by contrast injection every 2–4 h.

Operations

ANGIOGRAPHY

Acute colonic haemorrhage

Angiography is a quick and effective way to localize the site of lower gastrointestinal haemorrhage. It is important that the procedure is not delayed while resuscitation is carried out before the patient is sent to the radiology department, because gastrointestinal haemorrhage is often intermittent and the site will not be identified if the haemorrhage has ceased. Patient resuscitation can be performed during angiography if adequate skilled help is available. Emergency surgery in these patients carries a high mortality rate (20–50%), and accurate preoperative localization reduces this. Vasopressin infusion or transcatheter embolization may convert an emergency laparotomy into an elective resection.

A proctosigmoidoscopy should precede angiography to exclude a site of haemorrhage from the rectum or anal region. Acute lower gastrointestinal haemorrhage without haematemesis may be caused by bleeding below the oesophagogastric junction. Upper gastrointestinal endoscopy should precede angiography, but the occasional exception can be made if the haemorrhage is rapid. The three major abdominal vessels should be examined at angiography, and the site will be shown if the haemorrhage is greater than 0.5 ml/min.

Radionuclide studies have been disappointing except in those patients where haemorrhage is rapid, but may be helpful if angiography proves negative. Labelled red cells can be monitored over a 6-h period, although there is usually some free technetium released into the lumen of the gut which may lead to false positive identification of the site of blood loss.

The inferior mesenteric artery is injected first at a rate of 3 ml/s for 4 s as the distribution of the superior rectal artery can be obscured by a bladder that fills with excreted contrast medium; filming is continued for 12–16 s to include a full study of the venous phase.

The superior mesenteric artery is then injected at a rate of 8 ml/s for 5 s, and filming is performed for 16 s. Two separate injections may be required because the relatively small size of rapid sequence films may not be large enough to cover the distribution of the inferior and superior mesenteric arcades to include the splenic flexure.

The coeliac axis must always be examined (8 ml/s for 5 s) if the examination of the inferior mesenteric and superior mesenteric arteries proves negative.

Provocation angiography

The site of haemorrhage can be elusive and evade detection despite good quality angiography and

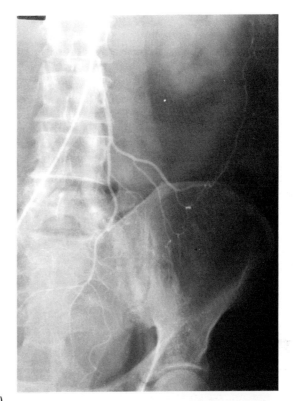

(a)

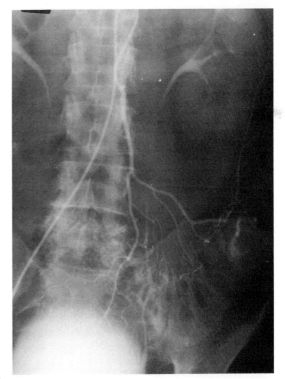

(b)

Figure 1   A 52-year-old man had had five large rectal bleeds in the previous 2 years, and a further bleed 24 h before angiography. (a) Initial angiography was normal. (b) Extravasation into sigmoid colon occurred after papaverine, 20 mg, and streptokinase, 5000 units for 4 h. Surgical resection then showed that the pathology was a bleeding diverticulum

radionuclide studies. The reasons are not clear, but intermittent vascular shutdown ('spasm') and clot formation when the systemic blood pressure is low contribute to negative angiographic findings.

Provocation angiography may be indicated. It is only performed with the full consent of the patient and his clinician. It is indicated in patients who have had repeated colonic bleeds requiring hospitalization and resuscitation and negative angiography, often on a number of occasions. It also may be indicated in those patients who require long-term anticoagulation, but who suffer repeated gastrointestinal bleeds without an identified cause.

The catheter is left in the artery that is thought to be the most likely supply vessel, i.e. inferior mesenteric or ileocolic vessel. A vasodilator is injected (papaverine, 20–30 mg or isosorbide dinitrate, 1–2 mg) and angiography is repeated. If this does not precipitate extravasation from the bleeding site, streptokinase, 5000 units/h for 4 h or tissue plasminogen activator, 0.5 mg/h is infused for 4–6 h and angiography is again repeated (*see Figure 1a and b*).

It must be emphasized that this procedure is only done with the full consent of the patient and full knowledge of a surgeon who may be required to perform emergency surgery if the resultant bleed cannot be controlled with vasopressin or embolization.

It is not effective or indicated in patients with chronic gastrointestinal bleeding or those that have not had an acute bleed in the previous 2–3 days.

EMBOLIZATION AND VASOPRESSIN

Vasopressin infusion is an effective method of controlling haemorrhage. It is not necessary to position the catheter highly selectively but it is left in the main trunk of the superior or inferior mesenteric artery. It is occasionally necessary to site the catheter in an aberrant middle colic artery which arises from the coeliac axis. It has been necessary to achieve more selective positioning in a few cases of postsurgical blood loss in the middle small intestine (anastomotic bleed) to achieve vasospasm.

Vasopressin, 100 units, is mixed with 500 ml of saline, (0.2 units/ml final strength) and then delivered at a rate of 30–60 ml/h. Angiography is repeated after 20 min, and if extravasation is still present the infusion rate is doubled to 60–120 ml/h or the concentration is doubled to 0.4 units/ml. If extravasation is still present after 20–30 min an alternative therapy should be undertaken. Further dose increases are unlikely to be of benefit. The infusion is continued for 24 h if good vasoconstriction is achieved.

Abdominal cramp is a sign of effective vasoconstriction, as vasopressin precipitates intestinal wall contraction which should subside after 20–30 min. If persistent, it is evidence of excessive vasoconstriction and the rate of infusion should be reduced.

The side effects of vasopressin are varied, but may be severe, particularly if manifest in the cardiovascular system (arrhythmias, severe hypertension, ischaemia of the legs). Development of intestinal ischaemia is rare, but recorded. Cerebral oedema may develop secondary to low serum sodium levels and all patients should remain on full monitoring and have regular electrolyte checks to avoid hyponatraemia. Local catheter complications (sepsis and haematoma) may also occur.

Transcatheter embolization of the intestine has been slow to be accepted because of the risks of resultant ischaemia. It is now, however, a real alternative, as the catheters can be removed and a long-term arterial infusion is avoided, thus minimizing patient discomfort. A definite end-point is also attained. It is a safe technique in the branches of the coeliac artery, but it is prudent for the catheter tip to be in a superselective situation.

There is evidence that selective embolization of the bleeding point in the intestine is a feasible therapy. It should only be performed when the catheter is superselective, which usually requires a coaxial system. Gelatin sponge plugs are used, though a single mini-coil may also be effective.

The incidence of symptomatic ischaemia is only 15% in published series, and fewer than 10% have required surgical intervention. Embolization may facilitate resuscitation of the patient and allow elective surgery to be undertaken. It can also be indicated in the patient in whom surgery is not feasible because of concomitant disease in other systems, for example severe cardiac or lung disease or irreversible clotting defects.

Acute haemorrhage (*Figure 2a–d*)

Acute haemorrhage at the site of a surgical anastomosis is effectively controlled by vasopressin. Severe blood loss from ischaemic colitis is also well controlled by vasopressin, but embolization is contraindicated.

The widespread use of sclerotherapy to control oesophageal varices has led to diversion of the portal venous blood to the superior and inferior mesenteric veins, and varices develop along postsurgical adhesions between intestine and parietes. They may present with lower gastrointestinal haemorrhage and can be controlled by vasopressin before surgical therapy or transhepatic portal vein embolization.

Angiodysplasia requires surgical resection, but acute blood loss can be controlled by vasopressin or embolization.

Tumours seldom present with acute blood loss and are normally diagnosed by other methods, but a small carcinoma in the caecum may be confused with angiodysplasia and may be overlooked at barium radiology or colonoscopy.

Vascular–enteric fistulae must always be considered when haemorrhage is severe particularly when a vascular graft is present. Colonic haemorrhage may

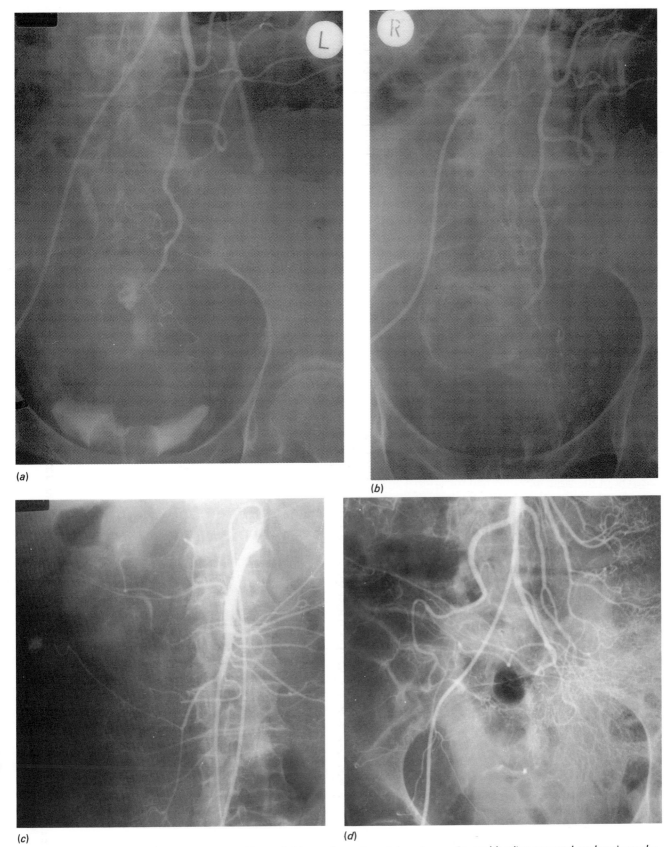

(a)

(b)

(c)

(d)

Figure 2   (a, b) In a woman aged 62 years, sigmoidoscopic biopsy showed a rectal carcinoma. Severe bleeding occurred, and angiography showed transection of the superior rectal artery. This was embolized with a surgical gelatin sponge plug and bleeding ceased. (c) In a man aged 72 years, injection of the superior mesenteric artery produced extravasation from a branch of the ileocolic artery, due to a bleeding diverticulum. (d) A woman aged 74 years suffered severe rectal bleeding. Injection of the superior mesenteric artery produced extravasation into the pelvic caecum. Surgical resection showed Dieulafoy's disease.

result if the iliac limb of a vascular graft erodes into the sigmoid or descending colon.

Haemorrhage after biopsy or polypectomy is usually simply managed by selective embolization.

Diverticular haemorrhage is usually more severe from the right colon than from the left and can be controlled with vasopressin, but embolization is quicker as a prelude to elective surgical resection.

Irresectable arteriovenous malformations of the rectum can be managed with repeated embolization.

Chronic colonic blood loss

Angiography is indicated in patients who have persistent anaemia with positive occult blood testing, and in whom other methods of investigation have failed to uncover the source of blood loss.

The three major intestinal vessels are examined as described in the previous section, but extravasation of contrast medium into the intestinal lumen will not be seen, the lesions being localized by their abnormal vascular pattern.

Leiomyomas and leiomyosarcomas are well defined, hypervascular and contain irregular tumour vessels. Carcinoids show a characteristic stellate distribution of the central vessels or may distort the root of the mesentery by an associated desmoplastic reaction.

Arteriovenous malformations may demonstrate large dilated tortuous feeding vessels, but these may be undetectable without good-quality venous phase films. A venous arteriovenous malformation can involve a long segment of the large intestine, and the arterial anatomy may be normal. The large number of tortuous, irregularly draining veins opacify poorly (up to 40 s after injection) and may fill after the normal venous drainage has cleared.

Angiodysplasia is regarded as an acquired condition and is predominantly seen in patients over 60 years old. The demonstration of early opacification of a draining vein alerts the angiographer to examine the antimesenteric border of that segment of intestine. Clusters of small arteries may be visible, but if very small an arterial abnormality may not always be detected. Most are detected in the right colon opposite the ileocaecal valve, but they may be found throughout both large and small intestine.

If angiography demonstrates an arteriovenous malformation or angiodysplastic lesion in the small intestine preoperative selective catheterization is indicated. Methylene blue, 1–2 ml, is injected through the catheter in the operating theatre to identify the appropriate small intestine segment. The specimen must be left intact and the artery injected to enable the pathologist to take sections of the appropriate area. A small angiodysplastic lesion or arteriovenous malformation will be missed if a strict protocol is not observed.

Meckel's diverticulum may be diagnosed by angiography if it is either distended with blood or associated with an elongated and straightened distal ileal branch of the superior mesenteric artery.

Carcinomas of the caecum, if small, may closely mimic the angiographic appearances of angiodysplasia, and the tumour vessels can be overlooked. Colonoscopic evaluation is advised in all patients, and angiodysplasia may be successfully treated with electrocoagulation or laser therapy at the same session.

EMBOLIZATION AND CYTOTOXIC THERAPY FOR HEPATIC METASTASES

The results of conventional treatment of hepatic metastases are poor; the response rate to 5-fluorouracil, for example, is less than 20%. A number of adjunctive therapies have been developed, including percutaneous injection of 70% alcohol, intermittent ischaemia and injection of radioactive agents. Embolization or chemoembolization employing simultaneous cytotoxic drugs and particulate agents is being assessed.

Although there is a dual blood supply to the liver (portal vein, 75%; hepatic artery, 25%), liver tumours are predominantly supplied by the hepatic artery, which is accessible to percutaneous catheterization.

Iodized oil fluid injection angiography (*Figure 3a* and *b*)

Iodized oil fluid injection angiography has rendered smaller tumours visible, particularly if vascular, and is indicated if metastases have been identified in one liver lobe and resection is being considered. The technique involves direct infusion of 6–8 ml of iodized oil fluid (Lipiodol) into the main hepatic artery (peripheral to the gastroduodenal) with follow-up CT scan after 14 days. The iodized fluid oil is cleared from the liver parenchyma by the reticuloendothelial system, but persists in the abnormal circulation around the tumour where lymphatics are absent. It will demonstrate tumours of 2–3 mm in diameter. The effectiveness of cytotoxic agents depends on the degree of extraction and the level of concentration within the liver. It is attractive to assist the cytotoxic contact time by direct arterial injection attached to iodized oil fluid.

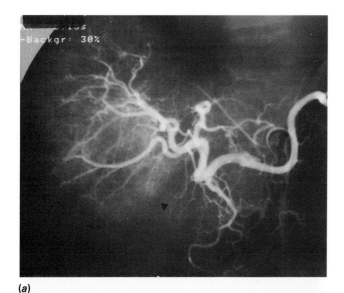

(a)

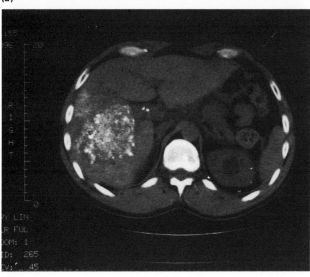

(b)

Figure 3   Iodized oil fluid injection angiography. (a) Coeliac axis injection shows a large vascular tumour in the right lobe of the liver (arrowed). (b) An injection of 6 ml into the hepatic artery followed by a CT scan after 10 days shows residual iodized oil fluid in the tumour in the right lobe, but the left lobe is clear of other metastases

Tumour embolization (Figure 4a–d)

The role of concurrent embolization is uncertain, but much evidence suggests that devascularization and consequent anoxia is an effective method to induce tumour necrosis. In the experience of the author, the more vascular the tumour, the greater the response to particulate embolization.

There is much uncertainty and dispute as to whether chemotherapy should be combined with particulate embolization. It is the author's practice to perform particulate embolization in all patients who undergo chemotherapeutic infusion of metastases. This is followed by repeat angiography, chemotherapy and further embolization each month for 3 months. A vascular tumour is embolized with permanent particulate material and steel coils, and follow-up angiography is devoted to embolization of recanalized and collateral vessels inclusive of the extrahepatic supply, such as the lumbar or intercostal, inferior phrenic or right colic vessels.

No patient who is motivated to undergo treatment should be excluded, but caution should be exercised if the portal vein is thrombosed. It is the author's policy not to proceed to particulate embolization of both right and left lobes if the portal vein is thrombosed, but single-lobe embolization has been undertaken without detectable complication.

An intravenous line must be in place before the procedure to facilitate administration of sedatives, antibiotics and analgesics as required. The procedure is covered by antibiotics for 5 days, which has reduced the incidence of hepatic abscess and sepsis to 2%.

Coeliac and superior mesenteric angiography are performed to evaluate the blood supply of the liver and establish the patency of the portal vein. Common anatomical variants include the right hepatic artery arising from the superior mesenteric artery (25%) and the left hepatic artery arising from the left gastric artery (5%).

A coaxial system of catheterization (2.2-Fr within 5 Fr) may be required, but it is usual to attain superselective positioning of the 5 Fr catheter using available guidewires. A small number of procedures require a brachial approach if a large liver distorts the angle of the origin of the coeliac artery.

The most effective form of chemoembolization is under assessment at different centres. It is possible to repeat percutaneous chemotherapy and therefore administer regular doses, usually on a monthly regimen. Iodized oil fluid is now given in the same syringe, which aids retention in the liver and around the tumour mass.

The author's regimen is a monthly treatment for 3 months. CT is carried out before embolization, at 3 months, 6 months and at 1 year. Repeat chemoembolization is performed at 6 months, at 1 year, 6-monthly to 3 years and then annually.

Absolute alcohol (70%), 2 ml, iodized oil fluid, 8 ml, and mitomycin C, 20 mg, are infused, followed by gelatin sponge powder. Polyvinyl alcohol replaces gelatin sponge at the third treatment. Starch microspheres of mitomycin, cisplatin, doxorubicin hydrochloride and 5-fluorouracil may be considered as alternative agents.

The assessment of the response may be difficult. Decrease in the size of the liver on palpation (75 cm), decrease of the tumour size on CT (50%), or decrease in serum carcinoembryonic antigen are commonly measured parameters.

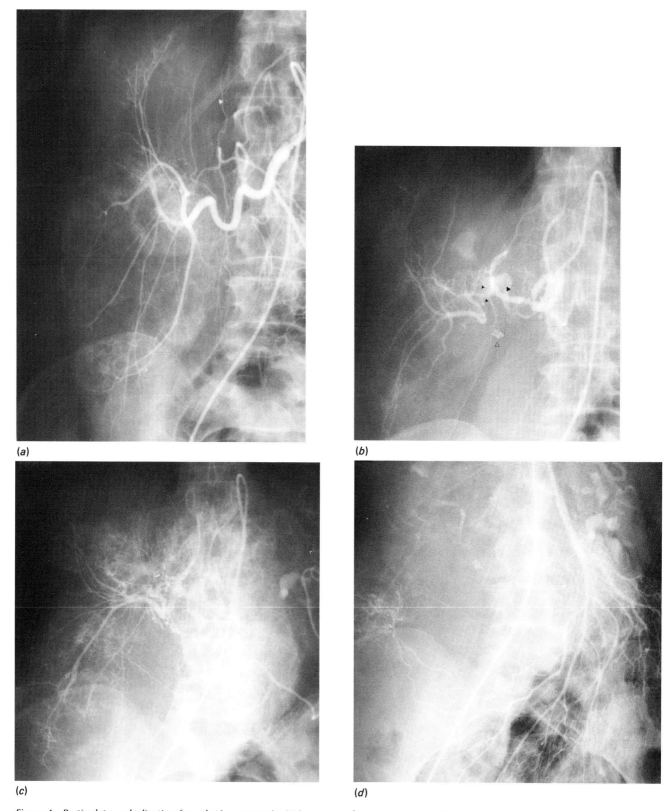

Figure 4   Particulate embolization for colonic metastasis. (a) Large vascular metastasis in right lobe; (b) 4 years after initial embolization, injection into the left hepatic artery (large arrowhead) shows cross-circulation into the right hepatic artery (small arrowheads). Note the residual tumour is much smaller but still perfused and the coil (open arrowhead) in the obstructed right hepatic artery stem; (c) and (d) the same, 4 years later. Multiple vascular metastases appear in the left lobe with enlargement of the original tumour. Injection of the superior mesenteric artery shows collateral supply from the right colic artery to the original tumour mass

Results

Comparison of the diameter of the mass underestimates the response, as there is a delay of 2–4 months before necrotic tumour is resorbed and metabolized. Clinical benefit may be evident without objective confirmation.

Assessment of the true benefit of chemoembolization for colonic metastases is not possible, as there are no controlled clinical trials. In the author's personal experience, particulate embolization with mitomycin and iodized oil fluid has a response rate greater than 50%, with clinical benefit in more than 70% of patients. The response is related to the vascularity of the tumour on angiography (the greater the vascularity the better the response to particulate embolization), the histological grade of the primary tumour and the time of diagnosis of metastases after the original surgical resection.

Percutaneous tumour injection of alcohol

Ultrasound-guided percutaneous injection of alcohol can be used as adjunctive therapy. It is indicated for metastases that are small in number (up to five) and small in diameter (2 cm), but may be used if a single tumour is large (4 cm). The volume of absolute alcohol injected is related to tumour size.

Early follow-up and assessment of response has been promising.

PERCUTANEOUS BIOPSY AND ABSCESS DRAINAGE

Percutaneous abscess drainage is now standard therapy, and laparotomy is very seldom performed.

Ultrasonic guidance is quick and effective, but occasionally lack of a 'window' due to overlying gas indicates other forms of imaging. It is important that the relevant images, whether fluoroscopic, ultrasonographic or computed tomographic are correlated before drainage is undertaken to avoid drainage of a necrotic tumour or asymptomatic haematoma.

Indications and imaging

It is not necessary to arrange for a surgical team to be on stand-by. An abscess can be drained even if there is enteric communication, if it is multilocular, or it is shielded by overlying structures.

It may be prudent to aspirate with a fine needle (22 Fr) and perform a Gram stain or cytology in a doubtful mass lesion before embarking on dilatation of a tract into the abscess cavity.

It may be necessary to insert more than one drainage tube in a large multilocular cavity or when the septa cannot be broken down by a catheter and wire combination.

Drainage is performed in the ultrasound suite and fluoroscopy is seldom required. If the cavity cannot be clearly visualized, it may be necessary to move the patient to the CT scanner and identify a suitable tract. Fluoroscopy is used at follow-up tubography to establish the presence (or absence) of an internal communication and to document healing of the cavity.

Percutaneous drainage is now routine for hepatic and renal retroperitoneal collections and peritoneal abscesses in subhepatic, subphrenic and paracolic spaces (see Figure 5a–c). The lesser sac and deep pelvic spaces (paravesicular and pararectal fossae) may require a CT scan as a diagnostic method to plan the safest and most suitable route of approach.

Technique and equipment

Several systems are used, and the choice is usually made on personal preference. The safest method is to guide a fine needle (20 Fr) into the cavity and insert a 0.18-inch diameter flexible-tip guidewire with a stiff shaft. The tract can then be dilated to 5 Fr with an angled dilator with an end hole and an additional side hole through which a larger diameter J-tip guidewire (0.35 inch) exits. The tract is then dilated to the required diameter before introduction of the drainage catheter.

'Pigtail' catheters, 8.5 Fr in diameter, are large enough to drain fluid collections and cysts, but thick pus, necrotic pancreatic abscesses and empyemas will require 14-Fr catheters with large side ports. Very occasionally, 20 Fr may be required. It is wise to utilize pigtail catheters with a locking device, usually a suture that fixes the pigtail into a loop in addition to skin sutures.

The cavity is irrigated and aspirated with saline at a low pressure to avoid sepsis. The radiologist should see the patient daily, and follow-up tubography under fluoroscopy is arranged for 48 h later. The tube is removed when the radiological criteria of closure of cavity and the clinical criteria of a normal leucocyte count, normalization of temperature and no drainage are met. The tube is only removed after discussion with the clinicians concerned. A simple abscess seldom requires drainage for more than 7 days.

Pericolic abscess drainage

Drainage of abscesses associated with local perforation of the colon, such as periappendicular or peridiverticular abscesses, or those associated with Crohn's disease, do not require percutaneous drainage if it is preferable to remove the abscess and the abnormal colonic segment at one surgical procedure. Drainage of a diverticular abscess, however, may permit a single elective surgical resection and anastomosis instead of a two-stage surgical procedure. Furthermore there is debate as to whether the appendix requires removal

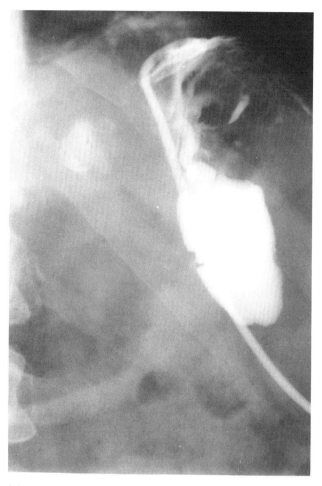

(a)

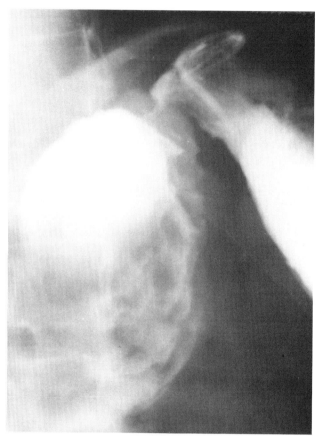

(b)

after drainage of an appendicular abscess and Crohn's disease abscesses may be drained without resort to surgical resection if no enteric communication is present.

Pericolic abscesses are best drained under CT guidance as they are intimately related to the intestine. In the pelvis drainage may be achieved by direct rectal or vaginal puncture and tract dilatation using the same techniques if imaging demonstrates intimate contact.

Diverticular and appendiceal abscesses often require a longer period of drainage (2 weeks) if an enteric connection is present. Successful drainage and closure of fistulae is achieved in more than 90% of cases.

Haematomas may be simply aspirated, but if they contain clot and fibrous tissue they may not drain. No haematoma should be formally drained unless it is painful or is causing obstruction, to avoid introduction of secondary infection.

DILATATION OF STRICTURES

Benign anastomotic strictures of the rectum and sigmoid colon are easy to catheterize using 'arterial'

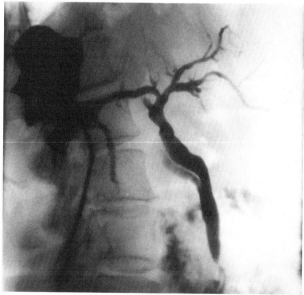

(c)

Figure 5   (a) Drainage of an abscess with enteric connections. (b) Drainage of a left subphrenic abscess after a perforated sigmoid diverticulum, showing communication with the gastric fundus. Spontaneous closure occurred after 4 weeks of catheter drainage. (c) Drainage of a hepatic abscess (secondary to diverticulitis). Spontaneous rupture to right bile duct occurred. Spontaneous closure occurred after 3.5 weeks of catheter drainage

techniques and equipment. More proximal strictures are best approached by colonoscopy.

Dilatation of these strictures is possible with balloon catheters that inflate to 2–3 cm in diameter. Prolonged expansion is required, but the inflation pressure is usually insufficient to eliminate the narrowed segment. It is a procedure that is at best temporary and the symptoms and the stricture usually recur within 1 month. Repeated dilatations may be undertaken.

PERCUTANEOUS CAECOSTOMY (*Figure 6a–c*)

Obstruction of the colon is treated by surgical means, but percutaneous caecostomy may be indicated in those patients who are unfit for anaesthesia or in the frail, elderly patient with pseudo-obstruction.

The technique is identical to that for drainage of an abscess. Percutaneous enteric drainage kits are available for introduction of gastrostomy tubes, but these are not normally required for drainage of a large dilated caecum.

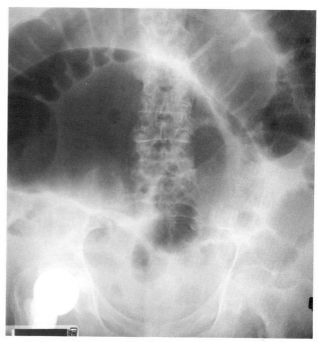

(a)

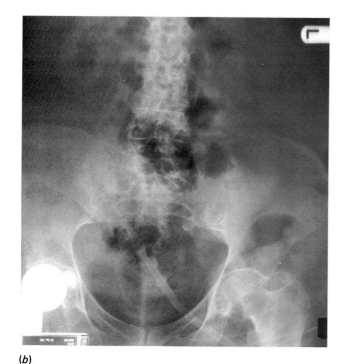

(b)

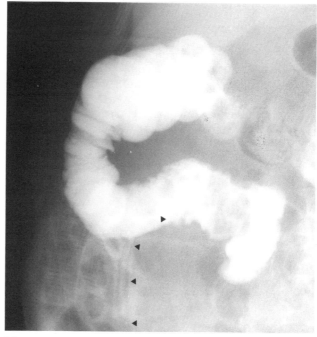

(c)

Figure 6   A women aged 91 years suffered repeated episodes of pseudo-obstruction of the sigmoid colon. (a) Gross dilatation of the caecum and colon to the sigmoid colon region. (b) At 24 h after percutaneous caecostomy, resolution of the dilated colon was demonstrated. (c) Injection of contrast through a balloon catheter 24 h after insertion. (With acknowledgement to Dr L Murthy, Freeman Hospital).

Illustrations by Gillian Lee

Operating on the immunosuppressed colorectal patient

Timothy I. Davidson ChM, MRCP, FRCS
Lecturer in Surgery, Westminster Hospital, London, UK

Timothy G. Allen-Mersh MD, FRCS
Consultant Surgeon, Westminster Hospital, London, UK

Patients with suppressed cell-mediated immunity are susceptible to opportunistic infections and atypical malignancies. Once the T4 lymphocyte count (normally $>500/mm^3$) falls below $200/mm^3$ viral, fungal, protozoal or bacterial infection is likely. With the advent of the acquired immune deficiency syndrome (AIDS), surgeons dealing with colorectal disorders in immunosuppressed patients will, in the main, be treating patients with AIDS. Surgical practice in these patients requires additional precautions to protect the surgeon and operating staff, additional measures to protect the immunosuppressed patient, an awareness of AIDS-related colonic problems which may require abdominal surgery and a knowledge of AIDS-related anorectal surgical conditions.

Additional measures to protect staff

Preoperative screening

The preoperative identification of patients with human immunodeficiency virus (HIV) disease remains controversial and routine preoperative testing for HIV has not yet become practice in the UK or USA. Patients known to be HIV positive and those in high-risk categories require treatment with additional precautions during surgery. However, a negative HIV antibody test does not exclude the possibility that a patient has been infected after the test was performed, nor that a patient may have CDC stage 1 infection (HIV-antigen positive but not yet HIV-antibody positive) at the time of testing. Because of these difficulties the Centers for Disease Control (CDC) have advocated exercising *universal precautions* for all patients whether or not they have known risk factors, are HIV positive or have AIDS[1]. These have been adopted as standard practice in centres with a high prevalence of HIV but in most surgical units they are not considered practical or financially viable.

Extent of risk

Available data indicate that the risk to the clinician following exposure to HIV is small. The estimated risk of seroconversion following a single needlestick or sharps injury whilst operating on an HIV-positive patient is 1 in 275 or roughly 0.4%[2] (the risk of transmission of hepatitis B via the same route is 20 times greater). Mucous membrane exposure has very rarely been implicated in occupational exposure and it is unlikely that HIV can be transmitted via intact skin. There is no evidence for spread of HIV via faecal–oral or droplet inhalation. Special precautions are considered unnecessary when dealing with faeces, sweat or urine, but are recommended when dealing with peritoneal, pleural or pericardial fluid, semen, vaginal secretions or any fluid containing visible blood.

Precautions in the operating room

For their own protection operating room staff must be informed that a patient with known or suspected HIV is an 'inoculation risk' patient and the operating list should be annotated accordingly. HIV-infected patients need not be scheduled to undergo surgery in separate operating rooms nor at the end of the operating schedule[3]. Procedures on HIV-infected patients should be performed by fully trained medical and nursing staff since medical students and trainee nurses are more vulnerable to sharps injuries and should not assist. Staff with abrasions on their hands should likewise not assist. Staff should be immunized against hepatitis B.

Protective clothing

Disposable gowns with plasticized fluid-resistant reinforcement of sleeves and anterior body areas are recommended. Blood soak-through means that conventional linen gowns do not provide an adequate barrier to the patient's blood. Plastic aprons should be worn under gowns. Rubber boots offer better protection than clogs against blood spillage and fenestrated footwear should not be worn because of the risk from a falling sharp instrument. Eye protection is necessary and operating staff should wear a visor, safety glasses or goggles. Eye protection must be disposable or must be cleaned and disinfected after use.

Intact surgical gloves provide an adequate mechanical barrier to HIV[4]. Wearing a double layer of gloves has been adopted in many centres to reduce the incidence of hand contamination. Double-gloving does not reduce the incidence of needlestick injuries but does reduce skin exposure through inadvertent glove perforation. As soon as a perforation of one or both layers is recognized, the surgeon should change gloves.

Surgical technique

1 While operating, attention must be given at all times to the handling and disposal of sharp instruments and operative techniques should be modified. Sharp instruments (such as scalpel or mounted needle) should *not* be passed from hand to hand but placed into and retrieved from a dish. A 'no touch' technique should be used and tissues should be supported with forceps (not fingers) when placing sutures. Hand-held needles should not be used and when tying sutures by hand the needle should first be removed. Transmission of HIV via aerosol or smoke inhalation during the use of cautery or laser diathermy has not been recorded but an efficient smoke evacuator should be used to scavenge aerosol or smoke into a filtration system.

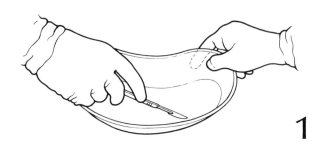

1

Precautions on completion of surgery

At the end of the procedure the patient drapes, surgeons' gowns, overshoes, gloves and safety glasses, masks and visors are collected for disposal in sealed bags as the staff leave the operating room. Instruments are cleaned in soap and water and then placed in a clearly marked autoclavable bag. Blood and body fluid spillages on the operating table or floor are cleaned with sodium hypochlorite (bleach) or sodium dichloroisocyanurate in concentrations of 10 000 p.p.m. available chlorine. Immersion of biopsy specimens in formaldehyde or formol saline rapidly inactivates HIV. Unfixed tissues should be handled with the same precautions as blood and the pathology department informed before unfixed tissue is dispatched.

Procedures following exposure to HIV

In the event of exposure to blood or body fluids from a patient with HIV, the degree of risk should first be assessed.

With *low-risk exposure* (mucous membrane or skin splash onto unbroken skin) no specific treatment is advised apart from standard irrigation.

Following *high-risk exposure* (deep or intramuscular sharps injury, hollow needlestick injury, or inadvertent injection of the patient's blood) immediate prophylactic zidovudine (AZT) should be considered in a dose of 1 g orally without delay followed by 200 mg orally every 4–6 h for 4 weeks[5,6]. Zidovudine carries dose-related side effects and its long-term toxicity is not known. Seroconversion has been documented despite zidovudine prophylaxis and the drug is unlikely to be of benefit if there is a delay of more than 6 h in starting therapy.

For the exposed clinician the personal and professional implications of undergoing subsequent HIV testing must be addressed. An initial negative HIV test followed by documented seroconversion within 3 months of exposure would indicate occupationally acquired HIV.

Additional measures to protect the patient

Major surgery and general anaesthesia in immuno-competent patients are associated with transient depression of cell-mediated immunity, which does not affect outcome. Data on the long-term immunological response of patients with AIDS or other forms of immunosuppression to surgery are not available; however, there has been concern that surgical intervention may accelerate the progression of AIDS[7], giving further reason to avoid unnecessary surgery or anaesthesia in these patients.

Immunosuppressed patients undergoing colorectal surgery should be given systemic antibiotic prophylaxis at induction of anaesthesia to prevent bacteraemic complications. The antibacterial spectrum should cover anaerobic and Gram-negative organisms. Fibreoptic endoscopes should be immersed for 1 h in glutaraldehyde 2% before use to reduce the chance of transmission of opportunistic organisms such as *Mycobacterium tuberculosis*, atypical mycobacteria or cryptosporidia[8].

Impairment of wound healing after anorectal surgery[9] and following laparotomy in patients with AIDS has been reported. Patients with AIDS-related immune thrombocytopenia may require perioperative platelet cover or steroid therapy.

Pneumocystis carinii and cytomegalovirus (CMV) pneumonia may be present in AIDS patients undergoing colorectal surgery and consideration must be given to reducing respiratory complications (for example the use of total intravenous anaesthesia with propofol). Patients may be wasted and experience discomfort during lengthy procedures without general anaesthesia. Special attention must be given to pressure areas. Finally, care must be taken with regard to the psychological needs of these, mainly young, patients with a fatal disease in whom colorectal surgery may, at best, achieve only temporary palliation.

AIDS-related colonic problems requiring abdominal surgery

Although one in eight patients with AIDS experiences abdominal pain, the majority of these are managed conservatively and only 5% of patients with pain require surgery. The causes of the acute abdomen are different from those in immunocompetent patients and most are AIDS-related. The most common disease process among AIDS patients undergoing emergency laparotomy is acute CMV colitis[10].

CMV toxic megacolon

The development of CMV toxic megacolon or colonic perforation may necessitate surgical intervention. Clinical diagnosis is based on increasing abdominal pain, distension, peritonism and general toxaemia. Radiological features are similar to those of megacolon in ulcerative colitis. CMV usually causes a pancolitis with extensive mucosal ulceration and the treatment is total colectomy with formation of ileostomy and rectal mucous fistula. With more limited ileocolitis right hemicolectomy may be appropriate.

Colectomy for CMV toxic megacolon may restore the patient with AIDS to a period of relatively good health with weight gain and improved haemoglobin and T4 lymphocyte levels. Worthwhile palliation may be achieved, and the patient may survive for more than 6 months; some patients have been well enough to undergo ileorectal anastomosis several months later[11].

A small number of patients present as CMV toxic megacolon, but histology of the resected colon shows features of Crohn's colitis or ulcerative colitis in addition to CMV, and the role of CMV as a cofactor is unclear. Colonization of the gut by CMV is present in almost all HIV-positive homosexuals and CMV colitis may occur despite anti-CMV therapy. Multiple opportunistic organisms, including salmonella, cryptosporidia, mycobacteria and herpes virus, are commonly isolated.

Other AIDS-related conditions

AIDS patients with non-Hodgkin's B cell lymphoma of the intestine may present with intestinal obstruction or perforation. The most common site of involvement is the ileum but colonic lymphoma, usually of the right colon, or multifocal lesions have been reported. Intestinal resection may achieve macroscopic clearance but lymphoma in these immunosuppressed patients often runs an aggressive course, with death within 3 months of laparotomy. Other conditions encountered at emergency laparotomy are appendicitis (with CMV a causative agent in some) and infection with *Mycobacterium avium-intracellulare* (MAI) causing enlargement of intra-abdominal nodes, liver and spleen (*see Figure 1*).

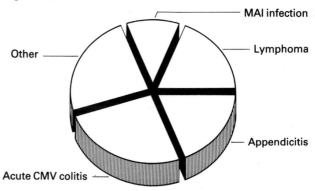

Figure 1

When abdominal pain occurs in the presence of an intra-abdominal mass (lymphoma, MAI) every effort should be made to avoid laparotomy by establishing the diagnosis with needle biopsy guided by computed tomography scan or by ultrasound. However, the AIDS patient with clinical and radiological evidence of toxic megacolon, bowel perforation or peritonitis should be offered laparotomy. With antibiotic cover, correction of bleeding disorders, and parenteral nutritional support, patients with AIDS may survive major abdominal surgery despite the presence of sepsis or toxaemia.

Colonic problems in other immunosuppressed groups

CMV colitis and toxic megacolon do occur in other groups of immunosuppressed patients (e.g. renal, cardiac and hepatic transplant recipients) with T4 cell counts $<50/mm^3$. In patients with aplastic anaemia or acute leukaemia undergoing high-dose chemotherapy, *neutropenic colitis*, or typhlitis, which primarily involves the caecum, may present with bloody diarrhoea, increasing toxaemia, abdominal distension and tenderness localizing to the right lower quadrant. This should be managed with bowel rest, nasogastric suction, systemic broad-spectrum antibiotics and parenteral nutrition. Overt perforation, massive haemorrhage or abscess formation require surgical intervention, usually by right hemicolectomy, ileostomy and mucous fistula, taking care to remove all necrotic tissue.

AIDS-related anorectal disease

Patients who are immunosuppressed by HIV develop an atypical spectrum of anorectal disease compared with the non-HIV population (where haemorrhoids and anal fissure predominate). The incidence of anorectal disease in HIV-positive homosexual males is over ten times greater than that in the general adult population and is the most common reason for surgical referral[12]. The most frequently encountered conditions are anal warts, anorectal ulceration, perianal sepsis and neoplasia. The large excess of anorectal disease is best explained by the combination of homosexual behaviour (anoreceptive intercourse) with immunodeficiency (*see Figure 2*).

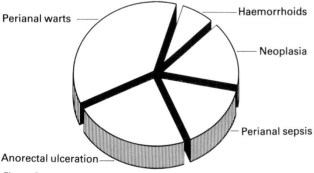

Figure 2

Anal and perianal warts

Perianal warts can be treated with podophyllin or, if extensive or involving the anal canal, by excision. Healing is slower and in over half the patients follow-up examination at 1 month reveals the need for re-excision. Warts in the HIV-positive population tend to be more dysplastic and aggressive than in HIV-negative patients and are often associated with human papillomavirus subtype 16. The association of squamous carcinoma *in situ* with warts underlines the need for histological examination of wart-bearing tissue and is an argument against treatment with podophyllin or electrocautery. Where dysplastic or *in situ* changes are identified, regular follow-up is advised but the additional workload of repeated anoscopy with aceto-white staining in these patients must be balanced against the overall poor prognosis from AIDS progression.

Anorectal ulceration

Ulceration may be confined to the rectum or the anal verge, or may be extensive and penetrating and involve both the anal canal and rectum. Swabs or biopsies may show CMV or herpes simplex virus (HSV), as well as cryptosporidia and other opportunistic organisms. Ulcers associated with HSV infection may respond to oral or topical acyclovir. The more chronic types of anal or anorectal ulcers are frequently adjacent to an oedematous skin tag. They appear more broad-based than a chronic anal fissure and are not restricted to the midline. Chronic anal ulceration is unlikely to respond to acyclovir but about half will heal after excision of the ulcer and skin tag.

Perianal sepsis

Perianal sepsis may be florid with multiple and complex perianal and submucous abscesses. Following laying open and drainage of the abscesses, healing is slower than in the normal population. Superficial fistulae may be laid open in the usual way but deep or high fistula tracks should be treated more conservatively, particularly in patients with advanced AIDS where healing is unlikely. Opportunistic infection with mycobacterial (e.g. MAI) or fungal organisms must be excluded. Histological examination is mandatory to exclude concomitant tumour such as Kaposi's sarcoma, non-Hodgkin's lymphoma or squamous carcinoma. Lymphoma in particular may present as perianal sepsis, with the diagnosis apparent only after histological examination of the abscess wall.

Neoplasia

Non-Hodgkin's lymphoma in the perianal region progresses rapidly and excisional surgery is unlikely to achieve tumour control. A defunctioning colostomy may be indicated for symptomatic palliation or to facilitate local radiotherapy. Kaposi's sarcoma seen on sigmoidoscopy is often asymptomatic and requires no treatment, but may present with rectal bleeding. The incidence of anorectal dysplasia, carcinoma *in situ* and squamous cell carcinoma of the anus is increased in immunosuppressed patients and human papillomavirus is considered a causative agent[13]. The value of screening HIV-positive patients by anoscopy to detect squamous cell carcinoma is unclear because the risk and interval of progression to invasive disease are unknown.

Haemorrhoids

Haemorrhoidal disease represents a relatively small proportion of anorectal complaints and injection sclerotherapy is as effective as in the immunocompetent patient. Haemorrhoids must be differentiated from Kaposi's sarcoma of the anal canal. Haemorrhoidectomy, anal stretching and lateral sphincterotomy are not preferred methods of treatment because of the tendency to diarrhoea, minor faecal incontinence and slow healing in immunocompromised patients[14].

Anorectal disease is the most common reason for surgical referral of HIV-positive patients and the surgeon must be aware of the opportunistic infections and neoplastic conditions that can arise. Careful examination under anaesthetic of the anal canal and rectum with biopsy of suspicious lesions is indicated in immunosuppressed patients with anorectal symptoms.

References

1. Centers for Disease Control. Guidelines for prevention of transmission of human immunodeficiency virus and hepatitis B virus to health care and public safety workers. *Morb Mortal Wkly Rep* 1989; 38: (Suppl. S6).

2. Cochrane JPS, Wastell C, eds. *The Impact of HIV on Surgical Practice.* London: Royal College of Surgeons, 1992.

3. Gazzard BG, Wastell C. HIV and surgeons. *BMJ* 1990; 301: 1003–4.

4. Dalgleish AG, Malkovsky M. Surgical gloves as a mechanical barrier against human immunodeficiency viruses. *Br J Surg* 1988; 75: 171–2.

5. United Kingdom Department of Health. *Guidance for Clinical Health Care Workers. Recommendations of the Expert Advisory Group on AIDS.* London: HMSO, 1990.

6. Centers for Disease Control. Public Health Service statement on management of occupational exposure to HIV, including considerations regarding zidovudine postexposure use. *Morb Mortal Wkly Rep* 1990; 39(RR-1): 1–14.

7. Konotey-Ahulu FID. Surgery and the risk of AIDS in HIV-positive patients. *Lancet* 1987; ii: 1146.

8. Working Party of the British Society of Gastroenterology. Cleaning and disinfection of equipment for gastrointestinal flexible endoscopy: interim recommendations. *Gut* 1988; 29: 1134–51.

9. Wexner SD, Smithy WB, Milsom JW, Dailey TH. The surgical management of anorectal disease in AIDS and pre-AIDS patients. *Dis Colon Rectum* 1986; 29: 719–23.

10. Wexner SD, Smithy WB, Trillo C, Hopkins BS, Dailey TH. Emergency colectomy for cytomegalovirus ileocolitis in patients with the acquired immune deficiency syndrome. *Dis Colon Rectum* 1988; 31: 755–61.

11. Davidson T, Allen-Mersh TG, Miles AJG et al. Emergency laparotomy in patients with AIDS. *Br J Surg* 1991; 78: 924–6.

12. Miles AJG, Mellor CH, Gazzard B, Allen-Mersh TG, Wastell C. Surgical management of anorectal disease in HIV-positive homosexuals. *Br J Surg* 1990; 77: 869–71.

13. Frazer IH, Medley B, Crapper RM, Brown TC, Mackay IR. Association between anorectal dysplasia, human papillomavirus and human immunodeficiency virus infection in homosexual men. *Lancet* 1986; ii: 657–60.

14. Gottesman LG, Miles AJ, Milsom JW, Northover JM, Schecter WP, Stotter A. The management of anorectal disease in HIV-positive patients (clinical conference). *Int J Colorectal Dis* 1990; 5: 61–72.

Endoscopy and laparoscopic techniques: introductory comment

L. P. Fielding MB, FRCS, FACS

Chief of Surgery, St Mary's Hospital, Waterbury, Connecticut and Clinical Professor of Surgery, Yale University School of Medicine, New Haven, Connecticut, USA and Visiting Clinical Scientist, St Mary's Hospital, London, UK

Investigative endoscopy and minimally invasive therapeutic endoscopic surgery are the most rapidly developing subjects in abdominal surgery. This rate of change and development is likely to continue throughout the 1990s and is the reason for bringing these chapters together into a single section of this operative text.

Improved light sources in the 1950s, the discovery and exploitation of flexible fibreoptics in the 1960s, the consolidation of electronic circuits in the 1970s, and the eventual miniaturization of the television camera in the 1980s, form the backdrop and have been the prerequisites for this very rapid expansion in surgical technology.

Techniques

This section starts with the traditional approach to the investigative methods of the gut with proctosigmoidoscopy and colonoscopy. These basic techniques are no less important because of the newness and 'glamour' of endoscopic surgery. Care in bowel preparation, gentleness of technique and avoidance of complications are essential ingredients for these procedures. The idea that intraoperative endoluminal endoscopy may be of help in some operations where the abdomen is either 'open' or 'closed' is another powerful argument in favour of specialised abdominal (colorectal) surgeons being capable of carrying out their own investigative endoscopy.

Lasers

Although lasers are in quite wide clinical use in the USA, the cost of the machines as well as the fibres and 'scalpel' tips have prevented their more widespread use.

The application of lasers in colorectal surgery has been relatively slow to develop because the laser beam has been used largely to replace the scalpel or the electrocautery machine. Very few randomized studies have been carried out comparing these techniques, and relatively unimpressive differences in favour of lasers have been observed. However, these results have as much to do with the methods of assessment of the outcome as with the relative lack of differences between traditional and laser techniques.

It is clear that, from the biological point of view, lasers can provide a more precise localization of tissue injury than electrocautery and, when used as a scalpel, laser energy is useful in preventing haemorrhage and tissue exudation. It is likely, therefore, that improvement in laser systems will continue, but at a relatively slow pace when compared with endoscopic procedures.

The role of laser energy as a modality of choice in certain conditions has yet to be established. Nevertheless, the treatment of anal condyloma acuminata and irradiation proctitis and photodynamic therapy for certain tumours are certainly candidates. Carefully conducted trials will be necessary to explore these possibilities.

Training

In the rush to endorse new endoscopic (laparoscopic) operations, we must temper our enthusiasm with a few words of caution. First, we must accept the need to establish guidelines for technical training, particularly for those who are already established surgeons. If surgeons proceed to operate on patients with these new methods after having attended a lecture or watched a film on them, long learning curves will result with the inevitable associated complications and occasional unnecessary and tragic patient death. Like justice itself, we must not only 'do the right thing' but we must 'be seen to be doing the right thing', and hence the need for training guidelines.

The four components of training are: (1) a thorough theoretical background knowledge of the instrumentation, the equipment, and the solution of the more common functional problems; (2) practical experience in a laboratory environment where the feel of the new instruments and the hand–eye coordination through a video monitor can be obtained; (3) experience on tissue in a well-equipped animal facility; and (4) supervised clinical experience in humans.

As this subject develops, the need for animal experience will diminish for at least two reasons. First, with time, initial experience will occur in the normal development of surgical experience in training programmes. Secondly, the development of computer technology will give rise to virtual reality systems specifically designed to train surgeons in a simulated environment.

It is of some importance for the surgical colleges around the globe to assist in the development of this technology and to set standards of training and not merely to reserve the right to criticize and to regulate. The colleges have the influence to promote high levels of performance and to encourage the simplification of the systems to bring down the cost of this technology so that it can be used in both the developed and less developed parts of the world in a cost efficient manner.

Future directions

There is little doubt that within a few years of the publication of this text the instruments for endosurgical procedures will be quite different. Nevertheless, the editors were not dissuaded from the mission to discuss the current 'state of the art' in this rapidly developing

area. Perhaps we will look back in some years and recognize that the instruments for these procedures represented our first steps towards robotic surgery. Be that as it may, today's instruments function reasonably well. However, the smoothness of function, handgrip design, fingertip controls, combined or composite instruments, and instrument balance are all in a state of development. Electromechanical safety will improve, and the ability to view tissues in three dimensions to achieve depth perception will occur.

Surgeons who are interested in developing their skills after basic and advanced laboratory training should take every opportunity to treat patients who require exploratory laparotomy using laparoscopic techniques. In some of these patients the diagnosis will become apparent, and may prevent open laparotomy; in others the pathology might be treatable by the laparoscopic technique (e.g. appendicitis and some forms of acute cholecystitis). As experience is gathered, more advanced dissections can be undertaken with increased confidence. It is important for those surgeons developing their skills to recognize that, at first, the goals should be to add technical experience slowly and safely and not to push to complete the procedure endoscopically if difficulties arise. Indeed, the construction of an anastomosis extracorporeally through a small 5-cm incision should, at present, be considered to be the norm because it does not detract from the advantages of endoscopic bowel mobilization, but appears to be the safer procedure. Extracorporeal intestinal anastomosis is certainly quicker, more exact, and therefore safer than intracorporeal techniques at present.

The reader of a chapter in this section is advised to review all these chapters on minimally invasive endoscopic procedures at one sitting because there are some differences between the authors in terms of their technique and some chapters have more details in their descriptions than others. It is clear that it will be some time before we develop a consensus concerning the tricks of the trade in this rapidly expanding and exciting field of surgery.

Illustrations by Peter Cox

Proctoscopy and sigmoidoscopy

J. D. Hardcastle MA, MChir, FRCS, FRCP
Professor of Surgery, University Hospital, Queen's Medical Centre, Nottingham, UK

Principles and justification

Indications

Proctoscopy is used to inspect the region of the anorectal ring and anal canal. The diagnosis and treatment of haemorrhoids (injection or banding) and other minor anal problems can be carried out through a proctoscope of adequate size.

Sigmoidoscopy is part of the routine examination of patients complaining of symptoms suggestive of rectal or colonic disease. It is indicated in all patients with rectal bleeding or a change of bowel habit. It should be performed before barium enema examination. Flexible sigmoidoscopy may also be indicated to confirm any biopsy lesions seen on barium enema examination and in the follow-up of patients who have had previous rectal or left colonic resection for colorectal cancer. In patients with rectal bleeding over the age of 50 years, flexible sigmoidoscopy should be performed to exclude polypoid lesions in the distal colon.

Contraindications

Anal stenosis or an acute anal fissure rendering proctoscopy painful are contraindications. These will be detected by preliminary digital examination of the anal canal.

A severe degree of anal stenosis may make it difficult to pass a rigid or flexible sigmoidoscope. When this is present, it is usually possible to dilate the stricture sufficiently to pass either a small-calibre rigid sigmoidoscope or a flexible fibreoptic sigmoidoscope. The incidence of perforation with flexible sigmoidoscopy is very low, but the examination should terminate if the patient complains of severe discomfort, and particular care should be taken in patients with acute inflammatory bowel disease.

Preoperative

No special preparation is required for proctoscopy.

Bowel preparation and medication for sigmoidoscopy

Rigid sigmoidoscopy can be performed without bowel preparation, but in many patients faeces present in the rectum will obscure the view and possibly limit the distance to which the sigmoidoscope can be passed. Examination without bowel preparation has the advantage that it enables the contents of the upper rectum to be inspected. For flexible sigmoidoscopy, a single phosphate enema provides adequate bowel preparation in the majority of patients, a second enema being only very occasionally necessary.

Sigmoidoscopy may be carried out in the outpatient department. After explanation, the patient undresses, puts on a gown and is given a phosphate enema. The patient should not be examined for at least 30 min, preferably after the bowels have been opened twice. This results in adequate clearance of the left side of the colon. Neither sedation nor analgesia is required, and antispasmodics have been shown to be of no help. The procedure should be terminated if severe pain is experienced.

In patients with artificial joints and valvular heart disease, prophylactic antibiotics should be given, as transient bacteraemia has been reported.

Operations

PROCTOSCOPY

Position of patient

1, 2 The left lateral position as described for sigmoidoscopy is satisfactory; however, the knee–elbow position is sometimes preferred and can most conveniently be achieved by the use of a purpose-built tilting examination couch.

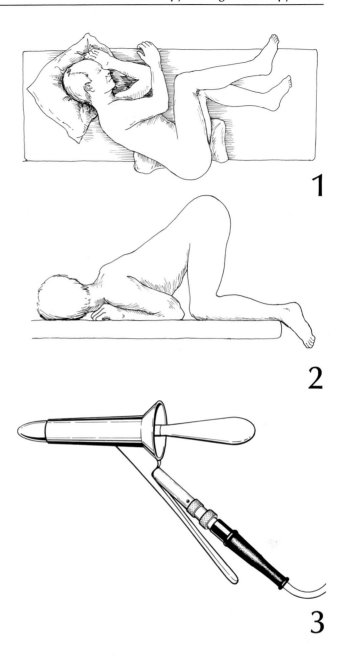

Instruments

3 Proctoscopes of many different sizes and types are available. The simple tubular proctoscope illustrated is useful for routine proctoscopy. Satisfactory disposable instruments are available. A 20-cm (8-inch) pair of non-toothed dissecting forceps is essential for cleaning the rectum with soft cotton-wool swabs. A fibreoptic light source is preferred because of its greater reliability and intensity of light.

Insertion and examination

The lubricated proctoscope with the obturator in place is passed with firm pressure into the anal canal in a direction toward the umbilicus. As the instrument is felt to enter the rectum, it is directed more posteriorly and passed to the full extent. The obturator is withdrawn and the light adjusted. The proctoscope is held steady in the rectum with the left hand, leaving the right hand free for carrying out necessary manipulations such as swabbing away any excess mucus, and for injection of haemorrhoids. The lower rectum is inspected by gentle rotation of the instrument so that the whole circumference of the wall can be seen; as the instrument is slowly withdrawn the mucosa becomes darker as it enters the upper anal canal and the mucous membrane closes over the end of the instrument. Haemorrhoids, if present, may prolapse into the proctoscope, especially if the patient is asked to strain. The lower end of the anal canal should be inspected for evidence of fissure. If it is decided to pass the instrument again it should be withdrawn completely and the obturator replaced.

RIGID SIGMOIDOSCOPY

Instruments

4 A number of instruments is available. The most useful for diagnostic purposes is the 25-cm Lloyd-Davies sigmoidoscope (internal diameter, 19 mm), which is available in lengths of 30 cm and 20 cm and is particularly useful if polypectomy is to be performed. Instruments with a distal circumferential light source are available with attachments, making it possible to perform polypectomy and other manipulations while maintaining inflation of the rectum. An insulated distal end of the instrument is advisable when performing polypectomy in order to avoid accidental burning of the rectal mucosa. A plastic disposable instrument is also available, which is satisfactory for routine diagnostic work.

Cup biopsy and grasping forceps are necessary together with a supply of soft cotton-wool swabs, so that fluid can be removed from the rectum. A long suction tube is particularly helpful in patients with fluid rectal contents.

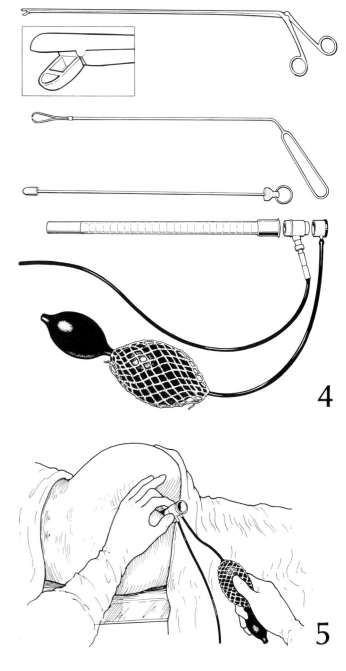

4

Insertion

5 Patients should be warned that during the course of sigmoidoscopy they will experience a desire to defaecate. After lubrication of the anal canal during digital examination of the rectum, the instrument is inserted pointing towards the umbilicus with the obturator in place, care being taken not to damage the anterior rectal wall. When the instrument is felt to enter the lower rectum, it is directed posteriorly and the obturator removed. The rectum is then gently inflated with air to allow the sigmoidoscope to be advanced through the lumen. Further passage may require depression and anterior movement at the proximal end of the instrument in order to find the intestinal lumen. Discomfort may be experienced as the instrument is passed into the lower sigmoid colon.

Unless the lumen of the sigmoid colon is clearly seen, the sigmoid colon has not been entered; the instrument can only be advanced by further stretching of the upper rectum. Inspection of the whole mucosa can be achieved by rotating the instrument during removal, taking care not to miss lesions hidden behind the mucosal rectal valves or rectal folds. Throughout the whole of the examination, the instrument is held in the left hand while the right hand holds the inflation bellows and bulb, which can be gently squeezed between the thumb and index finger to control the degree of inflation. The instrument should be passed with the minimum degree of inflation as this is one of the main factors causing discomfort and may make negotiation of the rectosigmoid angle more difficult.

5

Biopsy of neoplasms

The sigmoidoscope is manipulated so that the lesion is at the end of the instrument. The glass window is then removed, and although this causes deflation of the rectum, if the sigmoidoscope has been correctly positioned the lesion remains within view. Biopsies can then be taken under vision and should never be performed blindly. Excess bleeding at the site can be controlled by pressure from a cotton-wool swab or occasionally 1:1000 topical adrenaline. An instrument that allows a biopsy to be taken while maintaining inflation of the rectum may, at times, prove valuable.

Polypectomy

6 Polyps with a stalk can be removed with a diathermy snare technique. The polyp is grasped by polyp-holding forceps which have previously been passed through the loop of the diathermy snare. The snare is then passed over the polyp, care being taken not to take an excess of normal mucosa into the snare by excessive traction on the forceps; if this is done there is a danger of perforation of the intestine. Closure of the snare during application of diathermy will slowly coagulate the stalk of the polyp which can then be removed by the holding forceps.

Instruments that have facilities for polypectomy while maintaining inflation of the rectum are in some cases easier to use, as this makes more accurate placement of the snare possible without the use of polyp-holding forceps. After polypectomy the patient should be re-examined to make sure that the intestine has not been perforated and to inspect the coagulated area for bleeding; if necessary, the area can be coagulated with the small ball electrode.

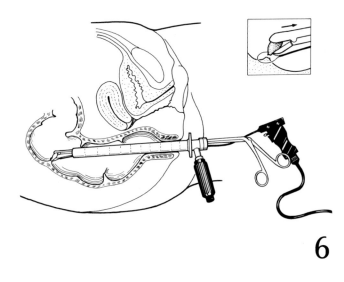

6

FIBREOPTIC SIGMOIDOSCOPY

Insertion

Patients should be placed on a couch or bed, initially in the left lateral position. A rectal examination should be performed to exclude a low anal or rectal lesion and to slightly stretch and lubricate the anal canal. Local anaesthetic gel is helpful if the digital examination is painful.

7 The tip of the sigmoidoscope should be well lubricated and inserted 'sideways' with slight finger pressure for a distance of 4–5 cm.

Initial inspection usually reveals a red blur as the tip of the instrument is against the rectal mucosa; the rectum should be gently inflated and the instrument withdrawn slightly, adjusting the flexible end until the lumen is in sight. The focus control should be adjusted and any residual fluid or faeces sucked out. The sigmoidoscope may then be advanced along the lumen of the rectum to the rectosigmoid junction.

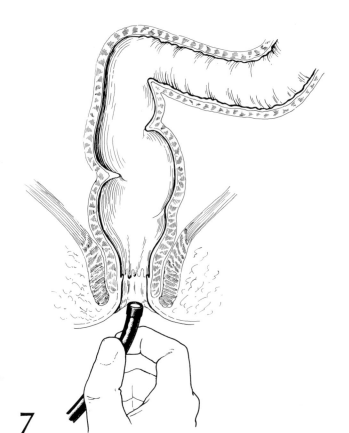

7

Negotiation of the rectosigmoid junction

8 An attempt should be made to pass around this corner under direct vision with minimal insufflation of air, by angling the tip of the instrument at about 15 cm. In patients with an acute angulation of the rectosigmoid region, it may not be possible to keep the lumen in sight. In this case the tip of the instrument should be gently advanced across the mucosa but without causing it to blanch. If, as the instrument is inserted, movement across the mucosa is not seen the sigmoidoscope should be withdrawn until the lumen comes into view again and a further attempt made to advance the instrument, angulating the tip in the direction of the lumen. It may help to twist the shaft of the sigmoidoscope during the manoeuvre to bring the tip into the correct position rather than to use the instrument control. If the tip becomes fully deflected the instrument will not advance further and it will again form a loop. Care must be taken to insufflate only small volumes of air to prevent an increase in the acuteness of the rectosigmoid angle and discomfort for the patient.

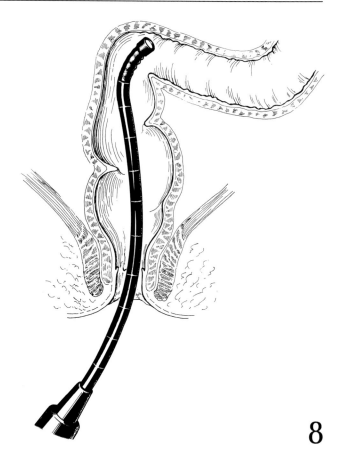

8

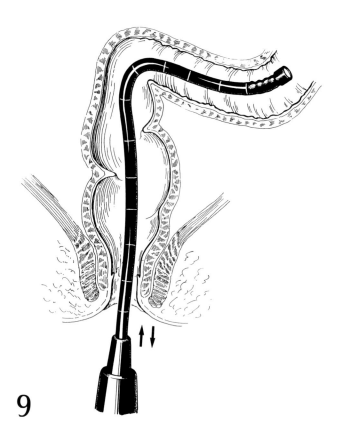

9

Negotiation of the sigmoid colon

9 By a combination of manipulation of the tip of the sigmoidoscope and twisting of the shaft, it is possible to reach the sigmoid colon in most patients. If a large loop forms, this can be reduced by withdrawing the instrument and at the same time rotating the shaft in a clockwise direction. This results in a straightening of the sigmoid colon and allows further advancement. If the tip does not advance rapidly along the sigmoid colon, short advancement and withdrawal movements of the shaft will cause the sigmoid colon to 'concertina' over the instrument.

More complicated procedures such as the 'alpha' manoeuvre (as described in the chapter on pp. 130–141), should be reserved for the experienced colonoscopist and are seldom necessary with flexible sigmoidoscopy.

Many patients experience discomfort as the sigmoid colon is negotiated, and this can be eased by the patient or assistant pressing on the abdomen at the site of discomfort. Alteration of the patient's position to prone may assist the angulation of the sigmoid colon, particularly if a mobile tumour is present.

In patients who have had an anterior resection or sigmoid colectomy, the sigmoidoscope can be passed more rapidly through to the descending colon.

Full insertion and withdrawal

Occasionally, the instrument tip may reach the splenic flexure with a characteristic view of the triangular transverse colon. In the majority, however, insertion is only possible to the descending colon and, furthermore, only part of the lumen is usually visualized in this direction. The main examination of the colon should be undertaken under slow instrument withdrawal, keeping the lumen *in view all the way*. If the instrument has a ratchet tip control, this should be used to prevent rapid passage around acute angles and for careful examination of the sigmoid colon. Biopsy or removal of samples for cytology of a lesion should be done during withdrawal – the lesion may be cleaned by injecting water down the irrigation channel. Polypectomy can also be performed, and the technique for this is described in the chapter on pp. 130–141.

During withdrawal of the instrument, as much air as possible should be aspirated in order to increase the patient's comfort.

Care and disinfection of flexible sigmoidoscopes

An assistant or nurse should be trained in the care, cleaning and disinfection of the equipment according to the manufacturer's instructions.

Immediately after use, instruments should be washed in fresh detergent solution, any adherent debris brushed away, and fresh detergent flushed through all hollow components. Instruments should then be cleaned in an ultrasonic cleaner, rinsed in tap water and disinfected with 2% alkaline glutaraldehyde. Some disinfectants give rise to skin reactions, and staff should be aware of the danger and wear gloves. Adequate ventilation should be provided in the area where glutaraldehyde is used for disinfection.

Postoperative care

No special postoperative observation is necessary after routine sigmoidoscopy. If the patient has had a snare polypectomy performed, however, a warning should be given that bleeding may occur after the operation and if this is excessive, medical aid should be sought. Barium enemas should not be given for several days after a biopsy because of the risk of extravasation of barium.

Colonoscopy and polypectomy

Christopher B. Williams FRCP
Consultant Physician, St Mark's Hospital for Diseases of the Rectum and Colon, St Bartholomew's Hospital and King Edward VII Hospital for Officers, and Honorary Consultant Physician, The Hospital for Sick Children, London, UK

Principles and justification

Indications

After clinical assessment, proctosigmoidoscopy or flexible sigmoidoscopy, and sometimes barium enema, colonoscopy is indicated when the clinical problem has not been resolved, when radiology demonstrates a possible or definite lesion requiring removal or biopsy, and when there has been bleeding or anaemia. Colonoscopy should replace diagnostic laparotomy for most patients with suspected disease of the colon or terminal ileum. Examination through a stoma is technically relatively easy and is usually preferable to contrast studies, which are often difficult to perform and interpret. Therapeutic possibilities include laser photocoagulation, sclerotherapy and stricture dilatation. Colonic snare polypectomy is the procedure of choice for removal of almost all colonic polyps.

Contraindications and complications

There are few contraindications to colonoscopy, but there are occasional serious complications (1 in 2500 perforation rate, 1 in 10 000 mortality rate) so that the procedure should not be undertaken or vigorously pursued without good clinical reasons. Colonoscopy can provoke cardiac arrhythmias and should not be undertaken after recent myocardial infarction. Bowel perforation can occur and colonoscopy is, therefore, contraindicated or should only be performed with great caution and expertise in any form of acute colonic disease where perforation is likely (e.g. very severe acute ulcerative colitis, Crohn's disease and ischaemic colitis). It is similarly contraindicated in the acute phase of diverticulitis.

Chronic severe diverticular disease or a colonic stricture may make the examination difficult and more likely to weaken the instrument, but the results of successful examination may avoid surgery. Postoperative adhesions (e.g. after hysterectomy) may make the colon fixed and result in a traumatic insertion. Use of a small diameter paediatric instrument (colonoscope or gastroscope) may help in all these conditions.

Preoperative

Bowel preparation

For limited colonoscopy (flexible sigmoidoscopy) a 100-ml phosphate enema without dietary preparation should give an adequate view except in patients with stricturing or diverticular disease. Otherwise bowel preparation for colonoscopy must be rigorous and the reasons for this should be explained to patients to obtain their full cooperation. Iron tablets and constipating agents are stopped 4–5 days before the examination but other medications are continued.

In purge regimens a clear liquid diet is started 24 h before colonoscopy and an aperient (senna or bisacodyl) is given on the afternoon or evening before examination. A further dose of high-volume aperient (magnesium citrate) or large-volume cleansing enemas are given on the day of colonoscopy. Nasal tube lavage using warmed isotonic electrolyte solution infused at a rate of 2–3 l/h for 3 h will produce a perfectly clean colon without enemas. Oral lavage involves drinking 3–4 litres of balanced electrolyte–polyethylene glycol solution over 2–3 h and is a highly effective preparation for those who can tolerate the volume and salty taste.

There is a risk that an explosive gas mixture will form after preparation with mannitol or other carbohydrate-based agents; these should not be used before polypectomy unless the risk is eliminated by the use of carbon dioxide insufflation. The use of carbon dioxide has the added advantage of leaving the patient less distended at the end of the procedure when compared with air insufflation.

Medication

Premedication is unnecessary before colonoscopy except in highly nervous patients or children. If a gentle endoscopic technique is used, sedation during the procedure may also be unnecessary, especially in confident and motivated patients or those known to be easy to examine – such as after resection of the sigmoid colon. Intravenous diazepam, 5–10 mg, or midazolam, 2–5 mg, combined with pethidine, 25–50 mg, makes the procedure easily tolerated by the patient (half dosage for elderly patients). Benzodiazepines alone contribute amnesia but are only weakly analgesic. Additional doses of pethidine can be given when necessary and can be completely reversed by intravenous or intramuscular naloxone. Antispasmodics are not routinely used by all endoscopists but if there is spasm intravenous hyoscine butylbromide, 40 mg, or glucagon, 0.1 mg, will help accurate examination on withdrawal of the instrument, or during insertion if there is severe diverticular disease.

General anaesthesia is generally contraindicated because pain supplies the only warning that the bowel or mesentery is being overstretched.

Choice of instrument

Shorter (130–140 cm) colonoscopes may have slight mechanical advantages over longer (165–185 cm) instruments in use and maintenance but, except in expert hands, will not always reach the caecum, especially if radiography shows a redundant bowel. Thinner and more flexible paediatric instruments are available and should be used both for children and when there is stricturing or fixation of the bowel causing problems with standard instruments.

Sterilization of the instrument requires rigorous measures, including perfusion of all channels and parts with glutaraldehyde solution or gas sterilization with ethylene oxide, particularly after examination of patients with mycobacterial infection or before those with immunodepression.

Is radiographic control needed?

Most examinations do not require radiographic screening control and most colonoscopists never use it. In the learning phase and for the less experienced, however, the extra information given can be invaluable, sometimes making difficult procedures quicker, safer and less traumatic. It will also help to localize obstructing lesions found unexpectedly at colonoscopy.

Technique

Position of patient

Most endoscopists start with the patient in the left lateral position and it is often possible to complete the examination without a change. If there are mechanical difficulties at any stage of the procedure, however, a change to the prone or supine position may alter the position of the bowel and make examination easier. The prone position helps to compress loops and also to reach the last few centimetres to the caecal pole; the supine position has the advantage of allowing palpation and visualization of the light transilluminating the abdomen. The right lateral position improves visualization of a fluid-filled descending colon and also greatly facilitates passage around the splenic flexure.

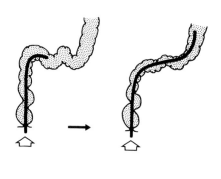

1

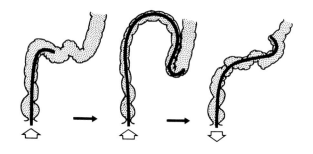

2

Insertion and passage through the rectosigmoid

1 The colonoscope tip and perianal region are lubricated, a digital examination of the rectum performed and the instrument is gently inserted. Initially there is no view because the tip is against the wall of the rectum and the instrument is withdrawn to disimpact it before a view can be obtained by insufflating air, angling the tip and rotating the instrument shaft as necessary.

In passing the many bends of the rectosigmoid the object is to distend or stretch the bowel as little as possible to keep it short, ideally passing almost straight into the descending colon. This is easier to suggest than to achieve, but is the ideal and is made more likely by observing the following points:

1. As little air as possible should be insufflated while keeping some view.
2. The bowel lumen should be followed accurately.
3. If the view is poor, even for a few seconds, the instrument should be withdrawn slightly and the direction reassessed.
4. Blind pushing should be avoided, although on acute bends this may be necessary for a few seconds, providing the general direction is certain.
5. If the tip will not angle round a bend the surgeon should try 'corkscrewing' by pulling back and twisting the shaft clockwise or anticlockwise.
6. The instrument should be pulled back repeatedly after passing any major bend and before starting each inward push. This straightens the colonoscope and shortens the colon, making insertion easier and more comfortable.

Sigmoid 'N loop': hook and twist manoeuvre

2 The most common situation on reaching the junction of the sigmoid and descending colon, in spite of all care, is for there to be an 'N loop', bowing up the sigmoid and resulting in a tip angulation which makes direct passage into the descending colon difficult or impossible. If the tip can be coaxed a short way round the bend, thus looking into the descending colon, it will be 'hooked' retroperitoneally so that the instrument can be withdrawn 20–30 cm to reduce and straighten out the loop. Because of the normal spiral configuration of the sigmoid loop, putting a strong (usually clockwise) twisting force (torque) on to the shaft of the colonoscope while it is withdrawn will help in straightening out this loop and keeping the tip in the descending colon. Occasionally, where the sigmoid colon is long or unusually mobile, an anticlockwise twist may work better because atypical looping can result when the descending colon is not fixed retroperitoneally in its usual left paravertebral position.

Sigmoid 'alpha loop'

3 Sometimes, especially in patients with a redundant colon, a loop is obviously forming but the tip none the less runs inwards without discomfort to the patient. This suggests that a spiral 'alpha' loop is forming (easily confirmed when fluoroscopy is used). If an alpha loop is suspected, the colonoscope should be pushed in as far as is comfortable for the patient, preferably to the splenic flexure, which uses about 90 cm of the instrument.

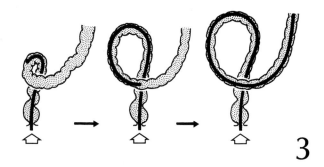

3

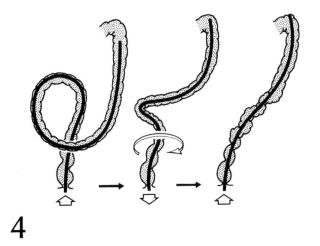

4

Straightening out loops

4 Having reached the upper descending colon or splenic flexure, a sigmoid loop should normally be removed, because loops create friction in the control wires, cause stress in the instrument and may hurt the patient. To remove the loop, the colonoscope shaft should be withdrawn firmly until the tip begins to slide or resistance to withdrawal is felt, usually at 45–50 cm insertion depth. When pulling back, the application of a clockwise twist often helps to prevent the tip of the colonoscope from slipping back prematurely.

Keeping straight or stiffening the sigmoid colon

5 Once the colonoscope is straightened, with its tip in the descending colon and the sigmoid colon convoluted and shortened, some care may be needed to prevent the sigmoid loop reforming. Continued clockwise (occasionally anticlockwise) twist on the shaft helps to keep it straight during insertion. Shaft insertion without tip movement (loss of 1:1 relationship) indicates relooping and the instrument is immediately pulled back again. Having an assistant push firmly in the left iliac fossa resists the tendency of the sigmoid loop to rise up from the pelvis.

In a few patients with a very redundant colon in whom unavoidable sigmoid looping occurs (but total colonoscopy is indicated), a 'stiffening' or overtube may be needed. This is a plastic tube which is placed in position over the colonoscope, lubricated with jelly and passed over the *straightened* instrument to stop it from flexing. Insertion of a stiffener is ideally carried out under radiographic control with to-and-fro rotary movement used to avoid catching redundant mucosa. A softer low-friction 'split' overtube is available which can be positioned over the endoscope after insertion (and taped over the split) which avoids having to withdraw the colonoscope and does not need fluoroscopy.

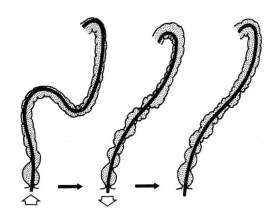

5

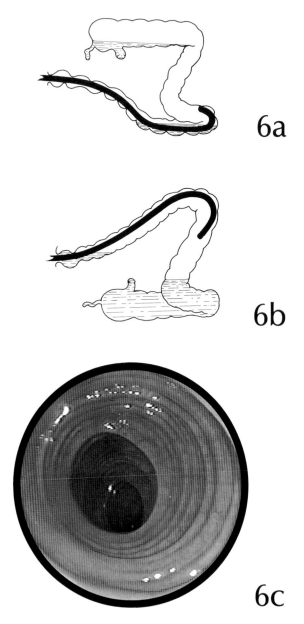

6a

6b

6c

Position and the splenic flexure

6a–c In the left lateral position the descending colon is deflated and filled with fluid. Changing the patient to the right lateral position not only improves the view in the descending colon (particularly important if there is blood or residual fluid), but also causes the transverse colon to flop down and open out the splenic flexure, making this point much easier to pass.

The instrument shaft should be pulled back and straightened out to 50 cm before tackling the splenic flexure or transverse colon; failure to do this accounts for most cases where the proximal colon is described as being difficult to pass. To prevent the sigmoid loop reforming, excessive tip angulation should be avoided, hand pressure by the assistant should be used over the left iliac fossa and a gentle clockwise twisting force maintained on the shaft while pushing gently inwards. Too rapid or aggressive pushing merely loops up the sigmoid.

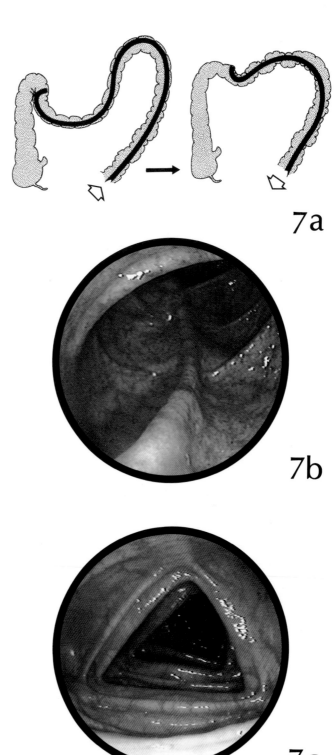

7a

Redundant transverse colon

7a–c The transverse colon may push down into a deep loop that makes it difficult and painful to reach the hepatic flexure. If this happens the correct procedure is to withdraw the instrument 30–50 cm to shorten the transverse loop; this withdrawal may need to be repeated several times, the tip advancing a few centimetres each time until the loop straightens. Deflation also helps to shorten the hepatic flexure, making it easier to reach and to pass. If the right lateral position has been used to pass the splenic flexure, the patient is changed back to the normal left lateral position when the proximal transverse colon is reached, thus facilitating insertion up to and around the hepatic flexure.

Difficulty in the transverse colon is often due to recurrent looping in the sigmoid colon, and continued abdominal pressure in the left iliac fossa may be more effective than trying to affect the transverse colon with pressure in the upper abdomen or left hypochondrium.

7b

7c

Passing the hepatic flexure

8 Having reached and deflated the hepatic flexure, and then angled around it into the ascending colon, the transverse colon loop may remain, making it difficult to pass the rest of the instrument into the ascending colon. Paradoxically, by withdrawing the colonoscope forcibly 30–50 cm, so straightening out the transverse loop, it becomes easier to pass it onwards.

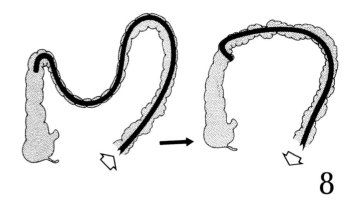

8

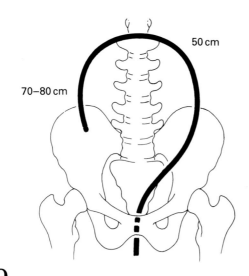

9

9 The hepatic flexure is a 180° hairpin bend and major angulation may be required, even though the view is imperfect. A combination of both control knobs and recurrent minor aspirations should be used to reduce the size of the flexure as far as possible to angle progressively around the hepatic flexure while simultaneously maintaining a limited mucosal view by pulling back if necessary. As soon as the ascending colon is seen it is deflated and shortened by aspiration and, while steering carefully to avoid further haustral folds, the colonoscope should spontaneously descend towards the caecum.

Reaching the caecum

If there is difficulty in reaching the caecal pole, changing the patient's position to prone or supine may be helpful. Excessive push pressure usually only loops up the sigmoid colon.

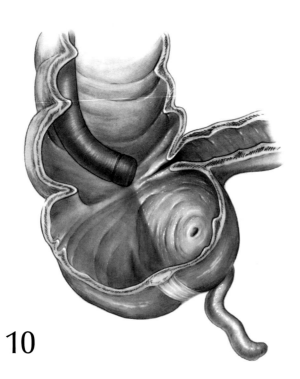

10

10 The colonoscope is known to have reached the caecum when the bulge and slit opening of the ileocaecal valve is seen or, 5 cm beyond this, the appendix orifice is identified at the junction of the taeniae coli. If these anatomical features are not obvious, and experience is sometimes needed to be sure, there is a danger of mistaking the hepatic flexure for the caecum. Transillumination should be visible in the right iliac fossa if the room is darkened and the instrument light is bright enough or a palpating finger can be seen indenting the bowel wall through the colonoscope.

The fully straightened colonoscope at the caecal pole is 70–80 cm from the anus, then during withdrawal the splenic flexure is at 50 cm and descending colon at 40 cm. However, during insertion and in cases where the caecum has not been reached, because loops invariably form, these distance rules do not apply and localization may be impossible without radiographic control, although transillumination and palpation may give some indication.

Entering the terminal ileum

11 The ileum joins the caecum through the variably shaped bulging or slit-like ileocaecal 'valve' on the first prominent haustral fold about 5 cm back from the caecal pole.

Deflation can help to locate the valve opening by making it bulge or bubble, but some valves may only be obvious after retroverting the instrument tip in the caecal pole to visualize a slit on the underside of the ileocaecal fold.

To enter the ileum the valve must first be identified, then the instrument straightened to 70–80 cm for maximum manoeuvrability. Ideally the valve should be placed at the top or bottom of the view for ease of entry using tip angulation with the up/down control. The caecum should be deflated slightly to make the region more supple, the tip angled towards the lower lip of the valve and (as seems appropriate) either pushed in or pulled back slowly so that the tip slips into the enveloping lips of the valve, with a 'red out'. Finally, the valve should be opened up by insufflation and passed into the ileum, which appears granular due to the villous surface seen in air (under water the villi show their characteristic frond-like configuration).

Examination

To some extent the colon is seen during insertion of the instrument but more active examination is normally undertaken during withdrawal of the colonoscope. Fastidious care is necessary to see behind folds, especially when the bowel has been convoluted by straightening the instrument.

Usually it is best for the endoscopist to control the instrument using a one-handed technique during

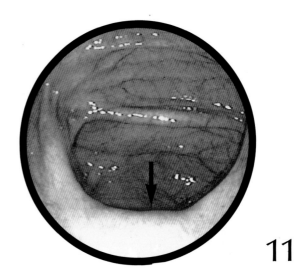

11

withdrawal, even if an assistant has helped with insertion. Very active manoeuvring of the controls, with corkscrewing rotation and to-and-fro movements of the shaft, may be necessary to avoid blind spots. Examination of the bowel on withdrawal may sometimes take as long as insertion of the instrument.

Postoperative care

In most cases no particular care is needed after colonoscopy apart from a few minutes of rest and some food and drink. If sedation has been used the patient must be warned not to drive a vehicle for 24 h. When the patient appears and feels well he or she can be safely discharged, preferably with an escort. Most examinations are performed on a day-care basis.

POLYPECTOMY

Safety

The principle behind colonoscopic polypectomy is to prevent bleeding by adequate electrocoagulation of vessels before transection, because the endoscopist operates 'single handed' without the surgeon's ability to use artery forceps or ligature should bleeding occur. On the other hand, avoidance of excessive heat damage is also essential to prevent necrosis of the colon wall, which can occur as a secondary phenomenon even when there has been little visible whitening at the time. This is the reason for a 'postpolypectomy syndrome' of peritoneal pain and fever, and also of secondary or 'delayed' haemorrhage due to damaged submucosal arterioles exposed by ulceration. Judgement is required as to the amount of current required – 'not too little; not too much'. Most experts use coagulating current alone with a relatively low power setting, relying on passage of time (usually 5–15 s) and applying progressive mechanical tightening of the snare during current application to cause first heating and whitening locally and then slow transection below the polyp tissue.

Adjusting the polypectomy snare

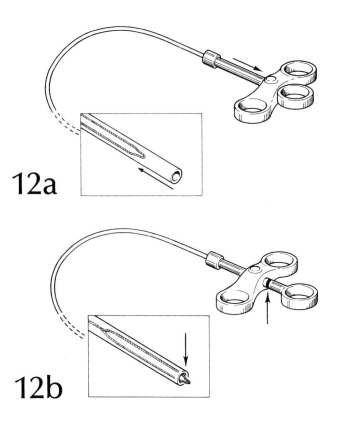

12a

12b

12a, b
For efficient electrocoagulation it is fundamental to 'neck' the stalk tissue to cause local current concentration, because heating increases as the square of current concentration and as the cube of snare loop tightening. Adjustment of the snare before the procedure is a necessary preliminary. The handle/wire assembly should be examined on a bench to ensure that it has an easy action with good 'feel', full opening and full closing. When completely closed (*Illustration 12a*) the tip of the wire should retract at least 15 mm, and preferably 20 mm, into the outer plastic sheath, to allow for inevitable crumpling of the sheath during forcible closure around a polyp stalk. Full closure is necessary for adequate necking and subsequent transection of a large stalk, which will greatly decrease the risk. Another invaluable safety measure (*Illustration 12b*) is to make an indelible mark on the snare handle at the point corresponding to the closure of the snare tip to the end of the plastic sheath. This mark on the handle indicates the correct snare closure point to the assistant, avoiding unintended mechanical 'cheese-wiring' through a small polyp, but also gives a measurable advance warning if the snare has entrapped the polyp head or if the stalk is unexpectedly large.

Small polyps

13 Polyps up to 5 mm in diameter are common but, because of their small size, can be disproportionately awkward to catch with the snare and troublesome to retrieve or aspirate for histology. Use of electrically insulated 'hot biopsy' forceps is an effective compromise, allowing electrocoagulation of the tented-up basal tissues of the small polyp while usually obtaining an adequate biopsy of the sample, which is protected from current flow within the jaws of the forceps. For safety, only the apex of the polyp is grasped and tented up towards the lumen by angling or twisting the instrument and pulling back the forceps slightly. Current is applied for only 2 s or less to cause localized electrocoagulation limited to the vasculature in the pseudopedicle – the 'Mount Fuji' effect of whitening at the apex of the small 'mountain' of pulled-up tissue.

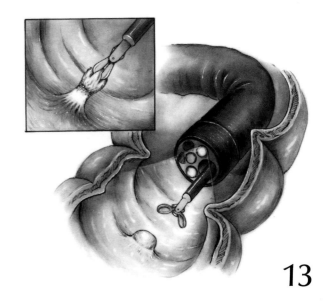

13

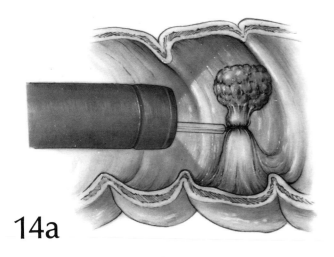

14a

Stalked polyps

14a, b The snare is manoeuvred over the polyp head and on to the upper part of the stalk, preferably leaving a short margin of normal tissue below the head for identification by the histopathologist. The snare loop is closed gently, correct closure of the handle to the previously made mark (*see* above) is checked and then the stalk is moved around for better visualization and to ensure that the colon wall has not been entrapped by the loop. Finally, continuous low-power coagulating current is applied, initially with quite gentle squeeze pressure on the handle but, as soon as visible swelling or whitening indicates local electrocoagulation, the squeeze is increased to sever the head. If any bleeding occurs (other than back-bleeding from the polyp head), the snare is quickly opened and the basal part of the stalk regrasped for a few minutes, with or without gentle extra electrocoagulation.

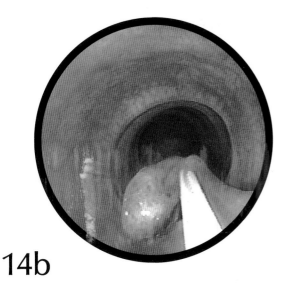

14b

Broad-stalked polyps

15 Semipedunculated polyps with bases or stalks over 1 cm in diameter present a problem in achieving sufficient depth of electrocoagulation to occlude all vessels in the feeding plexus. Basal injection with 1:10 000 adrenaline solution, 1–5 ml, with a long flexible sclerotherapy needle, can be used either before snaring or as an emergency measure should bleeding occur. Longer thick stalks can be preinjected in their mid-portion with 1 ml of a sclerosant–adrenaline mixture to ensure long-term effect, providing there is room to snare above the injection point which swells significantly.

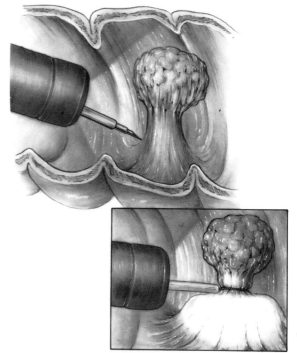

Large or sessile polyps (piecemeal removal)

16 Polyps over 2–3 cm in diameter without a compressible stalk are hazardous to snare in a single portion because the higher power current and longer application time required risk transmural heating and perforation. If such heating occurs, an unsedated patient will usually report immediate peritoneal pain which is an early warning to abandon the procedure (unless deflation suggests that the pain is actually due to distension of the colon). Piecemeal removal of larger sessile polyps (in up to 20–30 smaller portions, and in repeated sessions if necessary) keeps control of the procedure and provides a reasonable degree of safety, but allows removal of nearly any polyp if the patient can tolerate the long procedure time(s) involved. Snaring with the colonoscope tip in retroversion may be needed to entrap any part of a sessile polyp which is invisible on the proximal side of an acute haustral fold. Because some of these polyps will prove to be malignant, and surgery therefore possibly indicated, it is often wise to obtain initial histology by partial (80–90%) removal before repeating the procedure and removing the more risky basal parts of the polyp. Very fully informed patient consent of the risks involved are clearly essential before undertaking a hazardous polypectomy.

Making a nearby 1-ml tattoo injection of a 1:10 dilution of sterilized Indian ink facilitates follow-up examinations. The mark probably lasts for life, certainly for many years.

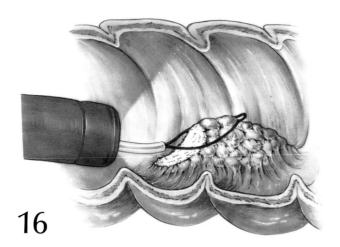

Retrieving polyps

The normal way to retrieve a snared polyp for histological examination is to catch the head with the polypectomy snare and pull it back with the endoscope. For very large polyps the patient may need to squat and then strain to relax the anal sphincter for successful final delivery. Multiple larger polyps may require multiple reinsertions of the endoscope for individual snare retrieval (an overtube can be used). Alternatively, 500–600 ml of tap water are syringe-injected through the instrument channel above the snared polyps or polyp fragments with additional air insufflation, and a disposable enema given after withdrawing the endoscope to stimulate spontaneous evacuation into a pan from whence they can be retrieved.

Follow-up

Judgement is necessary about the correct interval for follow-up. Some polypectomy sites heal completely within 2–3 weeks and are thereafter impossible to identify accurately. Thus, a malignant polyp site should be checked and tattooed within this time. On the other hand, a longer period is desirable to allow resolution of tissue damage before checking for regrowth of benign tissue after removal of benign sessile polyps.

Polyps can be missed at colonoscopy and it is sometimes justifiable to perform a check examination within a year. High-risk patients with multiple adenomas or malignancy need initial checks at 1–2 years but in many other patients examination at 3-yearly or even longer intervals is probably adequate.

Further reading

Cotton PB, Williams CB. *Practical Gastrointestinal Endoscopy*, 3rd edn. Oxford: Blackwell Scientific Publications, 1990.

Intraoperative endoscopy

Richard L. Whelan MD
Assistant Professor of Surgery and Director, Section of Colon and Rectal Surgery, Columbia Presbyterian Medical Center, Columbia University College of Physicians and Surgeons, New York, USA

Principles and justification

Intraoperative endoscopy is defined as the use of a flexible endoscope passed by mouth or by the anus to examine the stomach, small intestine, or colon, during a laparotomy. This is a relatively new procedure first described in the early 1970s[1], with indications that continue to be developed and modified. Intraoperative endoscopy can provide unique information not otherwise obtainable, but it should not be used as a substitute for routine upper or lower gastrointestinal endoscopy.

Although it is a very safe procedure, complications can occur. Furthermore, intraoperative endoscopy lengthens the operation, in some cases by up to 1 h, and often requires additional staff for its performance. Therefore, the use of intraoperative endoscopy should be limited to those situations where the examination cannot be performed before surgery or where there is a significant chance that the information obtained will alter the planned operation.

Established indications

Non-palpable lesions

1a, b Intraoperative colonoscopy is useful for locating lesions found on barium radiology or preoperative colonoscopy that are not palpable at the time of laparotomy. Similarly, small intestinal lesions detected on upper gastrointestinal contrast studies that are not palpable can be located by intraoperative enteroscopy.

Endoscopic localization allows the surgeon to perform a limited intestinal resection and should obviate the need for 'blind' resection. In some cases, careful, thorough and complete intraoperative endoscopy may rule out the presence of a suspected lesion, thus avoiding an unnecessary colotomy or resection[2].

Unsuspected intestinal lesions

Intraoperative endoscopy is quite helpful in confirming the presence and nature of intestinal lesions discovered on routine exploration during laparotomy for some other problem. This includes gastric, small intestinal, and colonic lesions.

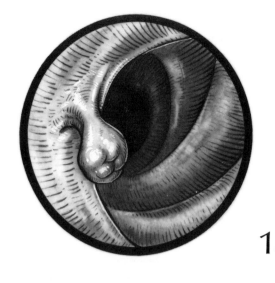

1a

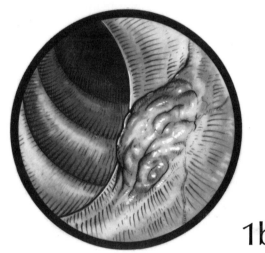

1b

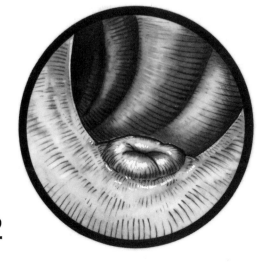

2

Malignant polypectomy localization

2 At laparotomy, it may be difficult or impossible to determine the location of a previously removed malignant polyp. Palpation and inspection of the intestine are usually not helpful. Intraoperative colonoscopy will in most cases allow identification of such polypectomy sites. This information allows the surgeon to perform an adequate, but limited, resection[3].

Alternative localization methods include tattooing of polyp sites and the use of fluoroscopy during colonoscopy, neither of which is widely practised.

Inability to complete a preoperative examination

It is reasonable to perform intraoperative colonoscopy in patients in whom routine colonoscopy has been incomplete and who come to surgery for some other reason. The intraoperative setting may provide the only opportunity for a complete endoscopic examination in these patients. The most common causes of incomplete colonoscopic examinations are adhesions and a tortuous intestine. At surgery, the adhesions can be lysed and redundant loops stented. These manoeuvres will usually enable the endoscopist to complete the examination, obtain biopsy material and carry out polypectomy.

An alternative to intraoperative colonoscopy is a preoperative barium enema because a negative contrast study (if of sufficient quality) would obviate the need for intraoperative colonoscopy. If the study revealed polyps or other lesions, however, endoscopy would be indicated to further investigate these findings.

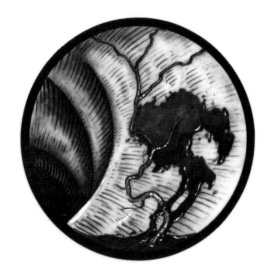

3

Gastrointestinal bleeding

The main goal of endoscopy in this setting is to localize the site of bleeding, so that a limited intestinal resection can be performed. Not uncommonly, it is necessary to perform both colonoscopic and enteroscopic examinations in these patients. It must be stressed, however, that the availability of intraoperative endoscopy does not obviate the need for a complete preoperative evaluation. Intraoperative endoscopy should be reserved for those patients requiring surgery whose bleeding site remains unknown despite an evaluation including radionuclide studies, upper and lower endoscopy and possibly angiography.

Intraoperative endoscopy for bleeding has been most successful in patients who undergo surgery because of chronic intermittent gastrointestinal haemorrhage of unknown aetiology. These operations are most often performed electively between bleeding episodes. This allows for a complete bowel preparation which greatly facilitates the endoscopic examination. These patients have usually received multiple blood transfusions and have undergone numerous complete diagnostic evaluations.

3 In this setting, angioectasias (i.e. arteriovenous malformations) of the small intestine or colon are the most likely cause of the bleeding. Although large angioectasias can be found on routine surgical exploration or endoscopy, the small lesions may escape detection.

Transillumination of the intestine during intraoperative endoscopy is a technique that allows identification of small angioectasias that might otherwise be undetected[4]. It is imperative that both enteroscopy and colonoscopy be performed on these patients, because these vascular lesions can occur in either the small or large intestine[5]. Based on the distribution and number of angioectasias, an appropriate surgical procedure can be selected. Treatment options range from simple oversewing of the lesions to a wedge resection or segmental resection of the intestine. Numerous studies have documented the efficacy of intraoperative endoscopy with transillumination in this clinical setting.

In the actively bleeding patient, intraoperative endoscopy has been less successful. It is very difficult to identify the source of haemorrhage in a blood-filled intestine. It is usually not possible to perform a preoperative bowel preparation in these patients. It has recently been shown that prograde lavage of the colon during laparotomy before endoscopy allows an excellent colonoscopic examination[6]. In several small series, this technique has been highly successful in localizing the site of haemorrhage.

Controversial indications

Crohn's disease

In patients with Crohn's disease who require surgery, intraoperative endoscopy may be of value in detecting small intestinal strictures and in determining the extent of active disease[2]. On occasion, usually in patients with a history of multiple abdominal operations, it may be difficult to determine the extent of mucosal disease based on the serosal appearance of the intestine. In these situations, intraoperative endoscopy is helpful in selecting the proximal and distal points of resection.

To identify the site of small intestinal strictures, most surgeons use a balloon-tipped catheter which is passed, deflated, through an enterotomy into the intestine. Once fully inserted, the balloon is inflated and the tube is withdrawn. The balloon will lodge at strictures that block its passage. Once identified, stricturoplasty (as described in the chapter on pp. 320–329) can be performed. Usually multiple enterotomies are required to examine the entire small intestine. Intraoperative enteroscopy is an alternative means of locating strictures that does not require an enterotomy. Furthermore, intraoperative enteroscopy permits mucosal inspection of the small intestine, which allows delineation between fibrous strictures and narrowing of the lumen caused by active disease.

Although these indications for intraoperative endoscopy are promising, it has not yet been demonstrated that they offer any advantage over the intraoperative methods currently in use.

Contraindications

Obstructing distal colonic lesions

In patients with obstructing lesions of the colon or rectum, a complete preoperative colonoscopy is not possible. If the surgeon was willing to perform an endoscopy across a fresh anastomosis, a complete examination could be carried out at surgery after resection and anastomosis. This, however, would subject the anastomosis to torque forces and the increased intraluminal pressures that result from insufflation. Thus, such an examination might damage the anastomosis, and in this setting intraoperative endoscopy is contraindicated. The risks to the fresh anastomosis far outweigh the potential benefits of the endoscopic examination. It is recommended that careful palpation of the proximal colon be performed at the time of surgery, and that a complete colonoscopy of the remaining intestine be performed 3–6 months after operation.

Routine screening examinations

Intraoperative endoscopy should not be performed in place of a routine preoperative examination. This is most often suggested for patients with a non-obstructing colonic malignancy who require colonoscopy to rule out a synchronous lesion. The advantages of an intraoperative examination, however, are that a single bowel preparation will suffice for both colonoscopy and intestinal resection, and that the patient will experience no pain.

There are several disadvantages to this type of examination. The intraoperative examination prolongs the operation, and on occasion is associated with complications. Furthermore, the pathology results of polyps sampled for biopsy or removed during the operation will not be available until after the surgery has been completed. This means that small sessile polyp cancers that may warrant intestinal resection will go unresected unless the clinical index of suspicion is very high. Preoperative endoscopy provides this information before surgery, which allows the operative plan to be altered if necessary. If colonoscopy is performed early the day before surgery, a single bowel preparation will suffice and the pathology results should be available before the operation.

Preoperative

With few exceptions, patients who are to undergo intraoperative endoscopy should have a standard mechanical large bowel preparation. If a colonic resection is planned, oral and/or intravenous perioperative antibiotics should be administered. Intraoperative endoscopy should be discussed with the patient before the operation and included on the operative consent form.

The operating room staff should be informed well in advance of the procedure, so that the necessary equipment will be available at the time of surgery. Appropriate stirrups should be available.

Anaesthesia

Provided that laparotomy is being performed under general anaesthesia, no additional medication or inhalational agents are required for the endoscopy.

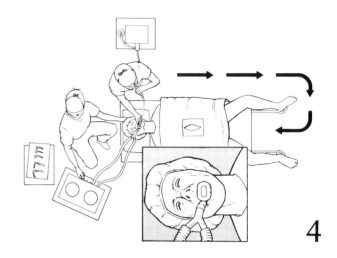

4

4 It is important to inform the anaesthetist before the operation if a transoral examination is planned. This will allow the anaesthetist to arrange his equipment to the right of the patient in order to provide space for the endoscopist at the head of the table. The endotracheal tube should be positioned and taped towards the right side of the mouth so that a bite block can be inserted.

A nasogastric tube or oesophageal stethoscope can serve as a guide to the endoscopist during insertion of the endoscope. It is recommended, however, that these tubes be removed once the endoscope has been successfully inserted, because they are likely to become entangled or dislodged when the endoscope is withdrawn. They can be reinserted once the endoscope has been withdrawn.

Operations

Equipment

The endoscopy equipment should be thoroughly checked by the surgical endoscopist before the start of the operation. The light source, suction unit, electrocautery unit and endoscope must all be functioning properly in order to perform a worthwhile examination. The electrical plugs of the endoscopy equipment may not be compatible with the operating room electrical outlets; therefore, adaptors may be necessary. An endoscopic snare, biopsy forceps and bite block must also be available. Although not essential, an endoscopic irrigating pump can be of great assistance.

Transanal examinations should be performed with a full-length colonoscope. Similarly, transoral entero-scopy also requires a colonoscope. Although a standard upper gastrointestinal endoscope is adequate for those few patients in whom a limited upper examination is planned (i.e. stomach and duodenum), the use of a colonoscope allows the examination to be extended if necessary. Some prefer a paediatric colonoscope for transoral examinations because this narrower instrument is more readily inserted. Children and patients with anal stenosis undergoing lower examinations may also require a paediatric colonoscope.

If panendoscopy is planned, it is recommended that the transoral examination be performed first, so that a single endoscope can be used for both examinations.

Position of patient

The patient must be positioned to provide the endoscopist with access to both the mouth and rectum if panendoscopy is anticipated. The necessary anaesthetic measures for transoral examinations have already been discussed.

5 The modified lithotomy position is most often used when intraoperative lower endoscopy is planned. The endoscopist performs the examination while sitting on a stool between the legs. A towel or drape is placed across the proximal thighs of the patient to prevent contamination of the operative field. Care must be taken to uphold the external portion of the endoscope because it is not otherwise supported.

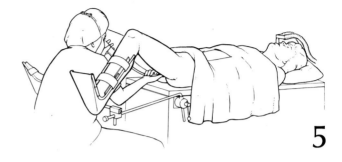

5

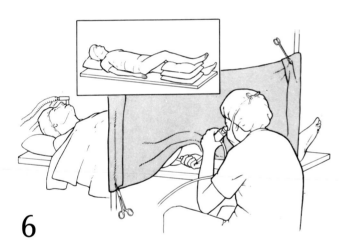

6

6 Alternatively, a modified supine position can be used for lower gastrointestinal examinations. Access to the rectum is provided by elevating the distal right thigh and lower leg with several pillows. When this position is used, it is important that the endoscope be introduced into the rectum and secured to the operating table before the patient is prepared, because the anus cannot be visualized once the patient has been draped. The endoscopist performs the examination from a sitting or squatting position to the right of the patient. An oblique drape across the pelvis and upper thighs is necessary to protect the operative field from contamination.

ENDOSCOPIC EXAMINATION

Once a thorough exploration of the abdomen has been performed, the endoscopic examination is commenced. Adhesions involving the intestinal segments to be examined should be lysed before endoscopy. This will allow the intestine to be straightened and facilitates the safe and rapid insertion of the endoscope.

7 It is most important that the terminal ileum is occluded with a non-crushing bowel clamp before insertion of the endoscope to prevent insufflation of the small intestine during colonoscopy and distension of the colon during transoral enteroscopy. If a limited examination is planned, the intestine should be occluded near the estimated point of furthest insertion.

As mentioned above, if panendoscopy is planned, it is recommended that the transoral examination is performed first. As for routine (closed abdomen) endoscopic examinations, the endoscopist advances the endoscope using a combination of insertion, withdrawal and torquing techniques. Working alone, however, the endoscopist will be unable to perform a complete intraoperative examination.

The surgeon and first assistant play a vital role in the performance of intraoperative endoscopy. With the abdomen open, the stenting effect of the intact abdominal wall is lost. This allows the formation of impressive 'loops' and 'bowed' segments of intubated intestine when the endoscope is inserted. Such loops not only make further advancement of the tip of the endoscope difficult, but may also damage the intestine. The mobile sigmoid and transverse colon are the most likely large intestinal segments to form loops. Loops may also form in a tortuous or redundant splenic flexure. Finally, large loops may form in the stomach and the small intestine when transoral intraoperative endoscopy is performed.

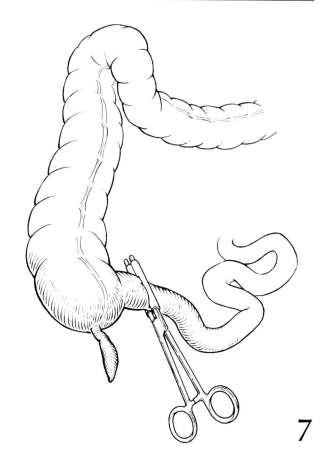

7

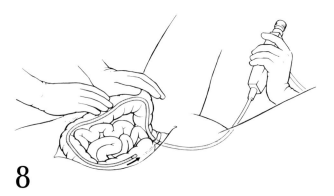

8

8 The surgeon prevents large loops from forming and facilitates further advancement of the tip of the endoscope by manually stenting the more mobile intestinal segments that have already been intubated while the endoscope is inserted further. At times, it may be necessary for the surgeon and first assistant to stent four separate areas simultaneously.

In the majority of colonoscopic examinations, the endoscopist does not need the help of the surgeon to direct the tip of the endoscope. On rare occasions, the surgeon can help to guide the tip of the endoscope through the fully mobile colonic segments (i.e. sigmoid and transverse colon). The surgeon, however, is of little help in directing the endoscope tip through the fixed portions of the large intestine (i.e. rectum, descending and ascending colon). Unless requested, the surgeon should avoid manipulating the colon near the endoscope tip, because this creates sudden and violent movements of the field of view that can be disorienting for the endoscopist.

9 Unlike colonic insertion, intubation of any significant length of the jejunum or ileum is impossible without guidance from the surgeon because of the great length and mobility of the small intestine. The surgeon manoeuvres the intestine onto the endoscope tip and shaft, while the endoscopist uses suction to decompress the intestine. This collapses the intestine, allowing it to 'accordion' onto the endoscope. At the surgeon's request, the endoscopist pushes the endoscope in further, so that additional intestine can be intubated.

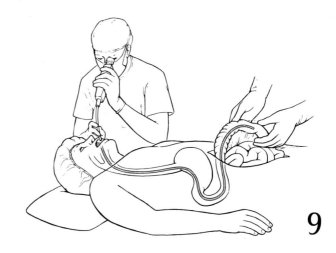

9

There must be frequent communication between the endoscopist and the surgeon for intraoperative endoscopy to be performed safely and effectively. For example, if the endoscopist notes that forward movement of the endoscope tip has ceased despite the insertion of additional lengths of endoscope shaft, he should ask the surgeon to examine for a new loop. The surgeon can then manually stent the 'bowed' segment, which will facilitate further insertion.

It is controversial as to when the detailed mucosal examination should be performed: during insertion or during withdrawal of the endoscope. During routine non-operative endoscopy, it is customary to perform the examination as the endoscope is withdrawn. The disadvantage of this approach is that minor traumatic mucosal injuries may result from insertion of the endoscope, particularly during enteroscopy where much manipulation of the intestine is necessary. It can be quite difficult to distinguish these traumatic injuries from small pathological lesions, such as angioectasias or polypectomy sites. For this reason, it is recommended that the examination be performed on insertion for those enteroscopies and colonoscopies being performed for gastrointestinal bleeding or to find a polypectomy site. When intraoperative endoscopy is being performed for other indications, the examination can be performed either on insertion or on withdrawal.

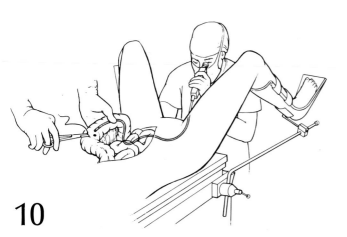

10

10 It is important that the surgeon marks the location of mucosal lesions that are identified endoscopically by placing a seromuscular suture at the level of the pathology.

Overinsufflation of the intestine should be avoided, because it makes intubation more difficult, may result in intestinal injury (i.e. serosal tears or perforations) and can cause a prolonged ileus. After withdrawal of the endoscope, care must be taken to suction all gas from the intestine. Failure to do this can make closure of the abdomen quite difficult. Decompression should be carried out segmentally, following examination of each portion of the intestine. After collapsing a segment, the non-crushing clamp can be reapplied just beyond the tip of the endoscope to prevent the proximal intestine from redistending.

SPECIAL TECHNIQUES FOR GASTROINTESTINAL BLEEDING

The technique of transillumination permits the identification of small angioectasias that might otherwise go undetected. With the room darkened, the light from the endoscope 'transilluminates' the intestine and outlines the vascular pattern of the intestinal wall. Examining the intestine from the serosal aspect, the surgeon can identify small angioectasias as dilatations or flat disc-like lesions situated along a vessel. Seromuscular sutures should be used to mark the location of the angioectasias that are found.

11 Prograde lavage of the colon during laparotomy and before endoscopy allows for an excellent colonoscopic examination in patients who are bleeding acutely. The lavage is performed through a catheter placed in the caecum at surgery. The effluent is drained through a rectal tube positioned before starting the operation. It is recommended that 4–6 litres of saline be used for lavage.

Postoperative care

Complications

Complications occur uncommonly; the most common is overdistension of the intestine, which can make abdominal closure difficult and can cause a prolonged postoperative ileus. Partial thickness intestinal wall injuries, such as serosal or mucosal tears, may also occur. Such tears may cause intramural haematomas and intra-abdominal or intraluminal haemorrhage. Frank perforations can also occur. Polypectomy and mucosal biopsy can very occasionally result in intraluminal bleeding. Splenic injury, resulting from excessive traction on the splenocolic ligament, can be the cause of significant intra-abdominal haemorrhage.

The surgeon must be aware of these potential complications and look carefully for them before abdominal closure. Similarly, the endoscopist should look for evidence of mucosal injury as the endoscope is being withdrawn. As with any surgical complication, prompt intraoperative recognition and early treatment may limit damage, curtail associated haemorrhage and prevent associated complications.

It should be stressed that, if performed carefully, intraoperative endoscopy can be carried out without complications in the great majority of patients.

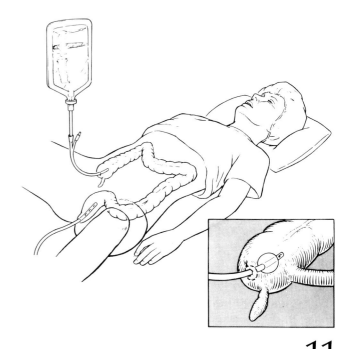

11

References

1. Espiner HJ, Salmon PR, Teaque RH, Read AE. Operative colonoscopy. *BMJ* 1973; 1: 453–4.

2. Whelan RL, Buls JG, Goldberg SM, Rothenberger DA. Intraoperative endoscopy: University of Minnesota experience. *Am Surg* 1989; 55: 281–6.

3. Cohen JL, Forde KA. Intraoperative colonoscopy. *Ann Surg* 1988; 207: 231–3.

4. Bowden TA, Hooks VH, Mansberger AR. Intestinal vascular ectasias: a new look at an old disease. *South Med J* 1982; 75: 1310–17.

5. Lau WY. Intraoperative enteroscopy – indications and limitations. *Gastrointest Endosc* 1990; 36: 268–71.

6. Campbell WB, Rhodes M, Kettlewell MG. Colonoscopy following intraoperative lavage in the management of severe colonic bleeding. *Ann R Coll Surg Engl* 1985; 67: 290–2.

Lasers in colorectal surgery

Brock M. Bordelon MD
Department of Surgery, University of Utah School of Medicine, Salt Lake City, Utah, USA

John G. Hunter MD
Department of Surgery, Emory University Hospital, Atlanta, Georgia, USA

History

Surgeons have been actively involved in the development of laser technology since its advent over 30 years ago. The role of lasers in surgery will continue to expand with the evolution of new wavelengths and new delivery systems.

The concept of *maser* (*m*icrowave *a*mplification by *s*timulated *e*mission of *r*adiation), was first introduced in 1955 by Gordon *et al.*[1]. The ruby laser was developed in 1960, and the neodymium yttrium–aluminium–garnet (NdYAG), argon, and CO_2 lasers were developed over the following few years[2,3]. The first surgical application of lasers followed soon thereafter[4], but it was not until the advent of flexible, thin quartz fibreoptic wave guides (laser fibres) in the 1970s that endoscopic application of laser energy became possible[5]. The argon laser was first used clinically in 1975 to control upper gastrointestinal haemorrhage[6,7].

Laser physics, tissue interaction, and safety

Overview of laser physics

When an electron is excited from its resting state to a higher energy state by the absorption of energy, it rapidly returns to its resting state spontaneously, releasing the absorbed energy as a photon. When this first photon encounters another excited electron it stimulates the release of a second photon, which is in phase temporally and spatially with the first photon. These two photons encounter two more excited electrons, causing a snowballing effect. This process is known as *amplification*, hence the acronym LASER (Light Amplification by Stimulated Emission of Radiation). A laser beam is a monochromatic (single wavelength) parallel column of light in which the photons are in phase across time and space (*Figure 1*).

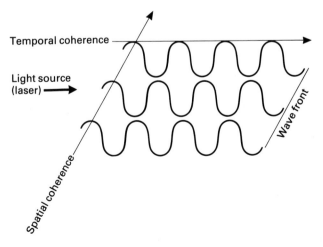

Figure 1

151

Such an arrangement is termed *coherent* light (a laser beam), which is then amplified between a pair of mirrors at either end of the laser medium and is emitted from a small hole in the centre of one of the mirrors. A lens focuses the beam upon the target or the end of a laser fibre.

Many lasers have been developed for medical use, each emitting light of a single wavelength from the infrared to the ultraviolet portion of the spectrum. A few newer lasers can be 'tuned' to emit light at several wavelengths.

Laser–tissue interaction

When laser energy interacts with tissue, it can be reflected, absorbed, scattered, or transmitted[8]. The amount of energy absorbed depends on the wavelength of the laser and the amount of chromophore in the tissue. The most common chromophores are water, haemoglobin, and melanin. Each wavelength is absorbed differently by each chromophore, yielding a predictable depth of tissue injury for each type of laser (*Figure 2*).

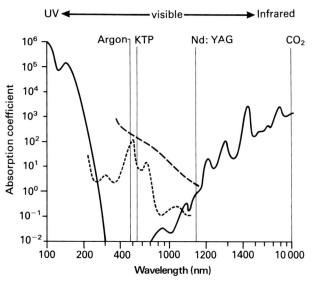

Figure 2. Absorption of light by chromophores: —— water; ––– melanin; ···· oxyhaemoglobin

Lasers destroy tissue by generating thermal injury, converting the energy of the laser beam into kinetic energy. The extent of tissue injury depends on the temperature achieved in the target tissue[9] (*Table 1*).

Types of laser

The lasers most commonly used in the clinical setting are the CO_2, argon, KTP and NdYAG lasers. Each has specific medical uses based upon its absorption properties.

Table 1   Thermal effects of laser–tissue interaction

Temperature (°C)	Tissue event	Tissue appearance	Outcome
45	Cell death, oedema, vasodilatation	Erythema, oedema	Cell death, inflammation
60–80	Protein coagulation, contraction of collagen and blood vessels	Tissue turns grey, white, or brown; blood turns black	Death, slough and ulceration, followed by repair
100	Tissue water vaporizes	Hole or ulcer in tissue	Tissue ablated
210	Dehydrated tissue burns	Black tissue glows and disappears; sparks may form	Tissue ablated

Carbon dioxide laser energy ($\lambda = 10.6\,\mu m$) is heavily absorbed by water, making it superb at cutting and vaporizing tissue, resulting in a depth of injury of $50–100\,\mu m$[10]. Unfortunately, transmission of CO_2 energy requires a bulky series of mirrors and an articulating arm, making it cumbersome to use in all but a few situations. There have been many attempts to develop a dependable fibre to deliver CO_2 laser energy but this goal has yet to be realized.

The argon laser ($\lambda = 488–514\,nm$) is heavily absorbed by haemoglobin and produces a uniform, shallow injury ($1\,mm$)[11]. This makes it especially useful for coagulation of vascular malformations and ablating benign mucosal lesions.

The KTP laser (Laserscope, San Jose, California) is a frequency doubled, or wavelength halved, NdYAG laser ($\lambda = 532\,nm$). Frequency doubling is performed with a potassium thionyl phosphate (hence KTP) crystal. The tissue effects of KTP laser energy are similar to those produced by the argon laser.

The NdYAG laser ($\lambda = 1064\,nm$) is less well absorbed by haemoglobin and water, penetrating deeper to produce thermal injury of $3–4\,mm$[12]. Thus, it is useful in treating bulky, space-occupying lesions such as colonic, rectal, and oesophageal malignancies. This is probably the most versatile and widely used laser in the clinical setting.

All of the above lasers can be used in the traditional non-contact mode or in a more recently developed contact mode. By sculpting the end of the quartz laser fibre to a fine tip (for vaporization) or a large orb tip (for coagulation), a variety of effects may be achieved using the same laser wavelength. The fibre tip is placed in direct contact with tissue, allowing more precise application of the laser energy. Contact laser surgery provides the surgeon with more tactile feedback, but delivers energy to a much smaller area and to a shallower depth of tissue, making ablation of large lesions more time consuming.

Safety

An important adjunct to the use of lasers is strict adherence to safety guidelines, including the use of protective eyewear, non-reflective surgical instruments, and non-flammable operating drapes. Furthermore, access to the operating room must be strictly controlled to avoid inadvertent eye injury. Video equipment must similarly be protected with a filter in-line to protect the video chip from the potent laser light. All commercially available endoscope cameras have infrared filters for use with infrared lasers, such as the NdYAG laser. It is essential that a central organization be in place in the hospital to ensure the proper and safe use of lasers.

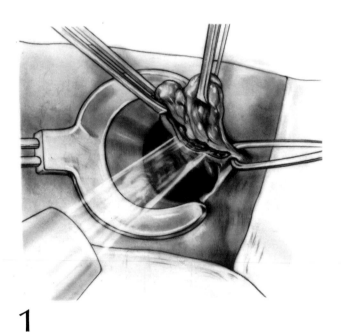

1

Application of lasers to colorectal surgery

Laser haemorrhoidectomy

The use of lasers in the performance of haemorrhoidectomy has become commonplace, but has yet to gain wide acceptance. In several studies, laser haemorrhoidectomy resulted in less pain, bleeding, urinary retention, and a shorter convalescence than conventional haemorrhoidectomy, cryosurgery, or rubber band ligation[12, 13]. Despite this, there remains much scepticism and there is at least one (unpublished) prospective, randomized trial demonstrating no benefit to laser therapy. In that trial, when contact NdYAG laser was used at energy levels greater than 15 W, an increased incidence of wound complications was seen (J. Nicholson, personal communication)[14].

Technique

1   The technique used by the authors for the excision of grade III and IV haemorrhoids is a conventional closed Ferguson haemorrhoidectomy, using the laser as a scalpel. The patient is placed in the prone jack-knife position under spinal or general anaesthesia (see page 49). A polyglactin (Vicryl) transfixion suture is placed at the top of the haemorrhoid column and the remainder of the column is grasped with Allis' clamps. The CO_2 laser, set at 5–10 W and focused to the smallest possible spot size, is used to vaporize the epidermis and mucosa distal to the ligature. Slight bleeding can be handled by defocusing the CO_2 laser beam (i.e. pulling it back), while more copious bleeding must be controlled with electrocautery because of the poor coagulating abilities of the CO_2 wavelength.

Essentially the same method is used for contact NdYAG laser haemorrhoid excision; a sapphire or quartz contact tip is employed, with a continuous power set at 5–10 W. Coagulation is better with a contact probe, and electrocautery is less frequently required. The mucosal defect is closed with a running Vicryl suture.

Grade I and II haemorrhoids may be treated with the NdYAG laser in a non-contact fashion. The patient should be lightly sedated and monitored for vasovagal reactions during treatment. With the NdYAG laser set at 40–60 W, the internal haemorrhoid is treated until the tissue blanches. This may be achieved directly through an anoscope, or through a retroflexed sigmoidoscope. The retroflex technique is a 'spot' technique, wherein the endoscope is moved in a circumferential fashion to coagulate the apex of each haemorrhoid column. This technique must be used cautiously, because the laser beam can easily damage the retroflexed endoscope.

Laser coagulation of grade I and II haemorrhoids offers no significant advantages over more commonly used 'tissue fixation' techniques. Significant sloughing occurs when utilizing direct NdYAG photocoagulation, which may result in large ulcers when too much mucosa has been coagulated. Rubber band ligation or infrared coagulation appears to give at least equivalent results.

Treatment of condylomas

Human papillomavirus infection, which is generally sexually transmitted, gives rise to genital warts that are difficult to eradicate. Treatment methods include use of topical podophyllin, cryosurgery, electrocoagulation and surgical excision (see pp. 806–813); all have high recurrence rates and produce unsatisfactory results. Perianal condyloma acuminata may be treated with laser techniques, most commonly using the CO_2 laser[14].

The laser treatment must extend to areas of normal-appearing epithelium surrounding the lesions because live virus can be found in the prickle cell layer up to 1 cm away from diseased areas. Baggish[15] has reported a 'brush' technique using the CO_2 laser to treat the regions surrounding grossly infected tissue that yields a 91% cure rate with a single treatment. He noted neither scar formation nor anal stricture.

Technique

Under spinal anaesthesia, the patient is placed in the lithotomy position (see chapter on pp. 47–50). With the CO_2 laser set at 5–10 W, all of the obvious lesion is vaporized. The laser is then defocused and the surrounding region is lightly 'brushed'; the outer layer blanches and then reddens with a reactive hyperaemia. Live papillomavirus can be found in laser plumes, therefore intense smoke evacuation is essential during this procedure.

Arteriovenous malformations

Laser therapy is particularly suitable for mucosal and submucosal vascular lesions. Scarlet arteriolar lesions absorb large amounts of argon and KTP laser energy; darker cavernous venous lakes may be better treated with the NdYAG laser. Since the first application of lasers to control gastrointestinal haemorrhage in humans, there has been great interest in their use to control bleeding for colonic vascular ectasias[7]. Unfortunately, there have not been any good randomized trials to compare surgical treatment with endoscopic laser treatment of vascular malformations anywhere in the gastrointestinal tract. Nevertheless, there is a substantial volume of clinical data detailing the effectiveness and safety of endoscopically directed laser therapy for arteriovenous malformations in the colon and elsewhere in the gastrointestinal tract[16].

Endoscopic treatment for lower gastrointestinal tract bleeding at the time of diagnostic colonoscopy is well accepted[17], and bipolar coagulation, monopolar coagulation with 'hot' biopsy forceps, heater probe coagulation, or lasers can be used through standard colonoscopes. Laser photocoagulation of gastrointestinal vascular ectasias offers several advantages over the use of electrosurgery. The depth of injury generated with the argon laser is easier to control and consistently shallower than monopolar electrosurgery injuries[11], which is of particular importance in the caecum, where there is a significant risk of perforation with the use of monopolar current[18]. Argon laser injuries heal rapidly and are re-epithelialized within 3–4 days of treatment. Furthermore, an unacceptable rate of perforation has been documented with the use of the NdYAG laser in this setting[16, 19]. For these reasons, the argon laser is the safest and most effective choice for the treatment of colonic vascular ectasias.

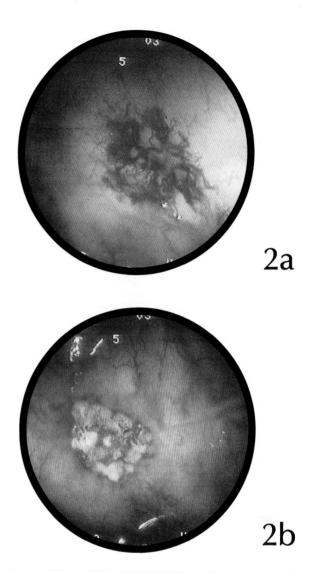

2a

2b

Technique

2a, b With the patient lightly sedated and in the left lateral decubitus position, the colonoscope is advanced to the diseased region. The argon laser, transmitted through a 600-μm sheathed fibre, is held 1 cm from the lesion. The gas in the colon is exchanged for CO_2 flowing around the fibre tip; this reduces the likelihood of intracolonic combustion. Power is initially set at 5 W, continuous, and is increased or decreased according to tissue response (vessel blanching). The likelihood of bleeding is diminished by first coagulating the surrounding feeding vessels. The entire arteriovenous malformation should be treated in a single session, and surveillance endoscopy must be performed to ensure ablation of the entire lesion. Although exceedingly rare, deep-seated arteriovenous malformations of the rectum may require treatment with the NdYAG laser to achieve adequate tissue penetration.

Radiation proctitis

Injury to the intestine is a well-known complication of radiation used in the treatment of neoplasia. Chronic radiation injury may be seen following treatment of gynaecological, prostatic, or urinary bladder malignancy and is associated with formation of fistulae, stricture, perforation, and blood loss. Bleeding occurs in 6–8% of patients with chronic radiation enteritis, and the rectum is a common site of injury because of its fixed location in the pelvis[20]. The common endoscopic appearance of radiation-injured bowel is a pale, friable, atrophic epithelium which may have multiple vascular ectasias. Severe chronic haemorrhage from the injured bowel may be refractory to conservative management and render the patient transfusion-dependent. Multiple approaches to this difficult problem have been tried, including steroid enemas, antibiotics, sulphasalazine,

and surgical resection. However, surgical procedures upon irradiated bowel are fraught with complications[20].

Endoscopic laser therapy is a promising way to treat the transfusion-dependent patient with radiation proctitis[21]. Argon therapy is well tolerated and is safer to use than the deeply penetrating NdYAG laser. Because of the significant morbidity and mortality rates associated with surgical management of this disorder, endoscopic argon laser management should be considered as first-line therapy.

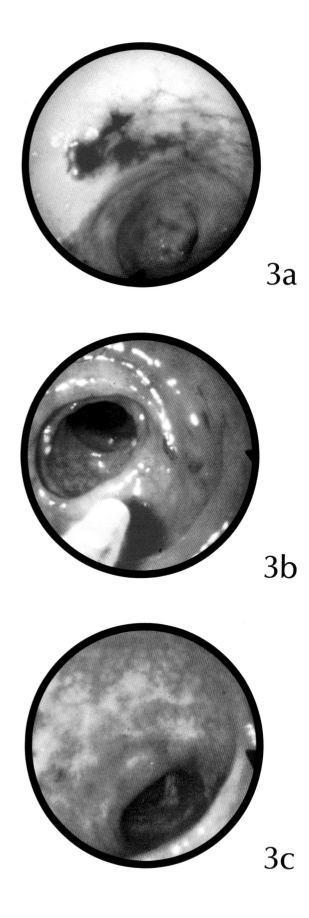

3a

3b

3c

Technique

3a–c Argon laser photocoagulation of radiation proctitis is undertaken in the same way as photocoagulation of arteriovenous malformations. Preparation of the rectum with a sodium phosphate enema is generally acceptable, and rectal gas must be exchanged for CO_2 before treatment. The initial power setting should be low (approximately 5 W). The laser is used in the non-contact mode in bursts of 0.5–5.0 s, until tissue blanching occurs. Liberal surveillance endoscopy should be employed to monitor this chronic condition. *Illustration 3a* shows a friable lesion in the proximal rectum; *Illustration 3b* shows the application of the argon laser fibre, which causes minimal scarring (*Illustration 3c*).

Adenomatous colorectal polyps

Laser photoablation of adenomatous polyps, although frequently employed in many centres, remains controversial. Histological examination of all polyp tissue is traditionally used to exclude the presence of invasive malignancy, but when laser energy is used to ablate adenomas, the ability to examine the tissue is lost, giving the potential of missing a carcinoma which could be resected curatively. Endoscopic laser treatment of colorectal adenomas should therefore be limited to a few well-defined clinical situations.

Treatment of familial polyposis involves either abdominal colectomy with mucosal proctectomy and ileoanal pull-through or subtotal colectomy with ileorectal anastomosis. The latter procedure leaves 10–15 cm of rectal mucosa at risk for development of polyps which must be periodically sought by endoscopic examination. Polyps found during surveillance can be eradicated using argon laser photocoagulation at 2–5 W after first obtaining histological specimens from the largest polyps in the rectal stump. This technique provides adequate surveillance and causes less scarring than extensive electrosurgical polypectomy. Laser therapy for control of adenoma in patients with familial polyposis following subtotal colectomy provides good control in most cases and does not produce the severe scarring that makes subsequent mucosal proctectomy and ileoanal anastomosis more difficult[22].

Successful NdYAG laser ablation of rectosigmoid villous adenomas has been reported by several centres[23], with a recurrence rate of 15–20%, and subsequent discovery of cancer in 5% of patients. Patients with adenomas encircling more than 50% of the lumen have significant risk of rectosigmoid stricture following laser treatment and a greater risk of developing carcinoma than do patients with smaller lesions, and should undergo excisional therapy if possible. Similarly, those lesions with high-grade dysplasia or invasive carcinoma should be surgically resected. Some of these lesions may be excised successfully with transanal endoscopic microsurgical techniques[24] (*see* pp. 228–239).

Technique

The patient is sedated and positioned as for routine diagnostic colonoscopy. Small adenomatous polyps are treated with the argon laser set at 2–5 W, continuous, until blanching is achieved. Larger villous adenomas should be debulked with a diathermy snare at an initial session, followed by treatment with the NdYAG laser approximately 1 week later. The entire lesion is coagulated (not vaporized) with 40–60 W of NdYAG laser delivered through a 600-μm gastrointestinal fibre. The adenoma is treated at intervals of 4 to 7 days to allow necrotic tissue to slough between sessions. Sodium phosphate enemas are usually adequate preparation, but the colonoscopist must exchange all rectal gas

with CO_2 to lessen the explosion risk. Surveillance endoscopy with biopsies should be undertaken at 3-month intervals for the first year following completion of treatment, every 6 months for the second year, and yearly thereafter.

Laser palliation of colonic and rectal malignancies

Colorectal malignancy is common, with three-quarters of afflicted patients undergoing resection for cure. However, there is a subgroup of patients who are too debilitated or are unwilling to undergo surgery. These patients should be considered for palliative measures to provide symptomatic relief.

A variety of palliative measures have been devised to treat the inoperable patient with rectal cancer. Cryosurgical treatment of bulky rectal tumours is associated with a 20% complication rate. Electrocoagulation, while effective, has been reported to have a complication rate of 21%. Radiation therapy rarely provides adequate palliation without the addition of surgical excision. Endoscopic laser therapy has the advantages of good patient tolerance, outpatient treatment, avoidance of general anaesthesia and operative risks, excellent control of bleeding and obstructive symptoms, and no dose limitation.

Elderly patients with early rectal carcinoma can be treated with a combination of NdYAG laser, transanal excision, and external beam radiation. The order in which these modalities are employed depends primarily upon the patient's symptoms. Laser treatment, when used as the initial therapy, rapidly alleviates troublesome bleeding. Patients with mild or no symptoms are probably best served by transanal excision and radiation, followed by laser therapy for tumour recurrence. Transanal endoscopic microsurgery may be appropriately used for some of these patients (*see* chapter on pp. 228–239).

Palliative treatment of advanced rectal carcinoma is readily accomplished with non-contact NdYAG laser therapy. In the authors' experience, exophytic lesions and those that are prone to bleeding respond best to this type of treatment, while circumferential lesions respond poorly.

Technique

The same technique as is used for villous adenomas is applied for rectal cancer. After exchanging all rectal gas with CO_2, the NdYAG laser is used to coagulate the entire lesion. Power is set at 40–60 W, and a 600-μm gastrointestinal fibre is used for laser delivery. Treatment continues at intervals of 4–7 days until the entire tumour has been ablated. Because of the significant fibrosis and deep invasion that may be associated with cancer, complete ablation is difficult to obtain for all but the most superficial cancers.

4a–f The appearance following treatment of rectal cancer with the NdYAG laser and transanal excision in a 66-year-old man is presented: before treatment (*Illustration 4a*); immediately after the first session (*Illustration 4b*); before the third session (*Illustration 4c*); after external beam radiation therapy (*Illustration 4d*); when transanal resection was complete (*Illustration 4e*); 16 months after transanal resection (*Illustration 4f*), the region is biopsy-negative for carcinoma.

The NdYAG laser may also be used to recanalize obstructing carcinomas in the left colon and rectum[25]. With the patient under light intravenous sedation, a Savary guidewire is advanced through the narrowed lumen under fluoroscopic guidance. The lumen is then gradually dilated with Savary dilators to allow insertion of a paediatric gastroscope to the proximal extent of the tumour. The NdYAG laser, set at 70–100 W, is fired in bursts of 0.5–1.0 s to ablate the tumour circumferentially in a retrograde fashion. Orthograde bowel preparation is then performed, and the patient avoids the complications attendant with resection in the face of unprepared bowel. This type of therapy is not necessary for obstructed tumours in the transverse and right colon, where a one-stage procedure is feasible.

Photodynamic therapy

Photodynamic therapy uses the principle of sensitizing selected tissue to a specific wavelength of light with a photosensitizing compound, then inciting destruction of the tissue with light of that wavelength. Many photoactive compounds, most notably the porphyrins, concentrate in neoplastic tissue; haematoporphyrin derivative is the most widely used photosensitizer. Application of light at the correct wavelength activates these compounds, generating a cytotoxic effect through the generation of singlet oxygen[26]. Laser light is useful in photodynamic therapy because it is intense and monochromatic; red light is generally used because it penetrates tissue and tumours more deeply than the shorter wavelengths.

To date, most of the experience gained with photodynamic therapy has been for palliation of oesophageal malignancy, but applications have expanded to include bronchogenic, gastric, bladder, and colorectal carcinomas[27]. Photodynamic therapy has several appealing aspects but also several problems that need to be overcome before it becomes more widely used. The ideal photosensitizer has yet to be found and most compounds cause severe cutaneous photosensitivity. After treatment with haematoporphyrin derivative, patients must remain covered from the sun and bright lights for a month to avoid full-thickness sunburn. The depth of tissue destruction is small, limiting the use of this therapy to superficial lesions and for palliative

measures. The development of tumour-selective photo-active compounds which are active at long wavelengths (>700 nm) and the further refinement of tunable dye lasers may make photodynamic therapy a useful tool in the future.

Technique

Photosensitization is achieved with intravenous haematoporphyrin derivative administration, given over 1 hour in a totally darkened room. The patient is kept away from direct light for 24–72 hours, after which time laser irradiation is performed. Most commonly, a tunable argon-pumped dye laser is used to deliver laser light endoscopically through a 200–400-µm quartz fibre. Straight-cut, spherical, or cylindrical fibre tips may be used, depending upon the desired pattern of light delivery. The fibre tip is placed 2–3 cm from the lesion, power is set at 300–400 mW, and each area is treated for 5 min. Light delivery to the surface of the lesion is fairly homogeneous with this therapy, but deeper penetration of laser energy is relatively poor. This problem may be partially overcome by interstitial insertion of a cylindrical or spherical fibre tip.

New wavelengths

Lasers currently in wide use have several problems which put the surgeon at a disadvantage: gas lasers (such as the argon laser) require frequent tube changes; most lasers require high power input and water cooling because they are very inefficient; dye lasers require expensive dye systems and frequent dye changes. Reliability, portability, and ease of use are paramount in the busy surgeon's practice. Thus the optimal laser would be solid-state and tunable over a wide range of wavelengths.

High-energy pulsed lasers, such as the erbium:YAG, holmium:YAG, excimer, and flash-lamp pumped-dye lasers, have several advantages over continuous wave argon or NdYAG lasers. With far shorter pulse durations and much higher peak power output, these lasers injure tissue with much less total energy, thereby creating less thermal injury to the region adjacent to the target tissue. The free electron laser converts an electron beam to a photon beam and can be tuned to any wavelength, but is expensive and far too large for clinical use.

Lasers that can be used as 'scalpels' have wavelengths in the ultraviolet or infrared portions of the spectrum, where absorption by water is prominent, delivering large amounts of energy and cutting tissue in a non-thermal manner. Excimer lasers such as the argon fluoride ($\lambda = 193$ nm) and the krypton fluoride ($\lambda = 248$ nm) are superb at non-thermal tissue cutting, but are not portable and require all of the maintenance of other gas lasers.

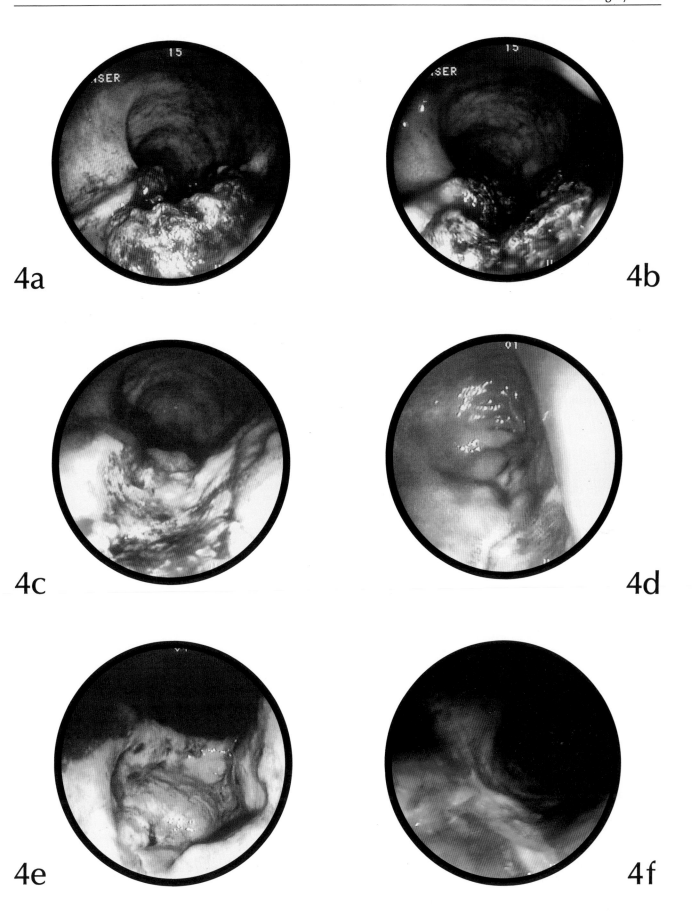

4a

4b

4c

4d

4e

4f

New procedures

Prevention of anastomotic leakage, occurring in approximately 4% of all colonic anastomoses, might avoid potentially fatal complications[28]. Experimental work on sutureless tissue welding has some promise but has yet to achieve the strength seen with conventional sutured anastomoses. More promising data come from studies of reinforcing sutured anastomoses. Low-power laser energy applied to experimental rat colon anastomoses has produced a significant increase in anastomotic strength[29].

Conclusions

Over the last two decades, lasers have grown from investigational tools to being widely used. The NdYAG and argon lasers are now a valuable part of the surgical endoscopist's armamentarium, providing effective and safe palliation of colorectal malignancy, control of haemorrhage from arteriovenous malformations and radiation-injured mucosa, and ablation of adenomatous polyps in selected patients. The role of lasers in the treatment of lower gastrointestinal tract disease will certainly expand with the development of new laser wavelengths and effective endoscopic photodynamic therapy.

References

1. Gordon JP, Zigler HJ, Townes CH. The maser – new type of amplifier, frequency standard, and spectrometer. *Physiol Rev* 1955; 99: 1264–74.

2. Maiman TH. Stimulated optical radiation in ruby. *Nature* 1960; 187: 493–4.

3. Patel CKN, McFarlane RA, Faust WL. Selective excitation through vibrational energy transfer and optical maser action in N_2–CO_2. *Physiol Rev* 1964; 13: 617–19.

4. McGuff PE, Bushnell D, Soroff HS, Seterling RA. Studies of the surgical applications of laser (light amplification by the stimulated emission of radiation). *Surg Forum* 1963; 14: 143–5.

5. Nath G, Gorisch W, Kiefhaber P. First laser endoscopy via a fiberoptic transmission system. *Endoscopy* 1973; 5: 208–13.

6. Dwyer RM, Haverback BJ, Bass M, Cherlow J. Laser-induced hemostasis in the canine stomach. *JAMA* 1975; 231: 486–9.

7. Frühmorgen P, Bodem F, Reidenbach HD, Kaduk B, Demling L. Endoscopic laser coagulation of bleeding gastrointestinal lesions with report of the first therapeutic application in man. *Gastrointest Endosc* 1976; 23: 73–5.

8. Fuller T. Fundamentals of lasers in surgery and medicine. In: Dixon JA, ed. *Surgical Applications of Lasers*. Chicago: Year Book, 1983; 11–27.

9. Hunter JG, Burt RW, Becker JM *et al*. Colonic mucosal lesions: evaluation of monopolar electrocautery, argon laser, and Nd:YAG laser. *Curr Surg* 1984; 41: 373.

10. Dixon JA. Current laser applications in general surgery. *Ann Surg* 1988; 207: 355–72.

11. Hunter JG, Burt RW, Becker JM, Lee RG, Dixon JA. Quantitation of colonic injury from argon laser, neodymium:YAG laser and monopolar electrocautery applied to flat mucosa and small sessile polyps of the canine colon. *Gastrointest Endosc* 1989; 35: 16–21.

12. Wang JY, Chang-Chien CR, Chen JS, Lai CR, Tang RP. The role of lasers in hemorrhoidectomy. *Dis Colon Rectum* 1991; 34: 78–82.

13. Sankar MY, Joffe SN. Laser surgery in colonic and anorectal lesions. *Surg Clin North Am* 1988; 68: 1447–69.

14. Scott RS, Castro DJ. Treatment of condyloma acuminata with carbon dioxide laser: a prospective study. *Lasers Surg Med* 1984; 4: 157–62.

15. Baggish MS. Improved laser techniques for the elimination of genital and extragenital warts. *Am J Obstet Gynecol* 1985; 153: 545–50.

16. Rutgeerts P, van Gompel F, Geboes K, Vantrappen G, Broeckaert L, Coremans G. Long term results of treatment of vascular malformations of the gastrointestinal tract by Neodymium YAG laser photocoagulation. *Gut* 1985; 26: 586–93.

17. Jensen DM, Machicado GA. Diagnosis and treatment of severe hematochezia: the role of urgent colonoscopy after purge. *Gastroenterology* 1988; 95: 1569–74.

18. Howard OM, Buchanan JD, Hunt RH. Angiodysplasia of the colon. *Lancet* 1982; ii: 16–19.

19. Gostout CJ, Bowyer BA, Ahlquist DA, Viggiano TR, Balm RK. Mucosal vascular malformations of the gastrointestinal tract: clinical observations and results of endoscopic neodymium: yttrium–aluminum–garnet laser therapy. *Mayo Clin Proc* 1988; 63: 993–1003.

20. Galland RB, Spencer J. Surgical aspects of radiation injury to the intestine. *Br J Surg* 1979; 66: 135–8.

21. Buchi KN, Dixon JA. Argon laser treatment of hemorrhagic radiation proctitis. *Gastrointest Endosc* 1987; 33: 27–30.

22. Hunter JG, Becker JM, Burt RW, Dixon JA. Colonic mucosal dissection following electrocautery or laser polypectomy. *J Surg Res* 1986; 40: 534–9.

23. Mathus-Vliegen EMH, Tytgat GNJ. The potential and limitations of laser photoablation of colorectal adenomas. *Gastrointest Endosc* 1991; 37: 9–17.

24. Buess B, Mentges B, Manneke K, Starlinger M, Becker HD. Technique and results of transanal endoscopic microsurgery in early rectal cancer. *Am J Surg* 1992; 163: 63–70.

25. Eckhauser ML, Imbembo AL, Mansour EG. The role of preresectional laser recanalization for obstructing carcinomas of the colon and rectum. *Surgery* 1989; 106: 710–17.

26. Gilbertson JJ, Dixon JA. Photodynamic therapy: basic aspects and tissue interaction. In: Jensen DM, Brunetaud JM, eds. *Medical Laser Endoscopy*. Dordrecht: Kluwer Academic Publishers 1990: 295–311.

27. Patrice T, Foultier MT, Yactayo S *et al*. Endoscopic photodynamic therapy with hematoporphyrin derivative for primary treatment of gastrointestinal neoplasms in inoperable patients. *Dig Dis Sci* 1990; 35: 545–52.

28. Mileski WJ, Joehl RJ, Rege RV, Nahrwold DL. Treatment of anastomotic leakage following low anterior colon resection. *Arch Surg* 1988; 123: 968–70.

29. Moazami N, Oz MC, Bass LS, Treat MR. Reinforcement of colonic anastomoses with a laser and dye-enhanced fibrinogen. *Arch Surg* 1990; 125: 1452–4.

Illustrations by Marks Creative Consultants

Basic laparoscopy and instrumentation

Karl A. Zucker MD, FACS
Professor of Surgery, University of New Mexico School of Medicine, Albuquerque, New Mexico, USA

Daniel T. Martin MD, FACS
Assistant Professor, University of New Mexico School of Medicine, Albuquerque, New Mexico, USA

Principles

Laparoscopy is a form of endoscopy in which the surgeon uses a rigid telescope to visualize the abdominal cavity. The goal of this form of endoscopic surgery is for the surgeon to diagnose and/or treat various intra-abdominal disorders without the need for larger, more disabling laparotomy incisions. Although laparoscopy has been used for several decades as a diagnostic tool by both surgeons and gastroenterologists, recent advances in television camera miniaturization and other instrumentation now make it possible to perform a multitude of therapeutic procedures.

Laparoscopic surgery differs from conventional surgery in several ways. Specific skills and instrumentation are required to perform laparoscopy in a safe and efficacious manner. The peritoneal cavity must be distended with carbon dioxide (CO_2) or other gases to provide the necessary exposure and space in which to operate. The use of a rigid laparoscope alters the surgeon's perspective and severely limits the field of view. In addition, most contemporary surgeons attach a specially designed video camera to the eyepiece of the laparoscope and visualize the peritoneal cavity with high-resolution video monitors. The advantage of this arrangement is that the entire surgical team can observe and participate in the operative procedure. The disadvantage is that video imaging lacks the depth perception on which most surgeons depend when performing abdominal surgery. In addition, the lack of tactile sensation when using laparoscopic instruments which are 30 cm or more in length is a limitation.

Despite these problems surgeons have found an ever increasing role for this minimally invasive form of surgery. Procedures such as cholecystectomy, appendicectomy, colonic resection, truncal and selective vagotomy and antireflux surgery are now performed in many community and academic medical centres. For the majority of these procedures many of the basic instruments and methods of establishing the pneumoperitoneum are similar. The following is a brief discussion of the basic manoeuvres that are used at the beginning of most laparoscopic procedures and the devices that are required.

Preoperative

Patients are prepared for laparoscopic surgery in an almost identical fashion as for conventional surgery, so that conversion from the laparoscopic approach to an open technique can be undertaken if the intra-abdominal findings preclude the minimally invasive technique or if there are complications. For most therapeutic laparoscopic procedures, a urinary catheter and a nasogastric tube are inserted to decompress the bladder and stomach, which will decrease the likelihood of their injury during the insertion of the insufflation needle or trocar, and will allow better visualization of the upper and lower abdomen[1].

Operations

In order to have space in which to manipulate the instruments and visualize the visceral structures, the peritoneal cavity must be distended with a gas. Early laparoscopists used room air infused into the peritoneal cavity with a hand-pumped syringe attached to a percutaneously placed needle[2]. The two most common gases now used are CO_2 and nitrous oxide (N_2O). The latter is used almost exclusively for diagnostic procedures because it has mild anaesthetic properties which makes it possible to perform the procedure using local anaesthesia alone. If electrocautery or lasers are to be used, N_2O should not be selected because this gas supports combustion.

The agent of choice for therapeutic laparoscopy is CO_2, because it suppresses combustion, is relatively innocuous to the peritoneum, and is readily available in most operating theatres.

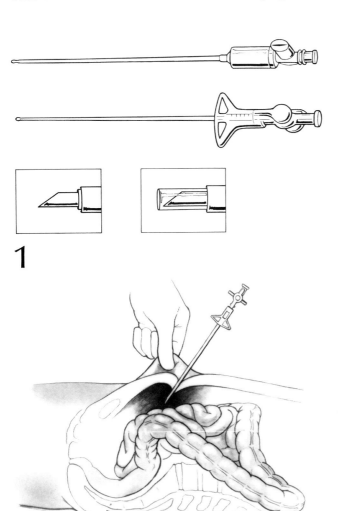

1

2

PNEUMOPERITONEUM: CLOSED METHOD

1 Initial access to the peritoneal cavity may be accomplished with a percutaneous approach using a specially designed needle (Verres needle). The sheath of this insufflation needle contains a blunt obturator which retracts over the sharp point after the tip has entered the peritoneal space.

2 The umbilicus is the most common site for insertion of the insufflation needle, because it is the thinnest portion of the abdominal wall and there is only one fascial layer to penetrate. A small incision is made in the upper or lower folds of the umbilicus and the abdominal wall is lifted upwards. This manoeuvre increases the surgeon's tactile sensation as the needle is guided into the peritoneal cavity. The needle is directed slightly caudad in the midline. This direction minimizes the likelihood of the needle injuring the aorta or iliac vessels. Many surgeons place the patient in a 15–20° Trendelenburg position to displace the small intestine and colon out of the pelvis, which reduces their risk of injury. The advantage of this manoeuvre, however, has never been convincingly demonstrated.

Several additional steps are then taken before commencing insufflation to ensure that the tip of the needle is positioned appropriately. A syringe is attached to the end of the needle, and the barrel is flushed with a few millilitres of saline to remove any tissue. The syringe is then aspirated and if blood, urine or intestinal contents are observed the needle should be removed and discarded. Most insufflation needle injuries are self-limiting and do not necessarily mandate an immediate laparotomy. The pneumoperitoneum can be established by inserting a second needle or, preferably, by the open technique. The site of injury can then be examined directly with the laparoscope and a decision made as to whether a laparotomy is necessary.

3   The next step is to place a small drop of saline over the hub of the insufflation needle and then pull upwards on the abdominal wall (sometimes referred to as the Palmer or saline drop test). This creates a relative negative pressure within the peritoneal cavity, and if the needle is in the proper location the fluid should be drawn through the barrel.

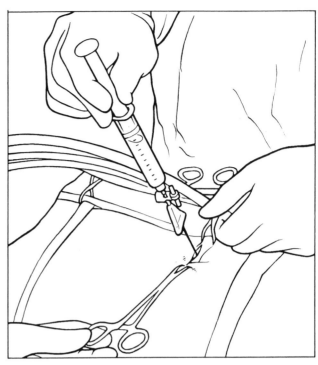

3

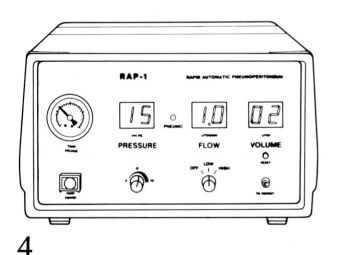

4

4   The final and most important step in confirming the proper location of the needle is measurement of the insufflation pressure. The hub of the needle is connected to an electronic insufflation device and gas flow (1–2 l/min) is commenced. Modern insufflation machines are capable of directly measuring the resistance to gas flow through the insufflation needle. If the tip of the needle is in the true peritoneal cavity, the gas will meet minimal resistance to flow and therefore the pressure should generally be less that 8.0 mmHg (which represents the resistance of gas flow from the tubing and the small barrel of the needle). If the needle is in a closed space, such as the prefascial space, omentum, or retroperitoneum, the gas flow will meet immediate resistance and the pressure will rise quickly.

After confirming the proper location of the needle the gas flow can be increased. Insufflators vary in their ability to pump gas into the peritoneal cavity. Most surgeons prefer a device with a maximum flow rate of 8–10 l/min, although machines capable of 15 l/min are now available. Insufflation devices also have automatic shut-off capabilities so that gas flow will cease once a preset level is reached. For most therapeutic laparoscopic procedures, this pressure should be set no higher than 14–15 mmHg. If the intra-abdominal pressure rises above this preset level, audible and/or visual alarms are activated. Higher pressures increase the likelihood of subcutaneous emphysema, pneumomediastinum, respiratory compromise and gas emboli.

5 After the abdomen has been adequately distended (usually 3–4 litres in a 70-kg adult), one or more laparoscopic cannulae are inserted through the anterior abdominal wall. These are specially designed sheaths with one-way valves that allow various instruments to be introduced into the peritoneal cavity without loss of pneumoperitoneum.

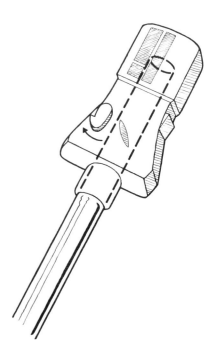

5

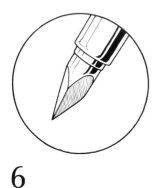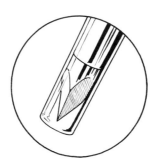

6

6 A sharp obturator placed through the length of the cannula is used to penetrate the abdominal fascia and peritoneum. These are available with either a conical or pyramidal shape. Laparoscopic cannulae are manufactured in both reusable (metal) and disposable (plastic) versions. The latter have become very popular in recent years because they are available with safety shields which retract over the sharp tip after the obturator has entered the peritoneal cavity[3].

The first cannula is generally inserted blindly through the umbilicus with the same care as was used with the introduction of the insufflation needle. If additional sheaths are desired, a laparoscope is placed through the initial sheath and used to guide the remaining cannulae.

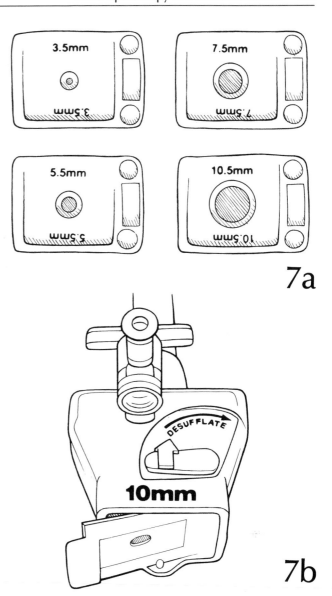

7a

7b

7a, b Laparoscopic cannulae are available in a variety of sizes ranging from 3 to 40 mm in diameter. The most common are 5 mm and 10/11 mm in diameter. Larger sized cannulae are used with specialized instruments with larger diameters, e.g. linear stapling instruments. Special adaptors or converters are used when a smaller sized instrument is inserted through a larger cannula.

Most laparoscopic cannulae also have an insufflation port in order to maintain the pneumoperitoneum.

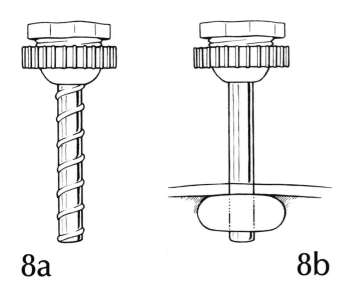

8a   **8b**

8a, b To minimize the problem of inadvertently pulling the cannula out of the abdominal wall, threaded sleeves (gripping devices) can be applied over the sheath. Other cannulae are designed with a balloon-like device which can be insufflated below the fascia.

PNEUMOPERITONEUM: OPEN METHOD

9a, b The open or Hasson technique is basically a mini-laparotomy performed over the intended site of primary cannula placement[4]. A somewhat larger (2.0–2.5-cm) incision is made in the folds of the umbilicus and the peritoneal cavity entered under direct vision.

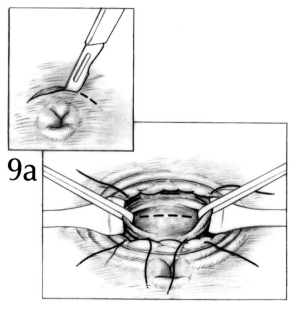

9a

9b

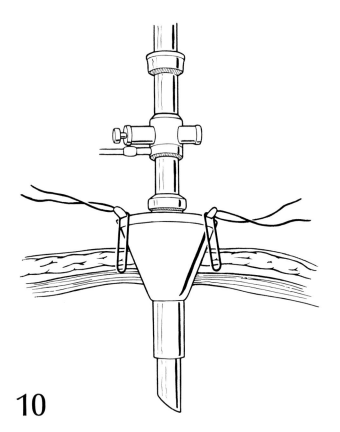

10

10 Specialized cannulae are available with cone-shaped sleeves to minimize any leakage of gas around this larger fascial opening. Large (0 or 2/0) sutures are placed through the edges of the fascial defect and secured to special wings on the sides of the cannula. These help prevent slippage or inadvertent removal of the cannula.

Many surgeons believe that this method of accessing the peritoneal cavity should be used routinely to avoid the risks of insertion of the insufflation needle[5]. Others use the open method only if there has been previous surgery near the umbilicus or if difficulty has occurred with the percutaneous approach[6].

Instrumentation

Laparoscopes and light sources

11 Rigid laparoscopes have undergone a number of major design changes over the past few decades. The most commonly used devices have the solid quartz rod design introduced by Hopkins in the 1960s for image transmission[7]. The light source is separate from the laparoscope, and most contemporary units use either a halide or xenon high-intensity light bulb. The power or light intensity of these machines varies from 100 W to 300 W. The term 'cold light source' is often used because only a fraction of the heat generated by the light bulb is delivered to the laparoscope. This heat is either blocked by specially designed shields or eliminated with high-speed fans within the light source. Light is transmitted from the source via a flexible light cord which is attached to the proximal portion of the laparoscope.

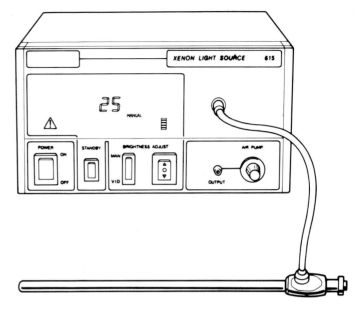

11

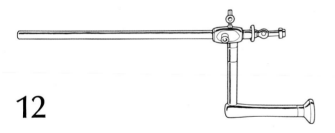

12

12 The most commonly used laparoscopes are either 5 mm or 10 mm in diameter, with the larger devices delivering a better image. Some rigid laparoscopes (often referred to as 'working laparoscopes') contain a working channel through the centre which allows the surgeon to insert various instruments without the need for an additional cannula. Because the optical channel is smaller, the image is inferior to that achieved with an 'operating laparoscope'.

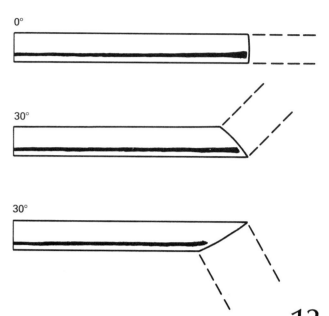

13 Both side-viewing and forward-viewing laparoscopes are available depending on the angle incorporated within the distal portion of the endoscope. The side-viewing laparoscopes allow greater versatility in visualizing the peritoneal cavity, but are more difficult to use. With these instruments the surgeon can look up, down, left or right by simply rotating the shaft of the endoscope.

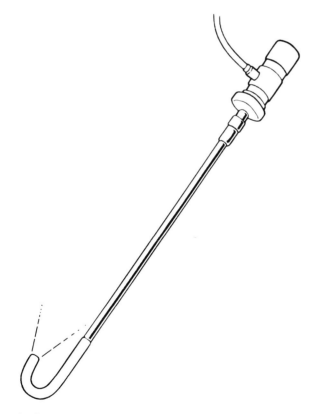

14 In an effort to improve on the concept of the side-viewing endoscope, semirigid laparoscopes with deflectable tips have been designed. These instruments offer the ability to see round solid structures within the abdomen. Unfortunately, the quality of the image transmitted is inferior to that obtained with traditional rigid laparoscopes.

Video cameras

15 In order for the entire surgical team to see the peritoneal cavity and participate in the operation, a video camera is attached to the eyepiece of the laparoscope. One or more video monitors are then positioned in the operating theatre, depending on the operative procedure and the preference of the surgeon. An end-viewing video camera transmits the entire image to the video monitors, while a split-beam camera is designed with an eyepiece so that the surgeon can look directly through the laparoscope as well as have a video image. With the latter configuration, the light from the operative field is split, and therefore the brightness and quality of the image is compromised. As most surgeons watch the video monitor(s) while performing laparoscopy, the split-beam design has not been popular.

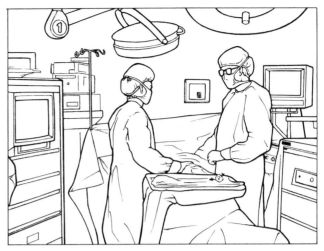

15

Although the clarity and sharpness of the transmitted image vary between different manufacturers, the quality of the picture will depend mainly on whether the camera is designed with one video chip (with approximately 450 lines of resolution) or three chips (700–800 lines). The latter clearly offers an advantage in picture quality and colour perception, but is considerably more expensive than the one-chip designs.

Certain features are common to all of these cameras. They must be capable of colour balancing or white balancing to reliably project an accurate image. This is important because colour perception is highly dependent on the quality of the light source. As the intensity of the light source may vary (as the bulb ages or with a different machine), it is important to calibrate the video

system each time so that it may accurately duplicate the entire colour spectrum without distortion. Before each use, the camera is directed at a white background and the camera calibrated.

Many video cameras adjust to variations in light sensitivity during use. This is usually by means of an automatic iris which measures the available light and adjusts the aperture accordingly. Some systems can also interact directly with the light source and the intensity.

All video cameras have a focusing mechanism, but many are also equipped with a zoom or magnification lens. An important consideration is the focal length of the lens system. Some laparoscopes require frequent focusing adjustments as they move in and out of the operative field.

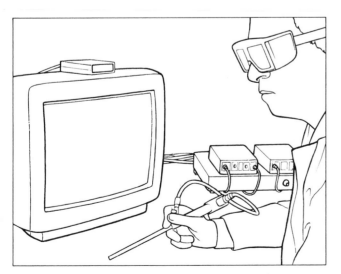

16 One of the most limiting aspects of operating with a video-projected image is the lack of depth perception. Three-dimensional video systems, which attempt to address this problem, are in the final stages of development.[8]

Two specially designed video cameras are connected to a rigid laparoscope, with the image processed through a computer and projected on a customized RGB video monitor. Depending on the type of system being employed, the user must wear either powered interactive or passive glasses with special filters and lens.

16

Energy modalities

A variety of different energy devices is available for tissue dissection and haemostasis. These include monopolar and bipolar electrocautery, lasers and the argon beam coagulator. Each modality has its own particular advantages and disadvantages.[9, 10]

The most familiar and popular energy source among general surgeons is the electrocautery device. These machines use microwave energy (500–750 kHz) to produce heat to dissect and coagulate tissues. Contemporary electrosurgical generators provide this form of energy in three separate waveforms: cut, coagulation and blend. Monopolar and bipolar electrocautery differ in the path of the electrical current. Monopolar current is applied through the tip of the surgical instrument and is then conducted through the body, exiting via a grounding pad. Bipolar devices are designed with both electrical contact points at the tip of the instrument. Therefore, the electrical energy, i.e. electrons, flows directly between these points interacting only with the tissue lying in this path. The result is that monopolar electrical energy is far less predictable than bipolar energy, because the flow of electrons will follow the path of least resistance through the body. Therefore, it is possible for tissues distant from the cautery tip to be injured. Although several manufacturers have attempted to develop laparoscopic bipolar instruments, the need to have both electrodes in close proximity has limited their application.

The safety of monopolar electrocautery during laparoscopy has recently been studied by several clinical investigators, and their work appears to support its safety when used with certain precautions[11, 12]. First, the insulation material on the instrument should be routinely inspected, and if damaged the device should be immediately repaired or discarded. The power settings used should be less than 25–30 W and the surgeon should apply only short bursts of energy. In addition, the tip of the cautery device should always be under direct visualization and kept well away from adjacent visceral tissues.

The argon beam coagulator (Birtcher Medical Systems, Irvine, California, USA) uses a gentle flow of argon gas to deliver a monopolar energy current. An advantage of this device is that the gas blows away blood from the operative field, which improves the coagulative effect. The depth of the thermal effect is reported to be approximately 0.5 mm at normal power settings.

The laser uses photons to dissect and coagulate tissue. The characteristics of the laser vary, depending on the wavelength of light used. The most commonly used lasers in laparoscopic surgery are the CO_2 (wavelength, 10 600 nm), the neodymium yttrium aluminium garnet (NdYAG; wavelength, 1064 nm) and the potassium titanyl phosphate (KTP; wavelength, 532 nm). Laser units are of two major types: free beam and contact. The effect of the CO_2 laser on tissue is almost exclusively vaporization and dissection with very little coagulative ability. For these reasons, the CO_2 laser has not been popular with most general surgeons. The KTP laser is a free-beam laser with an approximately 1.5-mm tissue penetration; it will coagulate vessels as large as 2.0 mm in diameter. The laser energy is delivered to the surgical site through a flexible catheter and can be used with various suction and irrigation probes. The NdYAG laser may be used either in contact-tip mode or as a free beam. The latter has a tissue penetration of approximately 5.0 mm and can coagulate vessels as large as 3.0 mm in diameter. In contact-tip mode, the laser energy is used to heat a synthetic sapphire tip which is then used to dissect and coagulate with a penetration effect of 0.2–1.0 mm.

The advantages of the laser are the very predictable nature of the energy effect on tissues and the lesser penetration or lateral tissue effect compared with electrocautery. The disadvantages are the cost of these systems (ranging from US $75 000 to US $125 000) and the fact that few surgeons have extensive experience with these devices in either conventional or endoscopic surgery.

Laparoscopic surgical instruments

Following the rapid and enthusiastic development of laparoscopic biliary tract surgery, there has been an unprecedented number of new and innovative instruments designed for this type of surgery. Various manufacturers have promoted disposable surgical instruments because of the problems of sterilization and instrument breakage with reusable laparoscopic instruments. In the near future, it is expected that instead of expensive single use, these 'disposable' instruments will be designated for limited use on a few occasions, which will help bring down the effective unit price.

In general, laparoscopic instruments fall into several categories:

1. Grasping forceps (to hold tissues).
2. Dissectors.
3. Retractors.
4. Cutting instruments.
5. Needle holders.
6. Knot tying devices.
7. Surgical clip appliers.
8. Automatic tissue staplers.
9. Various specialized instruments designed for one specific use.

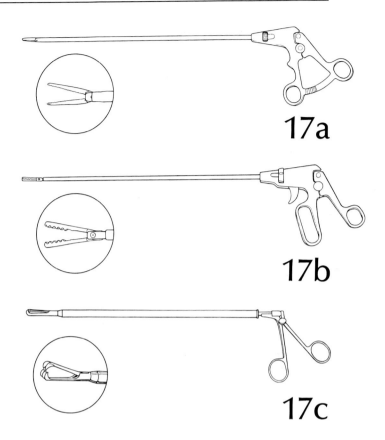

17a–c Grasping forceps are basically designed as either non-traumatic or traumatic. The former hold various tissues without injuring the serosa and are built with a non-crushing jaw. In addition, these instruments deliver less force as the jaws are closed. Laparoscopic bowel grasping forceps follow a similar design concept, except that the jaws are longer (30–60 mm) and are available in both 5-mm and 10-mm diameter sizes.

Traumatic grasping forceps are more useful as the smaller diameter instruments do not hold the small or large intestine well. Traumatic grasping forceps have sharp, penetrating teeth within the jaws and are used when there is less concern about injuring the tissue, such as with an acutely inflamed gall bladder. These instruments are also available in both 5-mm and 10-mm diameters.

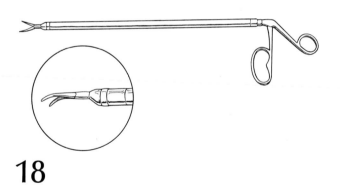

18 In the past, many different surgical devices were used to dissect tissues including curved clamps, Metzenbaum scissors, tonsil clamps, Kittners, and even the tip of the suction cannula. Many of the devices used in open surgery for this purpose have now been adapted for laparoscopic use. The first such instruments were simple straight dissecting clamps, which were soon replaced by angled forceps or the so-called Maryland dissector. Surgeons may now choose from a variety of such dissecting instruments, including right-angled and left-angled clamps and Mixter clamps.

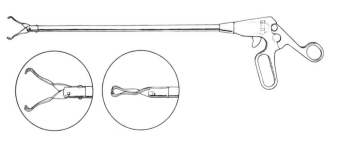

19 Laparoscopic versions of Allis' and Babcock clamps are used to grasp and retract tissues such as the colon, small intestine and stomach. These generally hold tissues better than the atraumatic bowel grasping forceps described earlier, but care must be taken in order to not injure the intestinal wall.

20 Disposable curved scissors are increasingly being used as dissecting instruments. Reusable laparoscopic scissors are difficult to keep sharp and as mentioned earlier are easily broken. Disposable scissors on the other hand are always sharp, and recent modifications in their design allow the jaws to rotate which has facilitated their use as a dissecting instrument.

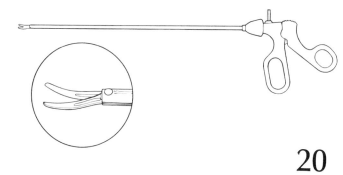

20

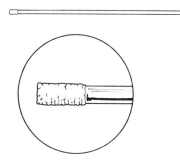

21

21 Unique blunt tissue dissectors based on the Kittner device used in open surgery have also been adapted for laparoscopic use. A small cotton pledget is firmly attached to a 5-mm shaft and inserted through a standard laparoscopic cannula.

22 Instruments for retraction are extremely important when performing any diagnostic or therapeutic laparoscopic procedure. These devices must be designed very differently from their counterparts in open surgery. Most of them can be incorporated within a 5-mm or 10-mm sheath and open up once inside the peritoneal cavity.

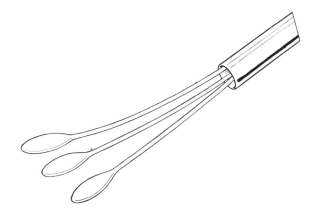

22

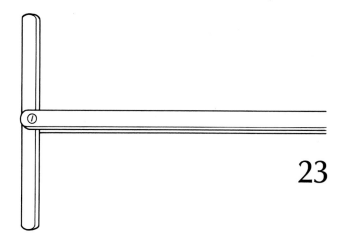

23 Another type of retraction device elevates the abdominal wall and is used to improve the exposure of the upper or lower abdomen in obese patients. The instrument is inserted through a standard 5-mm cannula and opened within the peritoneal cavity. The stiff T piece is then used to lift the abdominal wall.

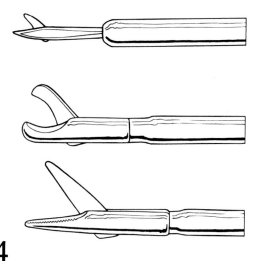

24 Several different types of cutting instruments have been adapted for laparoscopic use. Micro-scissors have small, usually curved, cutting surfaces with sharp tips for controlled, accurate incisions and not for dissecting through tissue planes or dividing sutures. Hook scissors are designed so that the tips of the jaws come together first, allowing the structure for division to be lifted away from the surrounding tissues to avoid adjacent tissue injury. Straight scissors are also available, but are seldom used except to cut sutures within the abdomen. As with any cutting instrument the tips of both jaws must be clearly visible before attempting to divide any structure.

25 Several new and improved laparoscopic needle holders are now available. The jaws of these instruments have been improved so that they can easily pick up and securely hold a straight or curved needle, and many have a curved jaw to facilitate these manoeuvres.

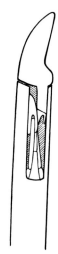
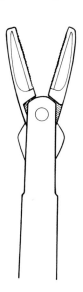
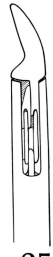

26 Other needle holders incorporate a cutting blade within the jaws so that the surgeon may divide the suture after completing the knot without the need to exchange instruments.

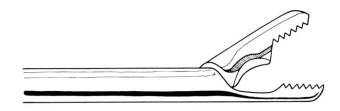

26

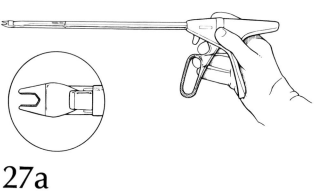

27a

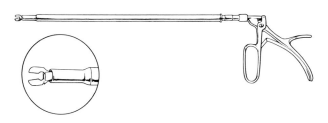

27b

27a, b Laparoscopic clip appliers initially became popular when surgeons used them to ligate the cystic duct and artery. Their ease of application and their effectiveness have persuaded surgeons to use them during other therapeutic procedures. Several different versions are available, including reusable single-loaded instruments and disposable appliers that hold as many as 20 titanium clips. Three lengths of staples are available: 6 mm, 9 mm and 11 mm.

28 The first linear stapling device similar to those used in conventional surgery (Endo-GIA) was designed with a 30-mm jaw which fired six rows of staples with a cutting blade through the centre. Two different staple configurations are available, one for intestinal applications and the other for dividing vascular tissues.

This device has been used successfully for such applications as dividing the appendix, small intestine and colon, cholecystoenteric anastomosis, enteroenteric anastomosis, dividing larger mesenteric vessels and controlling the splenic pedicle[13–15]. The limitations of the 30-mm staple cartridge have prompted the development of a 60-mm version.

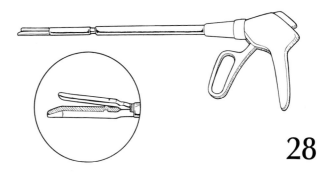

28

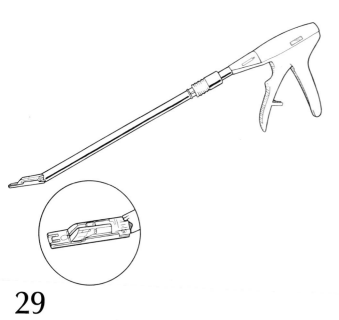

29

29 The 'hernia staplers' have penetrating staples that are used to firmly attach a prosthetic mesh to the pelvic fascia during laparoscopic herniorrhaphy[16]. They are built with an articulating jaw which facilitates proper placement of each clip. These stapling devices have also been used to secure mesh to the pelvic floor with the Ripstein repair for rectal prolapse[17].

Several innovative instruments have been developed for specific or unique laparoscopic applications and include such devices as cholangiography catheter fixation clamps, gall bladder extraction cannulae and sterile specimen removal bags.

30 An instrument that has proved useful while performing laparoscopic colonic surgery is the laparoscopic instrument holder. This device attaches to the operating table and can fix one or more laparoscopic cannulae in place. It was developed to reduce the number of assistants needed for the more complex laparoscopic surgical procedures and to avoid fatigue in those who needed to hold instruments in one position for extended periods.

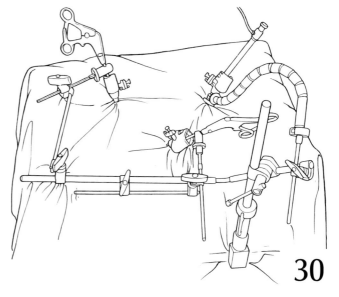

30

Conclusions

The recent developments in therapeutic laparoscopy represent one of the most exciting and dramatic changes in the area of abdominal surgery in the past 50 years. Without a doubt the indications for laparoscopic surgery will continue to expand as surgeons become more skilled and the instrumentation improves. The various devices described in this chapter represent only the basic instruments currently available. It is likely that laparoscopy instrument design will continue to evolve rapidly and will present the abdominal surgeon with the challenge of remaining knowledgeable and familiar with this developing field of technology.

References

1. Zucker KA. Laparoscopic guided cholecystectomy with electrocautery dissection. In: Zucker KA, ed. *Surgical Laparoscopy*. St Louis, Missouri: Quality Medical Publishing, 1991: 143–82.

2. Fillipi CJ, Fitzgibbons RJ, Salerno GM. Historical review: diagnostic laparoscopy to laparoscopic cholecystectomy and beyond. In: Zucker KA, ed. *Surgical Laparoscopy*. St Louis, Missouri: Quality Medical Publishing, 1991: 3–22.

3. Corson SL, Batzer SR, Gocial B, Maislin G. Measurement of the force necessary for laparoscopic trocar entry. *J Reprod Med* 1989; 34: 282–4.

4. Hasson HM. Modified instrument and method for laparoscopy. *Am J Obstet Gynecol* 1971; 110: 886–7.

5. Fitzgibbons RJ, Schmid S, Santoscoy R *et al*. Open laparoscopy for laparoscopic cholecystectomy. *Surg Laparosc Endosc* 1991; 1: 216–22.

6. Reddick EJ. Laparoscopic laser cholecystectomy. In: Zucker KA, ed. *Surgical Laparoscopy*. St Louis, Missouri: Quality Medical Publishing, 1991: 183–200.

7. Berci G. Instrumentation I: rigid endoscopes. In: Berci G, ed. *Endoscopy*. New York: Appleton-Century-Crofts, 1976: 74–112.

8. McFadyen BV. Three-dimensional video system: product review. *Surg Laparosc Endosc* 1992; 2: 273.

9. Hunter JG. Laser or electrocautery for laparoscopic cholecystectomy? *Am J Surg* 1991; 161: 245–9.

10. Easter DW, Moossa AR. Laser and laparoscopic cholecystectomy: a hazardous union? *Arch Surg* 1991; 126: 423.

11. Soderstrom RM, Levy BS. Bowel injuries during laparoscopy: causes and medicolegal questions. *Contemp Obstet Gynecol* 1982; 27: 41–7.

12. Saye WB, Miller W, Hertzmann P. Electrosurgery thermal injury: myth or misconception? *Surg Laparosc Endosc* 1991; 1: 223–8.

13. Moser KH, Schmitz R. Laparoskopische Appendektomie mit dem Multi-Fire Endo-GIA. *Chirurg* 1992; 63: 393–5.

14. Krasna M, Nazem A. Thoracoscopic lung resection: use of a new endoscopic linear stapler. *Surg Laparosc Endosc* 1991; 1: 248–50.

15. Goh P, Tekant Y, Isaac J, Kum CK, Ngoi SS. The technique of laparoscopic Billroth II gastrectomy. *Surg Laparosc Endosc* 1992; 2: 258–60.

16. Fitzgibbons RJ, Salerno G, Fillipi CJ, Corbitt J. Laparoscopic herniorrhaphy. In: *Surgical Laparoscopy – Update*. St Louis, Missouri: 1993.

17. Kusminsky RE, Tiley EH, Boland. Laparoscopic Ripstein procedure. *Surg Laparosc Endosc* 1992; 2.

Laparoscopic-assisted appendicectomy

Robert W. Bailey MD
Division Head, General Surgery, Greater Baltimore Medical Centre, Baltimore, Maryland, USA

Karl A. Zucker MD, FACS
Professor of Surgery, University of New Mexico School of Medicine, Albuquerque, New Mexico, USA

History

The recent introduction of laparoscopic cholecystectomy has had an enormous impact on the practice of general surgery. The advantages of this innovative procedure have been documented in several recent series[1,2]. Substantial reductions in the length of hospital stay, recovery period, postoperative discomfort and health care costs have led to its rapid acceptance. The first description of a laparoscopic incidental appendicectomy was in 1983 by Semm in Germany[3]. In 1987, Schrieber reported the first laparoscopic experience in a group of women with acute appendicitis[4]. He demonstrated the safety and efficacy of this approach in a clinical situation that is usually encountered by general surgeons. Several medical centres have subsequently adopted laparoscopy as the primary technique for the diagnosis and treatment of acute appendicitis.

Pier *et al.* recently published their experience with 625 consecutive laparoscopic appendicectomies[5]. Only 14% were histologically normal, and fewer than 2% of the patients required the procedure to be converted to an open laparotomy (most of these were in the first 50 cases). The operative morbidity rate was minimal, with only one case of appendiceal stump leakage and two patients developing intra-abdominal abscesses requiring interval laparotomy. They reported an operative time of less than 30 min and a wound infection rate below 2%[5]. Valla *et al.* have also shown the benefits of laparoscopic appendicectomy in a group of 465 paediatric patients with ages ranging from 3 to 16 years[6]. These and other reports have demonstrated that the appendix can be safely removed under laparoscopic guidance in the majority of patients, including those with extensive inflammation or atypical anatomy.

Principles and justification

Indications

A recent review of the literature suggests a possible role for incidental appendicectomy in patients between the ages of 10 and 30 years[7], but the indications are less clear for those of 30–50 years of age, and no benefit is apparent in those older than 50 years. As the risk of mortality from future acute appendicitis is so small and the benefits of a prophylactic appendicectomy are unconvincing, incidental appendicectomy, either under laparoscopic guidance or by open laparotomy, is not commonly performed at most institutions.

An appendicectomy performed solely as an incidental procedure, e.g. during elective gallbladder surgery, must be differentiated from the removal of a normal appendix during exploration for presumed appendicitis. Reasons offered for removal of a normal appendix following explorations for presumed acute appendicitis include: (1) the assumption by surgeons that any patient with a right lower quadrant incision has had their appendix removed; (2) to avoid future diagnostic confusion in any patient who may suffer from repeated episodes of lower abdominal pain, i.e. inflammatory bowel disease or gynaecological disorders; (3) failure to accurately determine the presence or absence of early acute appendicitis by gross inspection only; and (4) avoiding the risk of another anaesthetic in the future.

Although a conventional right lower quadrant incision is not made during laparoscopic appendicectomy, the growing popularity of this procedure may also result in possible confusion regarding the presence of an appendix. The remaining indications for removal of a normal appendix would apply regardless of the surgical approach. Because most surgeons agree with removal of a non-inflamed appendix during an open procedure, the authors' bias has been to recommend removal of a normal-appearing appendix during laparoscopic exploration for presumed appendicitis unless contraindicated by other intra-abdominal findings.

Contraindications

Absolute contraindications to attempting laparoscopic appendicectomy are few. Patients presenting with evidence of advanced intestinal obstruction, generalized peritonitis, or uncorrectable bleeding disorders should primarily undergo an open procedure. Although laparoscopic removal of the appendix may be technically possible in such circumstances, the operative time can be greatly increased.

Relative contraindications would include: previous lower abdominal surgery; evidence of localized abscess formation, i.e. a mass on palpation; suspicion of malignancy; or pregnancy. Whether such cases should be attempted will depend mostly on the capabilities of the surgeon. With increased exposure and operative experience, even the most difficult case can be successfully approached under laparoscopic guidance.

Potential advantages of laparoscopic appendicectomy

It is anticipated that many of the same advantages as with laparoscopic cholecystectomy will also be realized with laparoscopic appendicectomy.

Laparoscopic appendicectomy allows a more thorough exploration of the abdominal cavity than would be possible through a small right lower quadrant incision. This is particularly important in those patients presenting with evidence of lower abdominal peritonitis who appear to have a normal appendix. It also allows definitive treatment of other abdominal or pelvic pathology, as deemed appropriate by the operative findings. Conversion to a midline laparotomy may be avoided if the entire abdomen can be examined under laparoscopic guidance.

Laparoscopic appendicectomy shortens hospitalization and recovery periods[8,9]. Patients are generally able to leave the hospital 24 h after uncomplicated laparoscopic appendicectomy. Most are able to return to their normal activity within 2–3 days. Postoperative discomfort is also diminished. Although the pain following open appendicectomy is usually moderate to minimal, patients often complain of noticeable discomfort for 1–2 weeks and require oral narcotic analgesics. Almost no postoperative pain is experienced after laparoscopic appendicectomy.

Finally, the incidence of postoperative wound complications is reduced. Contamination of the wound is assumed following removal of a severely inflamed or perforated appendix through a traditional right lower quadrant or midline incision. During laparoscopic surgery the appendix can be removed without coming into direct contact with the fascia or subcutaneous tissues. In addition, the smaller less traumatic trocar puncture sites appear to diminish the incidence of wound complications such as abscess, cellulitis, dehiscence and necrotizing fasciitis[5].

Potential disadvantages of laparoscopic appendicectomy

The appendiceal stump may be difficult to mobilize and secure. Until recently, atraumatic intestinal clamps, angled forceps and curved scissors have not been available for laparoscopic surgery. In the past, methods of ligating the appendix were limited to pretied ligatures of plain or chromic catgut. Many surgeons were hesitant to rely on such sutures to close an appendiceal stump, particularly with inflamed tissues and a contaminated field. Recent refinements of laparoscopic suturing techniques and the development of endoscopic intestinal stapling devices have made closure of the appendiceal stump a simple manoeuvre.

Operative time can be expected to be increased during a surgeon's early attempts at any new laparoscopic procedure. Current reports from centres with extensive experience with this technique indicate that the length of a laparoscopic appendicectomy is comparable to the traditional method[5,6,8,9].

In some patients, atypical anatomy, extensive inflammation, dense adhesions, or abscess may necessitate abandoning the laparoscopic approach in favour of an open laparotomy. This will increase the length of the operation and may result in confusion if the patient believes that the need for conversion was the result of an intraoperative complication. Fortunately, the need to convert to an open technique is uncommon with increasing experience[5,6]. Patients should always be informed that any laparoscopic procedure may need to be converted to an open laparotomy and that this decision usually represents sound surgical judgement to minimize operative risk.

Preoperative

Preoperative evaluation and preparation for patients undergoing laparoscopic appendicectomy is nearly identical to that for patients undergoing traditional surgery. The basic guidelines for the safe performance of a laparoscopic procedure, e.g. stomach and bladder decompression, should be adhered to strictly. All other adjuvant measures, e.g. preoperative antibiotics, should be administered as for open appendicectomy.

Anaesthesia

Most therapeutic laparoscopic procedures require general anaesthesia. Regional anaesthesia, however, has been successfully employed on occasion for laparoscopic cholecystectomy[1]. With further refinement of operative and anaesthetic techniques, such options may become more readily acceptable in the future. Specific details concerning the use of anaesthesia during laparoscopic surgery have been previously published[10].

Operating room arrangement

1 The endoscopic imaging equipment, instrument table and energy devices, i.e. lasers and electro-surgery units, must be arranged to permit the surgical team to work comfortably in the lower abdomen. The video monitors should be placed near the foot of the table in clear view of the entire surgical team. Similarly, the insufflator should be positioned so that the surgeon can monitor the intra-abdominal pressure throughout the procedure. A basic laparotomy instrument set should be immediately available in the operating room.

The patient is positioned supine on the operating room table with both arms tucked-in at the side. If the arms are abducted they may hinder the ability of the surgical team to work in the lower abdomen and pelvis. The surgeon stands on the left side of the patient with the assistant standing directly opposite.

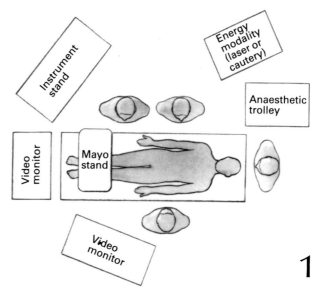

1

Operation

Establishment of a pneumoperitoneum

A pneumoperitoneum is established using currently accepted techniques (as described in the chapter on pp. 161–176). The patient is placed in a 10–20° head-down (Trendelenburg) position, and a 1.0–1.5-cm incision is made within the infraumbilical folds of the umbilicus.

2 A specially designed insufflation (Verres) needle is inserted into the abdominal cavity, and its position is confirmed by aspirating with an attached syringe and monitoring the insufflation pressure through the needle.

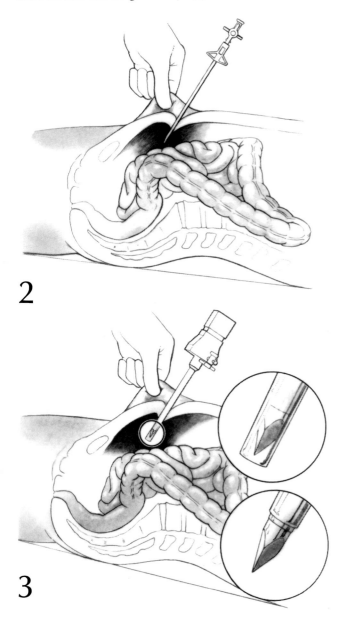

2

3 The peritoneal cavity is distended with carbon dioxide until a pressure of 12–15 mmHg is achieved. The needle is withdrawn and a 10-mm or 11-mm laparoscopic trocar and cannula are inserted through the same incision and into the distended abdomen.

3

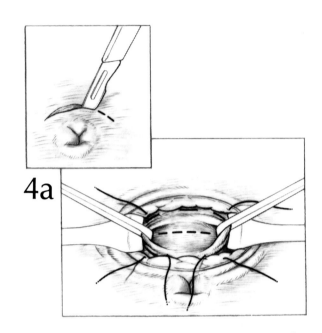

4a–c An alternative method of establishing the pneumoperitoneum is the open or Hasson technique[11]. A larger (approximately 2–3-cm) peri-umbilical incision is made, and the peritoneal cavity is entered under direct vision. A specially designed laparoscopic cannula with a blunt tip is guided into the abdomen and a purse-string suture closes the fascial opening around the sheath to create an airtight seal.

Diagnostic laparoscopy

A complete survey of the abdominal cavity is performed using a forward-viewing or side-viewing laparoscope introduced through the umbilical cannula. An angled telescope offers greater versatility in cases where the appendix is hidden from view, such as with a retrocaecal location. The diagnosis is confirmed, the extent and severity of the inflammatory process is determined, and the feasibility of a laparoscopic approach is assessed.

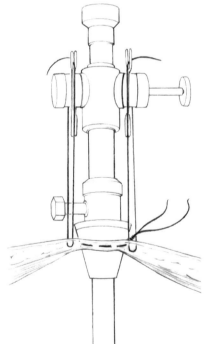

Accessory cannula placement

5 Insertion of additional trocars and cannulae is performed under direct laparoscopic vision. The locations of the epigastric vessels are identified and care is taken to avoid injury to them. Two accessory sheaths are often sufficient to complete the operative procedure; however, additional cannulae may be necessary to retract surrounding tissues. The two accessory sheaths are usually placed in the right anterior axillary line (at a site parallel or just cephalad to the umbilicus) and in the midline just above the pubic symphysis. In more complex cases with severe inflammation or atypical anatomy (i.e. retrocaecal appendix) a fourth cannula is often usefully inserted in the right upper quadrant of the abdomen.

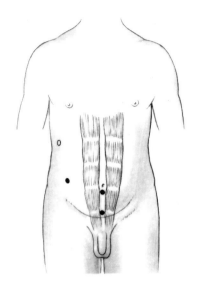

5

The sizes of cannulae used will depend on the technique and instrumentation employed. The most commonly used cannulae are available in diameters ranging from 5 mm to 12 mm. The authors generally use 10-mm sheaths so that a wide range of instruments, such as fan retractors and bowel-grasping forceps, can be introduced. The automatic intestinal stapler (Endo-GIA) requires a 12-mm cannula, and if its use is anticipated an appropriately sized sheath should be placed above the pubic symphysis. The additional trauma to the abdominal wall is negligible when using these larger devices, and difficulties are avoided that can occur when the surgeon is unable to introduce an instrument because an existing cannula is too small.

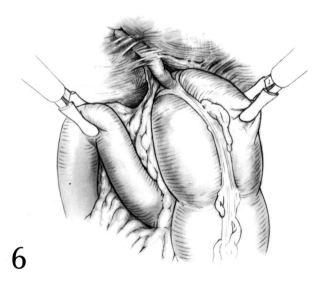

6

Identification and mobilization of the appendix and caecum

6 Following visual inspection of the abdominal cavity, the right colon and caecum are identified. The taeniae coli can be traced towards the caecum and appendix. Atraumatic bowel-grasping forceps are used to elevate the caecum and terminal ileum into the operative field.

7 Curved dissecting, i.e. Metzenbaum-like, scissors may be used to free the lateral and inferior peritoneal attachments of the appendix and/or the right colon. These scissors may be connected to an electrosurgery generator to deliver a monopolar current and facilitate haemostasis. Low-power settings (generally less than 30 W) and short bursts of energy should be used to avoid injury to surrounding structures. Alternatively, a free-beam or contact-tip laser device may be used for dissection in this area[12]. The appendix is identified and mobilized into the operative field.

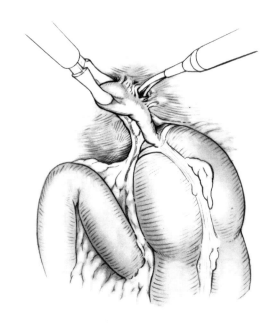

7

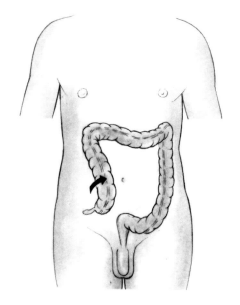

8 If the appendix is behind the caecum or deep in the pelvis, the ascending colon must be freed from its peritoneal attachments in order to retract it cephalad and towards the midline. This manoeuvre generally requires additional instruments and a fourth cannula is placed in the upper right abdomen.

8

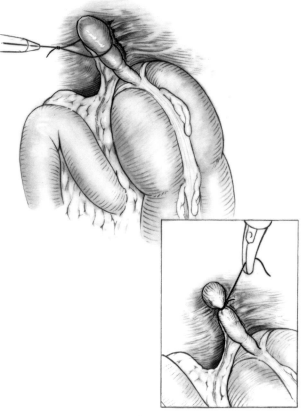

9 Once mobilized, the appendix is grasped at its tip with atraumatic forceps. If the appendix proves difficult to hold due to extensive inflammation or necrosis, a pretied laparoscopic ligature may be used to encircle the tip of the appendix. This suture may then be used as a point of retraction.

9

Dissection of the mesoappendix

The blood supply to the appendix may be divided in either a retrograde or an antegrade manner. Confusion exists, however, as to the distinction between a retrograde and an antegrade dissection. To avoid any such confusion, the subsequent narrative will refer to an antegrade dissection as that which originates at the junction with the caecum.

10 In the absence of significant inflammation, the appendiceal artery may be readily isolated at the base of the appendix with an angled dissecting forceps and controlled with either surgical clips or direct suture ligation.
   The remaining mesoappendix is then divided between clips or with monopolar or bipolar electrocautery.

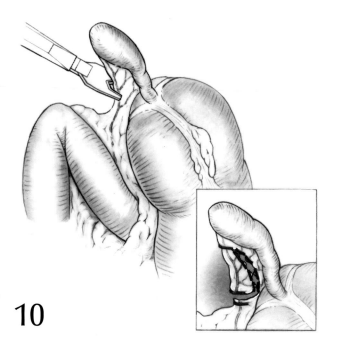

10

11a, b

Alternatively, the entire mesoappendix may be ligated and divided with an automatic stapling device using a vascular cartridge.

If the base of the appendix cannot be readily identified, then the blood supply can be sequentially ligated beginning at the tip of the appendix (retrograde dissection). The dissection should be continued until the base of the appendix and its junction with the caecum is freed from any adhesions or peritoneal attachments.

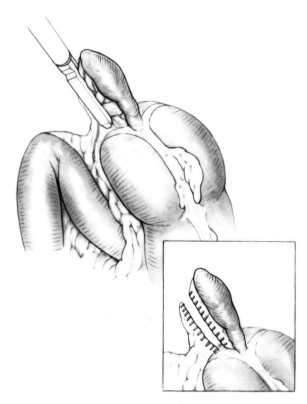

11a

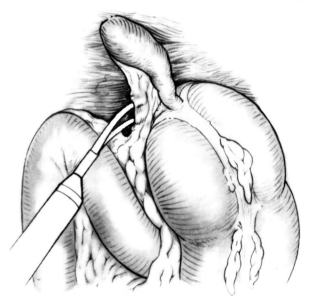

11b

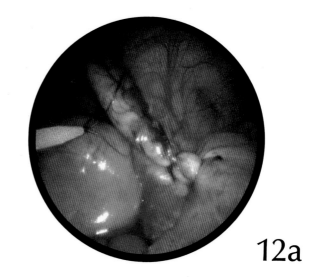

12a

Ligation and division of the appendix

12a, b Previously, the most common method of securing the appendix involved the use of pretied laparoscopic ligature made of 0 chromic catgut or synthetic suture. Two ligatures are placed near the junction with the caecum and a third placed on the proximal portion of the inflamed appendix. The appendix is divided, leaving the two ligatures on the caecum intact. The appendix may be sharply divided with a scissors, using monopolar or bipolar electrical current, or with laser energy. Many surgeons prefer to use an electrosurgery instrument in order to 'sterilize' the exposed mucosa. Extreme care must be taken to avoid burning the caecum, particularly when using monopolar current. This can lead to subsequent necrosis, sloughing of tissue and caecal fistula.

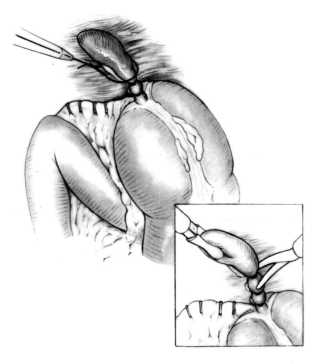

12b

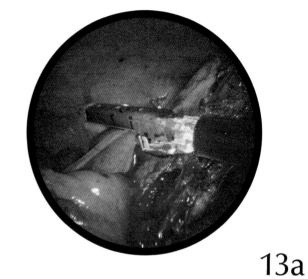

13a–c An alternative method uses an intestinal stapling device, which is fired across the base of the appendix, simultaneously dividing it between several rows of staples.

13a

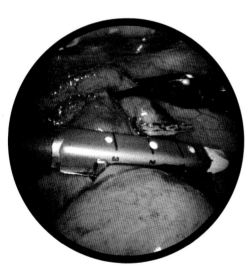

13b

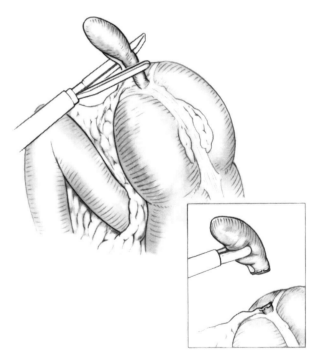

13c

14a–d With either of the above techniques, the base of the appendix remains everted. If desired, the apendiceal stump may be inverted or invaginated into the wall of the caecum with a purse-string or Z-type suture; however, few laparo- scopic surgeons have found this necessary. Recently, a large prospective trial involving traditional open surgery has shown no advantage with inverting the base of the appendix[13].

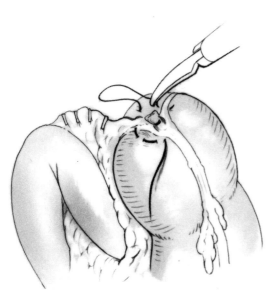

14a

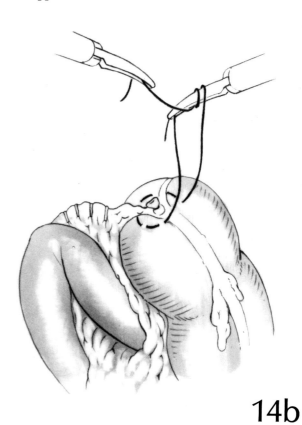

14b

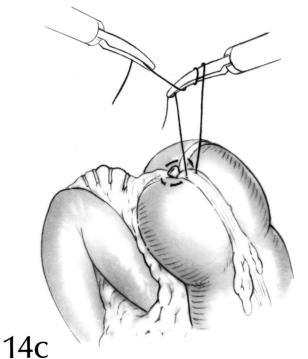

14c

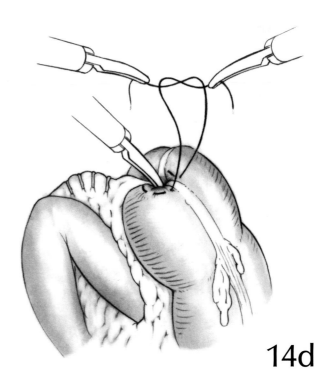

14d

Extraction of the appendix

15a, b An attempt should be made to remove the appendix and any other contaminated material without coming into contact with the anterior abdominal wall. This has been shown to almost eliminate the risk of postoperative wound infections[5,6]. If the appendix is not too enlarged, it can be first withdrawn into one of the 10-mm or larger accessory cannulae and then the entire sheath (with the enclosed specimen) removed from the peritoneal cavity.

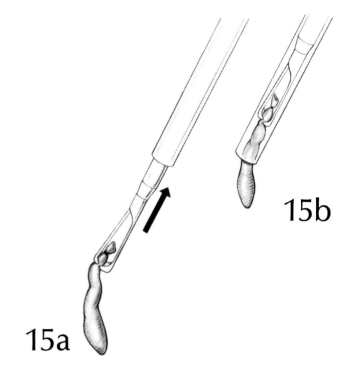

15b

15a

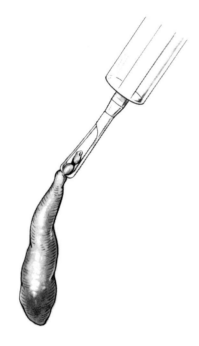

16

16 If the appendix will not easily pass through a 10-mm or 12-mm cannula, a 20-mm appendiceal extractor sheath can be exchanged for one of the sheaths already positioned (preferably at the umbilicus). The larger diameter of this conduit will permit the extraction of most appendices.

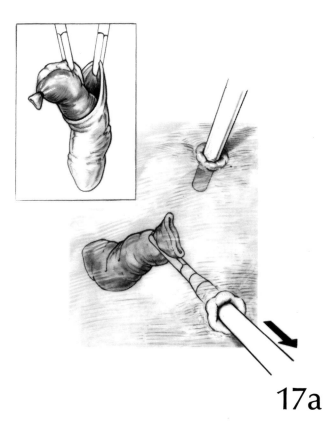

17a, b Another popular method involves placing a sterile condom (or the finger of a large surgical glove) into the abdomen and placing the appendix within this reservoir. The appendix is then removed through one of the cannulae or through an enlarged fascial opening without coming into contact with the abdominal wall. This technique is particularly useful for removing a necrotic or fragmented appendix. Commercially available 'bags' are also available which have incorporated a number of useful improvements.

17a

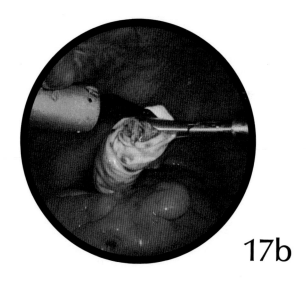

17b

Irrigation and drain placement

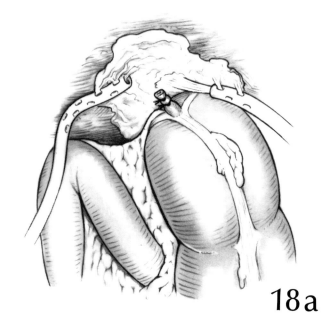

18a, b Once the appendix has been detached, the lower abdomen and pelvis are irrigated with large quantities of saline. Contaminated material and debris are removed with a pool-tip aspiration cannula or atraumatic forceps. The operative field is inspected for adequate haemostasis and the appendiceal stump re-examined to ensure proper closure.

Closed suction drainage catheters may be used in cases of localized abscess formation. The drains are trimmed to the desired length and placed into the abdomen through one of the larger laparoscopic cannulae. The drainage catheter is then held in place with a pair of forceps, and the external tip is brought out through one of the accessory cannulae. The entire sheath is then removed with the catheter and the drain is secured to the skin.

18a

Postoperative care

Postoperative care is similar to that following open appendicectomy. Patients undergoing laparoscopic surgery, however, generally experience a more rapid return of bowel function and earlier ambulation and discharge from hospital[8, 9]. The severity of the underlying inflammatory process, however, will continue to exert a major influence on the postoperative course of the patient. Antibiotics, analgesics and intravenous fluids are administered as are clinically necessary. The larger umbilical fascial defect should be closed with one or more synthetic sutures. The smaller accessory puncture sites generally do not require fascial closure. If a large (i.e. 12-mm) cannula has been used at one of these locations or if the fascial opening has been enlarged to extract the specimen, it should be closed in a similar fashion. The skin is approximated with either sutures or staples. Wound problems should be few with the avoidance of abdominal wall contamination.

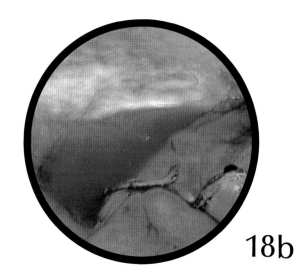

18b

Outcome

Experience with laparoscopic appendicectomy is growing. Current reports indicate that laparoscopic appendicectomy is indicated for all but a few patients,

provides definitive treatment of the underlying disease process, and can be performed with an acceptable incidence of operative morbidity and mortality. Recently published prospective randomized clinical studies comparing conventional appendicectomy with the laparoscopic method have demonstrated a shortened hospital stay and more rapid return to normal activity with the laparoscopic approach[8, 9]. Laparoscopy has the additional advantage of allowing examination of the entire abdominal cavity, and in many cases can be used to manage other disorders which may have mimicked acute appendicitis. It has yet to be demonstrated whether laparoscopic appendicectomy will decrease the incidence of long-term complications, such as pelvic adhesions or small intestinal obstruction.

References

1. Bailey RW, Zucker KA, Flowers JL, Scovil WA, Graham SM, Imbembo AL. Laparoscopic cholecystectomy: experience with 375 consecutive patients. *Ann Surg* 1991; 214: 531–41.

2. Spaw AT, Reddick EJ, Olsen DO. Laparoscopic laser cholecystectomy: analysis of 500 procedures. *Surg Laparosc Endosc* 1991; 1: 2–7.

3. Semm K. Endoscopic appendectomy. *Endoscopy* 1983; 15: 59–64.

4. Schreiber JH. Early experience with laparoscopic appendectomy in women. *Surg Endosc* 1987; 1: 211–16.

5. Pier A, Gotz F, Bacher C. Laparoscopic appendectomy in 625 cases: from innovation to routine. *Surg Laparosc Endosc* 1991; 1: 8–13.

6. Valla JS, Limonne B, Valla V *et al.* Laparoscopic appendectomy in children: report of 465 cases. *Surg Laparosc Endosc* 1991; 1: 166–72.

7. Fisher KS, Ross DS. Guidelines for therapeutic decision in incidental appendectomy. *Surg Gynecol Obstet* 1990; 171: 95–8.

8. McAnena OJ, Austin O, O'Connell PR, Hederman WP, Gorey TF, Fitzpatrick J. Laparoscopic *versus* open appendicectomy: a prospective evaluation. *Br J Surg* 1992; 79: 818–20.

9. Attwood SEA, Hill ADK, Murphy PG, Thornton J, Stephens RB. A prospective randomized trial of laparoscopic *versus* open appendectomy. *Surgery* 1992; 112: 497–501.

10. Hasnain JU, Matjasko MJ. Practical anesthesia for laparoscopic procedures. In: Zucker KA, ed. *Surgical Laparoscopy.* St Louis: Quality Medical Publishing, 1991: 77–86.

11. Fitzgibbons RJ, Salerno GM, Filipi CJ. Open laparoscopy. In: Zucker KA, ed. *Surgical Laparoscopy.* St Louis: Quality Medical Publishing, 1991: 87–97.

12. Saye WB, Rives DA, Cochran EB. Laparoscopic appendectomy: three years' experience. *Surg Laparosc Endosc* 1991; 2: 109–15.

13. Engstrom L, Fenyo G. Appendicectomy: assessment of stump invagination versus simple ligation: a prospective, randomized trial. *Br J Surg* 1985; 72: 971–2.

Laparoscopic-assisted right hemicolectomy

R. W. Beart Jr MD, FACS
Professor of Surgery, Mayo Clinic, Scottsdale, Arizona, USA

Henry Lee MD
Mayo Clinic, Scottsdale, Arizona, USA

Background

As the science of surgery progresses, less invasive means of performing operations are being sought. These allow more rapid patient recovery and can reduce the number of complications associated with large abdominal incisions. This more rapid recovery is well demonstrated after laparoscopic cholecystectomy and, at the time of the writing of this chapter, similar benefits can be achieved for patients undergoing colonic resection.

However, it must be recognized that these techniques are in a state of development, and new complications associated with the laparoscopic method must be avoided before we can state that these developments confer an overall advantage in patient management. The overall efficacy of a surgical procedure should not be sacrificed in the name of greater speed of recovery, and we must be certain that these methods are developed in a professional manner.

Principles and justification

Laparoscopic-assisted colectomy can be divided into two parts: first, the intra-abdominal portion of the dissection and, second, the bowel resection and anastomosis.

Intra-abdominal dissection

The dissection, mobilization and primary vessel ligation can take place intracorporeally. The advantage of this technique is that it minimizes the invasion of the abdominal cavity, resulting in a reduction of postoperative ileus (with its associated fluid shifts) and pain control requirements (with their associated effects on lung function and venous status). These features contribute to a shorter hospital stay.

Bowel resection and anastomosis

In contrast to bowel mobilization, the current techniques of achieving intra-abdominal bowel resection and anastomosis are cumbersome, they greatly lengthen the procedure and require leaving the bowel open within the abdomen for a lengthy period of time. These are significant disadvantages and, at the present, extracorporeal resection and anastomosis through a small abdominal wall opening would seem to be in the patient's best interest.

Indications and contraindications

The indications for a laparoscopic colectomy are essentially the same as for a traditional colectomy. It is important to note that the extent of resection must not be altered by the new technique. If at any point the effectiveness or the safety of the procedure is in question, the abdominal wall should be opened and traditional laparotomy performed. Similarly, it is inappropriate to prolong a surgical procedure unduly, and therefore, for all these reasons, the surgeon must be prepared to abandon the laparoscopic procedure if problems arise. Resection of the transverse colon is difficult by these new methods, and an extended right hemicolectomy to include the right transverse colon may be inappropriate.

Preoperative

Anaesthesia

General anaesthesia is recommended for overall patient comfort and to expedite open exploration should it become necessary.

Operation

1 The patient is placed in a supine position, and the preparation of the abdominal wall is performed as for open laparotomy. A urinary catheter and a nasogastric tube are used to decompress the bladder and stomach. Each member of the operative team must have an unobstructed view of a video monitor. The surgeon stands to the patient's left and the first assistant to the right.

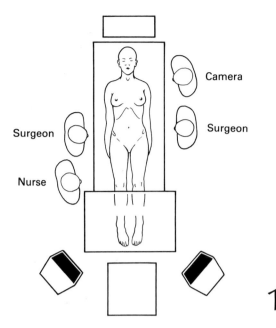

2 The camera (10-mm trocar) must be in a position to visualize the right lower quadrant and the hepatic flexure adequately, while not impeding the use of other instruments at the same time. The left upper quadrant is ideal for this purpose. An incision is made and the dissection carried out to the peritoneum. A Hasson introducer (*see* chapter on pp. 161–176) is placed into the peritoneal cavity under direct vision, and is held in place by fascial sutures which are inserted before cannula placement.

A pneumoperitoneum is established, and a 10-mm laparoscope is used to inspect the abdomen. Although a pressure of 15 mmHg is used for laparoscopic cholecystectomy, 10–12 mmHg is adequate for colon resection. This lower pressure reduces the retroperitoneal dissection of carbon dioxide, which can result in subcutaneous emphysema.

Three additional ports are needed, each being placed under direct vision using the laparoscope. A 5-mm port is placed in the left lower quadrant not far from the umbilicus; a second 10-mm port is placed in the midline in the suprapubic area; and a second 5-mm port is placed in the right lower quadrant lateral to the umbilicus in the anterior axillary line.

The patient is placed in the Trendelenburg (head-down) position and rotated with the left side down. This gains exposure to the right paracolic gutter.

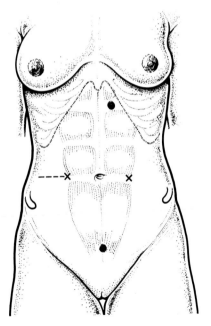

3 Dissection is similar to the open technique, with medial traction on the colon while the peritoneal reflection is divided laterally. Particular attention is given to the attachments of the terminal ileum. Once free from its lateral attachments, the colon can be reflected medially and the right ureter identified. This is best done with a paddle dissector because a hook dissector gets caught in the mesenteric fat. The paddle is used to reflect the colon bluntly.

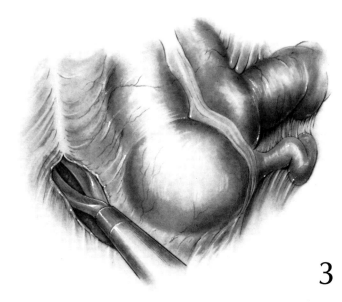

3

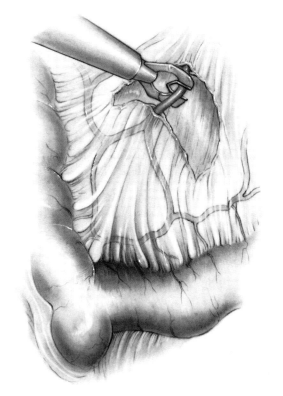

4

4 At this point the colon is replaced laterally and the mesentery is dissected with cautery and blunt dissection. The primary feeding vessels to the segment of colon involved are placed on traction and isolated. High ligation of these vessels not only constitutes a thorough cancer operation, but minimizes the need for dissection and clipping of multiple vascular branches. These vessels are then clipped. An Endoloop may be placed around these vessels for added security. Any vascular segment in the mesentery can be divided at this time to facilitate the eventual exteriorization of the bowel.

5   The bowel is then grasped through the right lower quadrant port and a small (5-cm) incision is made in this region. The bowel and dissected mesentery are brought out through this incision. The mesenteric dissection is completed on each side to the point where the bowel will be transected.

Bowel clamps are placed. The specimen is removed and an anastomosis (either hand-sewn or stapled) is performed extracorporeally (*see* chapters on pp. 51–73 and pp. 74–83). The bowel is then returned to the abdomen and the incision is closed in two layers. The abdomen is reinsufflated and inspected for haemostasis. After irrigation, the ports are removed under direct vision and the fascial defect of the larger trocar sites is closed by direct suture.

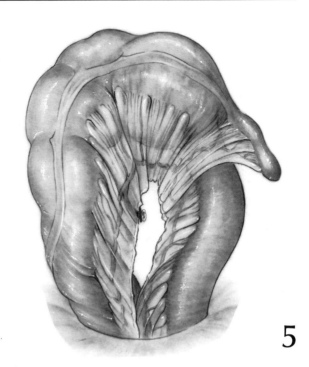

5

Postoperative care

Postoperative care is similar to other laparoscopic procedures. Patients may be started on a liquid diet after recovering from anaesthesia. A rapid progression to a regular diet can be expected. If there is any evidence of nausea or abdominal distension, oral intake is delayed. Most patients will show bowel activity with passage of flatus by the third postoperative day. Pain control with a passive cutaneous infusion pump is helpful, but is replaced with oral analgesics when the patient is receiving adequate oral intake.

Outcome

Our early experiences with laparoscopic-assisted colon resection in 50 consecutive patients who underwent colonic surgery, all of whom were considered for the laparoscopic technique, are as follows. Twenty-six patients did not have an attempted laparoscopic resection because of preoperative technical considerations or surgeon preference. Laparoscopic resection was attempted in 24 patients; the procedure was not completed in eight. Of the remaining 16 patients (32% of the original group and 67% of those in whom the technique was attempted), the intra-abdominal portion of the procedure was completed laparoscopically. In these 16 patients the mean time to oral intake was 1.1 days and the mean hospital stay was 3.6 days, which is shorter than in a comparable group of patients treated by traditional surgical techniques.

In conclusion, in a significant number of patients laparoscopic colectomy is a viable alternative which may offer lower morbidity rates and a shorter hospital stay than traditional open techniques. However, it is important that the surgeon develops laparoscopic skills in a controlled environment which includes both theoretical and practical training. Once this technology is used, the surgeon must be willing to abandon the laparoscopic procedure in favour of open surgery to avoid unnecessary prolongation of the operation and to maintain overall patient safety.

Laparoscopic-assisted left hemicolectomy

P. F. Leahy MB, MCh, FRCSI
Consultant Surgeon, Blackrock Clinic, Dublin, Eire

Preoperative

Assessment

The assessment of patients for major colonic surgery requires consideration of radiological contrast studies, colonoscopy, intravenous pyelography, ultrasonography and hepatic scanning, and blood markers to assist the management of those with colonic adenocarcinoma.

Preparation

Mechanical bowel preparation is undertaken with a hypertonic electrolyte solution such as GoLytely or Colyte, along with the non-absorbable intraluminal antibiotic neomycin. In the perioperative period, prophylactic antibiotics are used against Gram-positive and Gram-negative aerobic and anaerobic organisms. Deep vein thrombosis prophylaxis is achieved with calf compression boots or subcutaneous heparin, 5000 units twice daily.

Laparoscopic equipment

The following equipment is necessary for the four puncture technique (*see also* chapter on pp. 161–176): one 12-mm trocar, two 10-mm trocars, one 5-mm trocar, two intestinal grasping clamps, one Endo-Babcock tissue-holding device, an Endo-GIA, an Endo-clip apparatus, surgiwhips, surgities, and suture material to suspend the gut.

Operation

Position of patient

The shoulders and arms are securely fastened to the operating table, and a nasogastric tube and a urinary catheter are inserted. The patient is placed in the Trendelenburg (head-down) lithotomy position. The monitor of the video optical system is placed at the foot of the patient. Two monitors are preferred.

Trocar placement

1 In the four puncture technique, the initial trocar is inserted in the right upper quadrant. After a pneumoperitoneum has been created, a 12-mm trocar is inserted into this area, carefully avoiding the liver, gallbladder and colon. In the left upper quadrant a 5-mm trocar is inserted under direct vision using the laparoscope. In the left lower quadrant a 10-mm trocar is inserted for a laparoscope. In the right lower quadrant a 12-mm trocar is inserted so that an Endo-GIA stapler can be used through this port.

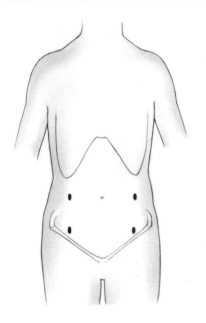

1

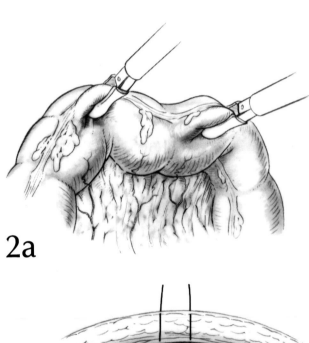

2a

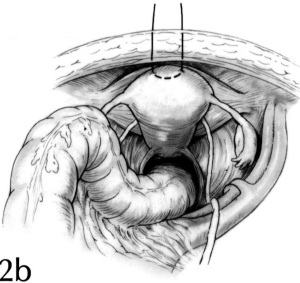

2b

Preparation of peritoneal cavity

2a, b An extensive examination and evaluation of the liver, colon and pelvis is performed and the degree of the Trendelenburg tilt is then increased. In women, it is imperative to suspend the uterus towards the anterior abdominal wall. This can be performed in two ways. A suture is placed one fingerbreadth above the pubic symphysis using a long Keith needle, which is inserted into the fundus of the uterus and is then passed out again to the anterior abdominal surface. When using this method, the uterus must be only lightly suspended because tightening the suture may cause extensive bleeding. Alternatively, a suture may be passed around the fundus of the uterus, clipped with an Endo-clip and attached to the anterior abdominal wall.

In patients in whom there are adhesions to the abdominal wall, these are dissected and divided. However, in some situations (e.g. after the patient has had a previous appendicectomy) the adhesions may form a 'shelf' behind which the small bowel may be lodged to facilitate dissection of the left colon.

If a left lower sigmoid colectomy is undertaken, it is sometimes beneficial to rotate the table away from the area of dissection by approximately 15°. A sigmoidoscope or colonoscope can be placed rectally and the lesion identified in the rectosigmoid colon by reducing the light intensity in the camera. This transillumination technique can help to identify the lesion, which is then marked with three Endo-clips in case one or two clips become dislodged during bowel mobilization.

Suspension of gut

3 A single suture is inserted through the abdominal wall into the peritoneal cavity, passed through the mesentery beneath the intestine, and brought up to the surface again. This suture is lightly clipped by a Mosquito clamp on the surface of the abdominal wall. It is important not to tighten the suture because it may transect the intestine. Thus the large intestine can be lifted up by the suture, freeing the grasping devices for further manipulation of the colon.

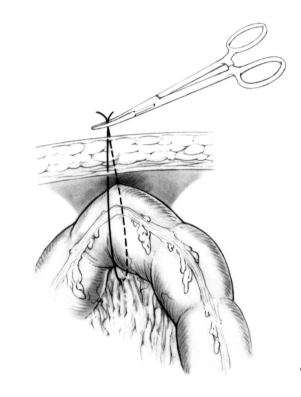

3

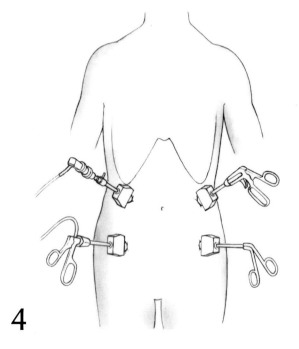

4

Bowel mobilization

4 A grasping forceps is now inserted through the left upper quadrant 5-mm surgiport. An Endo-Babcock tissue-holding device is inserted through the right lower quadrant 12-mm surgiport after the attachment of a 10.5-mm converter. The Babcock is used to exert countertraction on the intestine towards the right hand side of the patient. Similarly, the proximal aspect of the sigmoid colon is grasped by the first assistant using a 5-mm intestinal clamp. The lateral ligaments are identified. The surgeon replaces the 10.5-mm converter with a 5-mm converter and introduces an Endo-shears attached to a low power monopolar electrocautery. (It is advisable not to exceed mark 4 on the monopolar electrocautery device.) By a process of light coagulation followed by sharp dissection, the lateral attachments of the colon are divided.

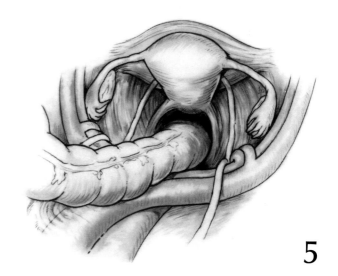

5 The closed blades of the Endo-shears are used carefully to retract the tissue by entering the avascular plane. The common iliac and internal iliac vessels are identified. The left ureter is also identified as it traverses these iliac vessels. The dissection is continued in a cephalad direction and also towards the pelvis.

5

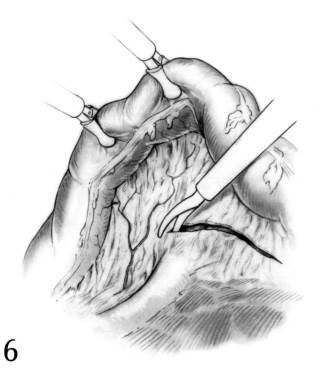

6 Once the ureter has been identified, the assistant surgeon changes the grasping device to a more proximal position, and the intestine is again placed to the right of the patient by exerting countertraction. This affords tension on the peritoneal reflection in the left paracolic gutter. The surgeon continues to dissect along this paracolic gutter in a cephalad direction. It is important not to overdissect in this area because uncompromising bleeding may occur if dissection enters the perinephric fat.

As the dissection continues, the colon, mesentery and lymph nodes are swept towards the right hand side of the patient, clearing away the mesentery, fatty tissue and lymph nodes from the underlying aorta.

6

7 At this stage, attention is directed to the splenic flexure, and the ligaments suspending this structure are divided. This step is imperative to avoid damaging the spleen and also to avoid excessive tension on the descending colon later in the procedure.

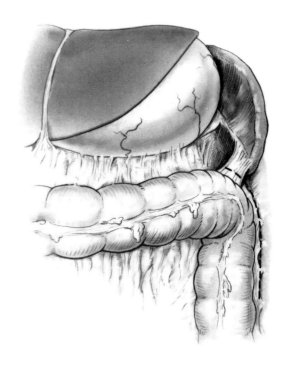

7

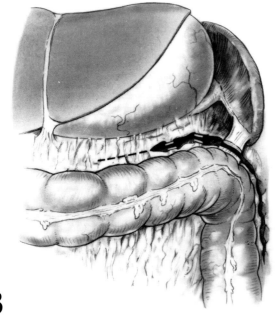

8

8 The omentum is detached. Individual vessels can be skeletonized and ligated using a 9-mm Endo-clip or a hand-suturing technique.

Attention is now directed to the peritoneum on the right side of the mesentery. The assistant surgeon grasps the proximal intestine and reflects the tissues towards the left hand side of the patient, thus causing tension on the peritoneum along the right hand side of the mesentery. This peritoneum is divided using dissecting scissors as previously described. This division is continued vertically downwards toward the pelvis and upwards toward the root of the mesentery. With careful meticulous dissection and retraction on the bowel, the mesenteric fat is retracted from the underlying vessels. It is not always necessary to identify the ureter along the right side, but in cases of carcinoma where extensive resections are to be used, it is preferred.

Transillumination of mesenteric arcades

9 A 10-mm telescope is introduced into the left hand side of the abdomen and placed adjacent to the mesentery. The intensity of the light source on the receptor camera is reduced, allowing transillumination of the mesenteric arcades. If the vessels do not transilluminate adequately, then it is necessary to skeletonize the vessels, removing the excess fatty tissue so that the vessels can be seen more easily.

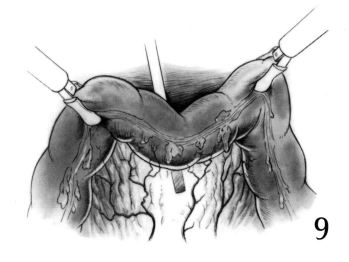

10 If difficulty is encountered at this stage of the dissection, a Doppler probe can be inserted through a 5-mm port in the right lower quadrant to confirm the position of the mesenteric vasculature.

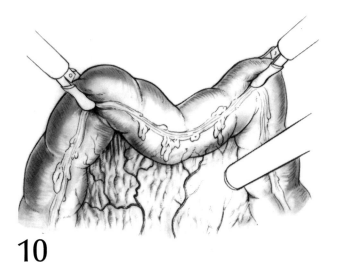

11 Once the mesenteric vessels have been identified, the inferior mesenteric artery is carefully selected. In cases of carcinoma, this must be ligated flush with the aorta. Several methods may be employed to ligate this vessel: a large Endo-clip, an Abslok clip, an Endo-GIA stapler or, alternatively, a hand suture technique using 3/0 chromic catgut.

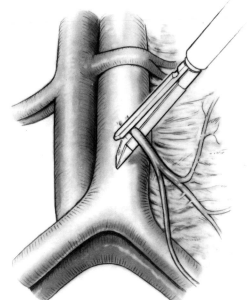

Extent of resection

12 When the inferior mesenteric artery has been transected, the remainder of the mesenteric arcade must also be resected, bearing in mind that a radical resection for cancer should involve removal of all the regional lymph nodes subtending the tumour for treatment and staging purposes. Should the vessels require individual ligation, skeletonization of the mesenteric arcade is necessary. This involves removing the fatty tissue using a combination of sharp dissection with light electric coagulation and aspiration using a suction irrigation device. The creation of windows using this technique can be time consuming and also has a high susceptibility to haematoma formation.

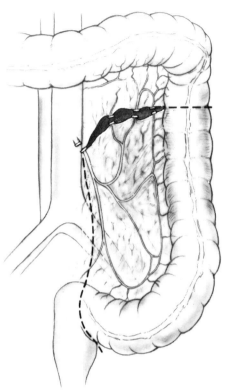

12

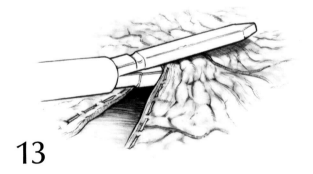

13

13 Alternatively, after ligation of the inferior mesenteric artery, the Endo-GIA device can be used to transect the distal colon and the thickened mesentery. This step should not be instituted until an Endo-gauge has been applied to the mesentery to determine its thickness and thus to determine the appropriate staple leg length. Either a 2.5-mm or 3.5-mm vascular cartridge staple length is usually suitable. The sequential application of the Endo-GIA is necessary for this step in the procedure. It is imperative that the Endo-GIA should be inserted into the 'V' of the previously divided staple rows. It may be necessary to fire three or four cartridges.

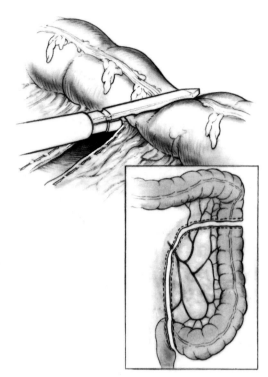

14 The intestine is transected both proximally and distally using the Endo-GIA, and the specimen is placed in the pelvis in preparation for removal. In cases of carcinoma where there is serosal involvement by tumour, an impermeable bag should be introduced into the abdomen and the specimen placed in it to prevent tumour contamination of the abdominal wall at the time of specimen removal.

14

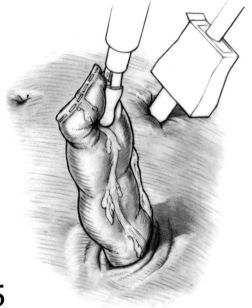

15

Opening the abdomen

15 The proximal staple line is grasped by a pair of atraumatic grasping forceps and brought to the left lower quadrant 10-mm port site. The skin incision is extended, the fascia divided, and the muscles split to fashion an incision of approximately 2.5 cm in length to allow the easy introduction of the anvil head of the stapling device and to remove the specimen.

Once the abdomen is opened, the specimen is removed.

16 The mobilized proximal segment of the bowel is exteriorized through the incision, a purse-string applicator is applied, and the excess intestine distal to the applicator is excised. An anastomosis sizer is introduced into the proximal bowel to determine which size anvil head should be used to fashion the anastomosis. An anvil of the appropriate size is inserted into the proximal bowel and the purse-string is snugly tightened, with inversion of the intestinal mucosa around the shaft of the anvil. The anvil and proximal gut are then replaced together into the peritoneal cavity towards the pelvis.

A purse-string polypropylene (Prolene) suture is applied to the peritoneum and fascia of the 2.5-cm incision, and the 12-mm trocar is introduced into this defect. The pneumoperitoneum is re-established.

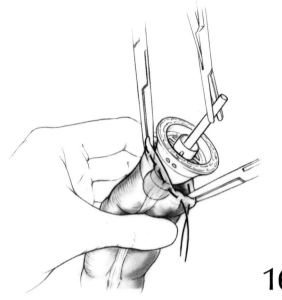

16

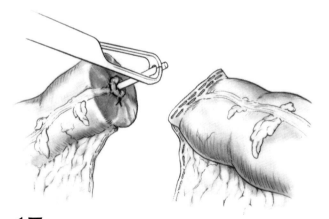

17

17 A specially devised grasping forceps is introduced into the right lower quadrant to grasp the shaft of the anvil, which is moved towards the rectal stump.

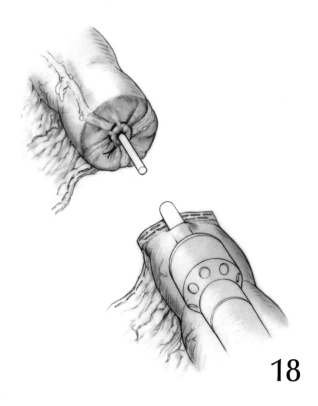

18 The assistant surgeon now places a Premium CEEA stapling device through the anus and advances the trocar 1 mm to the side of the staple line in the upper rectum. After penetration of the rectal stump, the trocar is removed with a specially designed pair of grasping forceps and is pulled out of the peritoneal cavity through the 12-mm port.

The grasping device is reintroduced into the abdominal cavity to grasp the anvil shaft, which is coupled with the locking mechanism of the circular stapler introduced through the anus. The stapling device is closed snugly, the mechanism unlocked, and the staples are fired. The stapling mechanism is opened, twisted two turns, and then gently removed from the rectum.

Saline is introduced into the pelvis and, using a colonoscope, air is insufflated into the rectum to determine whether there are any leaks from the anastomotic line. An excellent view is achieved with the colonscope to examine the anastomotic line endoluminally.

A drain is placed through one of the lateral ports in cases of inflammatory disease or after extensive dissection has been performed. A final inspection of the mesenteric defect and areas of dissection is carried out to determine whether there is any residual bleeding. A final irrigation of the abdominal cavity is performed using a pulsed irrigation system (Davol). The trocars are removed after decompression of the abdomen. The wounds are closed with 2/0 Maxon to the fascia and a 3/0 Maxon subcuticular stitch with Steri-Strips is applied to the skin. The nasogastric tube is removed at the end of the procedure.

Postoperative care

Routine postoperative measures are undertaken, including intravenous fluids and analgesics. Most patients can tolerate oral fluids from the second day, food from the fourth day, and can be discharged from hospital on the fifth day. The time to return to work varies according to the patient's preoperative condition and diagnosis. However, many patients can return to work after 14 days of recuperation.

Laparoscopic-assisted anterior resection and abdominoperineal resection of the rectum

G. H. Ballantyne MD

Associate Professor of Surgery, Department of Surgery, Yale University School of Medicine, New Haven, Connecticut, USA

Principles and justification

The application of laparoscopic techniques to resections of the colon and rectum is currently in a period of rapid evolution. Many of the instruments and techniques which will facilitate these operations in the future have not yet been developed. The goal of the laparoscopic surgeon should be to perform exactly the same operation using these new techniques as would be performed using traditional surgical techniques through large open abdominal wounds.

Indications and contraindications

Clinical experience with laparoscopic colorectal resections is limited. Consequently, empirical data that might indicate for which patients laparoscopic techniques will prove most suitable are not available. Moreover, patient selection for these procedures will vary with the experience of the individual surgeon. At present, the clinical indications for laparoscopic low anterior resection and abdominal perineal resection are the same as those for traditional open operations. Such factors as obesity and previous operations, however, may make the laparoscopic procedure more difficult.

Preoperative assessment and preparation

This is the same as for open operations. Indeed, it must be assumed that the operation may be converted to an open operation if laparoscopic techniques prove unwarranted or difficult. Preoperative pulmonary function should be assessed because insufflation of the abdominal cavity with carbon dioxide will increase the partial pressure of carbon dioxide in the blood. Patients should undergo standard mechanical bowel preparation and receive perioperative antibiotics. Information on the risk of abdominal sepsis or wound infections in patients who have undergone laparoscopic bowel resections is not currently available. A nasogastric tube and Foley catheter is inserted in all patients to minimize the risk of injury to the stomach and bladder during trocar insertion.

Setting up operating room

A large operating room is essential because laparoscopic surgery is a 'high tech' endeavour and the requisite equipment easily fills a large operating room. Consequently, laparoscopic colorectal procedures should not be attempted in a small suite.

The laparoscopy equipment is bulky. Custom-built cabinets to house this expensive equipment are well worth the investment. The carbon dioxide insufflator, light source and video camera should be stacked vertically. This saves floor space and also allows the surgeon to view all the settings on each component more easily. Separation of the electronic instruments with shelves improves air circulation and cooling. We have had difficulty with overheating of the video camera when it was stacked directly on top of the light source. The cabinet must be on wheels and be easily moved.

1 The proper distribution of equipment within the operating room will greatly facilitate the performance of the procedure. Two video monitors are required. One is placed just beyond the feet of the patient. This allows the surgeon, assistant surgeon and cameraman to view the pelvic dissection comfortably. A second monitor is positioned near the left shoulder or arm of the patient. This is used during mobilization of the descending colon and splenic flexure.

The techniques of laparoscopic colorectal resection have not been standardized as yet. As a result, a full array of laparoscopic instruments (*see* chapter on pp. 161–176) must be readily available. A cart which displays all the instruments is helpful.

Most lesions are identified and localized by intra-operative colonoscopy. The surgeon cannot palpate the lesion and only advanced lesions are visible. The endoscopy light source is placed near the patient's right leg. This light source can also be used for a second laparoscope.

Instruments

The operation is accomplished with a 10-mm 0° telescope. A second telescope is useful for transillumination of the mesentery or for photography. A 10-mm 30° telescope facilitates mobilization of the splenic flexure.

Surgeons will develop their own tactics for trocar selection and placement. Small trocars (5-mm) are used to introduce dissecting instruments. They do not, however, allow insertion of many of the recently introduced bowel instruments such as Babcock's tissue-holding forceps. The great advantage of 5-mm trocars is that they are easily removed and repositioned. Medium trocars (10- and 11-mm) offer flexibility. The telescope and most instruments can be interchanged among these ports. Reducing apertures are used with instruments of smaller diameter. Large trocars (12-mm, 15-mm and larger) are reserved for specific stapling devices. These are positioned to allow transection of the gut or mesentery with instruments such as the Endo-GIA 30 stapling device.

The dissection is accomplished with either cautery scissors or lasers. Reusable scissors are not adequate since they do not remain sufficiently sharp. While the surgeon uses a grasping instrument such as forceps, the assistant surgeon provides countertraction with two Babcock-type instruments.

The position of the patient is changed frequently throughout the procedure. The table must allow a very steep Trendelenburg position. It should also rotate left and right for elevation of either shoulder. An electric table expedites position changes.

Traditional surgical instruments must be readily available. Rapid conversion to open surgical techniques may be required for control of haemorrhage or other complications.

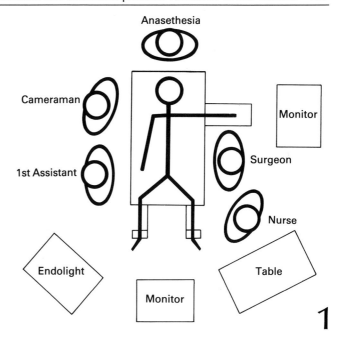

Operations

LAPAROSCOPIC ANTERIOR RESECTION
Position of patient

The patient's legs are placed in stirrups (*see* chapter on pp. 47–50). The thighs are not elevated but remain as straight as possible. Flexed thighs often impede the movement of the long surgical instruments used in laparoscopic operations. The legs are separated to allow access to the anus. This will allow introduction of the colonoscope for identification of the lesion and, subsequently, insertion of the Premium CEEA stapling device for construction of the anastomosis. A nasogastric tube and Foley catheter are inserted into all patients. This decreases the risk of perforation of the stomach or bladder during establishment of the pneumoperitoneum. The table is dropped into the deep Trendelenburg position before the pneumoperitoneum is established. During the operation the position of the table is frequently shifted. Deep Trendelenburg causes the small intestine to roll out of the pelvis. Reverse Trendelenburg exposes the transverse colon and splenic flexure. Rolling the right shoulder up shifts the small bowel and sigmoid colon away from the sacral promontory, right iliac vessels and right ureter. Rolling the left shoulder up exposes the left gutter, left iliac vessels and left ureter. Rotation and inclination of the table is the primary means of retracting the small intestine, omentum and other organs away from the operative field.

The abdomen is prepared and draped in the standard fashion. Access to the entire abdominal wall is necessary. Cables for the video equipment, carbon dioxide tubing, suction and irrigation tubing, and cautery wiring are bundled together and directed off the field. Slack must be left on the video cable so that the telescope can be moved from port to port.

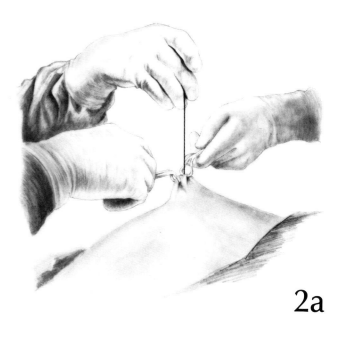

2a

Establishing the pneumoperitoneum

2a, b The table is in the deep Trendelenburg position, and the abdominal wall near the umbilicus is grasped either by hand or with two towel clamps and elevated. This creates a space between the abdominal wall and gut. A small skin incision about 1 cm in length is made just cephalad to the umbilicus. A Verres-type needle is inserted into the abdominal cavity, and the needle top is swung in a circle so that the needle subscribes a cone. Omentum or bowel stuck to the abdominal wall near the site of needle insertion blocks the excursion of the needle tip. If this should occur, the needle is removed and inserted elsewhere or an open technique of trocar insertion is used. Sterile water (5 ml) is injected through the needle and aspirated. If the needle is in the proper position there will be no return. The needle is removed if blood or enteric contents are aspirated. As the syringe is disconnected, the remaining fluid in the needle should drop rapidly into the abdominal cavity.

The carbon dioxide tubing is connected to the needle and insufflation is initiated slowly. The insufflator is set so that intra-abdominal pressure is limited to less than 15 mmHg. The initial intra-abdominal pressure should be low (less than 10 mmHg); if it is about 15 mmHg, the Verres needle should be withdrawn and reinserted. If the initial pressure remains high, an open technique of trocar insertion should be used. The low flow rate is continued until 1 litre of carbon dioxide has been pumped and then a high flow rate is initiated. Because of resistance, the Verres needle limits flow to a maximum of about 2.5 l/min. Carbon dioxide is pumped until an intra-abdominal pressure of 15 mmHg is achieved. This generally requires 3–5 litres of gas. The needle is withdrawn and a 10-mm trocar is inserted into the abdomen through the same incision. Rotation of the trocar aids in penetration of the fascia. The trocar must be sharp; consequently, disposable trocars are preferable to reusable ones. The carbon dioxide tubing is attached to the port. A high flow rate of insufflation is maintained throughout the remainder of the procedure. A 10-mm 0° telescope is immediately inserted down the port. The abdomen is inspected for evidence of injury inflicted by insertion of the Verres needle or 10-mm trocar.

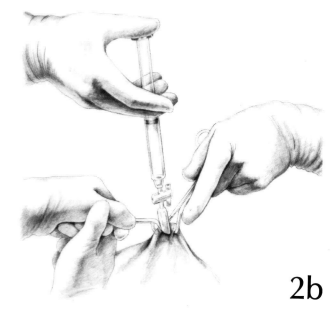

2b

Exploration

The abdomen is explored. The pelvis is first inspected because the patient is in the deep Trendelenburg position.

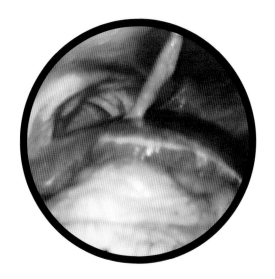

3

3 Adequate exposure of the liver is achieved only with the patient in the reverse Trendelenburg position. A 10-mm 30° telescope aids in visualizing the dome of the liver. Ultrasonographic equipment is available which can be introduced through laparoscopy ports. This can help in the identification of liver metastases.

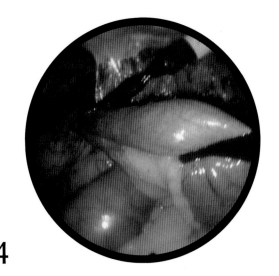

4

4 Complete exploration of the abdomen is achieved after introduction of additional ports. The entire small intestine is exposed with the aid of atraumatic grasping instruments. The right and left colon are exposed by rotation of the table.

Trocar placement

Strategies of trocar placement remain in a period of evolution. Introduction of new instruments which facilitate different aspects of the operation will continue to modify the sizes and positioning of ports.

5 At the beginning of the procedure, a 10-mm port is placed cephalad to the umbilicus for the telescope. Two 10-mm ports are placed lateral to the rectus sheath in the right lower quadrant and two in the left lower quadrant. This allows the surgeon on one side of the patient two instruments for dissection and the assistant surgeon on the other side of the table two instruments for retraction. A sixth port is often required at the level of the umbilicus on the right side for better exposure of the right side of the pelvis.

Retraction of the rectum out of the pelvis blocks the view of the telescope through the umbilical port. Generally, the caudal right lower quadrant port is replaced with a larger port when the mesentery and rectum are transected with an endoscopic stapling device. In very low procedures a suprapubic port may facilitate transection of the rectum.

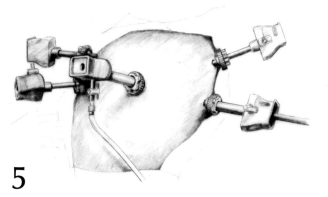

5

Mobilization

The patient is placed in the deep Trendelenburg position with the left shoulder rolled up. The dissection is viewed on the monitor between the patient's legs. Any adhesions between the small bowel and colon are divided with cautery scissors. The small bowel is pulled out of the pelvis with atraumatic grasping instruments. If the patient is sufficiently inclined, the small bowel will slide cephalad and remain out of the pelvis. Sometimes division of the retroperitoneal fixation of the caecum and terminal ileum is required to provide sufficient mobility so that these organs roll out of the operative field. In women, the uterus often obscures visualization of the distal rectum. Under these circumstances, the uterus is suspended from the abdominal wall with a heavy suture. A Keith needle is passed through the abdominal wall and the uterus, and is passed back through the abdominal wall. Alternatively, the uterus can be displaced anteriorly with a uterine elevator which is introduced transvaginally.

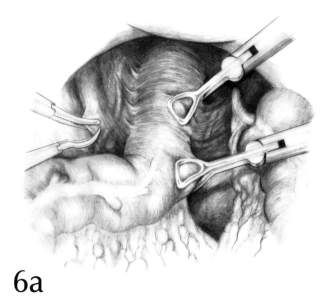

6a

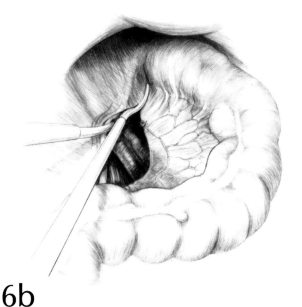

6b

6a, b Once adequate exposure of the pelvis is achieved, the rectosigmoid junction and the sigmoid colon are grasped by the assistant surgeon from the right side of the table with two Babcock clamps. Using cautery scissors and a grasping instrument, the surgeon frees the lateral attachments of the sigmoid colon.

The ureter is exposed over the iliac vessels. Illuminated ureteric stents can facilitate visualization of the ureter. When the intensity of the laparoscopic light source is turned down, the stents become visible.

7 The assistant surgeon (right side of table) grasps the rectum as low as possible with the Babcock clamp in the right hand. The rectum is pulled out of the pelvis, and the Babcock clamp in the the surgeon's left hand grasps the rectum near the other clamp.

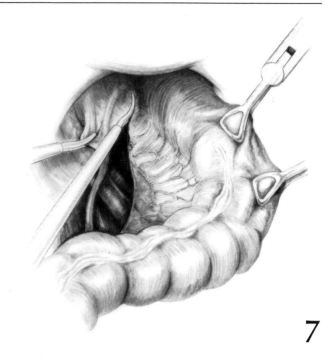

7

The Babcock clamp in the right hand is repositioned lower on the rectum, and this is retracted cephalad and ventrally. The surgeon incises the retroperitoneum along the pelvic brim medial to the iliac vessels. This further frees the left ureter. This is continued down into the anterior cul-de-sac. As the dissection continues down towards the anterior peritoneal reflection, the clamps may require repositioning for better exposure. The surgeon must maintain meticulous haemostasis in the pelvis. All tissues should be divided with cautery. Accumulation of even small amounts of blood will hinder dissection later in the procedure. Any pools of blood should be irrigated with heparinized saline (approximately 2000–3000 units/l) and aspirated. Even a few millilitres of blood appear like a large lake because of the magnification of the video system.

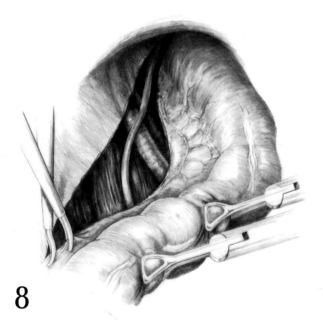

8

8 The assistant surgeon moves his Babcock clamps to the proximal sigmoid colon and distal descending colon, and provides medial and ventral retraction. The dissection is viewed on the monitor by the patient's left shoulder. The surgeon incises the white line of Toldt. The descending colon is then easily swept medially with the long shafts of the dissecting instruments. With the surgeon on the left side and the telescope in the umbilical port, the video image on the monitor is reversed. This impedes hand–eye co-ordination. Mobilization of the descending colon, however, is generally easily accomplished despite this impediment.

On the other hand, mobilization of the splenic flexure is much more difficult. When this is required, the surgeon should move to between the legs of the patient. Since the surgeon's instruments and the telescope are again aligned in the same direction, the image is no longer reversed.

The surgeon and assistant surgeon switch sides. The telescope is moved to the port at the level of the umbilicus on the right side. The table remains in the deep Trendelenburg position and is rolled so that the right shoulder of the patient is elevated.

9 The assistant surgeon, on the patient's left side, grasps the rectosigmoid colon with the Babcock clamp in the right hand and the mid-rectum with the other clamp. The rectum is retracted cephalad and ventrally. Tension is put on the mesorectum over the sacral promontory. Electrocautery scissors are used to enter the presacral space. The avascular plane between the fascia propria and Waldeyer's fascia is easily identified. If desired, the dissection can also proceed behind Waldeyer's fascia. The mesorectum is pushed away from the sacrum with the shaft of the surgeon's dissecting instruments. Again, all tissues should be divided with cautery. Some prefer a laser for this dissection. Even tiny amounts of blood stain the tissue and obscure the proper planes of dissection. The field is frequently irrigated with the heparinized saline and aspirated. The peritoneum is incised along the right pelvic brim medial to the ureter. Again, illuminated ureteral stents speed identification of the right ureter. The incision is continued until the incision on the left is reached in the anterior cul-de-sac.

Suspension of the rectum from the abdominal wall often improves exposure of the mesorectum and frees the assistant surgeon's instruments for other tasks. The assistant surgeon removes the Babcock clamp in his left hand, and retraction and elevation of the rectum is maintained with the other clamp. A dissecting instrument such as the Endo or Maryland dissectors is passed through the mesorectum near the rectal wall.

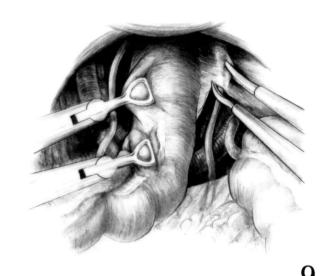

9

10 A long Kieth needle with a heavy suture such as 0 silk is passed through the abdominal wall just above the pubic symphysis. The needle is clasped by a needle holder, and most of the silk suture is pulled into the abdomen. The tip of the needle is grabbed by the dissecting instrument held by the assistant and pulled through the mesorectum; the needle is then passed back through the abdominal wall near its entry site. The suture is clasped with a clamp, and the rectum is pulled up to the abdominal wall by tightening the suture. Retraction on the rectum by the assistant is no longer required. He can now assist the surgeon with instruments introduced through the umbilical port or either of the left lower quadrant ports.

The suspended mesorectum divides the abdominal cavity and pelvis like a curtain. Introduction of a second telescope facilitates the remainder of the posterior pelvic dissection. Insertion of a second telescope through a left lateral port allows the surgeon constant visualization of the left ureter and the tips of his instruments as he connects the pelvic dissection on the right side with that on the left. In addition, the second telescope can be used to transilluminate the mesorectum and mesosigmoid. This aids the identification of the superior haemorrhoidal and inferior mesenteric vessels.

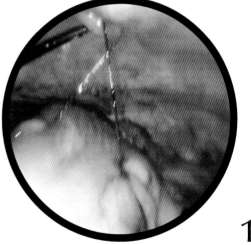

10

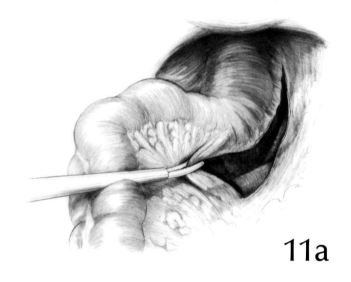

11a

11a, b The planes of dissection on the right and left are connected through the presacral space. The assistant surgeon can use flat instruments like the Endo-Grasp to push the mesorectum away from the sacrum as the surgeon extends his dissection deep into the pelvis. Similarly, the assistant can provide left lateral retraction on the mesorectum as the right suspensory ligaments are divided. This is usually accomplished with cautery scissors, but clips are sometimes required.

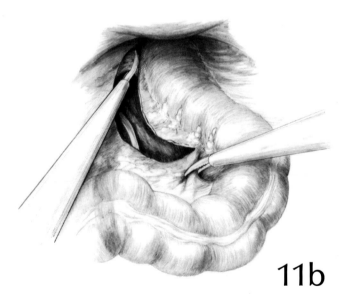

11b

Ligation of superior haemorrhoidal vessels

Early ligation of the superior haemorrhoidal or inferior mesenteric vessels decreases blood loss during the remainder of the pelvic dissection. Controversy about the advantages of high ligation of the inferior mesenteric vessels remains unresolved. As a general principle, surgeons should perform essentially the same operation using laparoscopic techniques as they do during open operations. With the mesorectum freed from the sacrum, transection of the superior haemorrhoidal vessels at the level of the sacral promontory is readily accomplished. The overlying fascia propria is incised.

12a–c An avascular window is generally found anterior to the superior haemorrhoidal vessel at this level, and this expedites the process. This window through the mesorectum is extended back to the take-off point of the last sigmoid branch. The thickness of this pedicle is calibrated with the Endo-Gauge and either the vascular (white) or bowel (blue) cartridge is selected. The port in the right lower quadrant is replaced with the 15-mm port. The Endo-GIA 30 stapling device is inserted into the abdomen. The jaws of the stapler are opened and slid over the vascular pedicle. The tips of the instrument are observed through the second telescope in the left lower quadrant. The assistant surgeon aids this process by opening the window in the mesentery with blunt instruments such as the Endo-Grasp. The Endo-GIA 30 is atraumatic and can be opened and repositioned many times without injury to the tissues. This device fires six rows of overlapping staples and divides the tissue with a knife, leaving three rows of staples on either side of the incision. The staple lines with the Endo-GIA 30 are 30-mm long, and with the Endo-GIA 60 are 60-mm long. Ligation of the vascular pedicle with a stapling device is rapid and secure. These advantages outweigh issues of cost because of the tedious and time consuming nature of traditional methods of vascular ligation when performed using laparoscopic techniques.

If desired, the inferior mesenteric artery can be ligated at its origin. The telescope is moved to a port in the right lower quadrant, and the surgeon faces the video monitor by the patient's left shoulder. The assistant elevates the mid-sigmoid colon with a Babcock clamp in his right hand. This maintains tension on the mesosigmoid. The assistant pushes the superior haemorrhoidal vessels dorsally with an atraumatic instrument in his left hand, and the surgeon dissects along the avascular plane between the inferior mesenteric artery and aorta with cautery scissors. The surgeon provides countertraction with a grasping instrument in his left hand. The artery is isolated, and the right lateral 10-mm port at the level of the umbilicus is replaced with a 12-mm port. The calibre of the vessel is measured, and the artery is divided with an Endo-GIA 30.

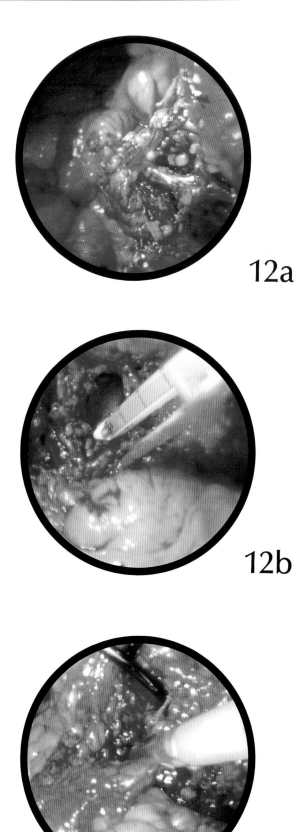

12a

12b

12c

Completion of pelvic dissection

Anterior mobilization of the distal rectum is difficult because instruments for anterior retraction of the bladder and prostate or vagina are not yet available. If the rectum is suspended from the abdominal wall, the suture is released. In women, a second assistant can help expose this plane by elevating the vagina with a finger. A second finger or a proctoscope in the rectum can provide countertraction. In men, a flat instrument such as the Endo-Grasp can be used to elevate the bladder and prostate once the anterior peritoneal reflection is incised. In the future, various retractors will be available which will facilitate this portion of the dissection.

Lesion identification

13a−c It is often impossible to visualize the lesion with a laparoscope. Consequently, the level of distal transection of the rectum which will provide an adequate margin of resection is not apparent. A colonoscope or rigid proctoscope is introduced into the rectum by an assistant. It is advanced to the distal edge of the lesion. As the intensity of the laparoscopic light source is turned down, the light of the colonoscope becomes visible through the rectal wall. A clip applier is introduced into the abdomen through a 10-mm port. The surgeon presses the jaws of a clip applier over the light of the colonoscope. The impression of the jaws as they are pushed against the rectal wall is conspicuously apparent to the colonoscopist, who can then direct the surgeon to move the clip applier up or down the rectal wall. Clips mark the distal edge of the lesion and also the planned level of transection of the rectum.

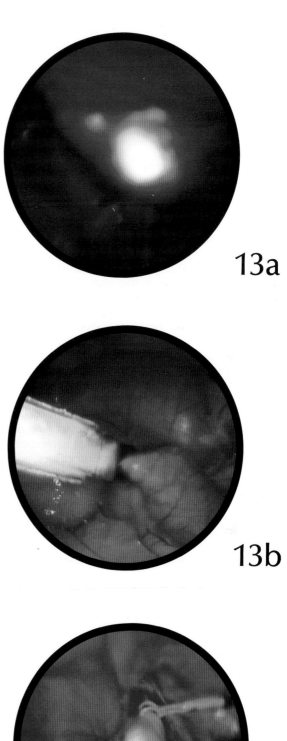

13a

13b

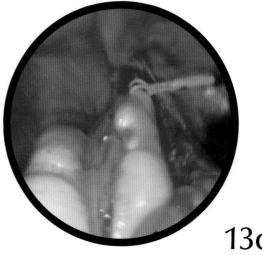

13c

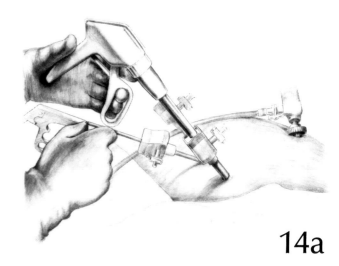

14a

Transection of rectum

14a–c The primary telescope is positioned through the right lateral port at the level of the umbilicus. The assistant retracts the rectum out of the pelvis with a Babcock clamp. The caudad right lower quadrant port is replaced with a 15-mm port if this has not already been done. Depending on the individual patient and the level of transection, insertion of the 15-mm port just cephalad to the pubis on the midline is sometimes preferable. The thickness of the rectal tissue is calibrated with the Endo-Gauge, and the rectum transected with the Endo-GIA 60 stapling device. The tips of the stapling device are observed through the second telescope which is positioned in a left lower quadrant 10-mm port. Sometimes, because of space constraints within the pelvis, it is easier to transect the rectum with multiple applications of the shorter Endo-GIA 30. Future modifications of laparoscopic stapling devices may facilitate positioning of these instruments deep in the pelvis. After transection of the rectum, the remaining mesorectum is divided with either cautery and clips or with an Endo-GIA 60.

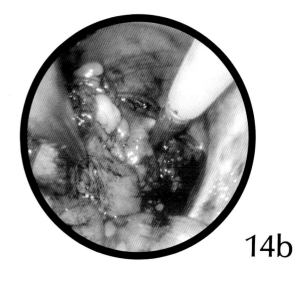

14b

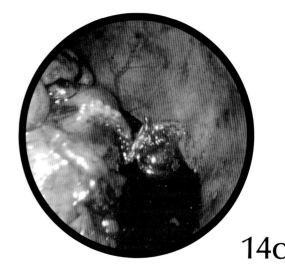

14c

Removal of specimen

15a–d The specimen is removed through a transverse muscle splitting incision in the left lower quadrant. The incision is often made through the site of the cephalad left lower quadrant port. The primary telescope is positioned in the right lateral port at the level of the umbilicus, and the surgeon is on the patient's left side. A Babcock clamp introduced from the right side of the table grasps the rectal staple line of the specimen. The surgeon pushes against the abdominal wall at the level of his planned incision. The specimen is elevated towards the indentation on the abdominal wall made by the surgeon's finger. If parts of the specimen are tethered, further mobilization is achieved. The surgeon makes a small transverse incision (2–4 cm) and the fascia is incised. Muscle layers are split along the course of their fibres. The surgeon's finger enters the abdominal cavity through a tiny incision in the parietal peritoneum; this manoeuvre maintains the pneumoperitoneum. A Babcock or Allis' clamp is inserted along the side of the surgeon's finger under direct visualization with the primary telescope. The staple line on the rectum is grasped by the Babcock or Allis' clamp. The laparoscopic Babcock clamp is released, and the incision is extended to the size necessary for delivery of the specimen. This is generally determined by the size of the lesion. The specimen is pulled through the incision onto the abdominal wall.

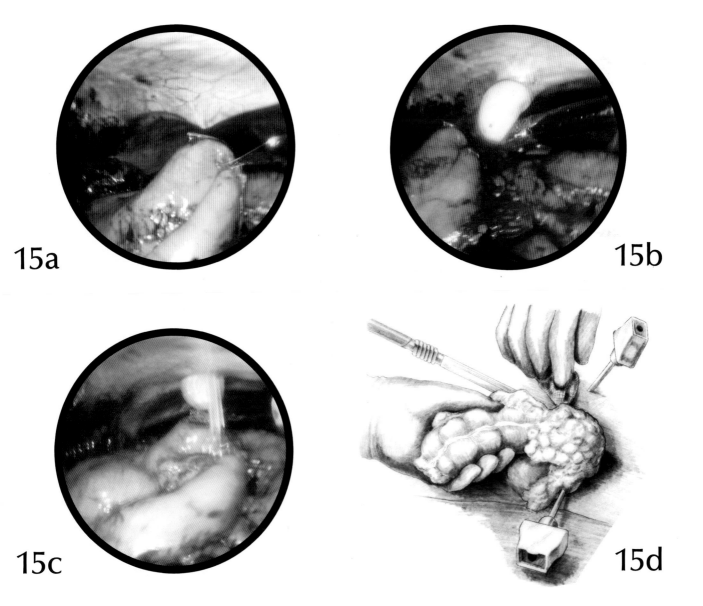

15a

15b

15c

15d

Proximal transection of specimen

16 The proximal level of transection of the specimen is selected. The remaining mesocolon is divided between clamps and tied with 3/0 silk. About 2.5 cm of the colonic wall is cleared of attached mesentery or epiploic fat tags. An automatic purse-string device is positioned and fired. A Kocher clamp is applied distal to the purse-string device and the bowel is divided. The specimen is handed to the pathologist, and is opened in the operating room. The distal margins are measured.

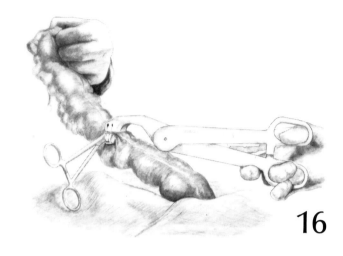

16

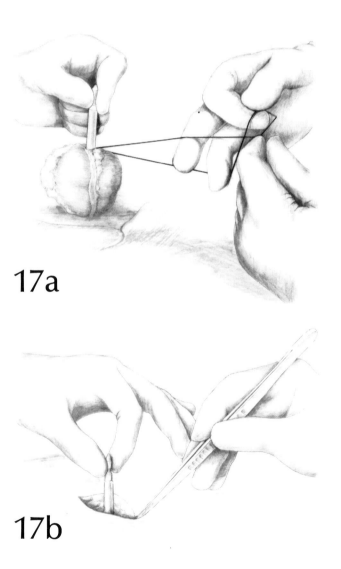

17a

17b

Placement of anvil

17a, b The lumen of the colon is sized and, if necessary, dilated with a finger or by distension of a 30-ml Foley balloon with water. It is preferable to use a 31-mm stapling device because of the potential of stricture of the anastomosis. The anvil and shaft assembly of the Premium CEEA stapling device is inserted into the colon. The purse-string is tied, and the abdomen and pelvis are liberally irrigated with warmed saline through the incision. Any clotted blood is removed with suction, and the colon replaced within the abdomen. The shaft of the anvil is positioned carefully in the pelvis with its tip pointing towards the rectal stump. Some surgeons find it helpful to tie a chromic suture around the shaft and leave a long tail. The long suture aids in identification of the anvil shaft assembly should it slide under the small bowel.

The incision is closed, and the pneumoperitoneum re-established. The shaft is immediately visualized with the laparoscope and grasped with a Babcock clamp. The shaft of the anvil is pulled down into the pelvis and positioned next to the rectal staple line. The colon should lie beside the rectal stump without tension. If necessary, further mobilization of the descending colon is achieved so that a tension-free anastomosis can be constructed.

Insertion of stapling device

The assistant sits between the legs of the patient. The anus of the patient is dilated to admit four fingers. The Premium CEEA stapling device is inserted into the rectum with the sharp spike withdrawn into the instrument. The assistant advances the stapling device up to the staple line on the rectal stump, and observes its advance on the video monitor at the patient's left shoulder.

18 The wing nut on the handle of the instrument is turned so that the spike penetrates the centre of the previous staple line. The spike is advanced until the orange collar of the instrument shaft is observed. The surgeon lassoes the spike with a pre-tied suture loop introduced into the abdomen through the 12- or 15-mm port. The spike is pulled out of the stapling device and retrieved through the port.

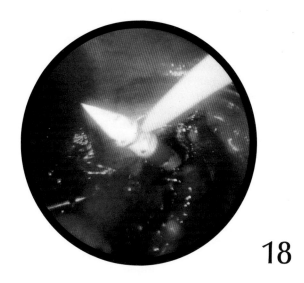

18

Docking of anvil shaft assembly into stapling device

19a, b The shaft of the anvil is seized with a Babcock clamp which is inserted through the suprapubic port or most caudad right lower quadrant port. If a Babcock clamp is not available, the large alligator-type clamp used for retrieving the gallbladder can be substituted, although accomplishing the manoeuvre with this instrument is very difficult. The axis of the Babcock clamp must run as close as possible to perpendicular to the axis of the stapling device. This maximizes the mechanical advantage for insertion of the anvil shaft assembly into the shaft of the stapling device. Recent modifications of the shaft of the anvil have greatly facilitated this manoeuvre. A groove has been machined into the shaft. The jaws of the Endo-Babcock fit snugly and securely into this groove. This task may be more easily achieved with the surgeon directing the Babcock clamp attached to the anvil with his left hand and the stapling device with his right hand. Insertion is only achieved when the shaft of the anvil perfectly aligns with the shaft of the stapling device in all three dimensions.

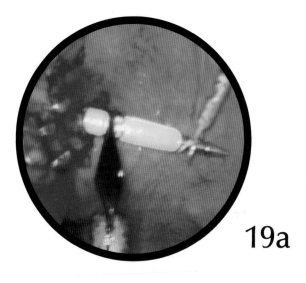

19a

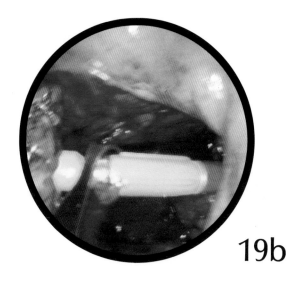

19b

Construction of anastomosis

Once the two parts of the stapling device are docked, the mesocolon is checked for rotation. The stapling device is screwed closed and fired and the wing nut is opened four half turns. The stapling device is rotated and rocked up and down and then withdrawn. Countertraction on the anastomosis is applied with an atraumatic grasping instrument. Two complete 'dough-nuts' of tissue should be found within the head of the stapling device. The outside of the anastomosis is visually inspected with the laparoscope. The pelvis is filled with saline squirted down a large port. The inside of the anastomosis is examined with a colonoscope or rigid proctoscope. The colon is grasped with an atraumatic bowel clamp proximal to the anastomosis. The rectum is insufflated until air escapes through the anus around the endoscope. Observation of bubbles surfacing in the saline filling the pelvis indicates an unsatisfactory anastomosis.

Closure

The saline in the pelvis is aspirated. Further irrigation can be accomplished through the large ports. If desired, a suction catheter is placed within the pelvis. A clamp which grasps the end of the catheter is passed down a port in the lower abdomen. The tip of the catheter is placed in the desired position under direct visualization with the laparoscope. A second clamp grasps the tip of the catheter, and the first catheter and port are withdrawn. The remaining ports are withdrawn under direct observation. The fascial defect from the 10-mm ports and larger should be closed with absorbable sutures such as 0 Dexon. Each closure is checked with the laparoscope to ensure that no bowel has been caught with a suture. After all other ports have been removed, the laparoscope is withdrawn. The pneumoperitoneum is deflated through the last port. The final port is removed and its fascial defect closed. The subcutaneous tissues are irrigated with a solution containing antibiotics. The larger skin incisions are closed with continuous subcuticular sutures such as 4/0 Dexon and the smaller incisions are closed with Steri-strips.

ABDOMINAL PERINEAL RESECTION

Setting up operating room and positioning of patient

The operating room is set out in the same manner as for anterior resection. A colonoscope or rigid proctoscope should be available for lesion identification and localization. The patient is placed in the modified lithotomy position (*see* chapter on pp. 47–50). The patient's thighs can be more flexed since less mobilization of the descending colon and splenic flexure is required. This will allow better access for the perineal portion of the operation. The stomach is intubated with a nasogastric tube and the bladder with a urinary catheter. Ureteric stents are particularly helpful for ureteric identification for the surgeon performing the perineal dissection.

Laparoscopic dissection

The abdominal portion of the operation is commenced first. Port placement and mobilization is identical to that described above for anterior resection. It is critical that, during the abdominal dissection, the ureters are identified and that they are freed from any attachments to the mesorectum. This will prevent traction of the ureters down into the pelvis and potential injury. In addition, initiation of anterior dissection between the rectum, bladder and prostate in men and vagina in women greatly facilitates identification of this plane from below.

Ligation of vascular pedicle

The superior haemorrhoidal and inferior mesenteric vessels are identified early in the procedure, and are divided at the desired level with an Endo-GIA 30 stapling device. This minimizes blood loss during the pelvic dissection. The mesorectum is mobilized off the sacrum, and the level of the lesion is confirmed. A decision is made as to whether a sphincter-saving procedure is appropriate.

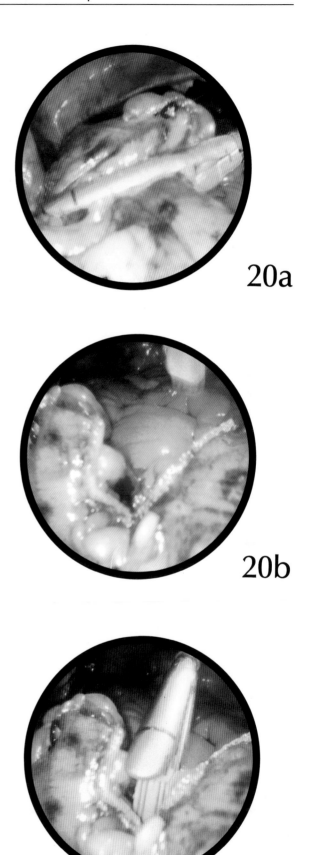

Transection of colon

20a–c The telescope enters the abdomen through the umbilical port. The surgeon is on the right side of the patient, and faces the monitor at the patient's left shoulder. The distal descending colon is grasped with a Babcock clamp which is introduced through the cephalad port in the left lower quadrant. The proximal sigmoid colon is grasped with a second Babcock clamp passed through the caudad port in the right lower quadrant. The cephalad 10-mm port in the right lower quadrant is replaced with a 12-mm port for the Endo-GIA 30 or a 15-mm port for the Endo-GIA 60 stapling device. The thickness of the colonic wall at the descending colon–sigmoid junction is calibrated with an Endo-Gauge. Generally, the blue (3.5-mm) cartridge is selected. The colon is transected with the stapling device; or even three applications of the Endo-GIA 30 may be required. In contrast, one firing of the Endo-GIA 60 usually transects the colon. The remaining mesocolon down to the level of the ligation of the inferior mesenteric vessels is divided with electrocautery and application of clips. Alternatively, the mesentery is divided by serial applications of a stapling device.

COMBINED LAPAROSCOPIC AND PERINEAL DISSECTION OF PELVIS

Once a decision has been reached to proceed with an abdominal perineal resection rather than a low anterior resection, the perineal portion of the operation is initiated. The laparoscopic surgeon performs as much of the pelvic dissection as can be easily visualized. Much of the pelvic dissection, however, is more easily accomplished by the perineal surgeon. The pneumoperitoneum can be maintained throughout the combined pelvic dissection.

Anterior dissection

21a–c Laparoscopic exposure of the plane between the anterior surface of the rectum and the vagina in women or the prostate and bladder in men is sometimes difficult. In men, the laparoscopic surgeon incises the peritoneum at the bottom of the rectovesical pouch on the base of the bladder. A finger in the rectum helps with posterior traction. The assistant retracts the posterior edge of the peritoneal reflection with a Babcock clamp. The seminal vesicles and vasa are pushed forward by the assistant with a flat instrument such as an Endo-Grasp. Denonvilliers' fascia is incised. Dissection is carried distally along the rectum as far as possible with cautery scissors.

In women, the anterior dissection is somewhat more easily exposed. The perineal surgeon provides posterior retraction of the rectum with a finger inserted through the anus. Similarly, a finger in the vagina aids with anterior retraction. The peritoneum of the rectovaginal pouch is incised over the vagina, and the posterior edge of the peritoneum is retracted as in men. The rectum is freed from the posterior wall of the vagina with a combination of blunt and cautery-assisted sharp dissection.

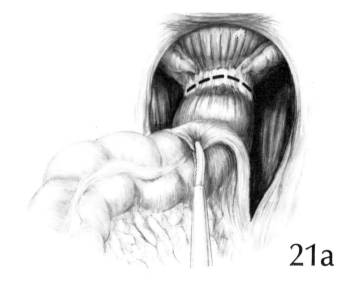

21a

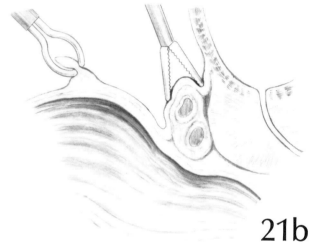

21b

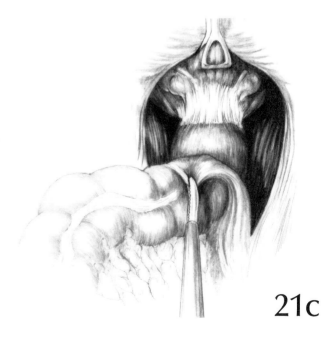

21c

Perineal dissection

22a–c The anus is sewn closed with a heavy suture. The perianal skin is incised down into the subcutaneous fat of the ischiorectal fossa, and the anococcygeal ligament is divided. The presacral space is entered ventrally to the coccyx. The surgeon pulls the levator muscles down with a finger and divides them at the desired level. The inferior haemorrhoidal vessels are divided with cautery or ligated. Alternatively, an intersphincteric dissection with preservation of the external sphincter can be performed. Preservation of the external sphincter, however, makes introduction of a hand into the pelvis more difficult.

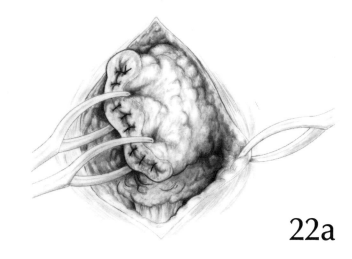

22a

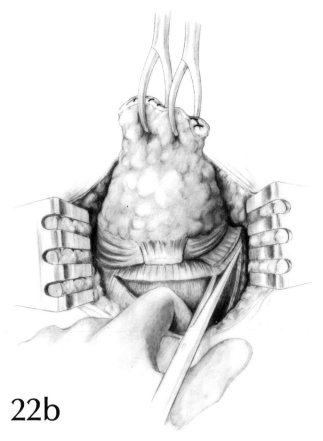

22b

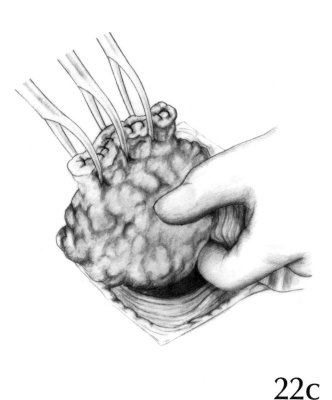

22c

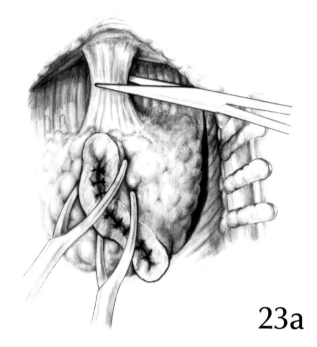

23a

23a, b After division of the anococcygeal ligament and the levator muscles, the superficial transverse perineal muscle is divided. The anterior surface of the rectum is freed in a plane at the posterior border of the deep transverse perineal muscle and the rectourethralis and puborectalis muscles are divided.

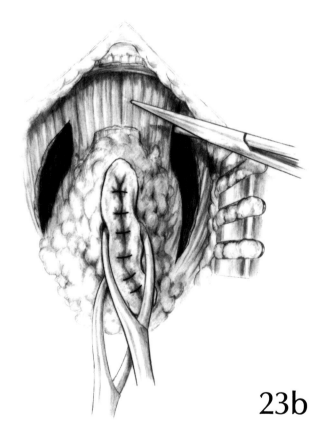

23b

Presacral dissection

24a, b The flat hand of the surgeon bluntly sweeps the mesorectum off the sacrum and off the pelvic side walls above the levator ani muscles. The surgeon advances his hand cephalad along the sacrum in the avascular plane between Waldeyer's fascia and the sacrum. The planes of laparoscopic and perineal dissection are initially connected posterior to the rectum. If Waldeyer's fascia has not been penetrated by the laparoscopic surgeon, it is tented up with the fingers of the perineal surgeon. Under direct observation, the laparoscopic surgeon incises Waldeyer's fascia with cautery scissors. The bulk of the perineal surgeon's hand and wrist maintains an airtight seal of the perineal wound. As a result, the pneumoperitoneum is maintained. Rotation of the hand around the posterior half of the pelvis frees the mesorectum from the pelvic side walls. The lateral suspensory ligaments, if not already divided by the laparoscopic surgeon, are retracted medially by the perineal surgeon. The laparoscopic surgeon divides these ligaments with cautery scissors under direct observation. If necessary, clips are applied to the middle haemorrhoidal vessels, again under direct visualization.

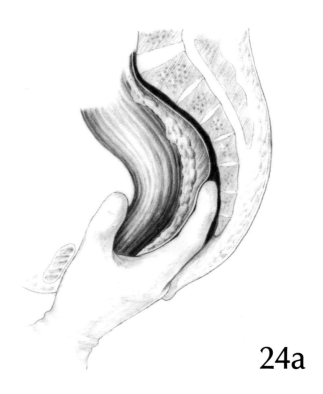

24a

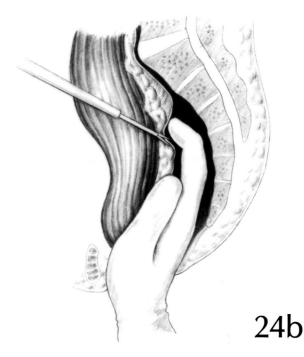

24b

Completion of anterior dissection by perineal surgeon

When exposure precludes completion of the anterior dissection by the laparoscopic surgeon, this plane is further developed by the perineal surgeon. The posterior and lateral dissections are first completed. The peritoneum of the rectovesical or rectovaginal pouch is incised. The perineal surgeon, with his palm behind the rectum, slides his fingers around the front of the rectum. The laparoscope projects this manoeuvre onto the video monitor which the perineal surgeon watches. If necessary, the laparoscopic surgeon opens the plane with retraction on the posterior edge of the incised anterior peritoneal reflection. The plane is bluntly dissected with the fingers of the perineal surgeon.

Delivery of specimen

25a, b The perineal surgeon passes his hand into the abdominal cavity through the perineal wound posterior to the mesorectum. He grasps the proximal end of the specimen and withdraws it out of the wound. The anterior surface of the rectum remains attached to the capsule of the prostate in men or the posterior wall of the vagina in women. With traction on the specimen, these attachments are easily divided.

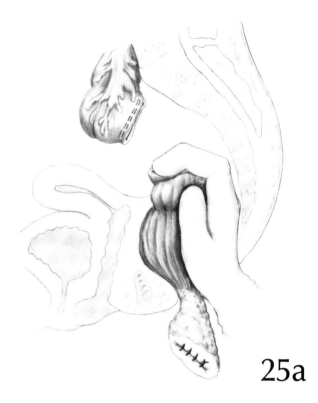

25a

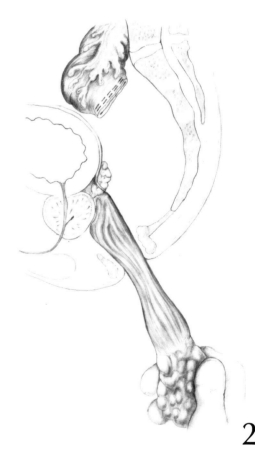

25b

Closure of perineal wound

The perineal wound is closed in the same manner as in a traditional abdominal perineal resection using open techniques. Two flat suction drains are introduced into the pelvis through stab wounds which penetrate the skin and levator ani muscles. The drains are positioned anterior to a line between the ischial tuberosities. Heavy silk sutures secure the drains to the skin. The edges of the levator ani are approximated with interrupted sutures of 2/0 Dexon. The skin incision is closed with a continuous suture of 4/0 Dexon.

Construction of end colostomy

The colostomy is best constructed at the end of the procedure. The pneumoperitoneum displaces the abdominal wall anteriorly, needlessly putting excess tension on the end descending colostomy. In addition, once the stoma site has been created, the pneumoperitoneum is lost. It cannot be re-established until the stoma site is made airtight by maturation of the colostomy. Furthermore, the port sites should be closed before the colostomy is matured.

The surgeon stands on the left side of the patient. A Babcock clamp, which is passed through the cephalad port in the left lower quadrant, grasps the proximal staple line on the descending colon. The assistant surgeon pushes a finger down on the abdominal wall at the previously selected stoma site. The Babcock clamps elevate the transected end of the descending colon up to the indentation of the abdominal wall caused by the assistant's finger. If necessary, further mobilization of the descending colon is achieved so that a tension-free colostomy is constructed. A Kocher clamp grasps the skin of the stoma site. A disc of skin with subcutaneous fat attached is excised down to the level of the anterior rectus sheath. A cruciate incision cuts through the anterior rectus sheath. A blunt curved clamp separates the fibres of the rectus muscle along their course. A finger is poked into the abdominal cavity through a small incision in the posterior rectus sheath and anterior parietal peritoneum. The finger plugs the hole and maintains the pneumoperitoneum. A Babcock clamp is passed into the abdomen, along the finger, and this elevates the transected end of the colon up to the colostomy site. Under direct vision through the laparoscope, the staple line is grasped by the Babcock clamp, which passes through the colostomy site. The incision in the posterior sheath is lengthened so that the end of the descending colon can be pulled out through the colostomy site. The pneumoperitoneum is lost. The ports are removed, and the fascial defects are closed as described for anterior resection. The staple line is excised, and the colostomy is sutured with eight sutures of 3/0 chromic catgut. Each stitch passes through the full thickness of the colonic wall and is anchored into the subcuticular layer of the skin.

Postoperative management

Management of patients after laparoscopic operations is similar to that following traditional operations. The patient is extubated in the operating room. The pneumatic compression stockings are left on the patient's legs and the nasogastric tube is generally left in place until the morning after the operation. The patient receives one dose of intravenous antibiotics in the recovery room. Intravenous fluids are continued until the patient is able to take liquids by mouth. Because of the extensive pelvic dissection required for treatment of malignancies, the urinary catheter is used to drain the bladder for 3–5 days. The patient receives intramuscular injections of morphine sulphate for pain; a patient administration system for analgesia is not recommended.

On the morning after operation the nasogastric tube is removed and the patient is allowed to take clear liquids if he desires them. Most patients tolerate clear liquids by mouth by the first or second day after the operation and advance to a regular diet on the second or third day. The patient is encouraged to ambulate on the day after the operation and the pneumatic compression stockings are removed when the patient is walking. Generally the patient suffers from only a moderate amount of pain and use of narcotics is minimal.

The patient remains in hospital until he is eating a regular diet and moving his bowels, both of which are usually achieved between the third and fifth postoperative day. The actual day of discharge is determined by additional factors which include the general condition of the patient and his social circumstances. Discharge of an elderly patient who lives alone may be delayed until additional support systems can be mobilized on his behalf. Similarly, after construction of a colostomy the patient remains in the hospital until he is able to care adequately for the stoma.

Endoscopic endoluminal rectal tumour resection

G. Buess MD, FRCSEd
Minimal Invasive Surgery, Department of Surgery, Eberhard-Karl University, Schnarrenberg Hospital, Tübingen, Germany

M. M. Lirici MD
Department of Surgery, La Sapienza University Medical School, Policlinico Umberto I, Rome, Italy

History

Local excision of sessile adenomas and early carcinomas of the rectum have become standard procedures since 1885, when Kraske reported the preliminary results of rectal tumour resection through a posterior rectotomy. More recently, local removal has been attempted after division of the sphincters by d'Allaines[1] and Mason[2].

From 1980 to 1983, Buess developed the first minimally invasive procedure for local resection of rectal tumours, and the operation has been called transanal endoscopic microsurgery to differentiate this technique from operative endoscopy through a flexible endoscope[2,3]. Transanal endoscopic microsurgery requires special optical equipment, endoscopic instruments and ancillary units. The team that carried out the technical and clinical development of the technique at the University of Cologne consisted of Buess, Theiss and Hutterer. The operation entered clinical practice in 1983.

Principles and justification

The precise removal of rectal polyps is necessary both for treatment of early carcinoma and for prevention of malignant evolution of an adenoma. Local excision of stage T_1 and T_2 invasive rectal carcinoma within 6 cm of the anal verge has been reported, resulting in survival and local control comparable with those obtained after more radical and invasive resection[4]. Furthermore, a permanent colostomy is avoided and the postoperative mortality and morbidity rates are far lower than after abdominoperineal resection. A complete local excision of T_1 tumours up to the rectosigmoid junction is considered to be as curative as radical surgery.

Sessile polyps in the rectum and the rectosigmoid junction may be difficult to reach through a conventional transanal approach. The use of Mayo or Parks' retractors allows the surgeon to reach polyps of the lower rectum but sometimes obstructs the view of the tumours, resulting in a lack of precision during surgical excision leading to a high tumour recurrence rate after conventional transanal excision of rectal polyps[3]. Larger or higher polyps require more invasive operations, such as the Kraske or Mason procedures, with their high postoperative complication rates[3].

In contrast, transanal endoscopic microsurgical dissection of the rectum allows treatment of both benign and malignant tumours up to 20 cm from the dentate line with low morbidity and mortality rates, resulting in less postoperative pain and a low rate of tumour recurrence[5,6]. Specially developed instrumentation allows the surgeon to achieve a clear view of the rectal lumen throughout the procedure and to perform different operations, from mucosectomy to full thickness dissection with resection of the retrorectal fat.

Indications

Besides sessile adenomas, the following classes of rectal cancer can be considered for transanal endoscopic microsurgery:

1. Low-risk carcinoma (pT_1): the operation has a high probability of being curative.
2. Moderate-risk carcinoma (pT_2): the operation has a limited probability of being curative.
3. Palliation in advanced cancers.
4. Unsuspected or previously undetected cancers, e.g. small areas of malignancy in large adenomas.

Preoperative

Investigations

In addition to routine investigations, preoperative assessment usually consists of digital examination, rigid rectoscopy, barium enema, computed tomography and endoluminal ultrasonography. Digital rectal examination and endoluminal ultrasonography are the most reliable examinations in the assessment of tumour staging, and rigid rectoscopy permits the exact evaluation of tumour location and size, which are mandatory assessments. A definition of tumour position relative to the rectal circumference is needed for correct patient positioning on the operating table and for the choice of the safest excision technique. These tests should be considered mandatory in the preoperative assessment of the patient.

Informed consent

The transanal endoscopic microsurgery procedure, its advantages and limitations, should be explained during an interview and consent signed before operation. The patient should know the possibility of converting the procedure to open surgery if the tumour is not localized properly or it is not possible to suture the defect.

Patient preparation

Bowel preparation consists of orthograde lavage through a gastric tube with 10 litres isotonic saline or Ringer's solution the day before surgery. Antibiotic prophylaxis consists of a single dose of metronidazole and a second-generation cephalosporin administered at the time of surgery.

Anaesthesia

Transanal endoscopic microsurgery is performed under either general or regional anaesthesia. Because of uncontrolled movements of the patient caused by intraoperative pain, time-consuming interventions or operations conducted with the patient prone should be performed under general endotracheal anaesthesia after placement of a urinary catheter. In the Buess series, up to 25% of patients underwent transanal endoscopic microsurgery under regional anaesthesia.

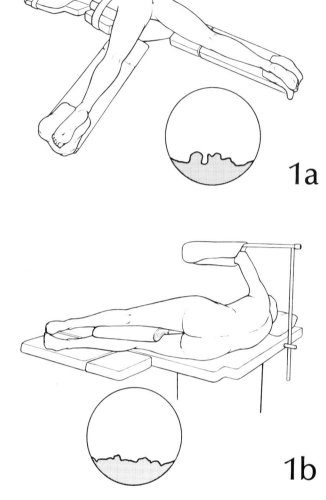

1a

1b

Operations

Position of patient and skin draping

1a, b As the rectal lesion must be situated at the bottom of the endoscopic field because of the angulation of the stereoscopic telescope, the patient is placed on the operating table in a lithotomy, prone, or lateral position, depending on the location of the tumour. Good padding of the brackets and frames of the apparatus is mandatory. With the patient in the prone position, the insertion of a roll between the patient's hips and the table, avoiding pressure on the abdominal wall, allows easier insufflation of the rectum. The perineal region is cleansed with alcoholic solution; skin shaving is not necessary. To isolate the operative field, a drape similar to that used for transurethral resection is applied to the skin.

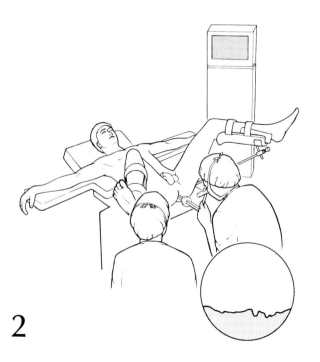

2

Operating theatre arrangement

2 The surgeon sits to operate through the rectoscope. The assistant sits on his left watching the operation on the television monitor. The scrub nurse stands to the surgeon's right and behind. The combined endosurgical unit for controlled automatic gas insufflation, rinsing and suction, and the electrosurgical unit are positioned on the left of the assistant. The video and camera equipment is on the surgeon's right side.

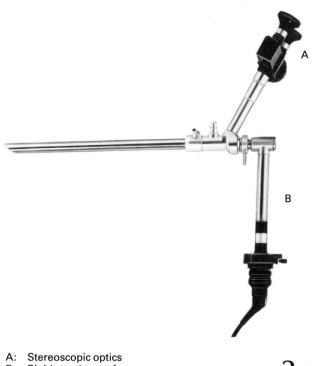

A: Stereoscopic optics
B: Rigid attachment for
    video monitoring

3a

Design of the operative system

3a, b The transanal endoscopic procedure is performed through a single access port: both the stereoscopic telescope and the endoscopic instruments are inserted through a 40-mm operating rectoscope. The rectoscope is provided with tubes of different lengths according to the distance of the polyp from the anal verge. The instrument has four ports, sealed by special sleeves and caps, for surgical instruments and one port for the stereoscopic optics.

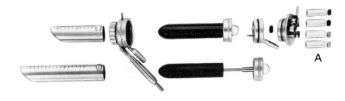

A: Sealing tubes and caps

3b

4 The handle, integrated with the basic element of the rectoscope, is fixed to the operating table by means of a double ball-jointed arm (D). The stereoscopic telescope allows a three-dimensional view of the operating field. An additional rigid optic for video monitoring can be introduced into the system. Specially designed instruments are necessary for transanal endoscopic microsurgery: high-frequency knife; right-angled and left-angled graspers and scissors (A); suction–coagulation probe (C); needle holder (B); and clip applier. A light cable and camera and silicone tubes for gas insufflation, suction and irrigation are connected to the assembled rectoscope.

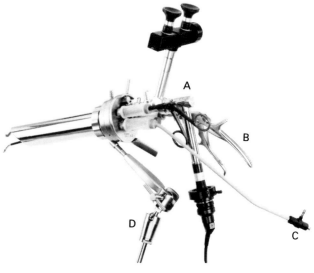

A: Grasping forceps
B: Needle holder
C: Suction–coagulation probe
D: Double ball-jointed arm

4

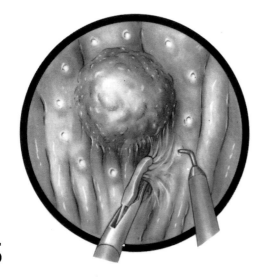

5

Definition of the margins of dissection

5 The operation begins with rectoscopy to localize the tumour and fix the 40-mm rectoscope to the table in the proper position. Carbon dioxide (CO_2) insufflation can then start, thus creating sufficient room for surgical manoeuvres. The resection safety margins should be at least 5 mm for adenomas and at least 10 mm for carcinomas. The ideal resection line is marked by several coagulation dots around the tumour with the high-frequency knife at the required distance.

MUCOSECTOMY

6a–c This technique is indicated for small polyps with no signs of malignancy and for larger polyps on the anterior wall in the intraperitoneal region more than 10 cm above the dentate line. The procedure should be carried out very carefully in order to avoid damage to the edges of the excised specimen. A fold of the mucosa distal to the polyp and just at a marking dot is lifted up, and the dissection starts using the high-frequency knife in the cutting mode. The incision is carried down to the muscularis mucosae from left to right. Magnification of the image is achieved by advancing the stereoscopic telescope towards the operating field. When bleeding occurs from small vessels, control is achieved by pressing and coagulating with the suction probe while sucking.

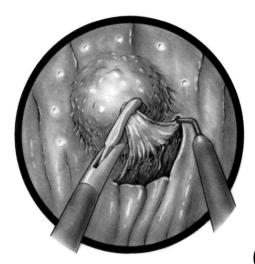

6a

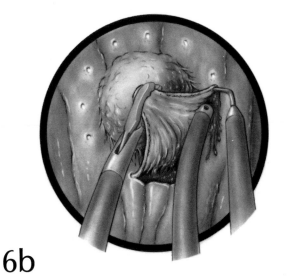

6b

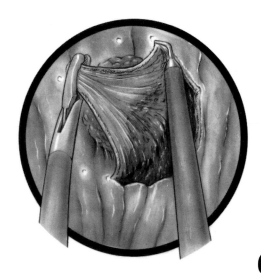

6c

FULL-THICKNESS EXCISION

Transanal endoscopic microsurgery performed with a full-thickness technique ensures an optimal depth during excision of T_1 carcinomas. Because of the high rate (20%) of preoperatively undetected cancers in sessile adenomas that have a diameter of more than 20 mm, this technique is indicated for such tumours in the extraperitoneal rectum. The full-thickness technique is only used in the extraperitoneal part of the rectum, hence it is the technique of choice for tumours of the posterior wall up to 20 cm from the dentate line, of the lateral walls up to 15–16 cm from the dentate line, and of the anterior wall up to 12 cm from the anocutaneous line.

7a, b The operation starts by grasping the rectal mucosa over a coagulation dot. The first stroke of the high-frequency knife divides the full thickness of the wall. Division is continued along the lower border of the resection. After completion of division of the distal margin, the incision is continued along the lateral aspects and then proximally. Hence, after lifting the transected margins upwards, the tumour base is exposed. In the case of an adenoma, the dissection is carried out between the outer longitudinal muscle fibres and the perirectal fat. The rectal wall division is accomplished when the divided upper margin is reached.

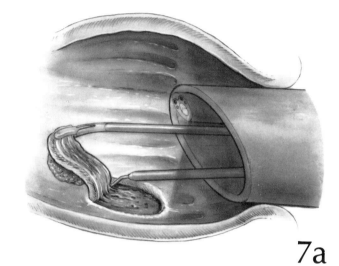

7a

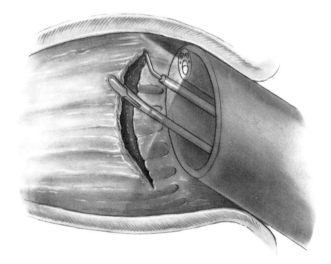

7b

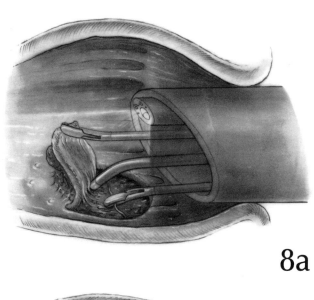

Coagulation

8a, b Bleeding vessels encountered during division of the muscular layer should be coagulated immediately because the light absorption of haematin greatly reduces the view. Vessels up to 1 mm in diameter are electrocoagulated using the suction probe. Larger vessels are grasped with the insulated forceps after preliminary compression with the suction probe and then coagulated. Bleeding may occur more often during dissection at the base of the polyp. A careful dissection is mandatory during this operative step, and vessels should be coagulated when encountered and before their division.

8a

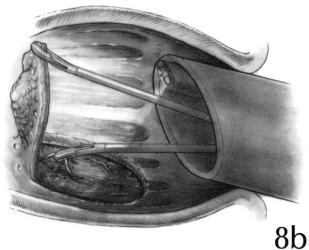

8b

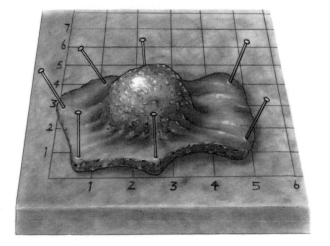

Management of the specimen

9 After removal of the specimen through the rectoscope, the polyp is pinned onto a cork board to properly evaluate the anatomical extent of the tumour and the clearance margins of the resection.

9

EN BLOC RESECTION OF RETRORECTAL FAT

En bloc resection of perirectal fat is possible for carcinomas located on the posterior and lateral rectal walls. Dissection of the retrorectal fat is performed down to Waldeyer's fascia. In such cases dissection to include lymph nodes is possible.

SEGMENTAL RESECTION

Segmental full-thickness resection of the rectum is possible for tumours of the middle third. Segments of the rectum up to 8 cm in length can be removed. Closure of the defect is achieved by a continuous end-to-end anastomosis. When segmental resection involves the intraperitoneal part of the rectum or the dentate line, full-thickness dissection should be avoided; a partial-thickness technique lessens the risk of opening the peritoneum and causing damage to the sphincter.

Suturing technique

10a–f The defect is rinsed with iodine solution, carefully checked and residual bleeding controlled. Closure of the defect is accomplished with a transverse continuous suture using 3/0 polydioxanone monofilament with a small half (Ethicon) needle. A silver clip (specially designed to not damage the thread when applied) is pressed onto the thread itself about 8 cm from the needle. The excess material is then cut. The needle held by the needle holder is inserted through the rectoscope and the running suture is started. The first stitch is directed from the luminal side towards the retrorectal aspect at the right corner of the defect. Additional silver clips are applied intermittently in order to reduce tension and maintain tissue approximation. Closure of a semicircular defect needs up to four 8-cm threads. The suture is finished by pressing a last silver clip onto the thread at the left corner of the defect.

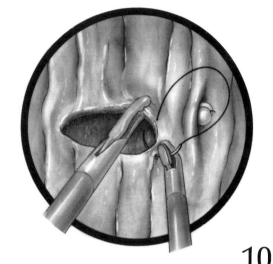

10a

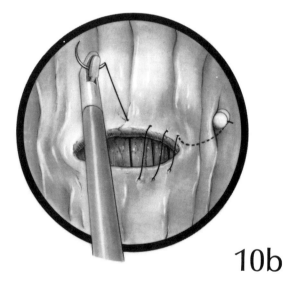

10b

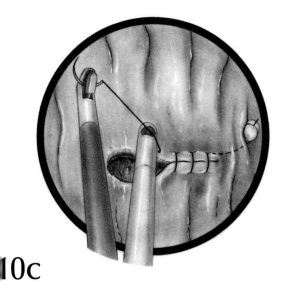

10c

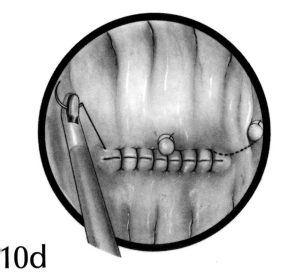

10d

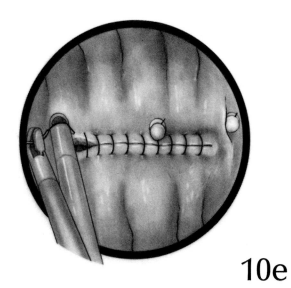

10e

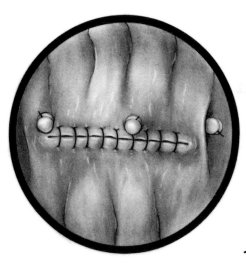

10f

Suturing extensive defects

11 In order to avoid tension while suturing large defects after resection of extensive longitudinal polyps or segmental resection, the insertion of temporary stay sutures is suggested. Several interrupted sutures are passed at a distance of 5 mm. Thereafter, the transverse running suture can be performed.

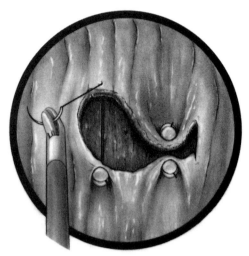

11

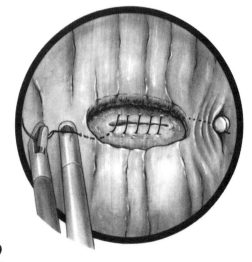

12

Closure of peritoneal defects

12 During resection of tumours within the intraperitoneal portion of the rectum, inadvertent peritoneal opening may occur, resulting in passage of CO_2 into the peritoneal cavity and a fall in the intrarectal pressure. Such a defect must be closed as soon as possible with a continuous 3/0 polydioxanone suture, otherwise the endoscopic view can be seriously compromised. The first suture starts from the rectal lumen returning back into the lumen where the thread is again secured with a silver clip.

Postoperative care

In most cases of full-thickness excision, postoperative management consists of 2 days of fasting with intravenous fluids; on the third day a full liquid diet is given. The patient can usually be discharged after the fourth day. After mucosectomy the patient is given clear liquid on the first day after the operation and regular meals from the second day; discharge from hospital is possible after the third day.

If severe pain occurs, usually encountered in patients who undergo resection of tumours close to the dentate line, the administration of oral analgesics is suggested.

Patients who undergo transanal endoscopic mucosectomy are mobile on the day of the operation. Micturition difficulties are often reported because of pressure trauma of the urethra which can occur while manipulating the rectoscope during the operation. Such problems usually last only 24 h. If these problems persist, urinary catheterization is indicated.

A transient pyrexia (up to 38.5°C) is common in patients who undergo a full-thickness resection. Such an increase in temperature disappears 2–4 days after operation and no antibiotics are administered. If the temperature rises above 38.5°C or lasts longer, wound dehiscence should be suspected and appropriate antibiotic therapy should be started promptly. In such patients, rectoscopy should be performed to evaluate the extent of the dehiscence. When needed, parenteral nutrition is started. The temperature usually drops within a few days. A loop colostomy may be necessary in cases of very large anastomotic defects, particularly after segmental resection.

If severe rectal bleeding occurs emergency rectoscopy is required. The source is usually the suture line or a mucosal tear. Careful coagulation with monopolar high-frequency current is indicated after detection of the bleeding source, taking care not to damage the continuous suture.

Follow-up after transanal endoscopic microsurgery for rectal cancer is performed at 3-monthly intervals, and for adenoma resection the first examination is after 3 months, with further endoscopic evaluation every year. The recurrence rate in patients with adenoma is 3%; the treatment in these cases consists of endoscopic excision by snare resection or hot biopsy.

Outcome

In our series of 386 transanal endoscopic microsurgery procedures performed at the University Hospitals of Cologne, Mainz and Tübingen from 1983 to 1991, 283 patients were suffering from rectal adenoma and 96 from carcinoma[5]. A full-thickness excision was performed in 70% of the cases operated for rectal adenoma.

The remaining cases underwent mucosectomy or partial-thickness excision. Segmental resection or retrorectal fat dissection was performed in 5% and 4% of cases, respectively. In patients with carcinoma full-thickness excision was performed in 85% of cases, and in 22% of cases the dissection of retrorectal fat was added.

The postoperative complication rate was about 9% and the mortality rate after transanal endoscopic microsurgery was less than 0.5%. The postoperative complications were mostly related to tension on the suture line; dehiscence (five patients) and fistula (three patients) occurred in the 191 consecutive procedures for adenoma. Stenosis caused by local wound healing problems occurred in five patients who all responded to dilatation. Other complications included bleeding, and one case in whom the peritoneum was opened for an anterior resection was followed by a pulmonary embolism.

Postoperative staging after transanal endoscopic microsurgery for cancer has to be considered so that the patient is correctly referred either to radical surgery or close follow-up[6]. All patients with pT_2 cancers should be referred to immediate radical surgery. In patients with pT_1 high-risk cancer, transanal endoscopic microsurgery is less curative than in patients with pT_2 low-risk carcinomas. Thirty-five of 55 patients with cancer in the 1985–1991 series who underwent the procedure without any further immediate more radical operation were suffering from pT_1 cancer: in the group of pT_1 low-risk tumours (30 cases), the recurrence rate was 3%; in the group of pT_1 high-risk patients the recurrence rate was 40%. Sixteen patients with pT_2 low-risk rectal cancer refused immediate radical surgery: in this group the recurrence rate at follow-up was 6%.

References

1. Nicholls RJ. Surgical treatment of adenomas. *World J Surg* 1991; 15: 20–4.

2. Buess G. Endoluminal rectal surgery. In: Cuschieri A, Buess G, Perissat J, eds. *Operation Manual of Endoscopic Surgery*. Berlin: Springer Verlag, 1992, 303–325.

3. Buess G, Kipfmüller K, Hack D, Grüsner R, Heintz A, Junginger T. Technique of transanal endoscopic microsurgery. *Surg Endosc* 1988; 2: 71–5.

4. Graham RA, Garnsey L, Jessup MJ. Local excision of rectal carcinoma. *Am J Surg* 1990; 160: 306–12.

5. Buess G, Lirici MM. Endoluminal therapy – TEM. In: Hunter JG, Sackier J, eds. *High Tech Surgery: the Minimally Invasive Approach*. New York: McGraw-Hill, in press.

6. Buess G, Mentges B, Manneke K, Starlinger M, Beckner HD. Minimal invasive surgery in the local treatment of rectal cancer. *Int J Colorectal Dis* 1991; 6: 77–81.

Stomas: introductory comment

H. Brendan Devlin MA, MD, MCh, FRCS, FRCSI, FACS
Lecturer in Clinical Surgery, University of Newcastle upon Tyne and Consultant Surgeon, North Tees General Hospital, Stockton-on-Tees, UK

History

The essential principles of stoma surgery have remained the same since Heister performed an enterostomy on battle casualties in Flanders in 1707[1]. In 1710 Littré demonstrated how a colostomy could overcome the obstruction on the corpse of a neonate with imperforate anus[2], and Dubois successfully performed this procedure on a 3-day-old child in 1783[3]. In 1756 Cheselden converted a strangulated umbilical hernia to a colostomy, allowing the patient to survive for many years[4]. Colostomy as part of a curative operation, as an alternative to purely diverting procedures, was introduced in the 1890s by Bloch in Copenhagen[5], Paul in Liverpool[6] and Von Mikulicz[7] in Breslau. In 1912 Brown advocated ileostomy for ulcerative colitis[8]. However, this operation did not become established until Crile and Turnbull in Cleveland unravelled disordered ileal function in 1952[9] and Bryan Brooke introduced his classic everted ileostomy also in 1952[10].

Principles of stoma surgery

Stomas remain as part of the colorectal surgeon's repertoire for 'diverting' the faecal stream in urgent cases of obstruction, or when there is some distal disease process to be rested or a distal operation site to be healed, or as 'permanent' stomas when the distal bowel is excised for ulcerative colitis, Crohn's disease, irreparable trauma or cancer. While these last four situations were confidently treated some 20 years ago with excision and permanent stoma, the disadvantages of a stoma are now well known, the world has moved on and stoma avoidance or the construction of 'continent' stomas and reservoirs is now the accepted mode of treatment. The number of permanent stomas constructed has fallen considerably[11] while at the same time, in the UK at least, there has been a shift away from temporary colostomy. If a temporary stoma is inevitable, an ileostomy is preferable to a colostomy[12]. If at all possible stoma formation should be avoided, so antegrade colonic lavage and immediate anastomosis is the preferred method when managing an acute left-sided colonic obstruction[13]. Because these techniques are more complex and call for greater skill than simple diversion, they are reserved for specialist colorectal surgeons. In recent years studies have confirmed the advantages of specialists in this field[14].

Stoma surgery demands skilled aftercare and patient rehabilitation. The contribution of stoma care nurses is essential, and the support of patient groups and ostomy clubs has been paramount[15]. For stoma surgery to be really successful there must be a partnership between the patient, the doctor and the rehabilitative agencies. The specialist colorectal surgeon should understand all these facets of patient care and should have the wisdom and skill to harness all these adjuncts to benefit the patient.

Choice of operation

The chapters in this section rightly concentrate on the indications for and the technical aspects of stoma construction. These contributions not only represent the 'gold standard' in the USA and the UK, but also illustrate differences in medical practice, and language, between these two para-Atlantic cultures.

In the UK, studies have indicated great advantages in postoperative management and rehabilitation when the loop ileostomy rather than the loop colostomy is chosen as the diverting stoma[16]. The loop colostomy became unpopular because of the unpredictable nature of its effluent and the difficulties with fitting a satisfactory appliance. It is also very prone to prolapse and herniae. Peristomal skin excoriation is a real problem, with poor appliance sealing and the aggressive nature of effluent from the right colon. The transverse colostomy can be difficult to close and this closure operation carries significant morbidity[17]. For these reasons the loop, temporary diverting ileostomy has gained preference in the UK where a simpler technique is used than that described by Fazio and Oakley. The proximal loop is marked before raising the stoma and the stoma sutured circumferentially only[11]. The need to suture the emergent ileal loop to the subcutaneous abdominal wall fat is usual in UK practice.

Selecting the stoma site

Selecting the site for the stoma before operation is important and should be emphasized. The author has always found tattooing the selected spot for the stoma on the skin most useful. It is even more useful if the tattoo needle is pushed more deeply so that an indelible mark is made on the anterior rectus sheath as well[18]. Using the tattoo for the opening in the rectus sheath to some extent obviates the problems of slippage of the abdominal wall layers after the abdomen is opened. Of course, if it is certain that a stoma is going to be formed, i.e. a permanent ileostomy and colorectal excision has already been decided upon, there are great advantages in making the stoma site incision before the laparotomy.

Early reconstruction

The chapter on colostomy should perhaps mention *early* reconstruction after Hartmann's operation for obstructing upper rectal carcinoma[19, 20]. This has been greatly facilitated by the intraluminal stapling device, the use of which allows an early reconstruction (within 14 days of the initial operation) that is certainly safe and is recommended (as described in the chapter on pp. 488–496).

Complications

While it is recognized that paracolostomy hernia and prolapse is very common (up to 50% is recorded with transverse colostomies[21]), the frequency of this complication with ileostomies should not be forgotten. Some paraileostomy herniation is found in 28% of patients with permanent end-ileostomy[22]. Computed tomography will often reveal this although the hernia is impalpable. The rate of paraileostomy herniation is similar, whether the stoma is constructed lateral to, or emerging through, the rectus muscle. The rate of development of paraileostomy hernia is unrelated to weight gain after surgery. The good news is that in one-third of patients with paraileostomy hernia there are no symptoms and there is no need for any surgical interference. Local repair with sutures through the aponeurotic abdominal wall is remarkably unsuccessful. The only satisfactory technique is an extraperitoneal repair with polypropylene mesh[21].

Recent technological advances

The new technologies available in surgery have made an immense impact on stoma management in the last 20 years. Plastic appliances and the use of hypoallergenic glues to fix the appliances have vastly improved patients' life-styles. Good management of stomas, the multiplicity of self-help guides available and, above all, the understanding by both patients and professionals of the partnership necessary for good stoma care, have dramatically improved matters[23–25].

The development of stapling is another great advance. Linear and intraluminal stapling to restore bowel continuity, and stapling through stomas to stabilize them, has enabled surgeons to deal easily with inaccessible problems of suturing.

Perioperative antibiotics are now available and their use is routine today. Deep sepsis and acute septicaemic shock are both largely eliminated by one dose of the appropriate perioperative antibiotic[26]. Metronidazole heralded this revolution in the 1970s and there are new and more powerful antibiotics available.

The revolution in sutures has made its mark. Biologically derived materials, with their inherent slowness of absorption and inhibition of healing, are no longer used. We forget that Lister introduced chromic catgut to delay absorption and counteract inflammation. The newer long-chain polymers, both absorbable and non-absorbable, have tremendous advantages for the healing of stomas.

Another recent technological revolution is engulfing us: the laparoscope[27]. Where this will lead stoma surgery is for the next edition of this text.

References

1. Richardson RG. *The Abominable Stoma: A Historical Survey of the Artificial Anus*. Queenborough: Abbott Laboratories, 1973.

2. Littré. *Diverses Observations Anatomiques. II. Histoire de l'Académie Royale des Sciences*. Paris: 1710: 36–7 (Edition published in 1732).

3. Allan. Rapport sur les observations et réflexions de Dumas, relatives aux imperforations de l'anus. *Recueil Periodique de la Société de Medecine de Paris* 1797; 3: 123.

4. Cheselden W. Colostomy for strangulated umbilical hernia. *Anatomy (Lond)* 1784.

5. Bloch O. Extra abdominal resektion of hele colon descendens og et stykke af colon transversum for cancer. *Hosp Tid Kjobenh* 1894; 4: 1053–61.

6. Paul FT. Colectomy. *BMJ* 1895; i: 1136–9.

7. Von Mikulicz J. Small contributions to surgery of the intestinal tract. *Boston Med Surg J* 1903; 148: 608–11.

8. Brown JY. The value of complete physiological rest of the large bowel in the treatment of certain ulcerative and obstructive lesions of this organ with description of operative technique and report of cases. *Surg Gynecol Obstet* 1913; 16: 610–13.

9. Crile G Jr, Turnbull RB Jr. The mechanism and prevention of ileostomy dysfunction. *Ann Surg* 1954; 140: 459–66.

10. Brooke BN. The management of an ileostomy including its complications. *Lancet* 1952; ii: 102–4.

11. Devlin HB. Colostomy: past and present. *Ann R Coll Surg Engl* 1990; 72: 175–6.

12. Etherington RJ, Williams JG, Hayward MW, Hughes LE. Demonstration of para-ileostomy herniation using computed tomography. *Clin Radiol* 1990; 41: 333–6.

13. Koruth NM, Krukowski ZH, Youngson GG, Hendry WS, Logie JRC, Jones PF *et al.* Intraoperative colonic irrigation in the management of left-sided large bowel emergencies. *Br J Surg* 1985; 72: 708–11.

14. Darby CR, Berry AR, Mortensen N. Management variability in surgery for colorectal emergencies. *Br J Surg* 1992; 79: 206–10.

15. Elcoat C. *Stoma Care Nursing.* London: Baillière Tindall, 1986.

16. Williams NS, Nasmyth DG, Jones D, Smith AH. Defunctioning stomas: a prospective controlled trial comparing loop ileostomy with loop transverse colostomy. *Br J Surg* 1986; 73: 566–70.

17. Aston CM, Everett WG. Comparison of early and late closure of transverse loop colostomies. *Ann R Coll Surg Engl* 1984; 66: 331–3.

18. Turnbull RB, Weakley FL. *Atlas of Intestinal Stomas.* St Louis: Mosby, 1967.

19. Roe AM, Prabhu S, Ali A, Brown C, Brodribb AJ. Reversal of Hartmann's procedure: timing and operative technique. *Br J Surg* 1991; 78: 1167–70.

20. Geoghegan JG, Rosenberg IL. Experience with early anastomosis after the Hartmann procedure. *Ann R Coll Surg Engl* 1991; 73: 80–2.

21. Devlin HB. *Management of Abdominal Hernias.* London: Butterworth, 1988.

22. Williams JG, Etherington R, Hayward MW, Hughes LE. Paraileostomy hernia: a clinical and radiological study. *Br J Surg* 1990; 77: 1355–7.

23. Devlin HB. *Stoma Care Today.* Oxford: Medicine Education Services, 1985.

24. Devlin HB, Plant JA, Griffin M. Aftermath of surgery for anorectal cancer. *BMJ* 1971; 3: 413–18.

25. Neale K, Phillips R. Living with a stoma. *BMJ* 1988; 297: 310–11.

26. Jensen S, Andersen A, Fristrup SC, Holme JB, Huid HM, Kraglund K *et al.* Comparison of one dose versus three doses of prophylactic antibiotics, and the influence of blood transfusion, on infectious complications in acute and elective colorectal surgery. *Br J Surg* 1990; 77: 513–18.

27. Lange V, Meyer G, Schardey HM, Schildberg FW. Laparoscopic creation of a loop colostomy. *J Laparoendosc Surg* 1991; 1: 307–12.

Ileostomy

John R. Oakley FRACS
Staff Surgeon and Head, Section of Enterostomal Therapy, Department of Colorectal Surgery, The Cleveland Clinic Foundation, Cleveland, Ohio, USA

Victor W. Fazio FRACS, FACS
Chairman, Department of Colorectal Surgery, The Cleveland Clinic Foundation, Cleveland, Ohio, USA

Principles and justification

Indications

The three types of ileostomy (end ileostomy, loop ileostomy and loop-end ileostomy) have differing indications.

End ileostomy

An end ileostomy is constructed under many varied circumstances:

1. At the completion of abdominal colectomy or after proctocolectomy performed for inflammatory bowel disease.
2. In patients with familial adenomatous polyposis in whom abdominal colectomy and ileorectal anastomosis is contraindicated because of rectal carcinoma, where a 'sea' of rectal polyps would make the future control of polyps difficult, or where restorative ileal pouch−anal anastomosis is not considered advisable or is not desired by the patient.
3. In the rare circumstances where multiple synchronous carcinomas are present in the large bowel.
4. A 'temporary' end ileostomy is sometimes constructed after ileal or ileocaecal resection for perforating Crohn's disease, ileocaecal trauma, obstructing right colonic lesions, or after complex fistula surgery. Subsequent removal of the ileostomy and reanastomosis of the bowel may be carried out.
5. Rarely in inflammatory bowel disease to allow the patient's general condition to improve before elective colectomy, but this is seldom advised.
6. When constructing an ileal conduit for urinary diversion.

Loop ileostomy

A loop ileostomy may be used to provide diversion (usually temporary) in the following conditions:

1. Above an ileal pouch−anal anastomosis for mucosal ulcerative colitis or familial polyposis.
2. Above an ileorectal anastomosis for inflammatory bowel disease.
3. Above a continent ileal reservoir.
4. Above enterocutaneous fistulae, before or after surgical resection.
5. Proximal to colorectal or coloanal anastomoses when a loop colostomy is judged to be technically difficult or undesirable.
6. In certain cases of ileocaecoappendiceal sepsis (such as perforating Crohn's disease).
7. To complement colonic decompression in certain cases of toxic megacolon.
8. Proximal to any distal bowel anastomosis where the anastomosis is tenuous because of radiation effects or malnutrition, or where it lies in proximity to a septic inflammatory 'nest'.
9. For certain cases of severe perianal Crohn's disease where proctocolectomy is not acceptable to the patient.

The advantage of a loop ileostomy is that the mesenteric vessels are not divided in its construction, so that ischaemia is virtually impossible. The major disadvantage is that the amount of ileal protrusion above the skin level is limited and with passage of time is more prone to recession than an end stoma.

Loop-end ileostomy

A loop-end ileostomy may be used as a primary procedure for the definitive stoma in patients with ileal urinary conduits or in obese patients with a thick abdominal wall where it would be difficult to maintain sufficient blood supply to allow the end of a divided bowel to reach beyond the skin level. Occasionally, a previous loop ileostomy may be converted to a loop-end stoma by transection and closure of the efferent limb of the ileum just inside the peritoneal cavity. In these patients, the mesenteric defect is not obliterated unless a loop-end ileostomy is constructed during a primary procedure.

Preoperative

The preoperative preparation required largely depends upon the underlying condition for which the ileostomy is planned. The surgeon, stoma nurse and sometimes also a trained lay ostomy visitor, should discuss the implications of surgery with the patient and his or her family, providing reassurance and encouragement. Most patients will benefit from reading pertinent literature available from local or national stoma associations.

Siting the stoma

1, 2 Rehabilitation of the patient begins before the operation, with selection of the optimal stoma site. It is preferable to mark a stoma site first with the patient seated, when any crease or fold of skin will become more prominent, and then to check the position with the patient supine.

The following rules apply:

1. Use the summit or apex of the infraumbilical fat mound.
2. The mark should be in the middle of, or at least within the surface marking of, the rectus abdominis muscle.
3. The mark should be at least 4 cm from the planned incision line.
4. The stoma site and the adjacent skin should be away from creases, scars, the umbilicus, any prominences and anticipated future incisions. Using a commercially available standard size template facilitates correct placement.
5. A site where the skin has been injured, e.g. from a skin graft, burn, or radiotherapy, must be avoided.

At the selected site a vertical line is marked downwards from the umbilicus, and a horizontal line is marked outwards from the lower border of the umbilicus.

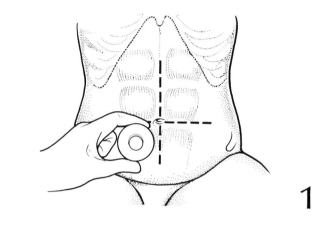

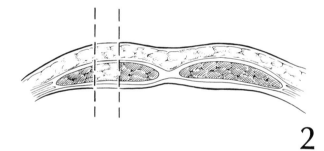

Marking the stoma

3 Once the position of the faceplate is determined with the patient seated, the patient is asked to lie down while the faceplate is held in position. An indelible mark is then made by placing a drop of India ink or methylene blue over the stoma site; a needle prick produces a tattoo which cannot be washed away during preoperative bathing or when preparing the abdominal wall with antiseptic solution.

Anaesthesia

General anaesthesia with relaxants and endotracheal intubation is used. Peroperative intravenous broad-spectrum antibiotics are given. A nasogastric tube is inserted after induction of anaesthesia and the bladder is catheterized if a bowel resection is contemplated.

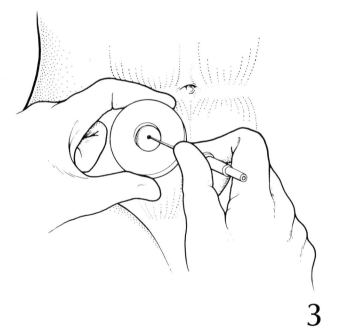

Operation

END ILEOSTOMY

Position of patient

A supine or modified lithotomy-Trendelenburg position is used, depending on whether a combined abdomino-perineal proctectomy is to be part of the procedure (*see* chapter on pp. 47–50).

Incision

The incision is made in the midline, skirting just to the left side of the umbilicus. If colectomy is planned, the incision is carried to the upper epigastrium to a point where the surgeon judges that the splenic flexure can be safely mobilized. Because of the possibility of future stoma revision and relocation (especially when operating for Crohn's disease), a midline incision is very much preferred over a paramedian approach so that the sites for possible future stomas are left intact.

Division of the terminal ileum

4 In the absence of ileal disease, the ileum is transected 7–10 cm from the ileocaecal valve unless a later ileal pouch–anal anastomosis is contemplated, in which case the terminal ileal division should be 1–2 cm proximal to the ileocaecal valve. To minimize contamination in the course of later delivery of the end of the ileum through the abdominal wall, a linear stapling instrument should be used.

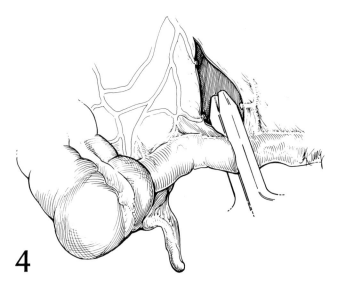

4

Ileostomy aperture

5 The cut edge of the linea alba and the dermis at the level of the stoma site are then grasped with Kocher (or similar) clamps and retracted medially.

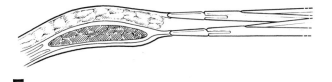

5

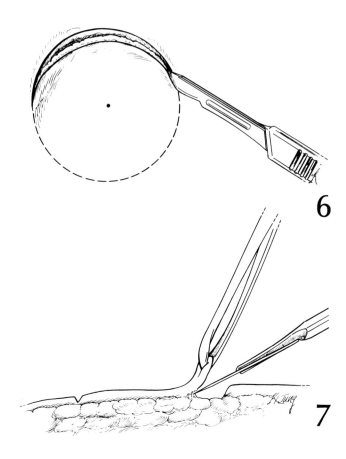

6, 7 A circumferential incision, 2–2.5 cm in diameter, is made around the previously marked stoma site. No trephine is made; only the skin disc is excised. The subcutaneous fat is preserved to minimize the chances of a dead space and accumulation of a parastomal seroma or abscess, and to add support to the stoma as it traverses the subcutaneous tissues. The sagittal view (*Illustration 7*) shows excision of the skin disc and preservation of the fat.

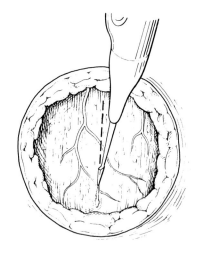

8 A vertical incision is made through the subcutaneous tissue. Any bleeding from the skin edge, which is usually minor, should be left to stop spontaneously, as coagulation could severely traumatize the skin and cause mucocutaneous separation.

9 An abdominal pack, or a sponge, is then placed within the peritoneal cavity behind the rectus muscle while the surgeon maintains medial traction on the wound edge to ensure that the rectus muscle does not slip laterally during the course of fashioning the ileostomy aperture. This manoeuvre is facilitated by the operator's hand pushing upwards from inside the abdomen over the area of the ileostomy aperture.

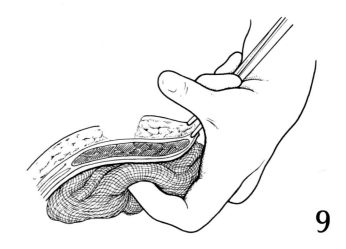

9

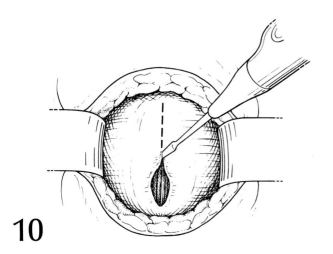

10

10 Scarpa's layer of fascia is incised and short right-angle retractors are positioned medially and laterally to display the anterior rectus sheath. The cutting cautery incises the sheath for 3–3.5 cm in a vertical direction; lateral cruciate incisions are not necessary.

11 An artery forceps is inserted perpendicularly down to the posterior sheath and the jaws gently opened in the horizontal plane, minimizing the risk of injury to the inferior epigastric vessels. Before the instrument is withdrawn, medial and lateral retractors are placed to prevent the vertical fibres of the muscle springing back and making identification of the site of rectus split difficult. A muscle splitting, rather than a muscle cutting, procedure is used to minimize the risk of postoperative hernia or prolapse of the ileostomy.

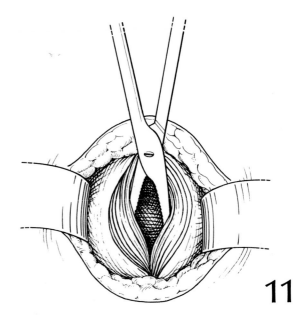

11

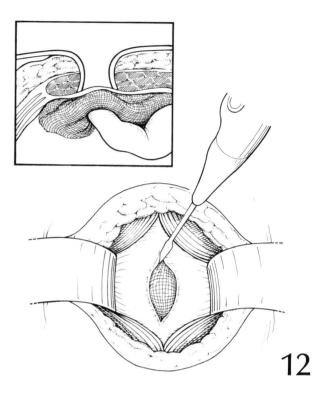

12 With an assistant maintaining lateral and medial retraction of the rectus muscle and exposing the posterior rectus sheath, and the surgeon pushing upwards from inside the abdomen, the posterior rectus sheath and peritoneum are divided in the vertical plane, cutting directly on to the sponge, which protects the operator's left hand.

12

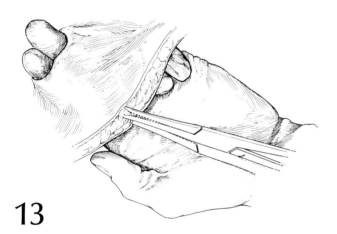

13

13 The aperture size is tested: for the surgeon who uses size 7 or 8 gloves, the optimal size corresponds to a snug two-finger aperture such that the distal interphalangeal joint of the middle finger and the pulp of the index finger can be seen. If the aperture is too large, prolapse or parastomal hernia may occur; if too narrow it may become obstructed.

14 Manipulation of the aperture may cause bleeding from the rectus muscle or tributaries of the inferior epigastric vessels. A large pair of Kelly forceps may be passed through the aperture and used as a retractor to check for any bleeding.

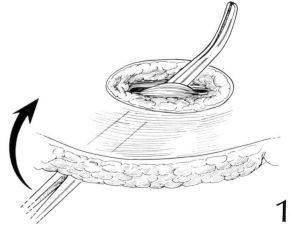

14

Fashioning the stoma

15 The terminal ileum is prepared for drawing through the aperture by dividing the mesentery 0.5–1.0 cm from the bowel wall so as to preserve a vascular arcade close to the bowel. This reduces the bulk of the mesentery and straightens the terminal ileum. Sufficient length of bowel should be prepared to pass through the thickness of the abdominal wall and to protrude 5–6 cm beyond the level of the skin. It is wise to suture ligate the divided vessels to ensure that the ligatures are not dislodged when passing the bowel through the stoma. Arterial bleeding from the distal mesenteric attachment confirms a good blood supply to the stoma.

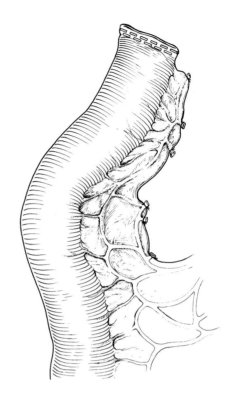

15

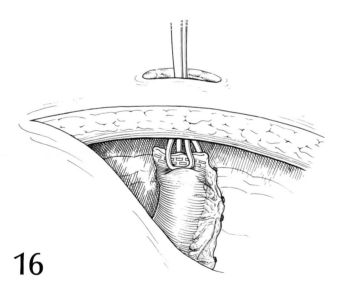

16

16 A Babcock clamp is passed through the stoma aperture, grasping the prepared ileum and drawing it gently through the abdominal wall so that the ileal mesentery lies in a cephalad direction to facilitate later obliteration of the mesenteric defect. A 6-cm length of exteriorized ileum is optimal.

17 Although some surgeons prefer to obliterate the mesenteric defect by suturing the cut end of the mesentery to the lateral abdominal wall, or by fashioning an extraperitoneal ileostomy, these techniques can be time consuming and technically difficult. The authors' preference, after completion of the colectomy, is to suture the cut edge of the mesentery to the anterior abdominal wall. This is achieved using interrupted or continuous 2/0 chromic catgut (or other absorbable material) sutures, starting at the mesenteric attachment to the bowel and suturing the free edge of the mesentery to the back of the abdominal wall approximately 2.5 cm lateral to the wound edge. At the cephalad end the suture is continued to the free lower edge of the falciform ligament. Residual transverse mesocolon or redundant lesser omentum may be included in the stitch. Care must be taken not to injure significant vessels in the free edge of the mesentery.

Stabilizing sutures of 3/0 chromic catgut, or absorbable sutures of 3/0 chromic catgut or Vicryl are usually placed between the seromuscular layer of the ileum and the peritoneum around the internal aperture. These sutures may be omitted in patients with Crohn's disease because they increase the risk of fistula formation, but if they are inserted carefully without taking deep bites into the bowel, the risk is reduced and they probably add another safeguard against ileal prolapse.

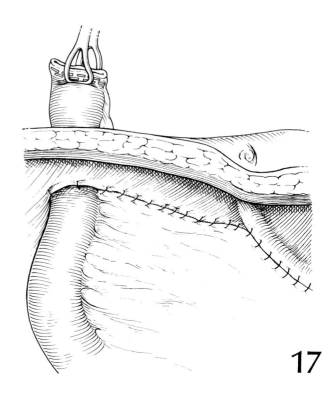

17

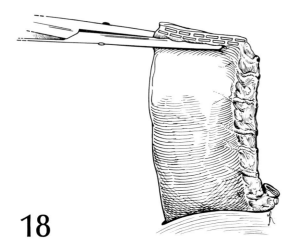

18

Maturing the ileostomy

18 The end of the ileostomy is opened after the main incision has been closed and is isolated with drapes to minimize bacterial wound contamination. Arterial or 'nuisance' bleeding from the cut end of the bowel is a sign of bowel viability.

19 One of the problems that confronts the surgeon and the stoma therapist is the late occurrence of a gully or 'moat' at the mucocutaneous junction of the stoma, which tends to occur as the patient gains weight, notwithstanding the initial satisfactory placement of the stoma. To minimize this effect, the skin edge can be everted by placing radial sutures of 3/0 catgut between the bowel wall and the subcutaneous fat. The sero-muscular bowel stitch is placed about 1 cm above the skin level and is sutured to the most superficial part of the subcutaneous fat, bringing the suture out at the fat–epidermis junction. As the suture is tied a slight concertina effect is produced, which reduces any tendency for formation of a parastomal gully.

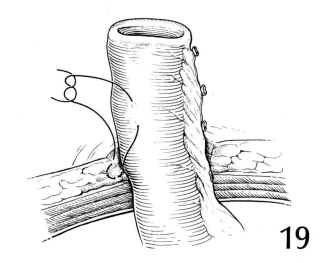

19

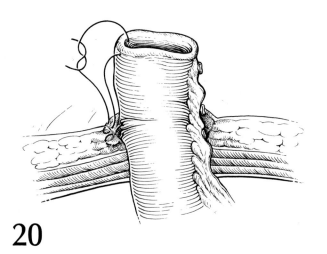

20

20 Radial sutures of 3/0 chromic catgut are placed at the four compass points of the stoma, through full-thickness bowel edge and sutured to the subcuticular skin. They should be placed vertically rather than tangentially or horizontally through the subcuticular skin, because minor degrees of vascular compromise here may cause separation of the mucosa and serositis of the exposed ileum. The sutures should not go through the external skin because of the risk of ileal mucosal island implantation, which may cause early separation of the stoma appliance.

21a, b Four additional sutures are then placed between the four compass-point sutures and the sutures are tied down, everting the stoma.

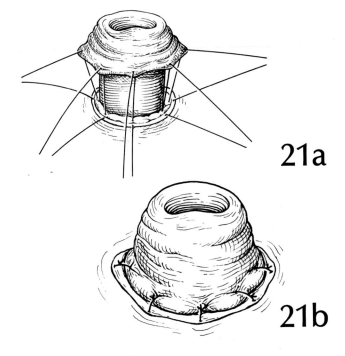

21a

21b

22 The maturing sutures may alternatively be inserted through full-thickness bowel edge and through the seromuscular layer of the bowel wall at skin level before passing through the subcuticular skin. This produces a three-point suture which helps to keep the stoma everted, especially in the patient with flabby subcutaneous tissue where there is little support for the stoma. This type of suture is best avoided in patients with Crohn's disease because of the risk of development of skin-level fistulae.

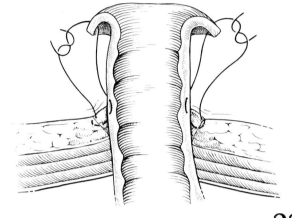

22

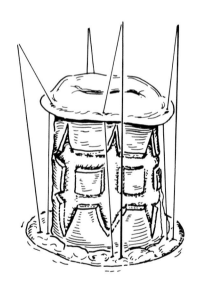

23

23 An alternative method of constructing the end ileostomy is to add a two-directional myotomy to the spout. This minimizes the risk of stoma recession and is appropriate for short stomas or in patients with a thick abdominal wall.

LOOP ILEOSTOMY

24 A midline incision is used. Positioning is as for an end ileostomy.

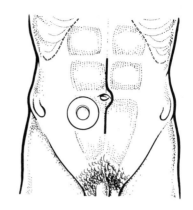

24

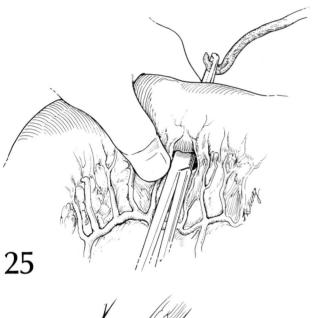

25

25, 26 When a loop ileostomy is being placed proximal to an anastomosis or for diversion above distal small bowel pathology, it should be created 15–20 cm proximally, depending on the thickness of the abdominal wall. The distance above an intact ileocaecal valve may be reduced to 10–15 cm. At the apex of the loop selected, a tape is brought through a small window made in the small bowel mesentery, to act as a retractor. It is important to be able to differentiate the proximal from the distal site of the loop, because as the loop is brought through the abdominal wall aperture, it may rotate and not be recognized. Therefore, each site should be tagged, adjacent to the apex of the loop, with sutures of different material, colour or length.

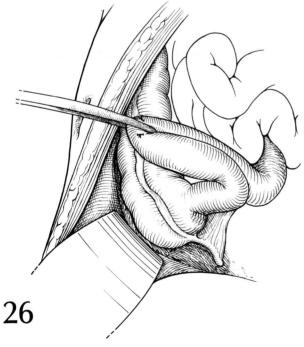

26

27a–e

The ileostomy loop is brought through the abdominal wall aperture using curved forceps to grasp the ends of the tape, and checking the orientation of the loop so that the proximal end is cephalad and the distal end caudad. An ileostomy rod is placed under the loop. Possible injury to the mesenteric vessels can be minimized by placing a Kocher clamp on one end of the tape and making several twists in the tape. As the tape is pulled through the mesentery, detorsion or rifling of the Kocher clamp will lessen the risk of damage by the clamp. The rod is grasped by one of its eyelets and gently brought through the mesentery to support the loop.

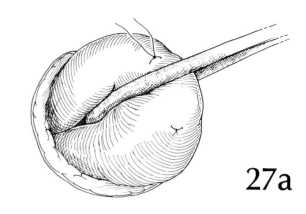

27a

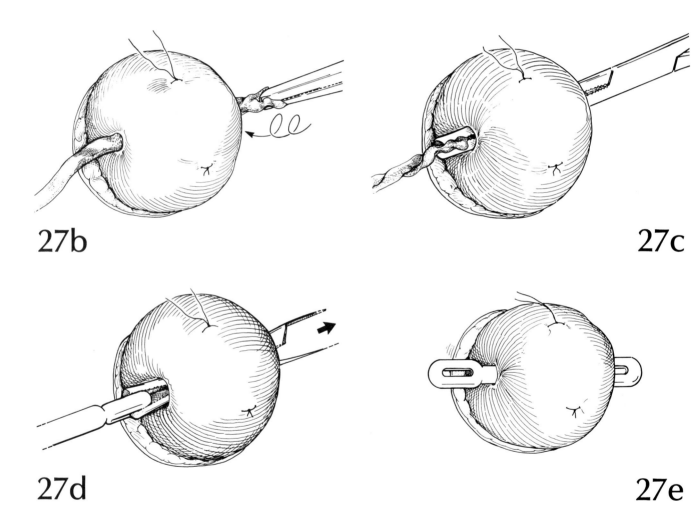

27b

27c

27d

27e

28 The abdomen is closed and the main incision isolated from the ileostomy with drapes. The identifying tags may now be removed. An incision is made in the loop on its caudad and distal side across 80% of its circumference approximately 0.5 cm above, and parallel to, the skin. If the incision is flush with the skin, mucus may escape from the recessive limb and cause a faulty seal with the appliance.

Bleeding may occur as the enterotomy is extended towards the mesenteric edges, and the incision should stop about 5 mm short of the mesentery on both sides. A useful technique to minimize bleeding is to make an initial seromuscular incision with scissors, allowing the submucosa to pout out. Selective light electrocoagulation of the visible submucosal vessels can then be performed before completing the enterotomy.

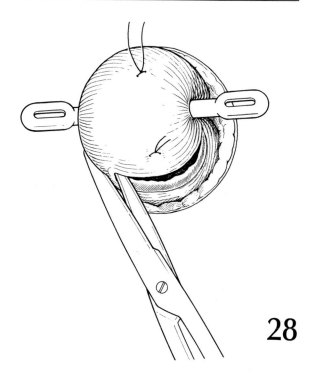

28

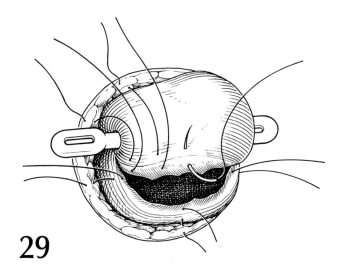

29

29 Sutures of 3/0 chromic catgut are then placed, for both loops, through full-thickness bowel edge and then through the subcuticular layer of skin. The sutures are tagged and not tied down until all have been inserted because it is difficult to place them with accuracy next to the rod. On the caudad, or lower, side three sutures are usually sufficient; one adjacent to the rod on each side and one centrally placed. Five sutures are usually needed on the cephalad side.

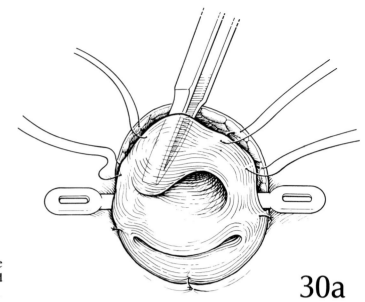

30a, b The caudad sutures are tied before the cephalad part of the bowel is everted with the help of the blunt end of a pair of tissue forceps.

30a

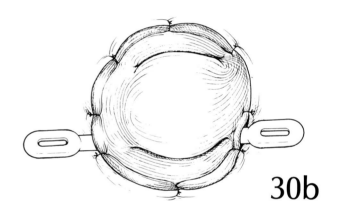

30b

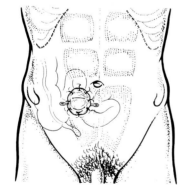

31

31 The completed loop ileostomy in the distal small bowel to divert the faecal stream from the colon is shown.

LOOP-END ILEOSTOMY

This may be performed at the time of colectomy or by conversion of a loop ileostomy to a loop-end ileostomy. In the latter instance, the distal limb is transected and oversewn just inside the peritoneal cavity. The following illustrations show the technique for construction of the loop-end stoma at the time of colectomy.

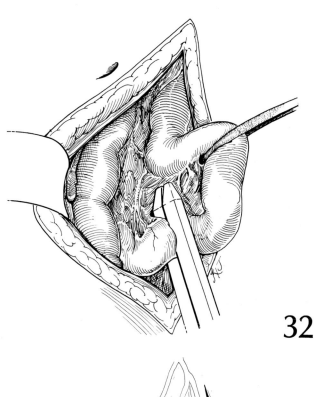

32

32, 33 The line of transection of the ileum is chosen close to the ileocaecal valve using hand sutures or a linear stapling device. A moist tape is placed around the ileum, passing through a small mesenteric window 7–10 cm above the transected bowel after judging the amount of small bowel that will be needed to traverse the thickness of the abdominal wall. The closed distal end should lie just within the peritoneal cavity.

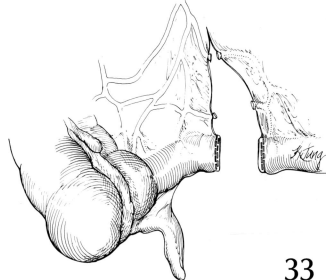

33

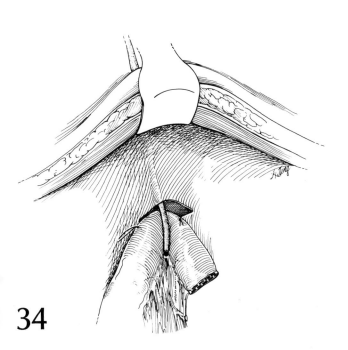

34

34 The abdominal wall aperture is made in the same way as for conventional ileostomy and the loop drawn through, after marking the proximal and distal ends with differing sutures as with loop ileostomy. The mesenteric defect is to be obliterated, and the functional end lies caudad and the non-functional end cephalad. This allows the cut edge of the small bowel mesentery to be aligned easily with the anterior abdominal wall.

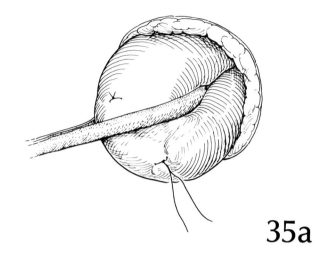

35a

35a, b Using the tape, the loop is drawn through the abdominal wall aperture until 2–3 cm protrude beyond the skin. The tape is replaced by a short plastic ileostomy rod. Stabilizing sutures of 3/0 chromic catgut may then be placed between the seromuscular layer of the loop and the subcutaneous fat to facilitate further eversion of the skin, but this manoeuvre is optional.

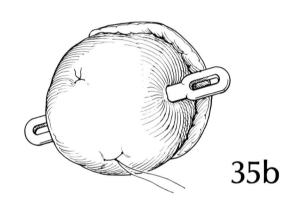

35b

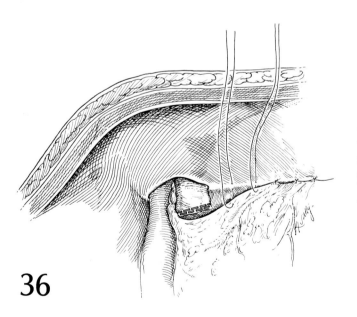

36

36 The mesentery of the small bowel is sutured to the anterior abdominal wall 2–3 cm lateral to the main incision using interrupted or continuous absorbable sutures. The suture line is carried cephalad up to and on to the free edge of the falciform ligament and caudad to the internal aspect of the abdominal wall aperture. Seromuscular sutures may also be placed between the limbs of the loop and the peritoneum of the ileostomy aperture.

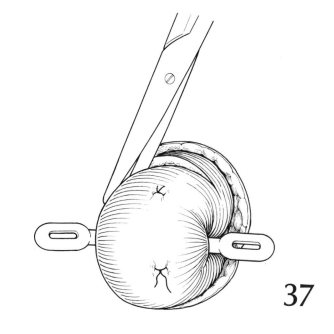

37 An enterotomy is made on the cephalad side of the loop across 80% of the circumference of the ileum, about 0.5 cm above skin level.

38a–c Sutures of 3/0 chromic catgut are placed through the full thickness of the cut edge of the ileum and sutured to the subcuticular layer of skin: three sutures are usually required on the defunctioned side and five on the functional side. The sutures should be placed so that the rod remains slightly eccentric and closer to the defunctioned side. As described for loop ileostomy, the sutures are not tied until all have been inserted. The blunt end of a pair of tissue forceps aids eversion.

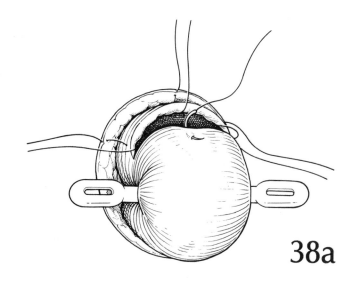

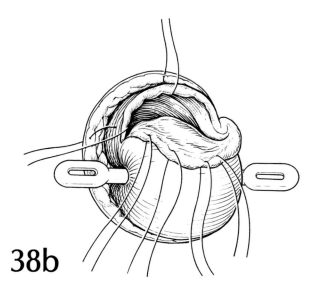

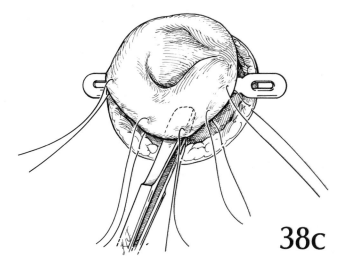

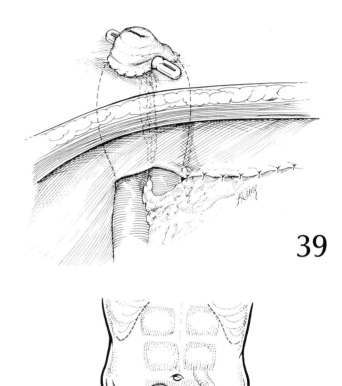

39, 40 The main incision is closed before breaching the ileal lumen, as for other types of ileostomy construction, but for clarity the completed stoma is shown with the incision unclosed.

Note

In cases of extreme obesity, the fashioning of an ileostomy, even a loop ileostomy, may be extraordinarily difficult. In such cases a generous (8–10 cm) incision is made in the peritoneum and posterior rectus sheath of the internal aperture so that the bowel can be brought through the abdominal wall easily. However, before delivering the bowel through the aperture, sutures of 1 Prolene are placed on both sides of the extended incision and left untied. After the bowel has been delivered to a length that satisfies the surgeon, these sutures may be tied, partly closing the defect; the surgeon should watch for any ischaemic effects on the bowel produced by these ties. This manoeuvre will help to reduce the possibility of formation of a parastomal hernia.

Postoperative care

Early management

A skin barrier is applied to the stoma in the operating room, the most suitable being a large karaya disc which can be applied over the ileostomy rod in the case of a loop or loop-end stoma. An open-ended transparent pouch with adhesive backing is attached to the skin barrier using hypoallergenic paper tape to secure the periphery of the pouch to the skin. The clear pouch allows easy inspection of the stoma in the postoperative period, with special attention being paid to stoma colour, skin separation and oedema. Two-piece pouches are available, the extra length of which rests in the bed next to the patient so that the weight of the contents does not cause separation of the pouch from the skin. One-piece units are also available, which have the advantage that they can be used by personnel who are less skilled in stoma management.

Approximately 3–5 days after surgery, the patient is instructed in the care of the stoma. Until that time the stoma therapist or nurse checks the pouch daily. Usually 3 or 4 days of careful instruction are required before the patient can confidently assemble and apply the pouch to the stoma.

Ileostomy equipment

The essential components are a *skin barrier* to which a *pouch* is attached. One-piece and two-piece appliances are available, the latter having detachable and disposable pouches. The barrier protects the skin and encourages irritated, denuded, and eroded skin to epithelialize. The most common barriers are karaya (which is available as a wafer, ring, paste, or powder) and gelatin–pectin based products (wafers, rings, powder, or paste) such as Stomahesive and Hollihesive. The skin barrier may be supplied with the opening precut to various sizes, or the patient may need to cut it to an appropriate size and shape. Almost all modern stoma equipment is disposable.

Many combinations of one-piece and two-piece systems, drainable and non-drainable pouches, precut and uncut skin barriers are available. Most appliances are self-adhesive, in some an in-built convexity of the skin barrier is useful to adhere to the skin around a recessive stoma or one located on a 'flabby' abdominal wall. Various skin sealants (gels, sprays, wipes, and liquids) are available as added protection to the surrounding skin.

Application of the pouch

The skin is prepared with a fat solvent such as non-medicated soap. The stoma diameter is measured, using calipers or a commercially available template, to obtain the correct aperture size, which should be slightly larger than the base of the stoma. The patient will need to cut the aperture to the appropriate size unless a precut barrier or faceplate is to be used. A gelatin–pectin based or karaya ring or a rim of paste may be added to the barrier, with or without a convex insert, in order to obtain a better seal around the base of the stoma. The faceplate is then placed centrally over the stoma and attached to the skin and secured with the in-built adhesive tape or by a 'picture frame' of microporous tape. It is advisable to protect the skin with a sealant before applying the tape. In a one-piece system the pouch will be supplied attached to the appliance, but in a two-piece system the pouch should be applied at this stage. A pouch cover made of cotton is useful in hot weather and for patients with vinyl sensitivity.

Home-going equipment

By the time of discharge from hospital most patients will be fitted with a 'permanent' appliance. The type selected will depend on the configuration of the stoma, the surrounding skin and the abdominal wall, and also on the patient's personal preference, type of employment and lifestyle. An experienced stomal therapist should fit the patient with the most appropriate form of pouch. Some trial and error may be necessary and a large order for equipment should not be placed until the time of the postoperative visit, several weeks after surgery.

Follow-up

The patient is seen in the outpatient clinic approximately 6 weeks after surgery when it is necessary to remeasure the stoma diameter because shrinkage has usually occurred. The patient's skin is checked, any problems are discussed, and further encouragement is given.

Complications

Mucosal slough

Slough of mucosa results from ischaemia or excessive tension, and if minor requires no treatment. Slough of part of the everted muscle as well, or mucocutaneous separation, may leave exposed serosa of the non-everted part of the ileostomy, delaying the maturation of the stoma.

Degrees of pseudo-obstruction may be encountered, and late stenosis at the skin level (Bishop's collar deformity) may be seen if the defect is significant. Early surgery and revision are not indicated except for the obviously necrotic stoma or where there is wide circumferential separation or ischaemia at the mucocutaneous junction.

High output

In the early postoperative period a watery green effluent may be noted. Caution should be exercised in interpreting this as a sign of return of normal bowel function: it may indicate pseudo-obstruction or ileus, which may be recognized by finding mucous clumps or strands which are grey-white in appearance. Oral intake should be withheld until a thicker brown effluent is noted.

After the patient resumes normal eating and drinking, the effluent may remain high in volume: codeine, diphenoxylate, loperamide, tincture of laudanum, or combinations of these may be used to reduce the output to 700–1000 ml/day. Psyllium seed derivatives sometimes help to thicken the stool.

Parastomal irritation

There are many causes of parastomal irritation, including a poor seal, candidiasis, parastomal ulceration, allergy to the pouch material or adhesive tape, folliculitis, trauma to the skin from frequent pouch changes, pressure ulcers, psoriasis and eczema. Most of these problems can be resolved by very careful stoma management, and the involvement of a stoma therapist is invaluable.

Ileostomy fistula

This may occur early as a result of suturing the bowel wall to the rectus fascia (as opposed to the peritoneum or subcutaneous fat), or late secondary to faceplate trauma or recurrent disease, particularly Crohn's disease. If it is symptomatic, surgical revision is required, but often the fistula opening is adjacent to the mucocutaneous junction and the fistula can be incorporated into the pouching system.

Paraileostomy ulceration

When extensive paraileostomy ulceration occurs requiring debridement which leaves a large raw area, a non-seal and non-adhesive appliance may temporarily be required to allow healing. A non-adherent dressing is applied over the ulcer and the pouch held in position by a belt, with the dressing being changed two or three times a day until the ulcer is small enough to allow a conventional pouch to be applied.

Ileostomy obstruction

Bowel obstruction after ileostomy may occur at any time because of adhesions, volvulus, or entrapment of the bowel in the fascial closure. Food bolus obstruction is also seen after this operation: ingestion of poorly digested food (string vegetables, corn, popcorn, peanuts, fruit skins) may produce a picture of bowel obstruction, especially in the first 3 months after surgery. Predisposing causes such as low-grade or partial obstruction by adhesions or recurrent Crohn's disease may exist.

Bolus obstruction should be treated conservatively; irrigation of the ileostomy by gentle lavage with 50–100 ml saline introduced through a small catheter, repeated at intervals until an adequate return is seen. The bolus should then break up and this is recognized by the presence of vegetable fibre in the returned irrigation fluids.

Ileostomy recession

Recession of the ileostomy may be treated by good stomal therapy techniques, particularly the employment of various degrees of convexity, either built in or added to the appliance. If this treatment is unsuccessful, stoma revision (usually without laparotomy) may be required (*see* chapter on pp. 292–306).

Ileostomy prolapse and hernia

Fixation of the mesentery and limiting the abdominal wall aperture will usually prevent prolapse. Prolapse may sometimes be managed by local revision of the ileostomy but relocation is often required. A small paraileostomy hernia beside a stoma where the bowel has been brought through the belly of the rectus muscle and the abdominal wall defect may be repaired and the ileostomy revised without relocation. However, if the hernia defect is large, or if it occurs with a stoma located outside the rectus muscle, local revision is unlikely to be successful and relocation is almost always required (*see* chapter on pp. 292–306).

Ileostomy closure
Timing of closure

Oedema and friability of the tissues, which occur early after ileostomy construction and persist for several weeks, increase the complications associated with closure. The operation should be deferred for at least 2 months, and preferably 3 months, after stoma construction.

Preoperative preparation

Before a loop ileostomy is closed, the integrity of any distal anastomoses or suture lines should be assessed in the distal bowel and distal obstruction or disease ruled out. This is usually achieved by standard endoscopy and by water-soluble contrast radiology.

Formal bowel preparation for ileostomy closure is not usually necessary, but administration of clear liquids for 12–24 h before surgery and preoperative enemas (to empty any residual colonic segment) are usually advisable. Broad-spectrum antibiotics are administered peroperatively.

Anaesthesia and positioning

General anaesthesia, with muscle relaxation to facilitate mobilization of the stoma from the abdominal wall and subsequent closure of the defect, is indicated. Surgery is usually performed with the patient supine, or in the modified lithotomy (Lloyd-Davies) position if other surgery is to be performed at the same time (*see* chapter on pp. 47–50).

Incision

41 A circumferential incision is made adjacent to the mucocutaneous junction, leaving a sliver of skin 1–2 mm wide attached to the bowel. Taking any additional skin results in an unnecessarily large defect with prolonged healing time and greater potential for distortion and puckering. It is not normally necessary to make transverse or vertical extensions of the circular incision, although the surgeon should not hesitate to do so later if there is any difficulty in mobilizing the stoma.

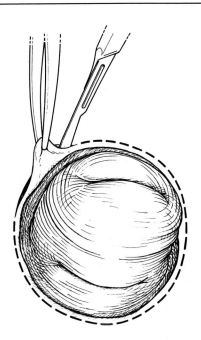

41

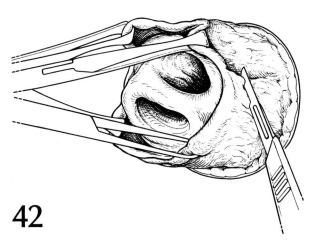

42

Mobilization of ileostomy from abdominal wall

42 The small rim of skin attached to the bowel is grasped by four Allis forceps and the subcutaneous tissue is freed from the serosal surface of the bowel by sharp dissection using a size 15 scalpel blade.

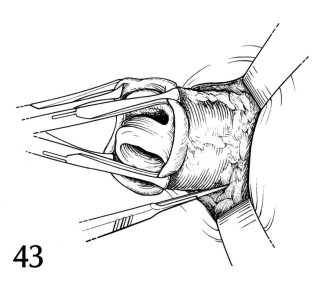

43 Gentle retraction with small right-angle retractors and countertraction on the bowel forceps facilitates the dissection, which should proceed around the circumference of the bowel, gradually deepening the dissection. It is necessary continually to move the retractors and to use deeper bladed retractors as the dissection passes deep to the anterior rectus sheath and to the fibres of the rectus muscle. Scalpel dissection with adequate retraction and appropriate countertraction will usually allow mobilization to the peritoneal level, but occasionally fine scissor dissection may also be necessary.

43

44 Once the peritoneal cavity is entered, an index finger can be placed deep to the posterior sheath, and the filmy adhesions attaching the bowel to the back of the abdominal wall can be broken down by gentle sweeping of the index finger around the circumference of the internal opening, combined if necessary with some sharp dissection under direct vision. The bowel, mesentery and any attached omentum must be freed from the abdominal wall for a distance of 2–3 cm from the internal opening.

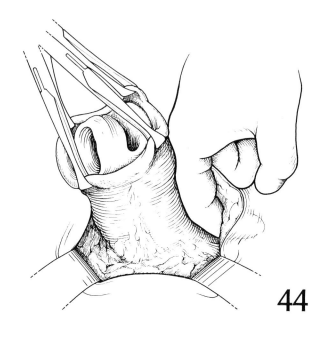

44

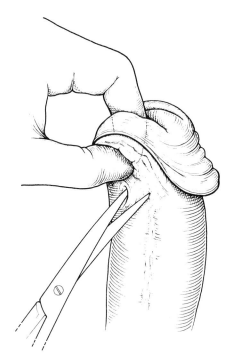

45

Preparation of the bowel for closure

45 The edges of the bowel which had been everted for the ileostomy construction are returned to their normal configuration by dividing the adhesions between the everted and adjacent segments of bowel wall. This is best achieved by scissor dissection against an index finger inserted into the functional end of the bowel, while gentle traction is applied to the rim of skin attached to the edge of the bowel.

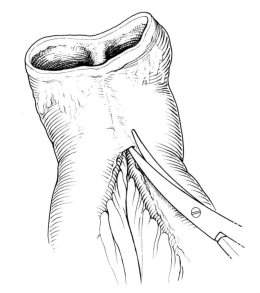

46, 47 After mobilization from the abdominal wall, the loops of bowel proximal and distal to the stoma will lie almost parallel to one another, with filmy adhesions maintaining this relationship. These adhesions need to be divided to straighten out the bowel and to prevent postoperative angulation and potential obstruction at the point of closure.

46

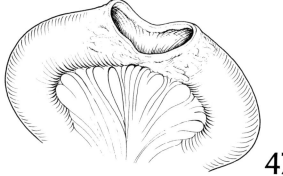

47

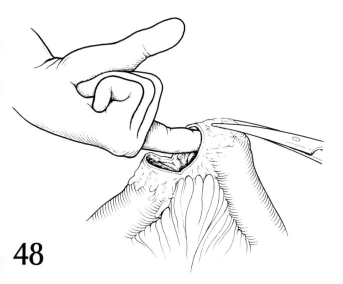

48

48 Any residual subcutaneous fatty tissue or fibrous scar is then excised from the bowel serosa.

49 The attached sliver of skin is trimmed from the bowel edges, leaving a soft, pliable, and freely bleeding bowel edge. It is important to excise all areas of fibrosis and scarring; these areas can often be located by feel more easily than by sight.

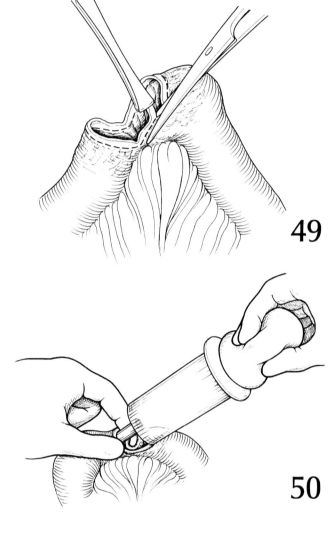

49

50 It is expedient to test each limb of the bowel for an unrecognized enterotomy by the instillation of a weak solution of coloured antiseptic such as povidone-iodine (Betadine).

50

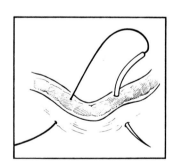

Closure of the bowel defect

51 The defect in the bowel is closed transversely with interrupted absorbable sutures of 3/0 Vicryl or 3/0 chromic catgut. The sutures are inserted through the seromuscular tissues and pass through the groove between the muscle and the submucosa of the bowel, rather than being full thickness. This assures accurate approximation of bowel layers and helps to maintain an inverted suture line.

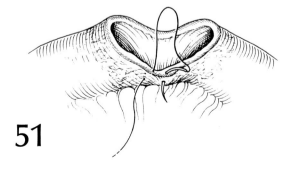

51

52 The initial two stitches are placed at the mesenteric ends of the defect, tied, and tagged to produce gentle lateral retraction. An antimesenteric stitch is then placed halfway between the two lateral stitches, and if there is discrepancy in the length of bowel on either side, intervening 'halfway' sutures can be placed to facilitate accurate bowel closure. These sutures are temporarily left untied and tagged with a small artery clamp.

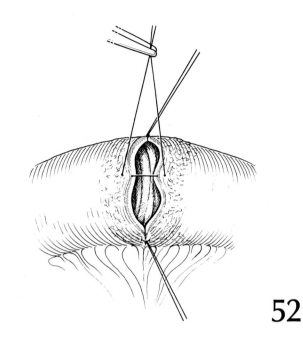

52

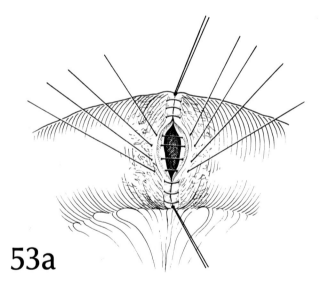

53a

53a, b Sutures are placed and tied from each end; the central four or five are placed and left untied until all have been inserted.

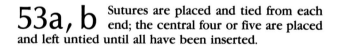

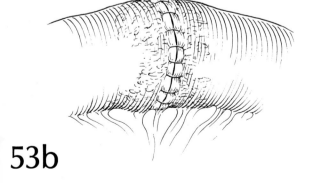

53b

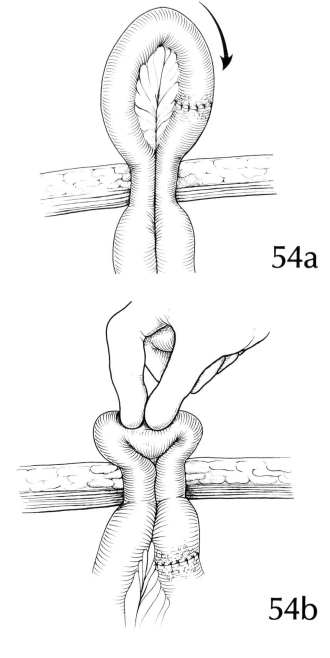

54a, b The closed bowel is irrigated with saline before being replaced into the abdominal cavity, which is best achieved by first replacing the bowel containing the suture line. Careful handling of the sutured bowel and gradual 'milking' of the remaining bowel back into the abdominal cavity using gentle finger compression prevents disruption of the suture line.

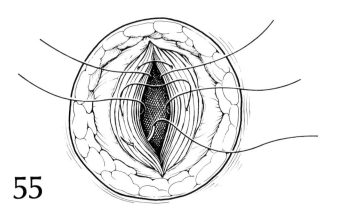

Closure of the abdominal defect

55 The defect in the abdominal musculature is closed parallel to the rectus muscle fibres by three or four full thickness sutures of strong absorbable material such as 1 Vicryl, with the knots placed deep to the posterior rectus sheath.

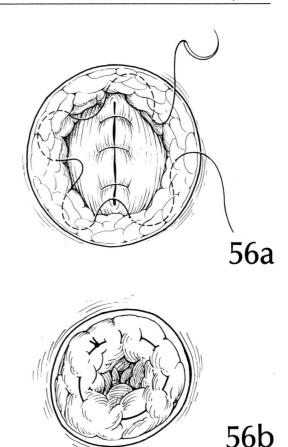

56a, b The depth of the subcutaneous wound is reduced by placing a purse-string suture of 2/0 chromic catgut approximately half-way between the fascia and the skin, but tied loosely so as not to distort or pucker the wound. Any residual defect is loosely packed with petrolatum (Vaseline) gauze and heals by secondary intention within several weeks. This produces a small, flat, undistorted scar which can be used again for a stoma site if necessary. Any attempts to primarily close the circular skin defect result in a puckered scar and are not recommended.

Postoperative care

The patient is maintained with postoperative fluids, and oral intake is restricted until bowel function resumes. Nasogastric suction is employed for about 24 h but is not continued routinely unless there are excessive amounts of aspirant. Peroperative antibiotics are not usually continued beyond the first 24 h.

The petrolatum (Vaseline) gauze packing is removed after 3 days, and a non-adherent dressing is applied and changed as necessary until the wound heals. The patient is advised to take a low-residue diet for 6–8 weeks to reduce the chance of a bolus obstruction at the ileostomy closure site where oedema persists for several weeks. Normal diet can be recommenced after 8 weeks.

Acknowledgements

Illustrations 2, 3, 5, 8–12, 15–17, 19–22, 24, 26, 28–31, 37, 38, 40–56 have been drawn from roughs prepared by Joseph A. Pangrace at The Cleveland Clinic Foundation.

Illustrations by the late Robert Lane

Tube caecostomy

Robin K. S. Phillips MS, FRCS
Consultant Surgeon, St Mark's Hospital for Diseases of the Rectum and Colon and Homerton Hospital, London, and Honorary Lecturer, St Bartholomew's Hospital Medical School, London, UK

James P. S. Thomson DM, MS, FRCS
Consultant Surgeon and Clinical Director, St Mark's Hospital for Diseases of the Rectum and Colon, London, Honorary Consultant Surgeon, St Mary's Hospital, London, Honorary Lecturer in Surgery, Medical College of St Bartholomew's Hospital, London, Civil Consultant in Surgery, Royal Air Force and Civilian Consultant in Colorectal Surgery, Royal Navy, UK

Principles and justification

Indications

Tube caecostomy procedures are now very uncommon, but can be used to achieve distal bowel gaseous decompression. However, this method does not divert the faecal stream and requires a considerable amount of nursing care to maintain its patency. After on-table colonic irrigation (*see* chapter on pp. 397–416), it is sometimes tempting to leave the irrigating catheter *in situ*, both to decompress the colon and to permit antegrade radiological examination of an anastomosis. However, the quality of such films is poor, and complications have been reported by leaving the tube *in situ*.

Caecostomy may be useful in the management of pseudo-obstruction but other techniques, such as colonoscopic decompression, are now available. Where there is impending caecal rupture, tube caecostomy cannot be relied upon as there may already be full-thickness necrosis of the bowel wall, thus mandating bowel resection.

Preoperative

Caecostomy is usually performed concomitant with another procedure and thus the preparation of the patient will be for the other procedure. When, however, it is used in a patient with a large bowel obstruction, the same efforts to optimize the patient's condition should be taken as for a more extensive procedure.

Anaesthesia

The operation can be performed under local or general anaesthesia depending on the condition of the patient.

Operation

Principles of technique

A large-bore balloon catheter, such as a 30-Fr Foley catheter, is inserted and secured in the caecum with its distal end directed towards the hepatic flexure. The caecum is in turn sutured to the anterior abdominal wall.

It is usual to remove the appendix, as it is theoretically possible for its lumen to be obstructed by the tube. Where the caecum is mobile the removed appendix stump may be a suitable site for the tube, but it is usual to place the tube in the anterior caecal wall to simplify the placement of sutures between the caecum and the anterior abdominal wall.

Caecostomy by mucocutaneous suture should not be undertaken, as the effluent is essentially ileal and, without a suitable spout, skin excoriation will develop rapidly. Furthermore, formal closure as opposed to tube removal would then become necessary.

Incision

1 When a tube caecostomy is constructed in association with a colonic anastomosis, a stab incision is made in the right iliac fossa. If caecostomy alone is performed, a small oblique incision some 6 cm in length is made over the caecum.

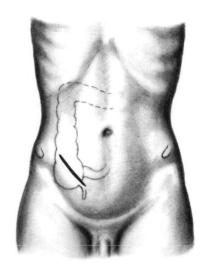

1

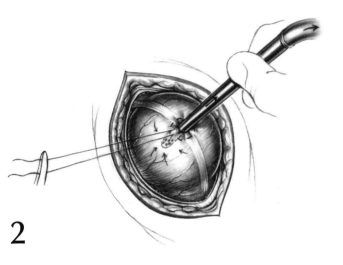

2

Opening the caecum

2 A purse-string 2/0 suture of soluble material is placed in the caecum at the site of the anterior taenia. If the caecum is grossly distended it may help first to aspirate the gas by puncturing the caecum with a large-bore needle attached to the suction tubing, thus allowing some of the tension to be relieved. This will allow a soft bowel clamp to be placed across a portion of the caecum so that when the caecum is opened and the Foley catheter is introduced there will be no spillage.

Insertion of caecostomy tube

3a, b The Foley catheter is introduced with the drainage end occluded to avoid spillage. The balloon is inflated and the purse-string pulled up against the tube and knotted. The soft bowel clamp can then be removed and suction applied to the Foley catheter if more decompression is required. It may be necessary to place a second purse-string suture at this stage to ensure a watertight fit.

Appendicectomy can then be performed.

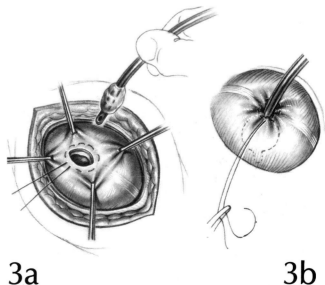

3a   **3b**

Securing caecum to anterior abdominal wall

4 Four 2/0 sutures of the same material are inserted one after another between the seromuscular layer of the caecum and the anterior abdominal wall. It helps if they are clipped but not tied until all four have been inserted.

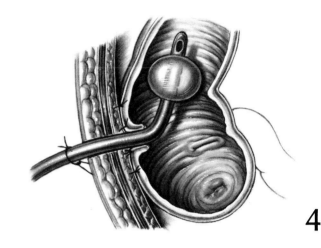

4

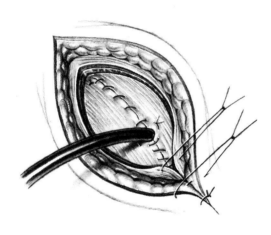

5

Wound closure

5 If an incision in the right iliac fossa has been made, then it should be closed.

Securing tube to anterior abdominal wall

6 The tube is secured primarily by a suture to the anterior abdominal wall. Undue pulling up of the Foley balloon catheter should be avoided as this may cause some ischaemic necrosis of the caecal wall against the anterior abdominal wall. The catheter is then secured to the abdominal wall with adhesive tape and attached to a urine drainage bag to create a closed system.

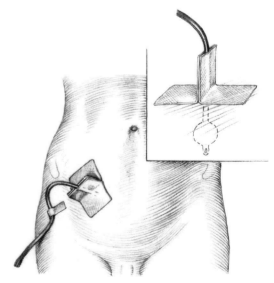

6

Postoperative care

Care of tube

After the first 36 h, the caecostomy tube is washed through every 6 h with 100 ml of physiological saline warmed to body temperature. At least the same volume should then be siphoned from the system. There is a theoretical risk of water intoxication if plain water is used, particularly if larger volumes are employed.

Removal of tube

A fistula between the caecum and anterior abdominal wall should be well established by the seventh postoperative day, depending on the nutritional state of the patient. The securing stitch on the abdominal wall should be removed and the balloon deflated. The catheter can be left to fall free spontaneously, which it usually does by the ninth day. Provided there is no distal obstruction in the bowel, the opening will close. Only very rarely is a formal closure required.

Laxatives

Mineral laxatives may increase faecal fluid, thereby keeping the fistula open; they should therefore be avoided.

Colostomy

Robin K. S. Phillips MS, FRCS
Consultant Surgeon, St Mark's Hospital for Diseases of the Rectum and Colon and Homerton Hospital,
London, and Honorary Lecturer, St Bartholomew's Hospital Medical School, London, UK

James P. S. Thomson DM, MS, FRCS
Consultant Surgeon and Clinical Director, St Mark's Hospital for Diseases of the Rectum and Colon, London,
Honorary Consultant Surgeon, St Mary's Hospital, London, Honorary Lecturer in Surgery, Medical College of
St Bartholomew's Hospital, London, Civil Consultant in Surgery, Royal Air Force and Civilian Consultant in
Colorectal Surgery, Royal Navy, UK

Principles and justification

Types of operation and indications

A colostomy diverts faecal flow onto the anterior abdominal wall and may be either temporary or permanent. A temporary stoma is sometimes used in a staged operation in the management of malignant large intestinal obstruction or with certain anal operations. A permanent colostomy is performed in association with operations to excise the rectum and sometimes for patients with idiopathic faecal incontinence.

The four main types of colostomy are:

1. Loop colostomy.
2. Double-barrelled colostomy.
3. Divided colostomy (Devine).
4. Terminal colostomy.

Loop colostomy

This is the most usually formed temporary colostomy. Its site depends on the reason for its construction and may be either in the transverse or in the sigmoid colon. In principle, a loop of colon is brought to the surface, secured by mucocutaneous suture and held in place by a rod until it becomes adherent (usually 5–8 days) when the rod can be removed.

Loop stomas are now less commonly constructed in cases of obstruction or complicated diverticular disease than in the past, as more surgeons embark on immediate intestinal resection in the treatment of these conditions. Thus, the majority of loop stomas are used to defunction

a distal anastomosis, but may be used with certain anal operations (some high anal fistulae or anal sphincter repair, particularly in cases of Crohn's disease).

The advantages of a transverse loop colostomy include its ease of construction and ease of closure. The disadvantages are: its site in the right upper quadrant (though there is nothing to prevent the surgeon from mobilizing the hepatic flexure so that the stoma can be sited in the more convenient right iliac fossa); its tendency to prolapse; and the vulnerability of the marginal artery during closure (and hence of the distal colonic blood supply if the inferior mesenteric artery has previously been ligated at its origin). Because of these disadvantages, some surgeons prefer to construct a loop ileostomy to defunction the distal intestine (as described in the chapter on pp. 243–269).

Double-barrelled colostomy

This is the type of colostomy used in the Paul–Mikulicz operation. A 'spur' is constructed between the two antimesenteric limbs of the colostomy, which can subsequently be divided using a linear cutting stapler. In theory the colostomy should then close spontaneously, but it is usual for a formal closure to be necessary. The operation is becoming obsolete, although it could be used in an unfit patient with a volvulus after resection of the sigmoid colon.

Divided colostomy

This colostomy is constructed in the usual way but with a tongue of skin separating the two limbs of the stoma. Because it is as easy to close the distal limb subcutaneously, and because a conventional loop stoma provides satisfactory bowel defunctioning, a divided colostomy has little place in current surgical practice.

Terminal colostomy

This end stoma is usually constructed in association with operations to excise the rectum (as described in the chapter on pp. 456–471) or Hartmann's operation (as described in the chapter on pp. 488–496). It may be necessary, however, in cases of irremediable faecal incontinence, when the operation can be performed without a laparotomy solely through a trephine incision, taking great care not to inadvertently close the proximal colon and secure the distal limb! The colostomy is formed from the sigmoid colon which is brought out through an incision in the left abdominal wall (as described in the chapter on pp. 284–291).

Closure of loop colostomy

A temporary loop colostomy is closed when there is no longer a need to defunction the distal intestine. If a colostomy has been constructed to cover a healing anastomosis, then it is essential that total healing of the anastomosis has occurred before undertaking the colostomy closure. This may partly be assessed endoscopically, when the bowel can also be seen to be healthy and not cyanosed or oedematous, but it is important to perform contrast radiology in addition because tracks may be overlooked with the endoscope. Anteroposterior and lateral films should be taken. Colostomy closure is easiest if undertaken at least 2 months after the original operation, and is most difficult if undertaken in the first month.

Preoperative

Bowel preparation

When circumstances allow, a full bowel preparation is preferable. Many of the conditions, however, for which a loop stoma is constructed are 'urgent' or 'emergency' in nature, which precludes bowel preparation. Perioperative systemic antibiotics are given against aerobic and anaerobic organisms.

Before colostomy closure, the proximal intestine should be prepared in the usual way, but taking into account that there is less intestine to empty. If the distal intestine contains any barium it must be washed out because the barium may solidify and cause intraluminal obstruction. Otherwise, distal loop washouts are unnecessary. The perioperative antibiotic regimen favoured by the surgeon for colonic surgery should be used.

Anaesthesia

General anaesthesia is preferred because traction on the mesentery causes pain and nausea. It is possible, however, to perform these operations under local or regional anaesthesia. Colostomy closure is best performed under general anaesthesia.

Operations

LOOP COLOSTOMY

Incision

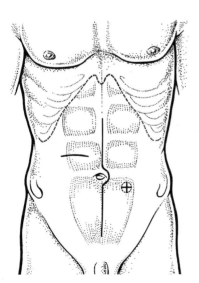

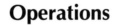

1 The sites of incision for a transverse colostomy and a left iliac fossa sigmoid colostomy are shown in *Illustration 1*. The ideal siting for a transverse colostomy is in the right iliac fossa, but the hepatic flexure must be mobilized in order to achieve this. If a transverse colostomy is to be performed, for example, as the first stage of a staged colonic resection, then the incision (usually 6 cm) must be in the right upper abdomen, midway between the umbilicus and the costal margin, and placed over the rectus abdominis muscle but extending just lateral to its lateral margin.

1

2 The incision is deepened through the anterior rectus sheath. The rectus abdominis may either be divided or split in the line of its fibres, and then the abdomen is opened.

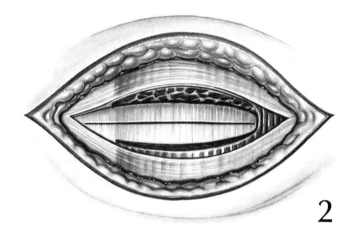

2

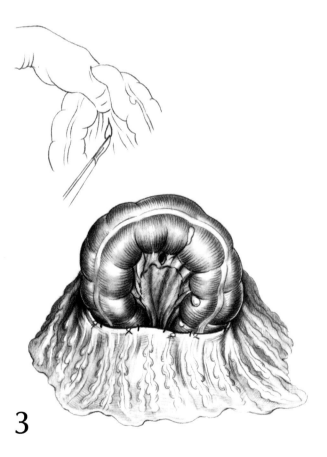

3

Preparation of the colon

3 A transverse colostomy may be prepared either by making a window in the omentum or by lifting the free edge of the omentum upwards and dissecting the intact omentum from its largely avascular attachment to the colon. A nylon tape is passed through the mesentery in order to draw the colon up to the surface where the tape is substituted with a plastic rod.

Opening the colostomy

4 The colon may be opened longitudinally or transversely. A transverse incision damages fewer of the encircling vessels in the colonic wall, is easier to secure and probably easier to close.

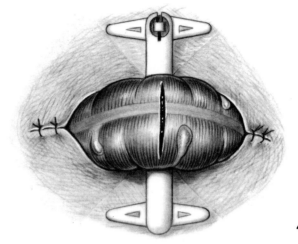

4

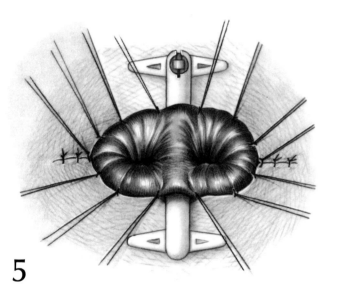

5

Mucocutaneous suture

5 Once open, the colostomy is sutured to the skin with interrupted sutures of 2/0 or 3/0 absorbable material mounted on a taper-cut needle, which penetrate the entire thickness of the intestinal wall but which pass through the subcuticular layer of the skin. The wound is cleaned and a stoma appliance is fitted immediately.

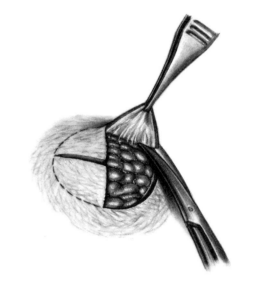

6a

TERMINAL COLOSTOMY

Incision

6a, b The exact site should be marked before the operation to ensure that an appliance will fit satisfactorily away from the umbilicus and the anterior superior iliac spine. A disc of skin approximately 2 cm in diameter is excised. This can be done most accurately using a cruciate incision and excising the four pieces of skin to complete the circle. The alternative of picking up a piece of skin and slicing it off with a knife results in a wound that is oval rather than round and which has edges that in places are only a partial thickness depth. When a laparotomy is also to be performed, a more satisfactory trephine incision is obtained when it is made before the main laparotomy incision.

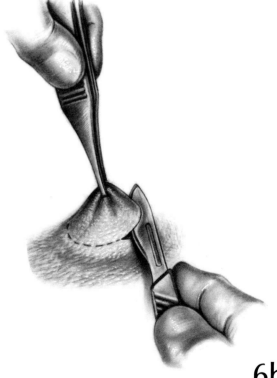

6b

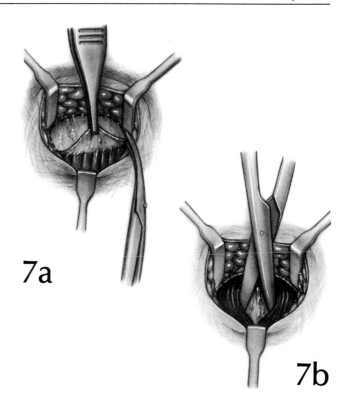

7a, b A cylinder of superficial fascia is removed, taking care to obtain good haemostasis. The dissection through the abdominal wall is aided by three equidistantly placed Langenbeck's or phrenic retractors. A disc of anterior rectus sheath is next removed, the rectus muscle is split, and the abdomen is carefully entered.

7a

7b

8

Delivery of colon through abdominal wall

8 The colon is delivered through the anterior abdominal wall. If it remains totally intraperitoneal, it is desirable for the space between the mesocolon and the abdominal wall (the lateral space) to be closed using non-absorbable sutures. This prevents the possible complication of internal herniation of the small intestine. Alternatively, the colon may be brought to the surface extraperitoneally.

Mucocutaneous suture

9 Before the main abdominal incision is closed, it is important to ensure, by adequate mobilization of the colon, that there will be no tension on the mucocutaneous suture line. Once the main abdominal incision has been sutured and dressed, the clamp on the distal colon is removed and a mucocutaneous suture is performed with 3/0 absorbable sutures placed into the dermal layer and through the muscularis serosal layers, avoiding mucosal penetration.

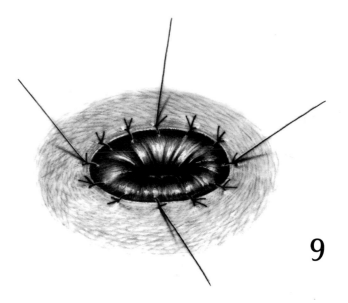

9

CLOSURE OF LOOP COLOSTOMY

A loop colostomy may be closed using one of two techniques:

1. Simple closure: after mobilization of the colon the opening is sutured (half-anastomosis).
2. Excision of the colostomy and anastomosis: the site of the colostomy is excised and the continuity of the colon is restored by end-to-end anastomosis.

In both these instances, the operation is conducted so that the colon is returned to within the peritoneal cavity. So-called extraperitoneal closure of the colostomy is seldom performed and is unsatisfactory because inadequate mobilization has been performed and the anastomosis is almost always under tension.

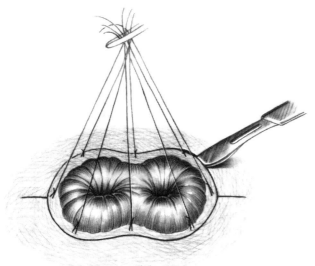

10

Mobilization of the colostomy

10 Between four and eight strong silk sutures are placed around the mucocutaneous junction of the colostomy allowing good control of the colon during mobilization. The incision is made around the edge of the colostomy taking a small fringe of skin approximately 2 mm wide. If necessary, the incision may be enlarged at either end of the colostomy in the transverse plane.

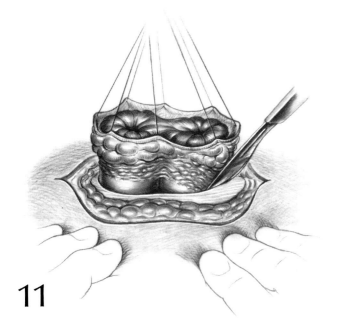

11

11 With traction applied to the colostomy using the stay sutures, the tissues of the anterior wall are freed from the colon. Great care must be exercised to remain in the correct plane and avoid damage to the colon. There is usually little blood loss during this procedure. If haemorrhage does occur, this suggests the surgeon is in the wrong plane.

Removal of the skin edge and unrolling of the colostomy edge

12 The rind of skin is removed and the edge of the colostomy is unrolled. Palpation of the proposed anastomotic edge between finger and thumb confirms when the unrolling is complete, and the colon is then ready for closure.

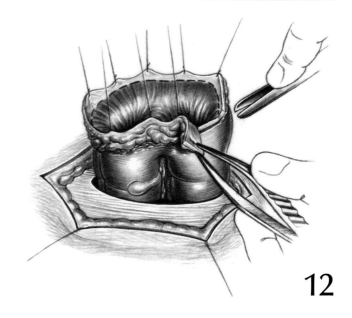

12

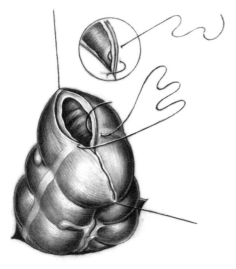

13a

Simple closure of the colon

13a, b This may be achieved in any way with which the surgeon is familiar (as described in the chapter on pp. 51–73): two-layer (usually a continuous inner absorbable suture and an outer interrupted non-absorbable layer); one-layer (usually an interrupted serosubmucosal stitch of either absorbable or non-absorbable material); or with the stapler (usually a functional end-to-end anastomosis; described in the chapter on pp. 74–83).

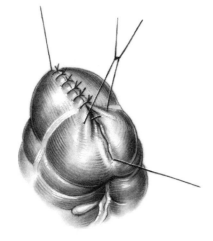

13b

Wound closure

14 A single layer of strong monofilament absorbable or non-absorbable sutures is inserted into all layers, taking large bites on either side of the wound. After all sutures have been placed they are then tied so that the edges of the abdominal wall are closely, but not tightly, approximated. The skin wound is closed, and if haemostasis is in any way in doubt a wound drain is employed.

Postoperative

General management

The general care of the patient will be largely determined by the indication for performing the colostomy. It is wise to maintain intravenous fluids until the patient has at least passed flatus.

It is important to check the viability of the intestine in the early postoperative period and also to make sure that it has not retracted.

It is unusual for the patient to require a nasogastric tube after colostomy closure. Intravenous fluids are maintained until flatus is passed and then a diet is gradually reintroduced.

Care of the colostomy

It is usual to fit an appliance as soon as the colostomy has been constructed. As the effluent from a transverse loop colostomy may be somewhat liquid, codeine phosphate, loperamide, or other constipating agents may be useful.

With a terminal colostomy, particularly in a younger and motivated patient, there is much to recommend colostomy irrigation for long-term management, after the patient has completely recovered from surgery.

Complications of colostomy

Delayed complications are described in the chapter on pp. 292–306.

Loss of viability

This will occur early in the postoperative course if the blood supply to the colostomy has been compromised.

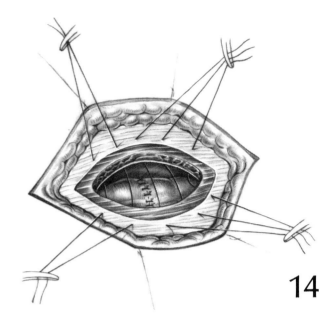

14

It necessitates reconstruction of the colostomy with viable colon. On occasion, however, only the last 1–2 cm of mucosa are ischaemic. As this will heal without intervention, it pays to examine the terminal few centimetres of the intestine endoscopically before deciding on revision.

Separation of the colostomy

This is usually the result of tension at the mucocutaneous junction, and if this occurs circumferentially the colostomy will need to be re-established. Partial separation may also be caused by tension or infection. It will usually heal spontaneously provided that less than half the circumference is involved.

Infection

Although surgery is performed in a potentially septic field, it is very rare for sepsis to complicate the construction of a colostomy. This does occasionally happen, however, with surrounding cellulitis, and there may be some separation of the edge of the colostomy. A haematoma surrounding the colostomy may be a predisposing factor, which emphasizes the importance of good haemostasis in the colostomy wound. Provided that there is adequate drainage, the colostomy will heal, but subsequent scarring might lead to some stenosis at the mucocutaneous junction.

Complications of colostomy closure

Wound infection

This is usually avoided if perioperative antibiotics have been employed and there has been no wound haematoma.

Wound hernia

Hernias do occur in these wounds, and occasionally they are complicated by strangulation.

Breakdown of the colonic suture line

This either results in a faecal fistula, which usually closes spontaneously, or peritonitis, which will require the colostomy to be re-established

Distal anastomosis abscess

If the colostomy is closed before satisfactory healing of the anastomosis has occurred, an abscess may develop at this site. This may also necessitate re-establishment of the colostomy. If the proper indications for performing colostomy closure have been observed, however, this complication should not occur.

Illustrations by Peter Cox

Trephine stomas

Philip F. Schofield MD, FRCS
Consultant Surgeon, Withington and Christie Hospitals and Honorary Reader in Surgery, University of Manchester, Manchester, UK

E. S. Kiff MD, FRCS
Consultant Surgeon, University Hospital of South Manchester, Manchester, UK

History

An end stoma may be created in association with an open operative procedure on the colon or rectum. The operation of creating a trephine stoma has been developed for those patients who require a stoma but not a laparotomy.

Principles and justification

Indications

A trephine stoma may be used in certain cases of faecal incontinence or chronic constipation. This technique is also useful if the intestine needs to be defunctioned for certain anorectal conditions that do not require laparotomy, such as inoperable rectovaginal fistula, or as part of the treatment of complex anorectal injury or sepsis.

Contraindications

An absolute contraindication to an end stoma would be intestinal obstruction, because a 'closed-loop' might be produced. Gross obesity is a relative contraindication.

Preoperative

Bowel preparation

Mechanical bowel preparation to empty the segment of gut that will become the defunctioned distal intestine may be used, but is not obligatory. The preferred site for the stoma is marked on the abdominal wall (as described in the chapter on pp. 274–283).

Anaesthesia

General anaesthesia with muscle relaxation is preferred but it is possible to carry out the procedure under epidural anaesthesia or even a field block with local anaesthesia.

Operation

COLOSTOMY

Either the supine or the Lloyd-Davies position may be used (as described in the chapter on pp. 47–50).

1 With the patient in the supine position a rectal catheter or 24-Fr Foley urinary catheter is inserted in the rectum and connected to the bellows of the sigmoidoscope. The catheter is taped to the thigh and brought over one side of the operating table so that the rectum can be inflated with air during the procedure. In an incontinent patient, it may help to inflate the 30-ml balloon of the Foley catheter to prevent leakage of air from the anus. The Lloyd-Davies position is best in patients in whom it is difficult to inflate the intestine, such as in operations for palliation of rectovaginal fistula. Under these circumstances, intestinal inflation may be achieved using a sigmoidoscope or as described with a Foley catheter.

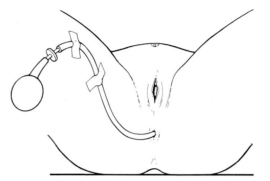

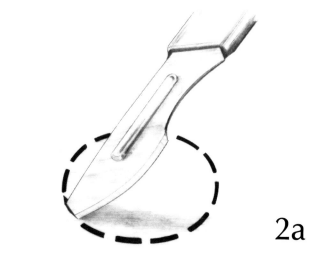

2a–e A 2.5-cm disc of skin and subcutaneous tissue is excised down to the rectus sheath. Two Langenbeck's retractors are used to expose the rectus sheath, which is incised in a cruciate manner. The rectus muscle is split by a pair of scissors in the line of its fibres. The peritoneum is picked up and opened between two forceps.

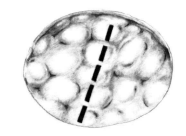

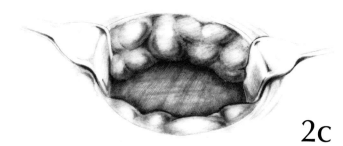

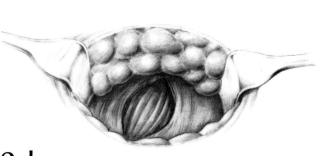

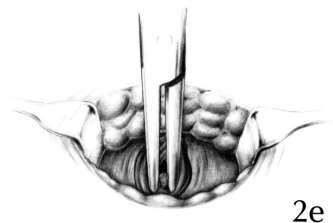

3 The left colon is located by identifying the most lateral intestine in the abdomen. The presence of taenia confirm that it is colon and the absence of the omentum excludes the transverse colon.

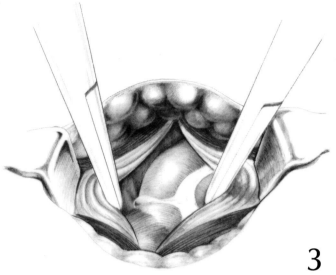

3

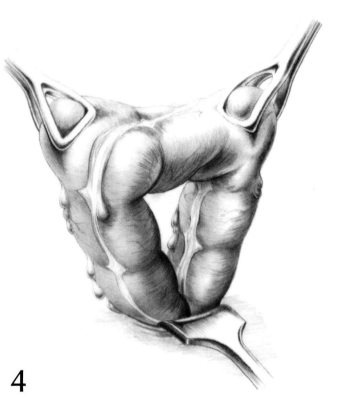

4

4 By using two pairs of Babcock's forceps, the left colon can be followed distally to a point where there is sufficient mobility to withdraw it through the wound. Occasionally, it is necessary to divide the peritoneum lateral to the colon to give adequate mobility free of tension.

5 Sufficient colon is drawn to the surface to allow a small window in the mesentery to be made which may require division of a single blood vessel. The intestine is occluded with either a soft clamp or a TA 55 staple gun applied across the apex of the loop of intestine.

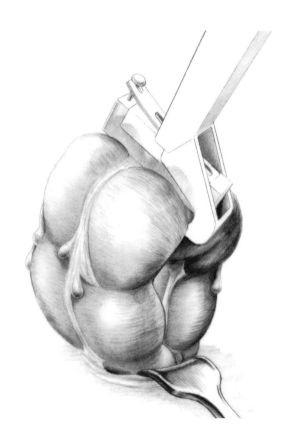

5

6 Air is insufflated into the rectum until the colon distends on one side of the occlusion. This identifies the distal side of the intestine. If an occlusion clamp has been used, it is replaced by a TA 55 stapler, which is fired, and the intestine is divided *proximal* to the stapler.

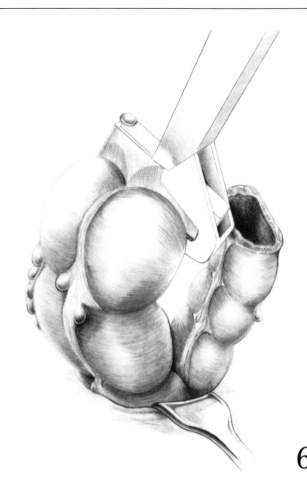

6

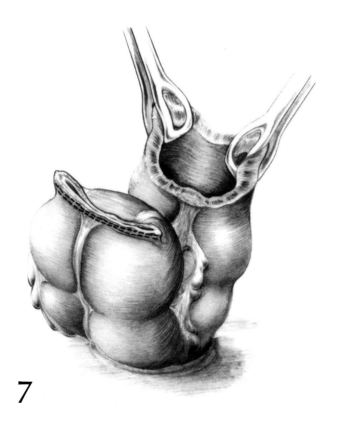

7

7 The TA 55 stapler is removed and the stapled end is folded back towards the abdominal cavity. As an alternative, the distal intestine may be closed with sutures rather than staples. The lateral space is not closed.

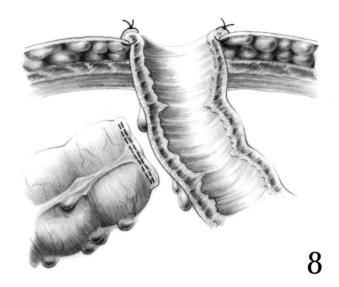

8

8 The proximal colon is sutured to the skin with eight 2/0 chromic catgut mucocutaneous sutures. The stoma appliance is fitted immediately.

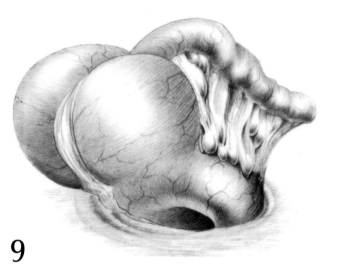

9

ILEOSTOMY

9 The trephine is made at the elected site in the right lower abdomen (as described in the chapter on pp. 243–269). The technique used to enter the peritoneal cavity is as described for trephine colostomy. The caecum is delivered through the abdominal wall, which allows identification of the ileocaecal junction. The caecum is returned to the abdominal cavity, but the terminal ileum is retained.

10 A position approximately 12 cm from the ileocaecal valve is selected where the mesentery can be divided for 6–7 cm.

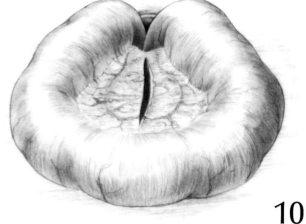

10

11 The TA 55 stapler is placed across the intestine and fired. The intestine is divided *proximal* to the stapler.

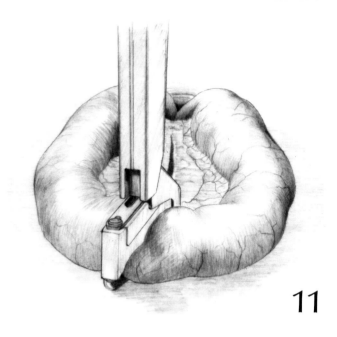

11

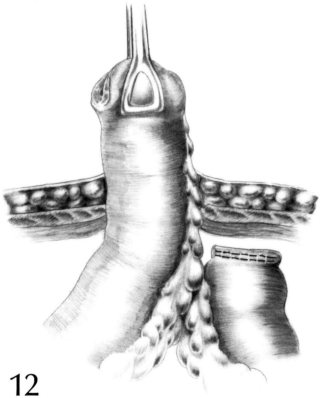

12

12 The stapler is removed and the stapled ileum is pushed back towards the peritoneum. No attempt is made to close the lateral space, but the mesentery is sutured to the rectus sheath with a single stitch of 2/0 polyglactin (Vicryl).

13 The ileum is formed into a spout ileostomy with catgut sutures placed in the muscular submucosal deep dermal position (as described in the chapter on pp. 243–269). After cleansing the area and drying the skin, a stoma appliance is fitted immediately.

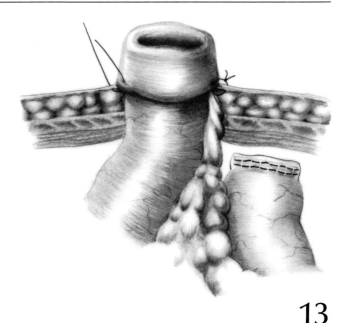

13

Postoperative care

The absence of a major abdominal wound makes postoperative care simple, because the appliance is easier to fit, there is less postoperative pain and little requirement for sedation, and there is minimal or no postoperative ileus, so that normal eating and drinking will usually be resumed within 24–48 h. Trephine stomas are suitable as short hospital stay procedures provided there is adequate stoma care service support for training the patients in stoma management.

Outcome

It is possible to carry out a trephine colostomy in about 90% of cases where it is attempted. There are few complications, but occasionally the mucocutaneous sutures separate in part and lead to cicatrization and colostomy stenosis in the longer term, which may then require revision (as described in the chapter on pp. 292–306). This problem can be prevented by sufficient mobilization of intestine to provide for a proper 1-cm stomal spout, which will help to prevent stomal retraction and stenosis.

Complications of ileostomy and colostomy

Hasse Jiborn MD, PhD
Associate Professor, Department of Surgery, Malmö General Hospital, University of Lund, Malmö, Sweden

Göran R. Ekelund MD, PhD
Associate Professor and Chairman, Department of Surgery, Malmö General Hospital, University of Lund, Malmö, Sweden

General technical considerations

Surgery for stoma complications requires an atraumatic technique to avoid damaging the intestinal wall so that it can be used for reconstruction; accidental perforation might result in fistula formation. The skin around the stoma should be incised with a knife or diathermy (preferably with a needle tip) and the stoma mobilized using careful dissection by needle tip diathermy or by a fine pair of scissors; mobilization is best achieved when tissues are under some tension. For good results even these 'minor' operations should be performed only when adequate assistance is available.

1 To get good access for this 'keyhole' surgery appropriate retractors should be used, such as the Löfberg's type which was originally developed for surgery of the thyroid gland.

If the stoma site is going to be reused and the original size is appropriate, the skin should be incised immediately (about 1 mm) outside the mucocutaneous junction in order not to create too large a skin opening. If additional incisions are needed for access, care must be taken to obtain perfect alignment of the subcutaneous tissue and the skin to produce a smooth scar, which is essential for safe function of the appliance.

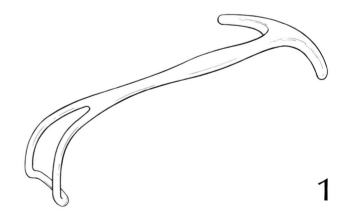

1

Suture material

The following suture materials are recommended:

Peritoneum and intestinal wall: 3/0 synthetic absorbable braided (e.g. Dexon, Vicryl) or monofilament (e.g. Maxon, PDS).

Fascia closure: 2/0 synthetic absorbable monofilament (e.g. Maxon, PDS) or braided (e.g. Dexon, Vicryl).

Mucocutaneous suture: 4/0 non-absorbable monofilament (e.g. Novafil, Prolene, Ethilon) or 3/0 synthetic absorbable braided (e.g. Dexon, Vicryl).

Skin suture: 3/0 non-absorbable monofilament.

Absorbable monofilaments may be preferred to braided sutures for parastomal hernia repair because they are less likely to maintain infection and they retain their strength longer than braided sutures. Non-absorbable suture material should be used only for deep sutures to secure any mesh grafts in repair of parastomal hernia.

Complications of ileostomy

Ileostomy complications are common. Most can be managed by experienced stoma care, but 30–40% require surgical revision[1,2]. The most frequent complications are obstruction, recession and prolapse; less common are parastomal hernias, fistulae, ulcerations and granulomas.

Obstruction

Obstruction may be caused by stenosis developing at skin and/or fascial levels. A food bolus is often the immediate cause of overt obstruction and this is usually managed by irrigation with 100 ml warm saline through a Foley catheter gently introduced into the stoma.

Intra-abdominal adhesion is another cause of obstruction. Recurrent disease must be considered in patients with Crohn's disease.

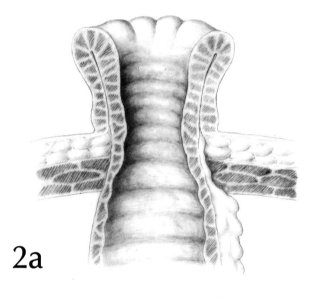

2a

Stenosis

Stenosis of the stoma can be managed by local repair.

2a, b The skin is incised around the stoma immediately outside the strictured zone; this should create a 2–3-cm wide (two-finger wide) opening in the skin. Care should be taken not to create a larger opening.

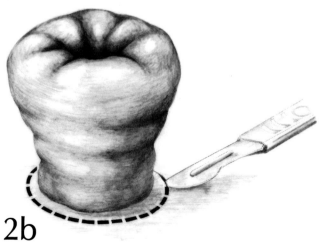

2b

3a, b The stoma is straightened, mobilized in the subcutaneous plane and the eversion reduced. The distal part of the ileum with the stricturing scar tissue is then excised.

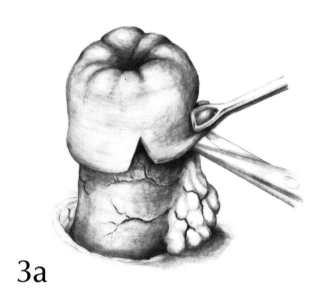

3a

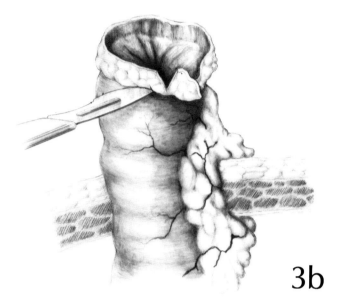

3b

4a, b The stoma is explored with a finger for any additional stricture at the fascial plane; if such a stricture is discovered, dissection is continued beyond the fascia. Part of the junction between ileum and fascia is opened and the fascia incised to create an adequate opening (not too large because of the risk of herniation).

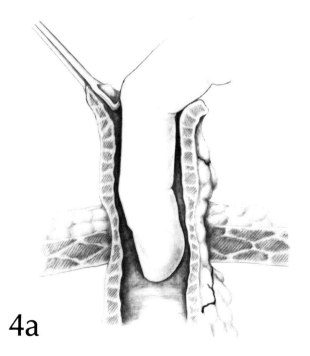

4a

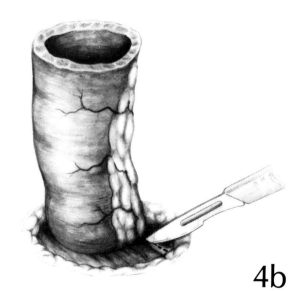

4b

5 The ileum is again everted and sutured to the skin with 4/0 non-absorbable monofilament: skin to seromuscular in the proximal limb at the skin plane; full thickness for the end of the ileum. The surgeon should be careful not to penetrate the bowel wall with the *seromuscular* bite because of the risk of fistula formation.

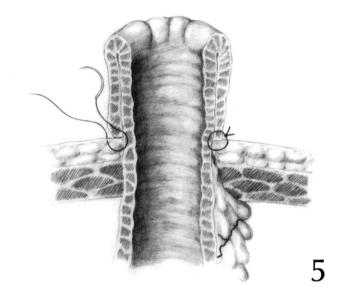

5

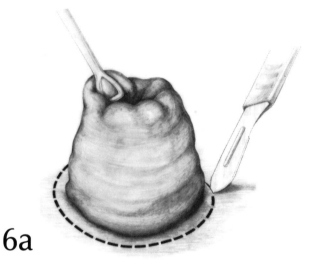

6a

Recession

Recession results from either too large an abdominal opening or inadequate fixation of the ileum at the fascial plane. Recession often occurs at night when the patient is lying down and may result in leakage because of impaired fitting of the appliance.

Local repair of stoma

6a, b The stoma is detached at the muco-cutaneous junction, straightened, the eversion reduced and mobilized down into the peritoneal cavity to gain extra length.

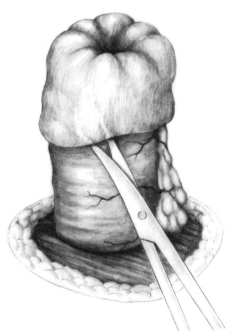

6b

7a, b The stoma is sutured to the peritoneum circumferentially with interrupted 3/0 absorbable sutures with seromuscular bites. If the opening in the fascia is too large, one or two interrupted sutures are placed in the aponeurosis to obtain an appropriate narrowing using 2/0 absorbable monofilament or braided sutures. The length of the ileum projecting outside the skin level should be 6–8 cm (if too long, the excess should be resected).

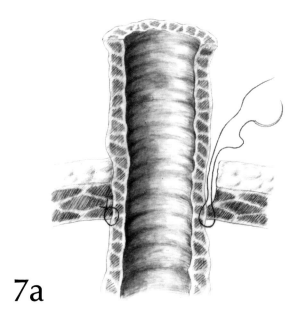

7a

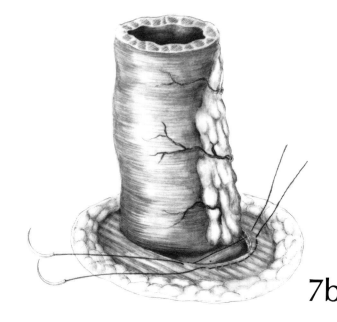

7b

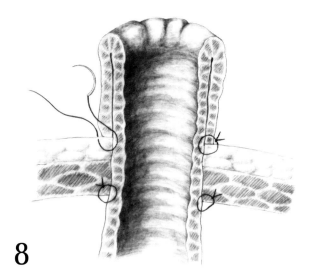

8

8 The ileum is everted and the mucocutaneous junction is re-established.

9a, b Too large a skin opening may be reduced by the Mercedes manoeuvre[3]. Two or three triangular skin excisions (with acute angles and the bases placed centrally) are made around the stoma and closed by non-absorbable monofilament sutures.

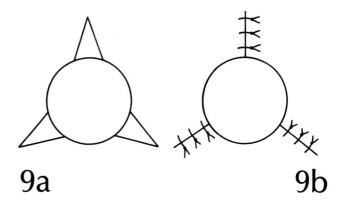

9a   9b

Local fixation of stoma with repair

Local fixation can often be achieved without detachment of the stoma.

10 The stoma is everted by grasping it with a pair of Babcock's forceps introduced into the stoma. The index finger is inserted into the stoma and interrupted 3/0 absorbable sutures are placed through the full thickness of the outer intestinal wall and the seromuscular layer of the inner wall, guided by the index finger to avoid penetration of mucosa in the inner layer and to lessen the risk of fistula formation.

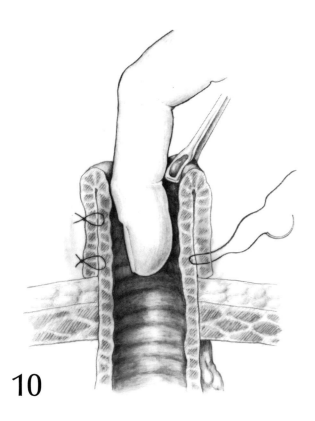

10

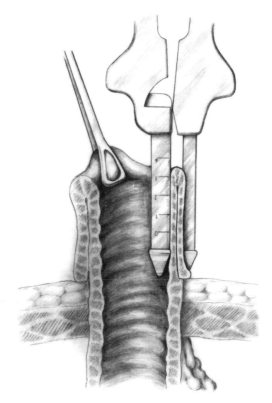

11 Another method of fixation is to use the GIA stapler *without* the blade instead of sutures. The retracted ileostomy is pulled out to a length of about 4 cm by inserting three pairs of Babcock's forceps 120° apart, one at the mesenteric region. The GIA stapler *without* the blade is placed towards the mucocutaneous junction between the forceps and fired. Three parallel rows of staples are created. Care should be taken to avoid placing the instrument over the mesentery since this may cause necrosis of the ileostomy. The stoma, even with correct placement of staples, is unsightly for about 6 weeks but gradually returns to a more normal appearance[4].

11

Retraction

Retraction (or fixed recession) is often caused by insufficient intestine being used for the construction of the stoma. By dissecting the stoma to the peritoneal level, sufficient intestinal length can often be mobilized to reconstruct the stoma with adequate length (2–4 cm). For operative technique, *see* section on Recession, page 295.

Recurrent Crohn's disease should be suspected when retraction develops and if this is in fact the case the problem should be managed accordingly, usually by radiological examination, endoscopy followed by laparotomy, resection and construction of a new stoma.

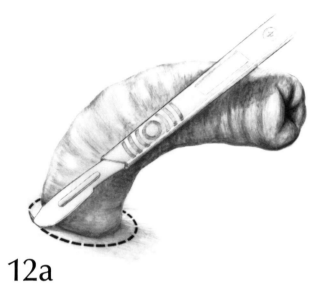

12a

Prolapse

12a–c The same operative technique can be used as described for recession, i.e. reduction of the eversion and mobilization of the stoma to the fascial plane. The base of the stoma is secured to the peritoneum (fascia) by interrupted seromuscular sutures, after which the abundant ileum is resected. The stoma is reconstructed with mucocutaneous sutures.

If the mesentery has been completely detached and an excessive length of ileum can be pulled out of the stoma site, laparotomy may sometimes be necessary to reattach it to the peritoneum using interrupted absorbable sutures. The stoma should then be reconstructed (*see* chapter on pp. 243–270).

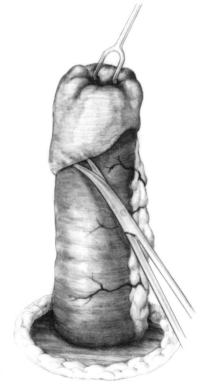

12b

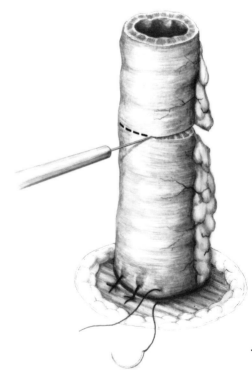

12c

Excessive length of stoma

A stoma which is too long is usually caused by misjudgement at the time of construction. The ileum should be detached at the mucocutaneous junction, eversion of the stoma reduced, amputated to the appropriate length, and resutured mucocutaneously (*see* section on Prolapse, page 298).

Parastomal hernia

Parastomal hernia is relatively rare in connection with ileostomy.

Local repair

13a, b The stoma is detached from the mucocutaneous junction and the ileum is mobilized to the fascial level. If access is necessary, a transverse 'help' incision may be made in the skin and subcutaneous tissue.

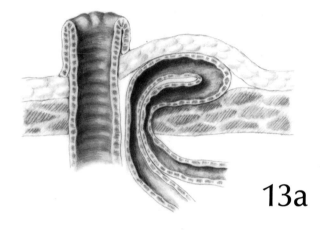

13a

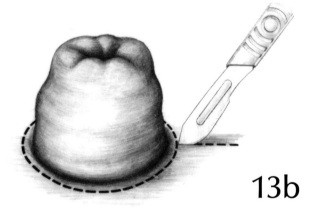

13b

14a–c The hernial sac is dissected free and excised. The aponeurosal defect is closed by interrupted 2/0 absorbable sutures through all layers, including the peritoneum, leaving an adequate opening for the ileostomy. This should be checked by the index finger in the stoma. The stoma is refashioned (*see* section on Recession, page 295). If a 'help' incision has been performed this is closed with interrupted subcutaneous sutures and skin sutures. Care must be taken to create a smooth scar.

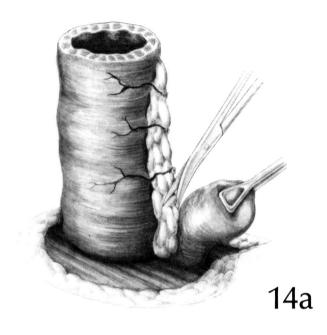

14a

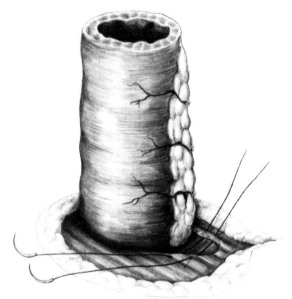

14b

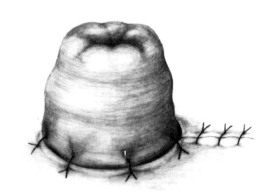

14c

Resiting of the stoma

In case of hernial recurrence the stoma may be resited by laparotomy. Before bringing the patient to surgery it must be ensured that the new stoma site has been selected appropriately (usually in the opposite lower quadrant), if possible with the aid of a stoma care nurse, and has been marked.

The stoma is detached at the mucocutaneous junction and dissected free down to the peritoneum. The stoma is dissected and closed at the end by staples or a running suture. Laparotomy is performed through a low midline incision (usually through the old incisional scar), the distal ileum and mesentery are detached and mobilized to fit the new stomal position.

Parastomal fistula

Fistulae may occur from trauma caused by pressure of the appliance flange and are thus located at skin level. Deeper fistulae usually arise from non-absorbable sutures having been placed too deep or too firmly in the bowel wall, and these fistulae usually originate at the fascial level. Recurrent disease must always be considered in patients with Crohn's disease and managed accordingly.

Preoperative assessment

The fistulous tract is assessed by a probe to search for the inner opening but probing must be performed with great care to avoid making false openings. Fistulography, enterography and ileoscopy are of value in locating fistulae and in the search for recurrent Crohn's disease.

Operative technique

Fistulae at the skin level may heal spontaneously after appliance correction.

Deeper fistulae require laparotomy, ileal resection and stomal reconstruction. If peristomal tissues in the bowel wall are not destroyed by the fistula and there is no gross infection, the stoma may be reconstructed at the original site, otherwise the stoma must be resited.

Ulceration

Peristomal ulceration is often due to recurrent Crohn's disease. If ulcerations are not accompanied by local recurrence in the ileum requiring resection, they usually heal if overhanging skin is excised and the ulcer is thoroughly curetted.

Granuloma

Granulomas in the stoma base are often caused by mechanical pressure by the appliance, which should be corrected if possible. Excision and cauterization are usually followed by recurrence. Granulomas may be an indication of fistula, which should be treated accordingly.

Complications of colostomy

Complications are also common with colostomies and have been reported in up to 50% of patients. Colostomy complications may occur early in the postoperative course (such as stomal necrosis) or may develop many years after operation (such as paracolostomy hernia[5]).

Necrosis

If necrosis of the stoma occurs, it appears early after operation. The disturbed mesenteric circulation, which is the cause of stomal necrosis, may be the result of too extensive mesenteric dissection, stretching of the colon in order to reach the abdominal wall or, sometimes, entrapment of the mesentery in the abdominal wall opening. Stoma necrosis is most common in obese patients and after emergency surgery with bowel distension.

15   Necrosis results in mucocutaneous separation of part of, or the entire, circumference of the stoma. The extent of mucosal necrosis is often not obvious but must be discovered. It can be judged using a glass test tube inserted gently into the stoma, illuminated with a torch. The mucosa is visible through the test tube and its condition can be judged[6]. If only partial and superficial necrosis is observed (well distal to the fascial plane) conservative treatment with repeated observations may be employed. If deep necrosis or total separation and retraction of the stoma has occurred, laparotomy with further mobilization of the colon must be performed and a new stoma established.

Stricture and retraction

Partial necrosis and mucocutaneous separation, if managed conservatively, often results in stricture formation and stomal retraction. A stricture and retraction of a colostomy should be managed surgically similar to that described for ileostomy complications.

Prolapse

Prolapse is most common in loop transverse colostomies and less common with end colostomies.

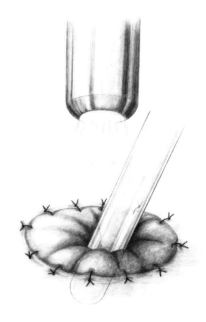

15

Loop transverse colostomy

Construction of a loop transverse colostomy should be avoided because of its significant complications and problems of management. Other methods should be considered, such as primary resection with or without a covering loop ileostomy (*see* chapter on pp. 397–415).

If, however, the prolapse of a loop transverse colostomy presents, conservative treatment can be used if the stoma is temporary and early further surgery considered. If the stoma is to be permanent, the transverse colostomy may be divided and transformed into a terminal end colostomy and a distal mucocutaneous fistula.

16a, b
The stoma is detached at the muco-cutaneous junction and mobilized to the peritoneum. The colon is transected at the stoma region and the distal part of the mesentery divided to allow separation of the two bowel ends. Any redundant colon is resected. The distal end is brought out as a mucocutaneous fistula via a separate stab incision to the left of the midline and secured to the skin by mucocutaneous sutures using 4/0 non-absorbable monofilament.

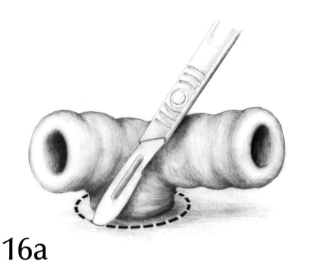

16a

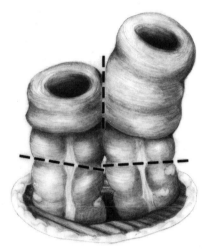

16b

17a, b
The proximal terminal colon is secured to the peritoneum by interrupted 3/0 absorbable sutures with seromuscular bites in the colon. If the fascia opening is too large it can be narrowed by one or two interrupted 2/0 absorbable sutures. The stoma is reconstructed by mucocutaneous sutures.

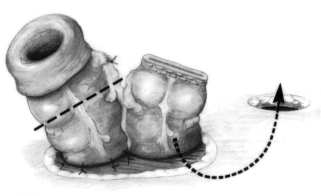

17a

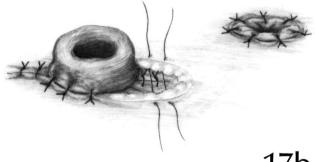

17b

End colostomy: local repair

18a–d A similar procedure as for ileal prolapse is employed. The stoma is detached at the mucocutaneous junction and dissected to the peritoneal cavity.

The redundant colon is pulled out. The mesentery and the colon are secured to the peritoneum by interrupted 3/0 absorbable sutures. The excess colon is resected 1–2 cm above the skin level and sutured to the skin.

End colostomy: resiting of stoma

If the prolapse is recurrent or is combined with a hernia, laparotomy and resiting of the stoma must be considered. The same technique as has been described for resiting of an ileostomy may be employed (page 301).

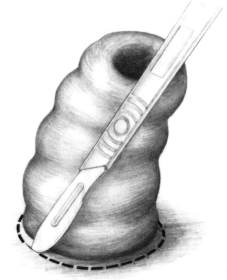

18a

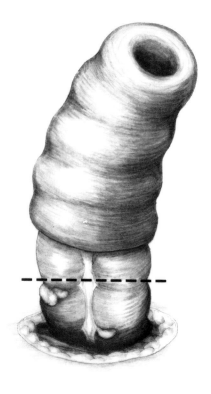

18b

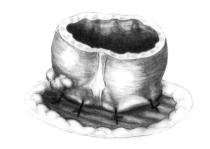

18c

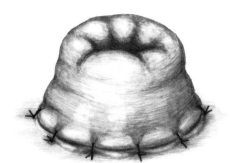

18d

Parastomal hernia

Some degree of parastomal hernia is common with end colostomies. Most should be managed conservatively with special care of appliances and girdles, because they are harmless to the patient, and the results of surgery are disappointing, with a high incidence of recurrence.

If the hernia is very discomforting (for example, it interferes with the wearing of an applicance, with irrigation of the colon, or causes unacceptable cosmetic problems), surgical correction must be considered. Symptoms are often aggravated if the hernia is combined with other complications such as stenosis or prolapse. Bowel strangulation may occur in a parastomal hernia but is rare and requires urgent surgery.

Two surgical options are available, local repair (with or without support of a synthetic mesh) and resiting of the stoma with closure of the abdominal defect at the original stoma site. Resiting of the stoma is often advocated, because local repair is accompanied by a high recurrence rate.

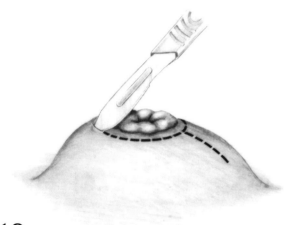

19

Local repair

19 The skin is incised circumstomally about 1 mm outside the mucocutaneous junction and then the stoma is dissected down to the fascia.

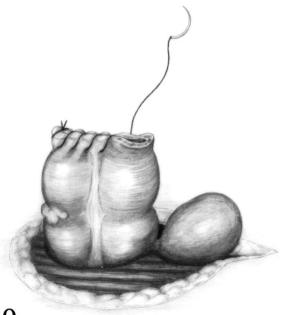

20

20 The stoma is closed by a running suture (e.g. non-absorbable monofilament). The hernia is identified and dissected to the peritoneal plane. A lateral transverse skin incision is often needed to expose the area.

21 The hernial sac is excised and the edges of peritoneum grasped with clamps. The stoma is now secured to the peritoneum by interrupted 3/0 absorbable sutures with seromuscular bites. The aponeurosal defect is closed by interrupted sutures through all layers, including peritoneum, using 2/0 absorbable monofilament leaving an adequate opening for the stoma. The transverse 'help' incision is closed by interrupted absorbable sutures in the subcutaneous layer and non-absorbable monofilament skin sutures (care must be taken to create a smooth scar). The distal margin of the stoma is resected and the mucocutaneous junction is restored (*see* section on Prolapse, page 298).

If necessary the aponeurosis may be reinforced by a sheet of synthetic mesh (e.g. Marlex, Gore-tex) sutured to the fascia with interrupted non-absorbable monofilament sutures. A more extensive method, raising a large skin flap and reinforcing the entire aponeurosal area surrounding the stoma, is described by Leslie[7].

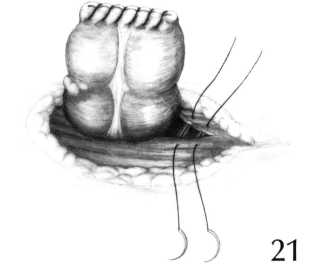

21

Resiting of stoma

The stoma and hernia are mobilized as above. Laparotomy is performed through a midline incision. The stoma is completely disconnected from its original site. The abdominal defect at the original stoma site is repaired in a routine fashion (the peritoneum is closed by a continuous 2/0 absorbable suture, the fascia by interrupted 2/0 absorbable sutures and the subcutaneous tissue and skin are left for secondary healing). The colon is mobilized to fit the new stoma site, the location of which must be carefully chosen before surgery. For details of the stoma construction, *see* chapter on pp. 274–284.

References

1. Carlstedt A, Fasth S, Hultén L, Nordgren S, Palselius I. Long-term ileostomy complications in patients with ulcerative colitis and Crohn's disease. *Int J Colorectal Dis* 1987; 2: 22–5.

2. Weaver RM, Alexander-Williams J, Keighley MRB. Indications and outcome of reoperation for ileostomy complications in inflammatory bowel disease. *Int J Colorectal Dis* 1988; 3: 38–42.

3. Todd IP. Mechanical complications of ileostomy. *Clin Gastroenterol* 1982; 11: 268–73.

4. Winslet MC, Alexander-Williams J, Keighley MRB. Ileostomy revision with a GIA stapler under intravenous sedation. *Br J Surg* 1990; 77: 647.

5. Allen-Mersh TG, Thomson JPS. Surgical treatment of colostomy complications. *Br J Surg* 1988; 75: 416–18.

6. Ekelund G, Hagenfeldt I. Postoperative control of newly established enterostomas. *Coloproctology* 1980; 2: 404–5.

7. Leslie D. The parastomal hernia. *Surg Clin North Am* 1984; 64: 407–15.

Small bowel surgery: introductory comment

W. Silen MD
Johnson and Johnson Professor of Surgery, Harvard Medical School, Boston, Massachusetts, USA

The past several years have seen some revolutionary changes in surgery of the small intestine, such as the emergence of stricturoplasty as an important component of our armamentarium for Crohn's disease. In addition, the treatment of other conditions of the small intestine has also been considerably refined. These advances are nicely covered in the ensuing four chapters.

Professor Alexander-Williams has made an extremely important contribution by clarifying and emphasizing the role of stricturoplasty in the treatment of Crohn's disease. He has clearly demonstrated the safety of this operation, a consideration which was widely challenged and questioned when it was first reported because of fear of disruption of a suture line in diseased intestine. The advent of stricturoplasty will surely save many patients with Crohn's disease from the ravages of the loss of long segments of small intestine, especially ileum. While it now appears that the incidence of symptomatic recurrences is not greater after stricturoplasty than that after resection, we are in need of even longer periods of follow-up to ascertain the natural history of the disease in the operated segment of intestine. From a theoretical standpoint, one might expect that bacterial overgrowth would be an important consequence of stricturoplasty. To date, however, little has been reported of this potential complication, and more time is required before the incidence and severity of this problem is known.

Both Alexander-Williams and Jackson have empha-sized that some strictures may easily escape detection at operation, a pitfall that needs to be emphasized. On a number of occasions, subtle intrinsic strictures have been overlooked or not treated, especially at the site of a pre-existing adhesion and particularly in cases of radiation enteritis. Jackson and Alexander-Williams have rightly emphasized the careful detection of such strictures by digital intraluminal palpation or by the use of calibrated balloon catheters, manoeuvres which previously had received little attention.

While technical details can always engender argu-ment and discussion among surgeons, there are few if any points with which to take issue. These four chapters present a sound compendium of techniques upon which the reader can reliably depend. However, a few personal observations might be useful. First, the almost universal recommendation of the midline abdominal incision needs re-evaluation in view of its much higher incidence of postoperative herniation when compared with the lateral paramedian incision. This is especially pertinent in patients with Crohn's disease who are likely to have numerous operative procedures.

Finally, the widespread use of muscle relaxants by our anaesthetist colleagues needs scrutiny because of the almost universal application of neostigmine to reverse the effects of these drugs. There is reasonable evidence that neostigmine causes violent contractions of the intestine which can hardly be regarded as beneficial to a fresh anastomosis or suture line, especially in intestine which is the site of Crohn's disease or prior radiation.

Resection of the small intestine for inflammatory bowel disease

Olle Bernell MD
General Surgeon, Department of Surgery, Huddinge University Hospital, Huddinge, Sweden

Göran Hellers MD, PhD
Chairman, Department of Surgery, Huddinge University Hospital, Huddinge, Sweden

Principles and justification

In most cases, small intestinal resection is an emergency procedure that is carried out in patients with intestinal obstruction, or less commonly, in patients with a vascular catastrophe or to remove a tumour. In such cases, neither the indications for, nor the technique of, intestinal resection pose any substantial problems. It is usually quite simple to identify the correct level for intestinal resection and to create a 'routine' end-to-end anastomosis (as described in the chapter on pp. 51–73).

In contrast, in patients with inflammatory bowel disease, the problems are different. The fate of the anastomosis is affected by the indications and the timing of surgery, and it is also more difficult to decide on the correct level for the resection.

In managing the intestinal lesion in Crohn's disease, it is therefore important to consider both the strategy and the tactics of the surgical approach. The most important strategic decision for an individual patient is to decide how soon into a period of medical therapy surgery might be undertaken. Surgery might be advised early in the natural history before serious complications arise in patients who are not doing well on medical therapy, e.g. those who require high doses or chronic use of steroids. In contrast, the surgical approach might be very conservative with surgery postponed until complications arise.

Once surgery is undertaken, the length of intestine affected by Crohn's disease, and therefore the amount to be resected, will have an impact on the likelihood of postoperative short bowel syndrome. Furthermore, the surgical plan must recognize that it is likely that patients with Crohn's disease will require a series of operations during the overall natural history of the condition. Thus, considerable clinical judgement is required to decide on the length of intestine to be resected in an individual patient.

From the tactical point of view, the timing of surgery and the preoperative and perioperative management of each operative procedure must be considered carefully. The aim here is to achieve safe anastomotic healing and to reduce the risk of immediate and late surgical complications.

Indications

Surgery for small intestinal Crohn's disease is performed either to achieve remission or to alleviate the symptoms of obstruction and/or septic complications. Surgery to achieve remission is carried out in patients who have active disease and in whom the symptoms cannot be controlled by medical treatment. Such patients are often malnourished and have a low serum albumin concentration because of the protein-losing enteropathy caused by the inflammatory process. These patients are often febrile (from local perforation and abscess formation) and have enteroenteric or enterocutaneous fistulae or extraintestinal manifestations of Crohn's disease, e.g. arthritis, ankylosing spondylitis or pyoderma gangrenosum. In addition, some patients may have small intestinal bacterial overgrowth caused by chronic intestinal obstruction, as well as intermittent colicky abdominal pain associated with this problem.

Preoperative

In patients with very active disease, it is often wise to postpone surgery for a few days to correct fluid and electrolyte imbalance. It is also advantageous to try to control the activity of the intestinal inflammation with short-term, perioperative, high-dose steroids. Small intestinal bacterial overgrowth should, if possible, be eliminated by nasoenteric intubation of the upper small intestine and direct administration of antibiotics. These antibiotics can be given both enterally and systemically using agents active against aerobes and anaerobic bacteria (as described in the chapter on pp. 41–46). Formal bowel preparation is advisable if there is a risk of fistulae into the large intestine or if there may be Crohn's disease of the large intestine which will require removal. In the absence of these possibilities, mechanical bowel preparation is unnecessary, and a few days on a liquid diet is sufficient. Perioperative steroid cover to prevent steroid crisis and subcutaneous mini-dose heparin to mitigate the risks of deep venous thrombosis and thromboembolic problems should be given.

Anaesthesia

Patients should be operated on under general anaesthesia supplemented by muscle relaxants. Continuous epidural block can be used for postoperative pain relief.

Operation

Extent of resection

Over the past two decades, there has been a major discussion about the possible benefits of extensive compared with conservative intestinal resection in Crohn's disease, and also about the use of frozen sections at the margins of resection to help to determine the extent of resection. It is now clear that extensive resection does not reduce the risk of recurrent inflammatory bowel disease in the residual small intestine. In addition, frozen sections have not been shown to be of value in deciding on the extent of resection, because in macroscopically normal intestine, which can be used for anastomosis, there are often histological features of Crohn's disease.

Thus, the selection of the site for intestinal resection rests with the judgement of the individual surgeon. It is recognized that surgeons should be 'conservative' in the amount of intestine resected because of the risk of recurrent disease requiring further resection, and also because some proximal intestinal thickening is secondary to obstruction rather than the ulcerative process *per se*.

Surgeons are advised to carry out a very limited resection and then immediately to open the specimen. If there is no major mucosal disease close to the resection margin, an anastomosis can be fashioned even if one or both ends of the remaining intestine is thickened. On the other hand, if the mucosal surface is severely ulcerated, an additional section of intestine can be removed.

In patients without obstructive disease, the intestinal wall is often much less oedematous, and the resection can be performed very close to the obvious Crohn's lesion. There is no reason to carry out a wedge resection of the mesentery associated with the intestine to be resected. The mesentery should simply be trimmed so that it can be easily closed.

Incision

In patients with inflammatory bowel disease, a midline incision should always be used, despite the greater risk of postoperative hernia formation, so that sites for stomas are not compromised. Exposure is greatly facilitated by extending the incision at least 5 cm above the umbilicus.

Suture material

One layer of interrupted absorbable sutures is sufficient, because it has been repeatedly shown that non-absorbable sutures do not offer any advantages and their persistence might be associated with fistula formation. The author's preference is 3/0 polyglactin (Vicryl).

Technique

1 After exploratory laparotomy, a pair of crushing clamps is used for each transection. The gut is 'shaved off' the crushing clamp on the healthy side of the intestine. The clamp should be narrow and firm, so that only 2–3 mm of gut is crushed within the jaws of the clamp. In Crohn's disease, the significantly diseased part of the small intestine most often has fat wrapping around the serosal aspect of the gut. The clamp should be placed across the intestine at a point where there is minimal fat wrapping, so that the ulcerated part of the intestine is excised.

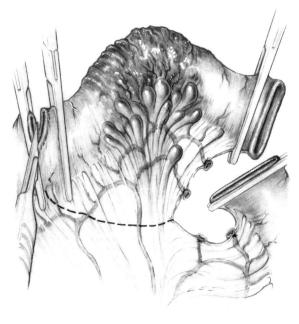

1

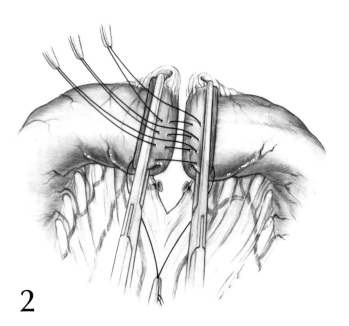

2

2 The crushing clamps are left *in situ* and a row of interrupted sutures is placed to fashion the posterior anastomosis. Once this row of sutures has been completed, they are tied serially and divided. The 'end' sutures are tied but are maintained as 'stay' sutures.

3 The part of the intestine that is closest to the anastomosis on both sides of the clamps is gently squeezed empty and a soft clamp is placed about 5 cm from the anastomotic site on each side. The area for the anastomosis is surrounded by warm, moist packs from the remaining part of the abdominal contents. The crushing clamps are removed and the intestinal lumen is opened on both sides. The inside of both ends of the intestine can be inspected. It is unnecessary to trim the 2–3 mm of crushed intestine because this zone provides haemostasis. If any bleeding points occur, they can be managed with diathermy.

If no linear ulcers are seen on either side, a second (anterior) row of interrupted sutures is placed. The sutures should be inserted about 3 mm from each other and placed through the serosa and muscle, taking in the submucosal plane but without penetrating mucosa. These sutures are then tied serially to complete the anastomosis.

The mesenteric defect is closed with a few interrupted absorbable sutures, making sure that there is no impairment of the blood supply to the intestine.

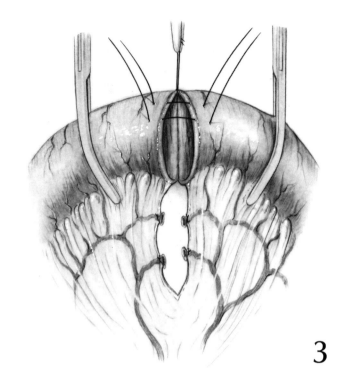

3

4 The soft bowel clamps are removed, and confirmation of an anastomotic lumen is obtained by gently palpating the anastomosis with the thumb and the index finger, making sure not to stretch or disrupt the suture line.

After completing the anastomosis, the area is washed with warmed physiological saline. The packs are removed, and the abdominal contents are again irrigated with significant volumes of warmed physiological saline. The abdomen is closed in the conventional manner. Drains are not necessary unless there is a chronic abscess cavity (an 'inflammatory nest') that requires drainage.

In patients with the unusual complication of free perforation from Crohn's disease with intra-abdominal sepsis, it is wise to consider construction of an end ileostomy and mucous fistula at completion of the resection. The intestine can be reconstructed at a later date when the patient has completely recovered (as described in the chapter on pp. 243–269).

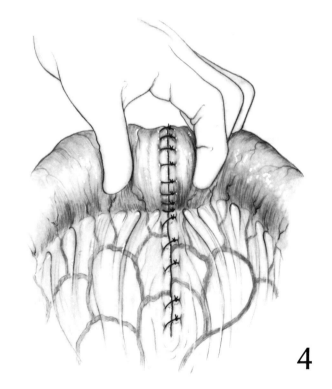

4

Postoperative care

The nasogastric tube is maintained until the patient is fully awake and then withdrawn as soon as possible. The patient is immediately mobilized. The postoperative feeding regimen is as follows. On the first day, 300 ml of liquid is a normal allowance; on the second day, the patient can usually take 500–1000 ml liquid by mouth; on the third day, it is usually not necessary to maintain the intravenous infusion, and a full liquid diet is usually tolerated; on the fourth day, the patient can usually eat normal, solid food.

Small bowel irradiation injury: prevention and management

Barry T. Jackson MS, FRCS
Consultant Surgeon, St Thomas' Hospital, London, UK

History

The first recorded instance of irradiation damage to the intestine was published in 1897, only 18 months after X-rays were discovered. During the first decade of the 20th century a syndrome known as 'roentgen-ray cachexia' became recognized. This comprised nausea, vomiting, bloodstained diarrhoea and loss of weight developing during, or shortly after, therapeutic irradiation of the pelvis or abdomen. By the early 1920s the condition of acute radiation enteritis was fully established.

The late, or chronic, effects of irradiation on the intestine were slower to be recognized. It was not until the 1930s that sporadic reports were published of small bowel strictures caused by radiotherapy; the first intestinal resection for this condition was described in 1935. After the Second World War an increasing number of authors reported late bowel injuries after irradiation which required surgical management. These were all accounts of small series until the effects of supervoltage radiotherapy on the gut became manifest in the 1960s. Since then a huge quantity of literature has accumulated, including collective reviews[1].

Nature of injury

Acute radiation enteritis is rarely the province of the surgeon. It is treated by medical measures, principally antidiarrhoeal agents, and usually subsides soon after treatment is stopped; it is not considered further in this chapter.

Chronic radiation injury is caused by progressive ischaemia of the bowel secondary to obliterative sclerosis of arterioles and small arteries.

Strictures

Narrowing of the terminal ileum causing subacute obstruction is the most common small bowel injury, with the median onset being 1–5 years after irradiation, although latent periods of up to 20 years or more are well recognized. The symptoms of intermittent non-specific abdominal pain, often without nausea or vomiting, are easily misdiagnosed as irritable bowel syndrome unless there is a high index of suspicion of irradiation injury.

Perforation

Mucosal ulceration which may progress to perforation is well recognized. The perforation may be free into the peritoneal cavity with associated peritonitis or walled off by omentum, causing a localized peri-ileal abscess.

Fistulae

Fistula formation may also occur, especially into the vaginal vault in women who have had a hysterectomy, but also to the urinary bladder and occasionally to the abdominal wall. All of these injuries may also involve large bowel, especially the rectosigmoid.

Prevention

Almost all intestinal irradiation injuries occur after pelvic radiotherapy given for malignancy of the uterus, ovaries, prostate, bladder or rectum. It is of paramount importance that an excessively high dose of radiation is avoided. The tolerance of the small bowel is generally believed to be less than 40–60 Gy, and a significant number of injuries will occur in patients who receive 50 Gy or more to the pelvis or abdomen. The greater the volume of intestine irradiated the greater the incidence of injury, and some radiotherapists therefore obtain small bowel contrast radiology before treatment to enable planning of radiation fields and dosage with knowledge of the patient's intestinal anatomy. The method of administration of radiation also seems to be related to the risk of subsequent injury. Intracavity caesium and remote after-loading systems of administration are implicated in many reports.

Some radiotherapists administer pelvic radiation with the patient in a head-down position to enable gravity to displace the small bowel out of the pelvis and thus out of the radiation field. However, patients who have undergone previous abdominal or pelvic surgical operations may have adhesions that anchor the small intestine in the pelvis and prevent upward displacement. It is generally accepted that previous abdominal surgery or pelvic sepsis increases the risk of radiation injury.

There have been several descriptions of Silastic prostheses being introduced by surgical operation into the pelvis before radiotherapy begins in order to exclude small bowel from the pelvis. Similarly the greater omentum, having been mobilized on a vascular pedicle, can be introduced into the pelvis, or the urinary bladder distended with saline to displace small bowel. However, these methods are mainly anecdotal accounts; none has yet been subject to controlled study, and the place of such techniques in preventing small bowel injury is uncertain. More recently there have been encouraging accounts of absorbable mesh slings being inserted at the level of the pelvic brim in order to partition the peritoneal cavity. It is possible that this technique may become the method of choice[2].

Elemental diets and various drug regimens given during radiotherapy treatment have also been reported, but the likelihood of these preventing chronic injury is doubtful.

Surgical management

Radiation enteritis is often progressive. Acute injury may become chronic, superficial mucosal ulceration may develop into full-thickness perforation, or mild radiation injury may become severe over a period of years. For these reasons, small bowel radiation injury with symptoms should normally be treated by surgical excision once the diagnosis has been made. Although intestinal bypass may relieve immediate symptoms, it will not prevent progression of radiation injury in the bypassed bowel which may necrose or fistulate many years later. Most surgeons experienced in this field believe that bypass operations should not normally be performed.

The main problem when operating on severely irradiated small intestine is in deciding how much bowel to resect. Too limited a resection may result in failure of the anastomosis to heal because of residual ischaemia of the cut bowel ends. Too extensive a resection may result in troublesome diarrhoea caused by short bowel syndrome. There is no easy answer to this problem. However, all authorities agree that an accumulated experience by the surgeon in managing radiation injuries is important. Some authors recommend wide excision to maximize the chance of completely removing the injured bowel and thus lessen the risk of anastomotic leakage while accepting the risk of severe intractable postoperative diarrhoea[3]. Other authors recommend a more limited excision but ensure that at least one of the two ends of bowel used for the anastomosis is outside the irradiated field[4]. However, in the case of ileal resection this necessitates sacrifice of the apparently normal right colon in order to use non-irradiated transverse colon for an ileocolic anastomosis. The present author has been progressively less radical with increasing experience and, by paying meticulous attention to surgical technique, has performed limited resections with ileoileal anastomoses in selected patients with good results. In a consecutive series of 60 patients operated on for intestinal radiation injury of varying type, there have been no clinical anastomotic leaks in 31 small bowel resections.

Preoperative

Small bowel contrast radiology will normally have been carried out before operation except in emergency presentations. It is advisable to examine the large bowel by contrast radiology or colonoscopy because concomitant colorectal irradiation injury may exist, especially in the region of the rectosigmoid. Water and electrolyte replacement is necessary in patients with subacute obstruction and parenteral nutrition is indicated for the patient who is chronically malnourished. It is essential that anaemia and hypoalbuminaemia be corrected before operation because failure to do so will increase the likelihood of anastomotic leakage. Vitamin deficiency must be corrected. Prophylactic antibiotics are given together with prophylaxis for deep vein thrombosis.

Anaesthesia

General anaesthesia with a muscle relaxant is used. It is essential that blood pressure is maintained throughout the operation and that excessive blood loss be replaced by transfusion in order to maximize oxygenation of the intestine at the site of the anastomosis. Failure to do so may increase the risk of anastomotic leakage.

Operation

Incision

A midline or paramedian incision is used, avoiding any areas of skin that show obvious irradiation changes which may predispose to poor healing.

Laparotomy

A full assessment of the peritoneal cavity and its contents is made with special attention to the possibility of recurrent malignancy, the ileum, and the rectosigmoid junction of the large bowel.

Recurrent malignancy may be obvious, but in the severely irradiated pelvis it may be difficult to distinguish with certainty between malignancy and dense irradiation fibrosis. Biopsy and frozen section histological examination may be helpful.

The whole of the small intestine should be examined carefully. It is likely that the maximum irradiation injury will be in the distal ileum but skip lesions are often present. The bowel must be handled gently at all times. Particular care must be taken if mobilization of the bowel from the pelvis is necessary; the friable irradiated bowel is easily damaged by rough handling, causing leakage of intestinal contents with the consequent risk of postoperative sepsis. Gentle finger mobilization is best. If the bowel is more than usually adherent in the pelvis, there is a possibility of occult fistulation into the vagina or urinary bladder. The small bowel may also be adherent to the rectosigmoid and, if so, careless handling may cause large bowel perforation.

The large bowel may be concurrently damaged by irradiation and should therefore be carefully assessed, particularly in the regions of the caecum and rectosigmoid, the sites most commonly damaged. Again, gentle handling of the bowel is essential.

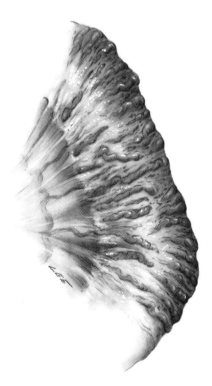

Assessment of irradiation injury

1 Areas of the intestine that have been damaged by irradiation may be obvious as evidenced by colour change, loss of sheen, thickening of the muscle wall and rigidity. With severe damage the colour is usually mottled red and white, but if the injury is less severe the colour may merely be paler than normal.

1

2 Localized strictures are usually obvious, not only by palpation of the thickened rigid area of the bowel, but also by the dilatation of proximal intestine caused by partial obstruction. It is important to check carefully for the presence of occult additional strictures in the collapsed distal segment before deciding on the limits of resection.

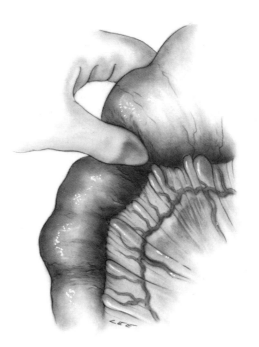

2

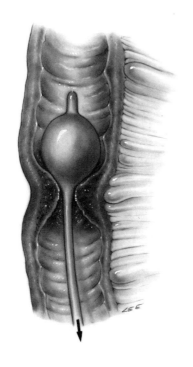

3

3 Sometimes a stricture is less obvious. If there is uncertainty as to the site, a Fogarty balloon catheter should be introduced into the lumen of the proximal intestine well away from the irradiated area. The bowel is threaded over the catheter with the balloon collapsed, the balloon is inflated and the catheter withdrawn. The balloon will impact at the site of an occult stricture which may then be marked with a suture. Remember that strictures may be multiple and the entire small bowel should be assessed.

Limits of resection

4   If there is a single localized stricture, deciding the extent of resection may be straightforward but if, as may be the case, the irradiation injury is extensive, the amount of bowel to be resected is difficult to judge. The appearance of the bowel should be noted, the texture palpated, and the small vessel blood supply to the bowel examined. If the operator is inexperienced in the management of radiation injuries it is best to err on the side of caution and resect generously.

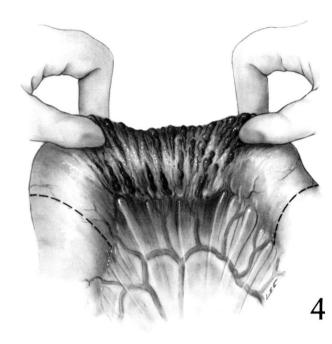

4

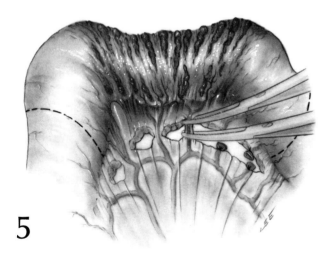

5

Resection

5   The limits of the resection are marked and the peritoneum of the mesentery divided with scissors, keeping close to the bowel to preserve as many mesenteric arterial arcades as possible.

6 The blood vessels close to the bowel wall are clamped using artery forceps, and are divided and ligated along the line of the peritoneal division.

It is essential that the blood supply to the anastomosis and the adjacent bowel is not compromised at any stage during the resection. *The anastomosis is therefore performed without the use of intestinal clamps.* A sucker is used throughout the operation to prevent contamination of the tissues by intestinal content.

Narrow intestinal clamps, such as Lang Stevenson's or Shoemaker's, are placed across the bowel to be removed at the sites of division and the bowel incised with the scalpel against the side of the clamp. Escaping bowel content from the unclamped lumen is simultaneously aspirated so that the bowel is empty when the transection is complete.

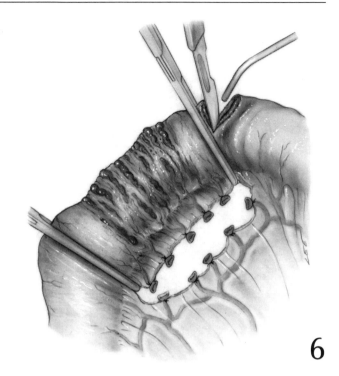

6

7 At the site of anastomosis a pulsatile blood supply to at least one cut end of bowel is essential. This is checked by deliberate division of the artery immediately adjacent to the cut end (inset). If pulsatility is not present the risk of anastomotic leakage is high and a further segment of bowel must be excised until pulsatility is obtained. (Ideally, there should be a pulsatile blood supply to both ends of the bowel.)

The anastomosis is normally performed using an end-to-end technique, but if there is undue disparity of size between the two lumens an end-to-side or side-to-side anastomosis may be considered (*see* chapter on pp. 51–73). Incision into the antimesenteric border of narrow bowel, or transection of narrow bowel obliquely, will give a wider lumen and enable easier and therefore safer end-to-end anastomosis. The technique of anastomosis is a matter of personal preference, but precision is essential. Some surgeons prefer interrupted extramucosal sutures while others prefer a continuous all-coats suture. The author's practice is to perform a two-layer inverting anastomosis using continuous suturing throughout. An absorbable suture such as 2/0 or 3/0 Vicryl or catgut is used. The material and method of suturing is less important than the precision of suture placement, and ensuring the correct degree of tension throughout. Bites approximately 3 mm deep are made into the cut ends of the intestine to prevent too large a cuff of bowel being turned in. The bites should be no more than 3–5 mm apart. The suture is pulled just tight enough to allow the two ends of the bowel to appose snugly. The suture must not be pulled too tight or the bowel within the suture line will strangulate, increasing the risk of anastomotic leakage. Two lengths of suture material are used, beginning in the middle of the posterior layer. Using an inverting technique each is

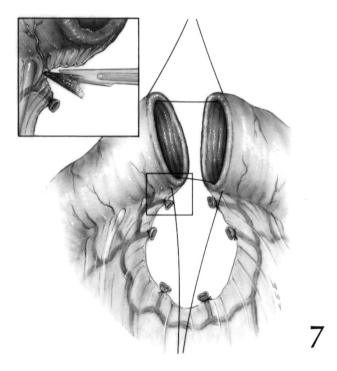

7

worked laterally so that they eventually meet in the anterior layer where they are tied together. This method turns in the corners of the anastomosis neatly. The second layer is now carried out, picking up only small bites of tissue to prevent narrowing of the anastomosis by excessive inturning of the bowel.

8 The defect in the mesentery is closed, taking special care that the blood vessels within the mesentery are not trapped by the suture, causing diminution of the blood supply to the anastomosis.

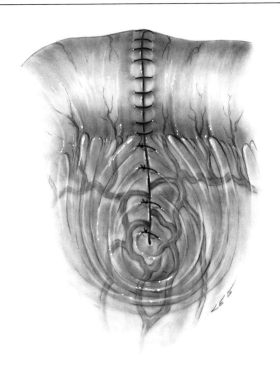

8

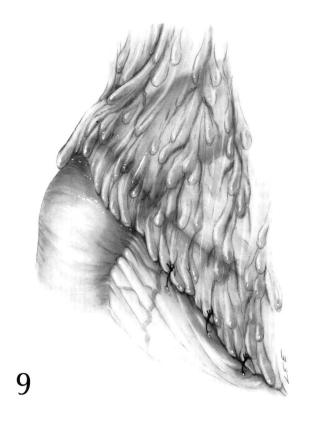

9

9 The greater omentum is wrapped around the anastomosis and lightly tacked to the mesentery to ensure that it does not become displaced.

A drain is unnecessary and is possibly harmful. A proximal loop stoma is unnecessary in uncomplicated cases provided that the anastomosis has been correctly performed. If there is doubt about the integrity of the completed anastomosis, a proximal loop stoma should be performed (*see* chapters on pp. 243–269 and pp. 274–283).

Postoperative care

Intravenous hydration, nasogastric aspiration and, if indicated, parenteral nutrition are continued until alimentary function has recovered sufficiently to allow adequate oral intake. No special immediate postoperative management is required.

The most serious postoperative complication is anastomotic leakage and signs of localized peritonitis must be sought on a regular basis. If leakage should occur the patient is returned to the operating room and a proximal stoma fashioned after antibiotic lavage of the peritoneal cavity (*see* chapter on pp. 93–104).

Late complications include vitamin B_{12} deficiency if extensive resection has been performed and diarrhoea which may respond to cholestyramine if it is caused by bile acid malabsorption.

Special situations

Bowel perforation

Preoperative

Energetic treatment of sepsis before operation is essential. Emergency surgery is indicated if the patient has generalized peritonitis, but if the perforation is localized by omental adhesions there is time to assess, resuscitate as appropriate and take the patient to the operating room electively. Ideally the patient should be transferred to a centre which has experience of bowel irradiation injuries.

Operation

The principles are as already described except that anastomosis should generally not be carried out because the risk of anastomotic leakage is particularly high in the presence of infection. The two ends of the intestine should be exteriorized as an ileostomy and a mucous fistula. However, it is still necessary to ensure a good blood supply to the two ends of intestine because failure to do so will result in either retraction or stenosis of the stoma. Reconstitution of intestinal continuity is carried out at a later date.

If an anastomosis is performed, a proximal loop stoma should always be established and not closed until contrast studies have shown the anastomosis to be soundly healed.

Enteric fistula formation

Preoperative

Small bowel fistulae caused by radiation will not heal by conservative management and always require surgery. Most commonly the fistula lies between a loop of terminal ileum and the vaginal vault at the site of a previous hysterectomy. Patients with this condition are likely to be severely debilitated by nutritional deficiencies and electrolyte abnormalities, and intensive preoperative preparation is particularly important.

Operation

The principles have already been described, but special care must be taken when mobilizing the ileum from the pelvis. Extensive dissection should be avoided because damage to the rectum, urinary bladder or ureters can easily be caused. Gentle blunt finger dissection is safer than sharp dissection, although in practice a combination of the two is usually necessary.

Although bypass of the fistula with exclusion will avoid difficult and potentially hazardous dissection, it leaves severely damaged bowel *in situ* with the risk that necrosis and sepsis might occur later. In general, excision of the fistula and resection of the diseased bowel is preferred. When associated sepsis is present a proximal loop stoma should be established (*see* chapters on pp. 243–269 and 274–283).

Concurrent large bowel injury

This is likely to be sited in either the caecum or the rectosigmoid junction. Caecal injury is normally treated by excision in continuity with the diseased segment of ileum as already described.

If the colonic injury is at the rectosigmoid, requiring surgical treatment, many authors believe that the operation of choice is a sleeve resection, preserving the middle and lower rectum, with a coloanal anastomosis. This obviates the need for deep pelvic dissection with the potential risks of injury to the urinary bladder and ureters. A temporary proximal stoma should always be performed.

Outcome

Historically, the results of surgery for irradiation injuries to the bowel have been poor because surgeons fail to appreciate that irradiated intestine heals poorly. Furthermore, as the condition is not common, relatively few surgeons have even moderate experience in the management of these often very ill patients. During the past decade, however, the reported results of surgery have been more encouraging as a consequence of better understanding of the underlying pathology, greater specialization and, especially, the referral of patients to surgeons with experience of irradiation injuries. This trend is to be strongly encouraged.

References

1. Smalley SR, Evans RG. Radiation morbidity to the gastrointestinal tract and liver. In: Plowman PN, McElwain TJ, Meadows A, eds. *Complications of Cancer Management*. London: Butterworth-Heinemann, 1991: 272–308.

2. Devereux DF, Chandler JJ, Eisenstat T, Zinkin L. Efficacy of an absorbable mesh in keeping the small bowel out of the human pelvis following surgery. *Dis Colon Rectum* 1988; 31: 17–21.

3. Schofield P. Treatment of radiation bowel disease. In: Schofield PF, Lupton EW, eds. *The Causation and Clinical Management of Pelvic Radiation Disease*. London: Springer-Verlag, 1989: 95–106.

4. Galland RB, Spencer J. General principles of surgical management. In: Galland RB, Spencer J, eds. *Radiation Enteritis*. London: Arnold, 1990: 206–14.

Intestinal stricturoplasty

John Alexander-Williams MD, FRCS, FACS
Professor of Gastrointestinal Surgery, The General Hospital, Birmingham, UK

History

For almost 100 years, stricturoplasty was used extensively for stenosis from peptic ulceration. Since the 1970s, it has been used for strictures as a result of tuberculosis after the disease has been controlled by drugs. In the 1980s, the operation was introduced for strictures in Crohn's disease[1, 2].

Principles and justification

Strictures of the intestine cause problems when they are so tight that they impede the passage of intestinal contents. If the contents are solid, as in the distal large intestine, a stricture can cause obstruction when it is 20 mm or less in diameter, whereas in the upper jejunum strictures as narrow as 10 mm can usually be passed by the thin, low-viscosity fluid. A critically narrowed area of gut usually needs widening because of obstructive symptoms or because the force needed to push the gut contents through is high enough to cause pressure necrosis (stercoral ulceration). The strictures can be dilated[3], resected, bypassed or widened by stricturoplasty[4, 5].

Causes of strictures

Strictures may be ischaemic after sewn or stapled intestinal anastomoses or after drug therapy with potassium salts or non-steroidal anti-inflammatory drugs[6]. They may also be due to chronic ulceration, in peptic ulcer disease, tuberculosis, bilharzia and Crohn's disease.

Indications

As there is no known cure for Crohn's disease, which has a constant rate of recrudescence, repeated resection of strictures may lead to a shortage of functioning intestine. Therefore, multiple and frequent recrudescence of strictures invites some conservative method of intestinal widening, such as stricturoplasty, in preference to repeated resection.

The presence of severe unremitting or recurrent symptoms of food bolus obstruction indicates the need for operation. Some patients who are only asymptomatic when they are taking steroids or a liquid diet would prefer operative or dilatation treatment to permit them the pleasure of a normal diet and the opportunity to stop steroids. Radiological appearances are *not* an indication for operation, although they may warn of impending problems.

Thus, the indications for stricturoplasty are: (1) multiple strictures, particularly of the jejunum; (2) skip lesions proximal to an area of severe disease that needs resection; (3) duodenal strictures where resection is not an option and where bypass would exclude the function of the pylorus; (4) anastomotic strictures that do not respond readily to dilatation; (5) where there has already been extensive loss of small intestine from previous resections.

Preoperative

Imaging of strictures

Strictures may be demonstrated on contrast radiographic studies, but it is often difficult to determine the luminal diameter or to differentiate fibrous strictures from spasm. Endoscopy may demonstrate an obvious stricture, but often strictures are inaccessible; multiple strictures usually defy intubation. The best demonstration of strictures is at laparotomy.

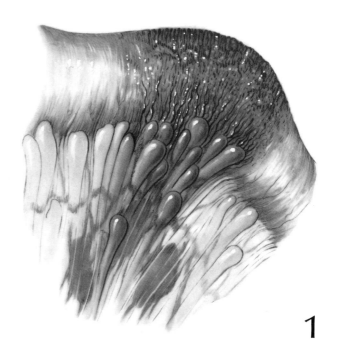

1

Operation

1, 2 The appearance of the serosal aspect of the gut is typical in active Crohn's disease. In quiescent disease it may be difficult to detect submucosal fibrous strictures from outside the gut.

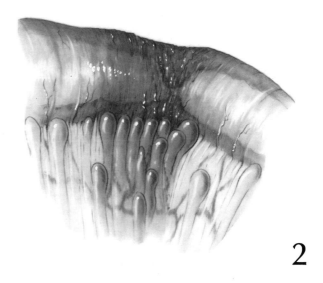

2

Incision

$3-5$ Usually at least one stricture site is obvious, and this is first opened by a longiitudinal diathermy incision, aided if necessary by dissecting forceps which spring apart once the lumen is open.

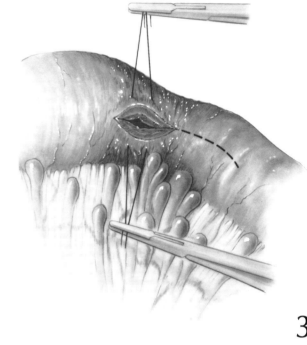

3

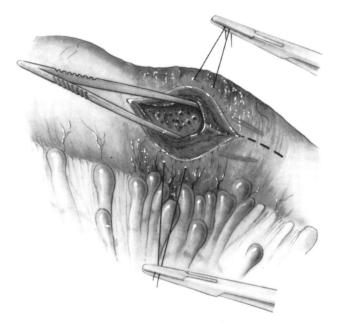

4

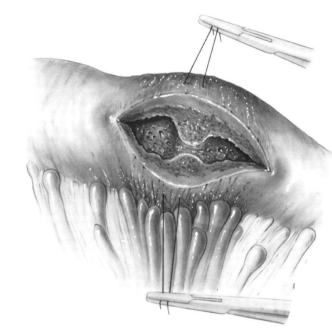

5

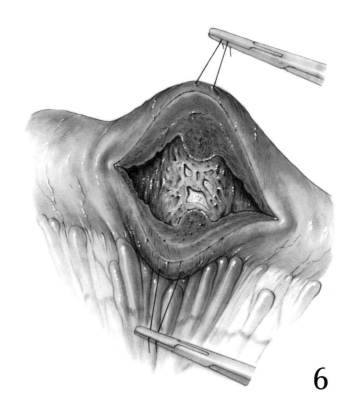

6 On the mesenteric side of the lumen, there is usually an ulcer at the site of the stricture.

6

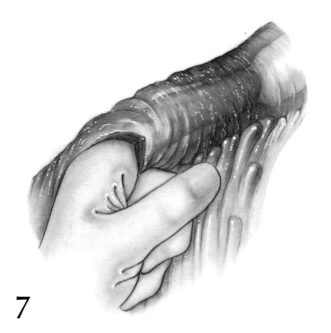

7

7 The index finger is then introduced into the lumen and the gut concertinaed onto it to search for other strictures within the adjacent 10 cm in both directions.

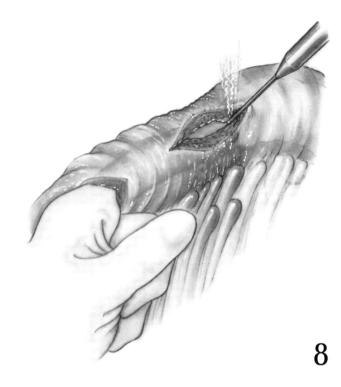

8 If another stricture is identified that is too tight to pass the finger, the intestine is incised with diathermy. Care must be taken that there is no hole in the surgical glove or a painful diathermy burn may be sustained.

To detect more distant strictures, a balloon 'pull-through' technique is used. A standard 18-Fr balloon catheter on an introducer is threaded along the intestine. Most of the small intestine can be concertinaed over one introducer, but sometimes a second enterotomy is needed. If another stricture is detected and incised, this becomes the new point of entry for the catheter. Once the catheter has passed up to the duodenum or down through the ileocaecal junction, the balloon is inflated with 8 ml water to give a balloon diameter of 25 mm. The balloon is then withdrawn and stopped wherever the lumen is less than 25 mm in diameter.

8

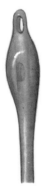 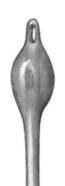 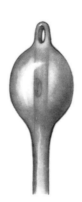

9

9 If necessary, the lumen can be sized by serial deflation of the balloon (8 ml = 25 mm; 6 ml = 20 mm; 4 ml = 10 mm). Most strictures 25 mm in diameter and all those 20 mm or less in diameter are incised longitudinally with diathermy. It is convenient to cut down onto the latex catheter but not onto the balloon itself which may be ruptured by diathermy.

Having identified all the strictures, attention is paid to each one. A cut is usually made at least 1 cm proximal and 1 cm distal to the stenosis. An index finger is then inserted into the gut lumen and the length of the incision is increased until the finger passes into the lumen without difficulty. Haemostasis is secured along the cut wall of the intestine using very fine dissection forceps and coagulating diathermy.

Wound closure

Three methods of closure are employed, depending on the length of the incision and the amount of thickening and oedema of the intestinal wall.

Short quiescent strictures

10 The simplest method is to insert the index finger through the incised stricture from an adjacent opened stricture. The presence of the finger stents the anastomosis and helps with eversion of the cut edges.

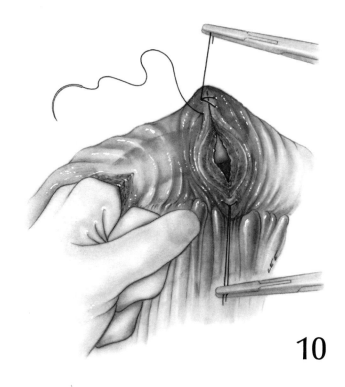

10

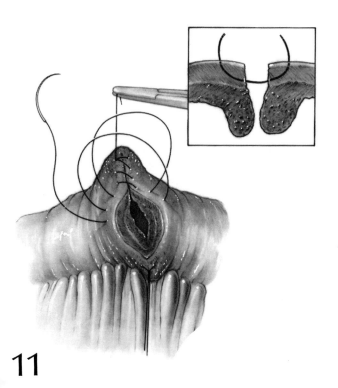

11

11 Starting furthest away and working towards the operator a 3/0 Vicryl (polyglactin) seromuscular suture is used, sparing the mucosa wherever possible. The distance between each bite in the continuous suture depends on the thickness of the intestinal wall; it is always thinnest in the centre of the suture line where there is also the most tension. The bites are usually placed 5–8 mm apart, with the gap preferably too large because it can always be reinforced with one or two sutures if the anastomosis is not gas-tight when tested. This simple suture method takes only a few minutes for each stricturoplasty, time economy being important when there are many strictures to repair.

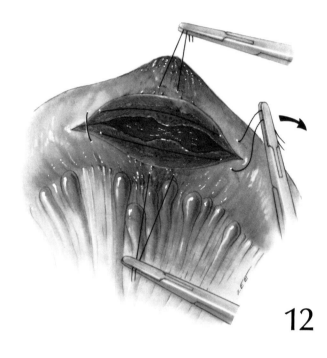

Longer strictures

12 A central mattress stay suture is used for longer strictures or when the intestinal wall is thickened and there is some tension at the centre of the suture line.

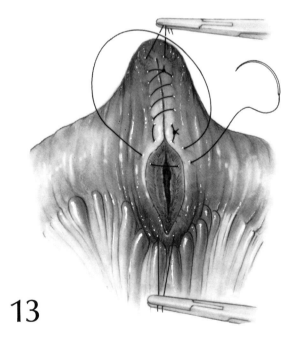

13 When this suture is tied, it indicates how much tension there is at the centre of the suture line and helps to hold the edges together while the seromuscular continuous suture is placed.

Long or multiple, confluent strictures

14 A technique is used that resembles the Finney side-to-side pyloroplasty for long or immobile peptic strictures of the duodenum. The intestine containing the stricture is cut longitudinally, often guided by the index finger in the lumen until normal diameter soft intestine is entered.

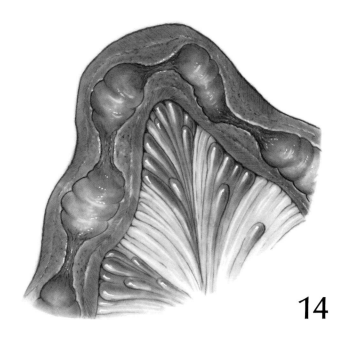

14

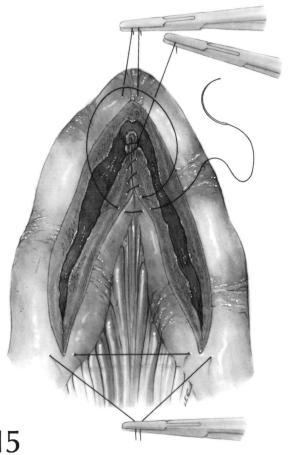

15

15 If the length incised is such that the edges cannot easily be brought together in the centre by a stay suture (as described above), then the length of incised gut is folded over into a loop and the 'posterior' wall is sutured.

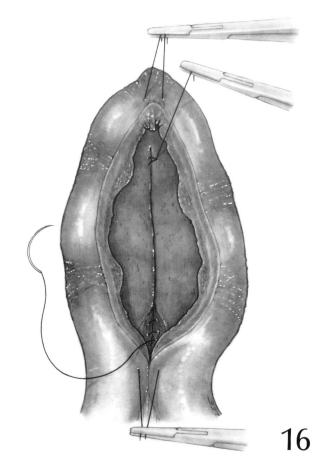

16

16 The wall is sutured until the central stay suture is reached and knotted to the running 3/0 Vicryl suture.

17 The anterior row is then completed with a continuous seromuscular suture.

17

Postoperative care

Complications

In the author's series, 229 stricturoplasties have been performed in 83 patients, with no deaths within 30 days of operation. The most serious complication was suture line leakage and fistula formation. The overall leakage rate was 6%, approximately twice the rate experienced in an overall series of resections for small intestinal Crohn's disease. Stricturoplasties, however, were often performed in poor-risk patients with multiple site disease after many previous operations, and such patients were often malnourished. A retrospective analysis of factors affecting leakage showed that the only significant factor was the presence of an intra-abdominal abscess before surgery; the leakage rate was 42% compared with 2% when no abscess was present[7]. All other factors (including anaemia, hypoproteinaemia and the administration of steroids) had no significant effect on the leakage rate.

Outcome

The relief of symptoms has been very successful. Stricturoplasty abolished or significantly improved the symptoms of food bolus obstruction in over 90% of cases and most experienced weight gain.

The need for reoperation has occurred at the expected rate of about 6% annually, as has been found for all operations on small intestinal Crohn's disease. A retrospective comparison of the site-specific recurrence rate per year in 41 patients having stricturoplasty was not significantly different from that in a matched series of 41 patients treated by small intestinal resection[8]. It has not proved possible, however, to mount a prospective trial to compare stricturoplasty with intestinal resection because the indications for the two operations are so different.

References

1. Alexander-Williams J, Fornaro M. Strictureplasty beim morbus Crohn. *Chirurg* 1982; 53: 799–801.

2. Lee EC, Papaionnou N. Minimal surgery for chronic obstruction in patients with extensive or universal Crohn's disease. *Ann R Coll Surg Engl* 1982; 64: 229–32.

3. Williams AJK, Palmer KR. Endoscopic balloon dilatation as a therapeutic option in the management of intestinal strictures resulting from Crohn's disease. *Br J Surg* 1991; 78: 453–4.

4. Alexander-Williams J, Allan A, Morel P, Hawker PC, Dykes PW, O'Connor H. The therapeutic dilatation of enteric strictures due to Crohn's disease. *Ann R Coll Surg* 1986; 68: 95–7.

5. Alexander-Williams J. How I do it – the technique of intestinal strictureplasty. *Int J Colorectal Dis* 1986; 1: 54–7.

6. Bjarnaston I, Price AB, Zanelli G *et al*. Clinicopathological features of nonsteroidal anti-inflammatory drug-induced small intestinal strictures. *Gastroenterology* 1988; 94: 1070–4.

7. Sharif H, Alexander-Williams J. Strictureplasty for ileo-colic anastomotic strictures in Crohn's disease. *Int J Colorectal Dis* 1991; 6: 214–16.

8. Sayfan J, Wilson DA, Allan A, Andrews H, Alexander-Williams J. Recurrence after strictureplasty or resection for Crohn's disease. *Br J Surg* 1989; 76: 335–8.

Small bowel tumours

Irvin M. Modlin MD, PhD, FACS, FRCSEd, FCS
Professor of Surgery, Yale University School of Medicine, New Haven, Connecticut, USA

Roger D. Hurst MD
Assistant Professor of Surgery, Yale University School of Medicine, New Haven, Connecticut, USA

Principles and justification

Small bowel tumours comprise a diverse collection of neoplasms. More than 35 different benign and malignant histological variants have been identified. As a group, these tumours are uncommon and represent at most 2% of all gastrointestinal tumours, although the small intestinal mucosa constitutes over 90% of the surface area of the entire gastrointestinal tract[1].

Benign tumours

Adenoma

Adenomas of the small intestine account for approximately 30% of all benign small intestinal neoplasms and are classified into three groups: adenomatous polyps; Brunner's gland adenomas; and villous adenomas. Adenomatous polyps generally exhibit a benign course and are most often discovered at post-mortem examination. Occasionally, they can cause obstruction or bleeding, or form the leading point of an intussusception. Brunner's gland adenomas originate from the submucosa of the duodenum. They are most often asymptomatic, but may very occasionally result in duodenal obstruction or haemorrhage. Villous adenomas of the small intestine are notable because of their propensity for malignant degeneration, and for this reason they should be resected[2].

Leiomyoma

Leiomyomas are benign, smooth cell tumours that arise from the wall of the intestine. They present with symptoms of haemorrhage or obstruction[3], and account for 20% of all benign small intestinal tumours. Erosion of overlying mucosa is common.

Hamartoma

Hamartomas of the small intestine usually occur as part of the Peutz–Jeghers syndrome. These mixed-cell polypoid masses are usually multiple and occur throughout the small intestine and occasionally in the stomach and colon. Intussusception with obstruction and haemorrhage are the most common presenting symptoms, and malignant transformation is rare[1].

Lipoma

Lipomas of the small intestine most commonly occur in the ileum. These benign tumours occasionally result in obstruction but seldom in haemorrhage. Small lipomas discovered as an incidental finding at laparotomy do not require resection. Larger small intestinal lipomas, however, should be removed[4].

Malignant tumours

Adenocarcinoma

Adenocarcinomas account for 35% of all malignant tumours of the small intestine. They are most often found in the proximal small intestine, with up to 70% of these lesions located in the duodenum and jejunum. They are locally invasive, and at the time of diagnosis have often metastasized to regional lymph nodes, liver, or peritoneal surface. Typical presenting symptoms include weight loss, vague abdominal pain, anaemia and intestinal obstruction. Perforation from small intestinal adenocarcinoma is uncommon[1].

Carcinoid tumours

Carcinoid tumours of the small intestine occur with a frequency equal to that of adenocarcinoma. These lesions originate from gut neuroendocrine cells and are capable of secreting a variety of bioactive peptides and amines. The majority of these lesions are submucosal and tend to grow slowly. Their malignant potential can vary, and over 70% are found within 60 cm of the ileocaecal valve. In general, carcinoids smaller than 1 cm seldom metastasize. The likelihood of spread beyond the confines of the small intestine increases with larger lesions. When metastasis to the liver occurs, carcinoid syndrome may develop, which can exhibit protean manifestations including diarrhoea, cutaneous flushing, bronchoconstriction and right-sided valvular heart disease[5].

Lymphoma

The small intestine can give rise to primary lymphomas or may be secondarily involved as part of a systemic lymphoma. Primary lymphomas of the small intestine most often occur in the ileum. The histological variants of primary small intestinal lymphoma are the same as those found in non-gastrointestinal lymphomas. Small intestinal lymphomas often present with signs of obstruction and ulceration. Additionally, perforation can occur in up to 25% of cases. Primary small intestinal lymphomas, like other small intestinal malignancies, should be resected[3].

Leiomyosarcoma

Leiomyosarcomas are malignant, smooth muscle cell tumours. They tend to be very slow growing, and by the time of diagnosis these lesions are often quite large. Leiomyosarcomas are locally invasive and metastasize haematogenously to the liver, lungs and bones[1].

Preoperative

Clinical course

The clinical course and presentation of small intestinal neoplasms can vary greatly. Most benign lesions are asymptomatic and are often discovered as an incidental finding at laparotomy or post-mortem examination. Malignant tumours, on the other hand, almost always produce symptoms, such as weight loss, abdominal pain, anaemia, acute gastrointestinal haemorrhage, or obstruction. If a malignant carcinoid tumour is suspected, urinary 5-hydroxyindoleacetic acid should be measured[1].

Diagnosis

The diagnosis of small intestinal neoplasms is most commonly made at the time of laparotomy for obstruction, haemorrhage, or abdominal mass. Preoperative diagnosis can often be made with radiographic contrast studies: either standard upper gastrointestinal series with small intestinal follow-through, or enterocolysis. Upper gastrointestinal endoscopy with standard endoscopes can readily identify lesions of the first and second portions of the duodenum. Additionally, specially designed endoscopes are available for examination of the distal duodenum and proximal jejunum. Abdominal computed tomography, though of limited value in identifying primary lesions, can be helpful in detecting liver and lymph node metastasis. Angiography can identify acutely bleeding lesions, haemangiomas, and highly vascularized lesions, such as leiomyosarcomas.

Preparation

The appropriate preoperative management of the patient with small intestinal neoplasms is tailored to the clinical symptomatology and presentation of the tumour. Thus, those patients presenting with intestinal obstruction require fluid and electrolyte resuscitation and nasogastric intubation before operation. Patients with bleeding tumours may require preoperative blood transfusions. Additionally, appropriate measures for replenishing nutritional deficiencies should be initiated early.

In each instance, the patient should be given nil by mouth before surgery. Appropriate prophylaxis against deep venous thrombosis should be administered. If right hemicolectomy is contemplated, the colon should be prepared with cathartics or enemas and antibiotic prophylaxis initiated 1 h before surgery. To avoid the intraoperative development of a carcinoid 'crisis', patients with malignant carcinoid tumours should be given octreotide, 100 µg subcutaneously, 1 h before surgery[6]. If not already present, a nasogastric tube is placed into the stomach after induction of anaesthesia.

Operations

Benign small intestinal neoplasms can usually be removed by local excision. Resection of malignant lesions of the duodenum requires pancreatico-duodenectomy. Malignant tumours of the ileum located within 10 cm of the ileocaecal valve require right hemicolectomy. Malignant tumours located elsewhere in the jejunum and ileum require small intestinal resection for cure or palliation. For lesions not amenable to surgical resection, enteroenterostomy should be performed to avoid or relieve obstruction.

Incision and exploration

After the skin is cleansed, and the surgical field draped in a sterile fashion, the abdomen is entered through an infraumbilical transverse incision. This approach provides excellent exposure and access to both the small intestine and mesentery. Alternatively, a midline incision extending approximately 12 cm above and below the umbilicus can be used.

Once the peritoneal cavity is opened, a thorough examination of the visceral contents is performed. As many small intestinal neoplasms are likely to have synchronous lesions, particular attention is given to the entire gastrointestinal tract, from the gastro-oesophageal junction to the proximal rectum. Additionally, the liver, spleen and lymph nodes of the mesenteric, portal, coeliac and periaortic regions are examined for possible metastatic disease. Intraoperative ultrasonography of the liver can be useful in the detection of occult metastatic disease.

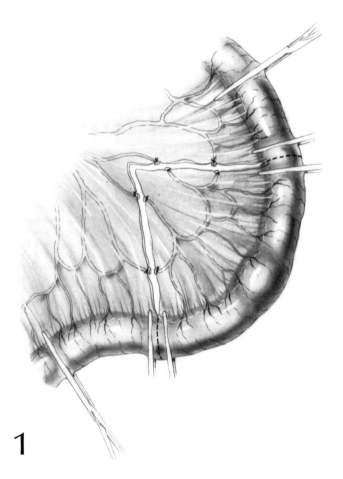

1

RESECTION

1 Malignant small intestinal neoplasms should be resected with a minimum margin of 5 cm proximal and distal to the gross lesion. Along with the segment of intestine, the accompanying mesentery and mesenteric lymph nodes are resected down to the main branch of the superior mesenteric artery. Both sides of the peritoneum covering the mesentery are incised along the line of resection. Blood vessels within the mesentery are individually ligated and divided. At the planned points of transection of the intestine, the mesentery is cleared from the intestinal wall for a distance of approximately 1.5 cm. Penetrating vessels entering the intestinal wall in this area are ligated with fine silk.

To prevent spillage of intestinal fluid, non-crushing intestinal clamps are gently applied a convenient distance proximal and distal to the portion of intestine to be resected.

At the points of resection, a pair of non-crushing intestinal clamps is applied to the intestine, which is divided between these clamps with either the scalpel or an electrocautery cutting current.

Hand-sewn anastomosis

This is described in the chapter on pp. 51–73.

Stapled anastomosis

This is described in the chapter on pp. 51–73.

LOCAL EXCISION OF BENIGN PEDUNCULATED TUMOURS

Detection of base and excision

2 To excise benign pedunculated tumours, the base of the tumour is identified by gently grasping the mass between the index finger and thumb and applying traction in the direction of the long axis of the intestine. This manoeuvre results in a dimpling of the wall of the intestine at the base of the polyp. After placement of non-crushing bowel clamps proximally and distally, a longitudinal elliptical incision encompassing the base of the tumour is made. Alternatively, if the base of the mass is located on the mesenteric border of the intestine, a longitudinal enterotomy is placed directly over the base. The base of the stalk is then suture ligated with 4/0 silk, and the tumour is excised.

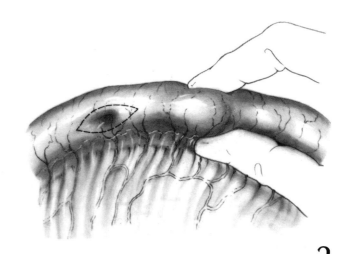

2

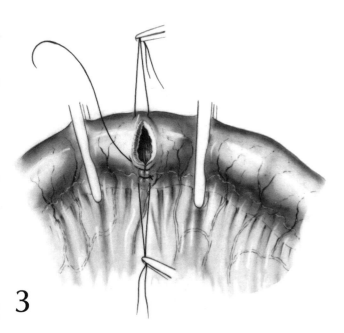

3

Enterotomy closure

3 The longitudinal enterotomy is closed transversely with two layers of interrupted 4/0 silk, and the bowel clamps are removed. All mucosal lesions removed by local incision are delivered to the pathologist for frozen section to rule out malignancy. If a malignancy is evident, small intestinal resection with wide surgical margins is performed.

REDUCTION OF INTUSSUSCEPTION

4 In those cases in which the small intestinal tumour forms the leading point for an intussusception, an attempt at manual reduction should be undertaken. This is done by gentle retrograde compression on the intussusceptum, squeezing it out of the intussuscipiens. Pulling on the intussusception with longitudinal traction should be avoided. Once the intussusception is completely reduced, the tumour can be managed as described above. If the intussusception does not reduce easily, small intestinal resection of the intussusception and tumour is performed.

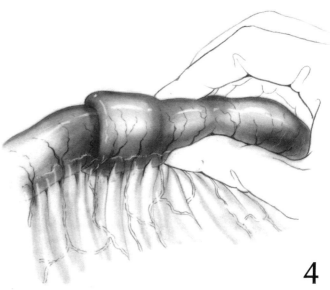

4

Postoperative care

After surgery the patient is hydrated with intravenous fluids and given nil by mouth. Nasogastric decompression is maintained until active bowel sounds are present. Following removal of the nasogastric tube, the diet is advanced as tolerated. In the absence of significant intraoperative contamination, continuation of antibiotics after operation is generally not necessary. Early ambulation and incentive spirometry is encouraged.

Outcome

The prognosis for small intestinal neoplasms depends on the histology of the tumour and the stage of the disease. Benign lesions in general carry an excellent prognosis. Patients with polyposis syndromes, such as Peutz–Jeghers syndrome, familial polyposis, or Cronkhite–Canada syndrome, are prone to develop new lesions, and therefore should be followed up as appropriate. Adenocarcinomas of the small intestine carry approximately the same prognosis as adenocarcinomas of the colon at the same stage. Adenocarcinomas of the small intestine, however, are usually discovered later in their course when intestinal wall penetration and lymph node metastases have already occurred. Hence, the overall 5-year survival for these patients is poor. Malignant carcinoid tumours and small intestinal lymphomas carry an overall 5-year survival rate of 50% and 45% respectively[1].

References

1. Ashley SW, Wells SA. Tumours of the small intestine. *Semin Oncol* 1988; 15: 116–28.

2. Bremer EH, Battaile WG. Villous tumours of the upper gastrointestinal tract. Clinical review and report of a case. *Am J Gastroenterol* 1968; 50: 135–43.

3. Herbsman H, Wetstein L, Rosen Y *et al*. Tumours of the small intestine. *Curr Probl Surg* 1980; 17: 121–82.

4. Wilson JM, Melvin DB, Gray GF, Thorbjarnarson B. Benign small bowel tumour. *Ann Surg* 1975; 181: 247–52.

5. Moertel CG, Sauer WG, Dockerty MB, Baggenstoss AH. Life history of the carcinoid tumour of the small intestine. *Cancer* 1961; 14: 901–12.

6. Hurst RD, Modlin IM. The therapeutic role of octreotide in the management of surgical disorders. *Am J Surg* 1991; 162: 499–507.

Intra-abdominal colonic surgery: introductory comment

T. G. Parks MCh, FRCSEd, FRCS(Glas), FRCSI
Professor of Surgical Science, The Queen's University of Belfast, Belfast, UK

Surgery of the colon is accompanied by significant rates of morbidity and mortality, particularly when operating on elderly patients in emergencies. If each patient is to have the best achievable outcome, it is vitally important that attention is paid to detail in the preoperative, operative and postoperative phases of management.

Preoperative

Preoperative assessment must focus not only on the extent and severity of the colonic disorder for which the operation is envisaged, but also on the coincidental or associated disorders which may have to be dealt with before, during or after surgery. The presence of correctable coexisting conditions, such as anaemia, malnutrition, dehydration or electrolyte disturbances, require attention. Even if impaired function cannot be completely eliminated, it is important that the best possible level of function in vital organ systems be obtained within a reasonable time.

Taking into account age and health status, preoperative evaluation should be made on the patient's fitness for operation and ability to cope with the implicit stresses which will occur in the postoperative phase. Consideration should be given to the potential technical difficulties inherent in the procedure and the main postoperative complications that may arise.

In patients undergoing elective colonic surgery appropriate endoscopic, radiological, haematological, biochemical and histological investigations should have been undertaken where indicated.

In emergency cases careful and intensive preoperative preparation of the patient is mandatory but investigative procedures may of necessity be more limited. In patients with shock due to colonic perforation, ischaemia or haemorrhage resuscitation must be prompt. Rapid extracellular fluid replacement and blood volume restoration are essential in order to achieve the best possible degree of stability before the induction of anaesthesia. Operation to control blood loss may be part of the resuscitative process because in some cases of massive colonic bleeding complete resuscitation may only be possible after 'the tap has been turned off'. When a diagnosis of intra-abdominal sepsis of colonic origin has been made, a course of antibiotics effective against aerobic and anaerobic organisms should be started forthwith and continued therapeutically after surgery.

For patients undergoing elective resection, bowel preparation by a regimen comprising a low residue diet for a few days and culminating in a liquid-type diet for 24 h before surgery is recommended, together with the use of a polyethylene glycol preparation (4 litres) taken orally on the day before operation. As with other methods of colonic preparation, special care is required in the elderly and in patients with stenosing lesions of the bowel.

If it is anticipated that the operation will include the formation of a stoma (ileostomy or colostomy) the surgeon should discuss details with the patient. The counselling services of a stoma care nurse are also most valuable. The site of the potential stoma should be accurately marked on the abdominal wall, and the temporary preoperative fitting of a reservoir appliance is advisable.

Prophylaxis against deep venous thrombosis is important in these patients. In addition to advice regarding cessation of smoking, the use of elastic support stockings, careful positioning of the patient on the operating table, early mobilization, etc., the prophylactic administration of low dose heparin is advisable for most patients undergoing colonic surgery. Heparin is given at a dose of 5000 units subcutaneously at the time of premedication and continued twice daily for 5 days.

Parenterally administered prophylactic antibiotics are advised in patients undergoing colonic surgery (as described in the chapter on pp. 41–46).

Operative phase

For a left-sided colonic resection the patient is placed in the lithotomy-Trendelenburg position (as described in the chapter on pp. 47–51). This allows access to the anorectum for irrigation before division of the bowel at the distal resection margin and permits a second assistant to be optimally positioned during the operation.

Catheterization of the urinary bladder is advised in most colonic operations involving extensive resection and in all colonic operations necessitating an anastomosis in the pelvis. It allows accurate monitoring of the hourly urinary output.

For most colonic operations (except appendicectomy and some stoma formation procedures) access through a midline incision of adequate length is preferred. This incision is rapidly made, is easily extended if necessary, and can be rapidly and securely closed by mass suture technique. Furthermore, all quadrants of the abdomen remain unscarred should it be necessary to create an intestinal stoma at the time of operation or subsequently.

On opening the peritoneal cavity the nature and extent of the specific lesion for which operation was indicated is confirmed, after which an orderly laparotomy is undertaken to exclude coexistent pathology. If infected fluid or a pocket of pus is encountered, specimens should be sent for bacteriological culture.

Gentle handling of tissues, careful sharp dissection, meticulous haemostasis, resection of the appropriate amount of intestine and, if indicated, removal of the relevant lymphatic drainage zones are time-honoured principles of surgery. Anastomosis should be performed between well vascularized pliable ends of bowel that are not under tension. In this respect, mobilization of the splenic flexure is often indicated for left-sided resection.

For colorectal anastomosis low in the pelvis the use of a circular intraluminal stapling device is convenient and gives results which are broadly comparable with those achieved by hand-sutured techniques. Controversy exists as to whether a single-layer interrupted technique is preferable to a two-layer inverted anastomosis. Excellent results are achievable by either technique.

In cases which are not emergencies, resection and anastomosis can almost always be safely achieved in one stage without a proximal stoma. Even in acute cases a one-stage operation is often feasible, e.g. in acute obstruction, where satisfactory conditions for colonic anastomosis can be achieved by orthograde on-table colonic lavage (as described in the chapter on pp. 397–415). However, in the presence of advanced sepsis in a poor-risk patient, as in perforated diverticular disease, while it is important to remove the septic focus and the source of contamination by resection it is often preferable to defer the anastomosis until a subsequent operation.

Irrigation of the peritoneal cavity is recommended at the end of colonic operations. This may be achieved using physiological saline alone but the addition of tetracycline, 1 g/l lavage fluid, seems to be advantageous. Krukowski and Matheson (1983) reported remarkably low incidence of wound infection and intraperitoneal abscess when this adjunct was part of meticulous surgical technique[1]. Routine use of drains is not advised but if a localized abscess has been noted the placement of a drain in that area is prudent.

Should a right transverse loop colostomy be judged necessary to protect a distal anastomosis, the supporting rod should always be placed to the right of the middle colic artery. After closure of the abdominal incision the exteriorized portion of the colon should be opened while the patient is still under general anaesthesia and direct mucocutaneous suture undertaken using fine interrupted sutures of absorbable material.

Postoperative care

Pain relief by efficient epidural analgesia speeds recovery after surgery and makes the postoperative period much less distressing for the patient. It helps in the avoidance of the respiratory depression which otherwise results from considerable doses of narcotic analgesics.

Careful attention must be paid to the monitoring of haemodynamic parameters and renal function, and to the control of fluid and electrolyte balance. Intravenous therapy is maintained until bowel function returns. The urinary catheter is kept *in situ* for approximately 4–5 days.

Intra-abdominal sepsis resulting from the primary pathological process or anastomotic dehiscence, if not identified and appropriately treated, may culminate in progressive deterioration, multiple organ failure and death. In an effort to prevent this downward spiral such patients require careful monitoring and energetic support of body system and vital organ functions. Abdominal radiology, ultrasonography, computed tomography and indium-labelled white cell scanning may each have a role in identifying a septic focus requiring local drainage and intensive systemic antibiotic therapy. Supportive therapy includes optimum oxygenation, adequate ventilation, maintenance of the composition of body fluid compartments and avoidance of malnutrition.

There can be no doubt that care and attention to detail at all times and in all aspects of management will significantly reduce the morbidity and mortality for which colonic surgery has long had an unenviable reputation.

Reference

1. Krukowski ZH, Matheson NA. The management of peritoneal and parietal contamination in abdominal surgery. *Br J Surg* 1983; 70: 440–1.

Illustrations by Jenny Halstead and Susan Hales

Open appendicectomy

Graham L. Newstead FRACS, FRCS, FACS
Senior Lecturer in Surgery, University of New South Wales and Associate Director, Division of Surgery, Prince of Wales and Prince Henry Hospitals, Sydney, New South Wales, Australia

Principles and justification

Differential diagnosis

The contradiction of appendicitis is that the classic history of central abdominal colic becoming constant right iliac fossa pain may occasionally be due to other pathology, yet acute appendicitis may present with a variety of subtle differences both in symptoms and signs. Any patient in whom appendicitis is suspected, however, should undergo appendicectomy, which may be preceded by laparoscopy. The suspicion of mesenteric adenitis should delay surgery only if signs are minimal and hospitalization allows continuous reassessment. This is particularly important in children, as progression to peritonitis may be rapid. Possible gynaecological pathology may warrant pelvic ultrasonography, consideration of laparoscopy and exclusion of pregnancy.

Recurrent mild right iliac fossa pain, not uncommon in children, should be treated by exclusion of other causes before consideration of interval appendicectomy, indicated in selected patients. A faecolith may be present within the lumen despite normal histology, yet its implication is uncertain.

Incidental appendicectomy for a normal appendix should be undertaken only in special circumstances. Appendicectomy to facilitate appendicostomy may be used for intraoperative colonic lavage in the presence of obstruction.

Masked diagnosis

Retrocaecal appendicitis may be more severe than apparent on palpation, due to the dilated caecum acting as a buffer between the inflamed appendix and the anterior abdominal wall.

Appendicitis in a long rectocaecal appendix or with a caecum situated high in the right hypochondrium may mimic acute cholecystitis. A long intrapelvic appendix may present as a pelvic abscess and be confused with tubo-ovarian pathology in women.

Particular care must be taken in assessing elderly and immunocompromised patients, in whom the clinical signs of appendicitis may be masked, as may the diagnosis.

Special situations

The presence of a mass does not preclude appendicectomy, as it may indicate a phlegmon and not an abscess. A chronic mass requires consideration of such factors as the patient's age and associated history. In the absence of acute signs, initial assessment of the caecum and terminal ileum by colonoscopy or radiology may be most appropriate. Appendicectomy during pregnancy is safest during the second trimester. If surgery is necessary, discussion with the patient's obstetrician and employment of a gentle surgical technique will usually avoid miscarriage or early onset of labour. At all times, early operation is preferable and safest.

Preoperative

An intravenous infusion should be commenced and a preoperative dose of broad-spectrum antibiotic is administered to all patients to cover aerobic and anaerobic organisms; it should be continued if there is significant peritonitis. A nasogastric tube should be inserted to empty the stomach in those patients experiencing excessive vomiting or who have definite peritonitis. The abdomen should be shaved (if required) in order to facilitate extension of an incision in the right iliac fossa or to accommodate a midline incision if needed. Informed consent should be obtained and advice given to the patient regarding prevention of deep vein thrombosis and postoperative deep breathing exercises. Consideration should be given to the use of subcutaneous calcium heparin and antiembolism stockings in adults, particularly if there is a history of previous deep vein thrombosis. An indwelling urinary catheter should be inserted in patients with peritonitis; all others should be encouraged to void before surgery.

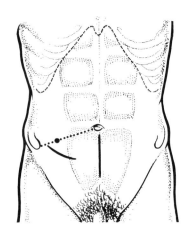

1

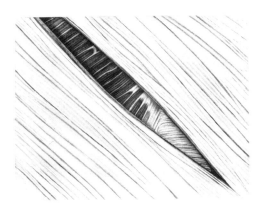

2

Anaesthesia

A fasting time of 4 h is preferred. After premedication, the patient is transferred to the operating theatre where general anaesthesia is induced and maintained with muscle relaxation and endotracheal intubation.

Operation

Position of patient

The patient is placed in the supine position. Calf compressors or muscle stimulators, if available, are used in adults and an adhesive diathermy pad applied to the thigh.

Preparation of abdomen

The entire abdomen is prepared with suitable antiseptic to allow extension or change of incision if required. The right lower quadrant is square draped to also allow access to the midline and the right flank above the anterior iliac crest.

Incision

1   The point of maximal tenderness elicited before anaesthesia should be compared with palpation of the abdomen following anaesthesia; muscle relaxation may facilitate palpation of a mass. These factors and concern for cosmesis will determine the area over which the incision should be centred. McBurney's point, being at the junction of the lateral third and medial two-thirds of a line passing from the antero-superior iliac spine to the umbilicus, is the classic surface marking for the base of the appendix, but the preferred incision may be somewhat transverse, keeping to the skin creases, initially to a maximum of 5 cm, but allowing lateral extension above the iliac crest if required.

A midline incision in patients with peritonitis and/or an indefinite diagnosis of appendicitis provides satisfactory exposure.

Splitting the aponeurosis of the external oblique muscle

2   The skin is incised, and the subcutaneous fatty and membranous layers of the superficial fascia are divided. The superficial circumflex and superficial epigastric veins may require ligation. The skin and fat are retracted, and a small incision is made in the lateral aspect of the fibres of the external oblique aponeurosis. A pair of scissors with the jaws opened a little is then pushed in the direction of the fibres, downwards and medially to their insertion into the anterior surface of the rectus sheath.

Splitting the internal oblique and transversus abdominis muscles

3 The fleshy muscle fibres of the internal oblique pass upwards and medially to insert into the anterior aspect of the lateral edge of the rectus sheath. An incision is made in the line of the most medial fibres, which are split by blunt dissection to separate them. At this point some small intermuscular vessels may be encountered which can be secured by diathermy. The tip of the forceps is angled laterally to split the deeper transverse fibres of the transversus abdominis muscle, which insert into the lateral edge of the rectus sheath. These muscle fibres are similarly split. The wound retractors are replaced to include these muscle layers.

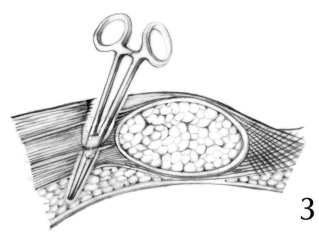

3

Opening the peritoneum

4 The extraperitoneal fat covering the peritoneum is gently cleared by blunt dissection and the peritoneum is grasped with an artery forceps. The tissue held by the forceps is inspected to ensure that no intestine has been trapped, and a second forceps is applied and further inspection made. The peritoneum between the two forceps is incised along the line of the skin incision for a small distance to allow inspection of the peritoneal cavity, again to ensure that no intestine has been inadvertently included. The incision is extended with scissors, the retractors are placed into the peritoneal cavity and the wound edges are elevated. A sample of any turbid fluid present is collected in a syringe and the air evacuated before it is placed in the container so that culture for both aerobic and anaerobic organisms may be undertaken. If there is a small amount of thick material, a little saline may be instilled to allow aspiration of a satisfactory sample.

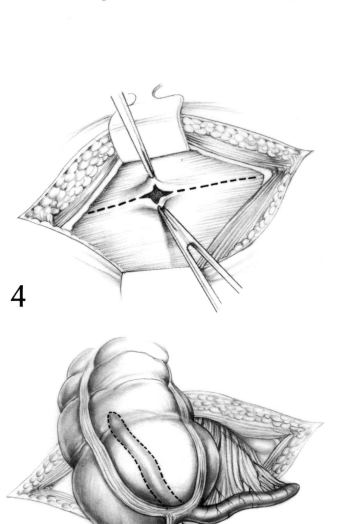

4

5

Identification of the appendix

5 If a taenia coli is immediately visible, it may be traced by index finger to the inferior pole of the caecum. The appendix may be immediately palpable and lie free, or it may lie behind the terminal ileum, pass down into the pelvis, or more commonly, pass superiorly behind the caecum.

Exploration of the peritoneal cavity

6 If the appendix is found to be normal, the index finger should be passed into the pelvis, particularly in women to examine the right fallopian tube and ovary. With wound retraction it may be possible to place a Babcock's tissue forceps on the round ligament to enable visual inspection. In smaller patients, the left fallopian tube and ovary may be digitally assessed. A gauze swab on a sponge-holding forceps should be used to exclude free blood or pus within the pelvis. The terminal ileum should be delivered, inspected and returned segment by segment until the distal 60 cm of ileum have been assessed to exclude ileal disease and a Meckel's diverticulum. The mesentery should also be checked for lymphadenopathy.

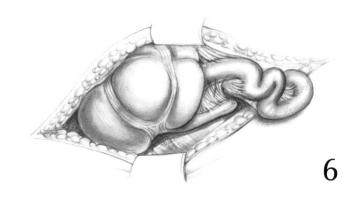

6

7

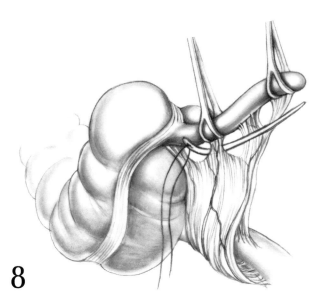

Delivery of the appendix

7 Retraction of the wound edges and easy palpation of the appendix may allow the application of Babcock's forceps to deliver the appendix into the wound, but perforation of an inflamed or gangrenous appendix must be avoided. If the appendix lies in the retrocaecal position, the caecum is grasped with non-toothed forceps and gently drawn inferiorly and then rocked up into the wound. This process can be gently repeated until the appendix base is visible. Scissors or diathermy may be used to divide any vascular adhesions covering the lateral aspect of the appendix as it lies adherent to the posterior aspect of the caecum. Retrograde appendicectomy may be required, necessitating lateral extension of the incision. Retrograde appendicectomy with medial extension of the incision may be required for a long fixed pelvic appendix (*see* later under '*Special circumstances*').

Division of the mesoappendix

8 The appendix is displayed between one pair of Babcock's forceps applied gently towards the tip and another near the base. Small windows are developed at the junction of the mesentery with the appendix using blunt forceps. The resultant pedicles containing the branches of the appendiceal vessels are ligated and divided. If the mesentery is thick, oedematous, or short, stitch ties may be required.

8

9 The appendiceal artery arises from a posterior branch of the ileocolic artery. It may be retrieved by inspecting behind the ileocaecal valve. The peritoneal fold beneath the caecum may need division to provide adequate mobilization if exposure is difficult. If the vessel is still unsecured, the wound incision may be extended medially or laterally as appropriate.

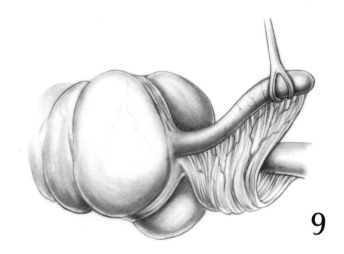

9

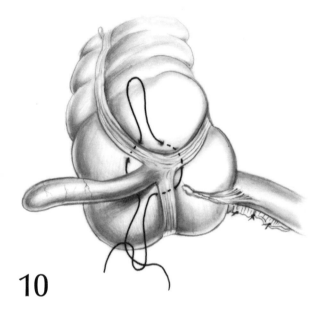

10

Insertion of purse-string suture

10 If invagination of the appendix stump is preferred, a circumferential purse-string suture is placed 1 cm away from the base of the appendix, gathering small seromuscular bites of caecal wall and ensuring that the line of the now divided mesenteric attachment is not picked up, thus avoiding a small recurrent branch of the appendiceal artery. The purse-string is left loose.

No purse-string suture is required if invagination is not intended.

Clamping, ligation, division and invagination of the appendix stump

11 The appendix is held somewhat vertically and crushed just above its base. A 0 chromic catgut tie is used to ligate the appendix base at this mark. The artery forceps is then applied to crush the appendix 5 mm above the ligature. A gauze swab is laid along the index finger and the appendix held along the index finger on the gauze by the thumb. An artery forceps is applied to the edge of the appendix between the ligature and the crushing forceps. The appendix is divided between the ligature and the crushing artery forceps. It is delivered to a dish, with the gauze swab and the crushing forceps, as 'unsterile'. The small remaining amount of mucosa visible outside the basal ligature may be scraped with a scalpel blade onto a further gauze swab, also placed into the waiting dish.

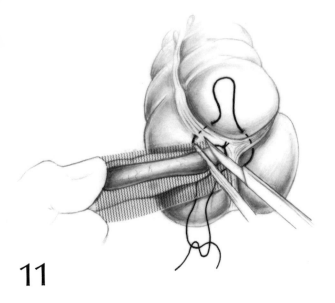

11

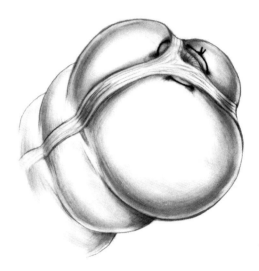

12 A decision to bury the appendix base requires that it be invaginated into the caecum and the purse-string suture is gently tightened and tied. If invagination is incomplete a further seromuscular bite to fully invaginate the stump may be obtained.

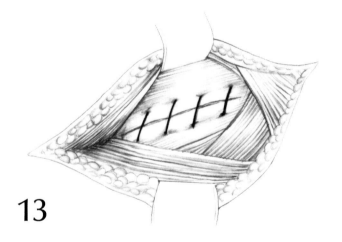

Wound closure

13 Warm normal saline should be poured into the right iliac fossa and pelvis and aspirated until the return is clear. Wound retractors are placed deep to the muscles and outside the peritoneum. Small artery forceps are placed at either end of the peritoneal incision and in the middle of its upper and lower edges. A continuous absorbable suture is inserted, ensuring at all times that intestine is not accidentally caught by the needle. An intraperitoneal drain should only be required if there is significant oozing or if a chronic abscess cavity has been opened.

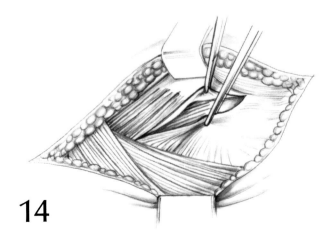

14 Further saline lavage is applied to the wound before muscle closure. The external oblique aponeurosis is retracted and interrupted absorbable sutures are used to loosely approximate the split layers of the transversus abdominis and internal oblique muscles without tension to avoid ischaemia, picking up the fascia of the internal oblique muscle rather than the muscle bundles.

15 A continuous absorbable suture is used to close the external oblique muscle, preferably burying the knot in thin patients. The membranous layer of subcutaneous tissue is approximated with interrupted absorbable sutures and the skin closed with interrupted or subcuticular sutures.

When significant pus has been encountered, it may be considered preferable to employ delayed wound closure, despite adequate intraperitoneal lavage. In such circumstances, interrupted absorbable sutures should be used in the muscular and aponeurotic layers. Loose approximating sutures are placed through the skin and subcutaneous layers for later tying.

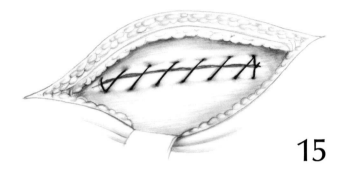

15

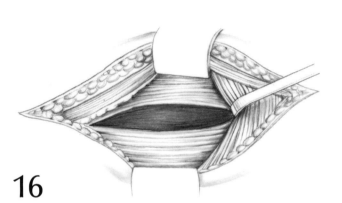

16

Special circumstances

Medial wound extension

16 By incising the lateral edge of the rectus sheath in the medial corner of the wound, the rectus muscle is exposed so that it can be further retracted medially. Care must be taken to avoid damaging the inferior epigastric vessels, which pass posterior to the rectus muscle. In the presence of peritonitis, the potential for infection in the rectus sheath space must be considered.

Lateral wound extension

17 This is necessary to deal with a high retrocaecal or subhepatic appendix. The skin incision should be extended above the iliac crest towards the lateral abdomen and flank. The muscle layers may be further split laterally, but fibres of the internal oblique and the transversus abdominis muscles may need to be divided to gain optimum exposure.

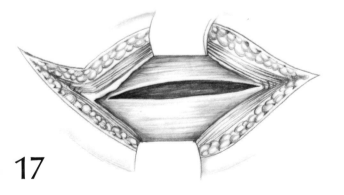

17

Retrograde appendicectomy

18 Having exposed the base of the appendix at its junction with the caecum, an artery forceps is passed through the mesentery and the appendix base is clamped, ligated, divided and invaginated with a purse-string suture in the manner described above. The mesoappendix is then secured from the base of the appendix towards its tip by serial clamping, division and ligation. At each stage the caecum is gently pushed superiorly within the abdominal cavity to give exposure to the portion of mesoappendix being ligated.

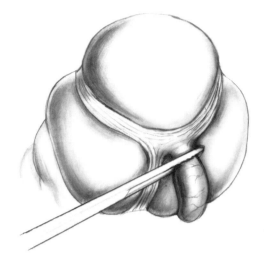

18

19 When it is necessary to extend the incision laterally for this purpose, incising the lateral peritoneum in the right paracolic gutter will allow the caecum and ascending colon to be gently pushed medially, thus exposing more of the elongated appendix.

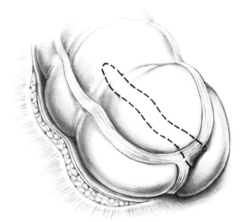

19

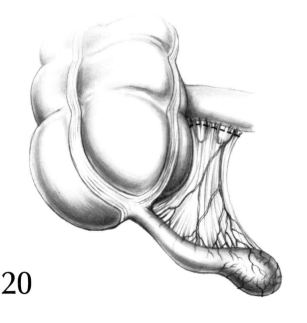

20

Appendiceal tumour

20 If the appendix contains a tumour less than 2 cm in diameter, near the tip and apparently confined to the appendix, appendicectomy should include as much mesoappendix as possible. Most of these tumours will be carcinoid tumours. If the tumour is greater than 2 cm in diameter, it should also be managed initially by appendicectomy, the need for subsequent right hemi-colectomy being determined by the microscopic features characteristic of carcinoid tumours and adeno-carcinomas.

Mass in the right iliac fossa

21 After incising the peritoneum, the caecum and appendix are inspected to ascertain the underlying pathology. If omentum is adherent it may be gently separated, thus delineating the aetiology. The terminal ileum should be inspected for evidence of inflammation, and obvious evidence of local tumour extension should be excluded. Extension of the incision may allow a more definitive assessment. If the appearance of the appendiceal inflammation suggests Crohn's disease that does not involve the caecum, the appendix may be removed, in which case care must be taken to ensure seromuscular apposition of the uninvolved caecum adjacent to the base of the divided appendix. If Crohn's appendicitis does involve the adjacent caecum, a modified right hemicolectomy may be required.

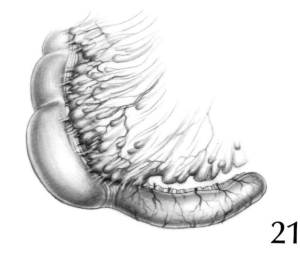

21

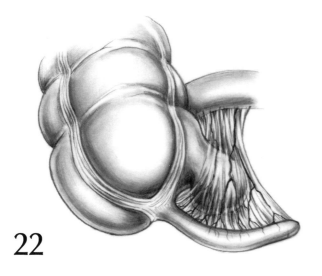

22

22 Localized diverticulitis of the caecum may occur, and if this can be confirmed by careful inspection, a decision on whether to close without resection or to carry out a segmental resection can be made. If the mass precludes a definitive diagnosis, it is reasonable to proceed as if dealing with a caecal tumour.

23 Tumours of the caecum may cause acute appendicitis. The caecum should be palpated carefully, and if an associated mucosal mass lesion is present, the wound may need to be closed and a midline incision made to allow an immediate right hemicolectomy to be undertaken.

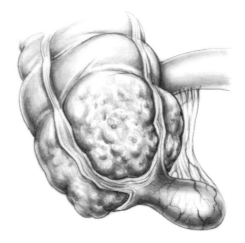

23

Postoperative care

After reversal of muscle relaxation and extubation, the patient is transferred to the recovery room and kept under routine observation until awake and stable. Suitable analgesia and antiemetics are prescribed. Intravenous infusion is continued until abdominal progress is satisfactory, and oral fluids are then introduced. Intravenous antibiotics are continued if peritonitis was present. Sutures remain for 1 week, but may be removed after 3 days and replaced by adhesive strips if desired.

Complications

Wound infection

After 24 h the wound dressing may be removed to allow frequent inspection. Minor cellulitis may be treated with appropriate antibiotics. Localized tenderness with fever may be treated by removal of a suture and probing to release accumulated pus.

Peritoneal abscess and septicaemia

This is relatively uncommon. Increasing abdominal or pelvic pain with diarrhoea after 1 week associated with fever may indicate the necessity for antibiotics after blood cultures have been taken. Other causes should be excluded. Computed tomography with needle aspiration of a collection may be considered.

Intestinal fistula

Conservative treatment is appropriate, and a small intestinal series, barium enema and perhaps colonoscopy may eventually be required, before consideration of re-exploration.

Further reading

Bak M, Asschenfeldt P. Adenocarcinoid of the vermiform appendix. A clinicopathologic study of 20 cases. *Dis Colon Rectum* 1988; 31: 605–12.

Cerame MA. A 25 year review of adenocarcinoma of the appendix, a frequently perforating carcinoma. *Dis Colon Rectum* 1988; 31: 145–50.

Engstrom L, Fenyo G. Appendicectomy: assessment of stump invagination versus simple ligation: a prospective, randomised trial. *Br J Surg* 1985; 72: 971–2.

Lewin J, Fenyo G, Engstrom L. Treatment of appendiceal abscess. *Acta Chir Scand* 1988; 154: 123–5.

Ruiz V, Unger SW, Morgan J, Wallack MK. Crohn's disease of the appendix. *Surgery* 1990; 107: 113–17.

Illustrations by Gillian Lee Illustrations and the late Robert Lane

Conventional colectomy

D. A. Rothenberger MD
Clinical Professor of Surgery and Chief, Division of Colon and Rectal Surgery, University of Minnesota Medical School, Minneapolis, Minnesota, USA

Principles and justification

Colon resections are performed for a wide variety of conditions including neoplasms (both benign and malignant), inflammatory bowel diseases, and other benign conditions such as colonic haemorrhage, procidentia or megacolon. Although the indication for colectomy will alter some of the technical details, the operative principles underlying the conduct of colon resections are well established. This chapter outlines these general principles and highlights some of the major alterations in technique designed to accommodate the specific demands of common variables such as malignancy, obstruction, inflammation and infection.

Preoperative

Patient status

Colectomy has become a safe operative procedure but remains a major undertaking with significant potential for morbidity. The surgeon must assess each patient for reversible risk factors such as anaemia, dehydration, electrolyte imbalance and malnutrition. Medical diseases such as diabetes, hypertension and cardiopulmonary problems should be optimally controlled. A detailed history of any pre-existing gastrointestinal dysfunction, especially of problems such as dumping syndrome, diarrhoea, irritable bowel symptoms or anal incontinence, must be obtained because such information may alter the extent of colectomy and the decision to perform a restorative anastomosis.

Disease status

Complete evaluation to determine the extent and nature of the primary colonic disease and to exclude other pathology is essential to proper planning of a colectomy. Several commonly encountered clinical problems deserve special consideration.

Carcinoma

The surgeon should anticipate potential problems which could affect resection of the primary lesion. For instance, a bulky, palpable lesion of the right colon may have invaded the duodenum or involve the ureter. Computed tomography might clarify the situation and facilitate planning of the operation. Before performing a colectomy for carcinoma, one must exclude synchronous lesions, preferably by colonoscopy examination or with an air contrast barium enema and proctoscopy. A search for distant metastases is worthwhile if the information would alter the operative approach. For instance, one may decide not to operate for a non-obstructing colonic cancer if there are extensive pulmonary metastases.

Obstruction

Colonic obstruction alters the usual preoperative assessment. The upper tract is decompressed with a nasogastric tube and the colon is evaluated with a water-soluble contrast enema to determine the extent, site, nature and degree of the obstruction. If the obstruction is partial and there is no evidence of impending perforation, the distal colon and rectum are cleansed with gentle enemas. Often, a limited oral bowel preparation becomes feasible and one can thus convert an emergency situation into a semielective operation in prepared bowel (as described in the chapter on pp. 397–415).

Inflammatory bowel disease

The surgeon must determine whether proctectomy should accompany colectomy for Crohn's disease or ulcerative colitis. Rectal function may be safely preserved by performing an ileorectal anastomosis if anal sphincter function is adequate, the rectum is compliant, the risk of neoplasm is not excessive, and the rectal disease is not severe.

Infection

Sepsis may dominate the clinical course of many patients with colonic pathology. Diffuse peritonitis obviously requires immediate laparotomy, but localized peritonitis secondary to a confined perforation and a walled-off abscess can often be controlled non-operatively by percutaneous drainage, guided by computed tomography or ultrasonography, and use of broad-spectrum antibiotics. Sepsis associated with colovesical, colouterine, colovaginal or colocutaneous fistulae often clears quickly after institution of systemic antibiotics. The goal is to convert an emergency situation to an elective operation on a prepared bowel as described in the chapters on pp. 369–386 and 387–396.

Genitourinary tract assessment

An intravenous pyelogram is not indicated routinely before a colectomy, but if the surgeon has reason to suspect retroperitoneal or genitourinary tract involvement, assessment of the ureters is indicated. This is probably best accomplished by a computed tomographic scan performed with intravenous contrast. If a retroperitoneal, periureteric or pelvic mass or inflammation is anticipated, ureteric stents placed via cystoscopy just before colectomy can be invaluable to avoid inadvertent injury to the ureters.

Stoma planning

The surgeon should anticipate those cases in which there is likely to be a need for a stoma, either temporary or permanent, and provide the patient with information regarding this possibility before the operation. Enterostomal therapy consultation before surgery is invaluable to select and mark a site on the abdomen for a stoma.

Bowel preparation

The majority of colectomies are performed electively and thus a complete bowel preparation is usually feasible. Standard bowel preparation may be conducted over a 24-h period and (in most instances) on an outpatient basis, allowing the patient to be admitted on the morning of surgery. The patient drinks only clear liquids for 24 h and consumes 4 litres of polyethylene glycol solution over 2–4 h in the afternoon the day before surgery. A sodium phosphate enema is given 2 h before surgery. Two doses of metronidazole and neomycin sulphate are given the day before surgery after the lavage preparation, and an intravenous second-generation cephalosporin is administered within 1 h before the incision is made. If patients anticipate they could not tolerate a large-volume oral lavage preparation, alternatives such as an oral sodium phosphate preparation or traditional cathartics and enemas can be substituted.

A nasogastric tube is usually placed to empty the stomach but is generally removed at the completion of the operation unless there was evidence of partial obstruction. For distal colonic lesions, the rectum is irrigated with sterile water through a proctoscope.

Anaesthesia

An epidural catheter for narcotic infusion is often used to supplement a general anaesthetic and to provide initial postoperative analgesia for 48–72 h. Once a general anaesthesia is induced, a Foley urethral catheter is inserted into the bladder.

Definition of terms

1   A variety of terms are used to describe different types of colectomy. These terms are somewhat misleading since they refer primarily to the portion of the colon resected and not precisely to the extent of mesentery or omentum resected with the colon. The mesenteric clearance technique dictates the extent of colonic resection. In general, a proximal mesenteric ligation will eliminate the blood supply to a greater length of colon and require a more extensive 'colectomy'. The mesenteric clearance technique used in a given instance is determined by the nature of the primary pathology (malignant *versus* benign), the intent of the resection (curative *versus* palliative), the precise location of the primary pathology, and the condition of the mesentery (thin and soft *versus* thickened and indurated). In general, the curative resection of a colonic malignancy is best accomplished by performing a radical mesenteric clearance with proximal vessel ligation and concomitant resection of overlying omentum. Resection of a benign process does not require wide mesenteric resection and the omentum can be preserved if desired.

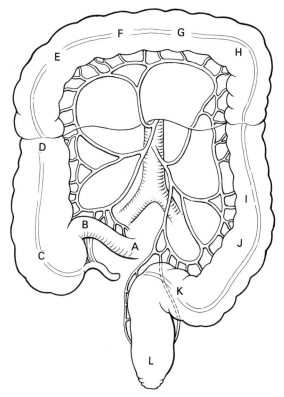

A → C	:	Ileocaecectomy
±A + B → D	:	Ascending colectomy
±A + B → F	:	Right hemicolectomy
±A + B → G	:	Extended right hemicolectomy
±E + F → G ± H	:	Transverse colectomy
G → I	:	Left hemicolectomy
F → I	:	Extended left hemicolectomy
J + K	:	Sigmoid colectomy
±A + B → J	:	Subtotal colectomy
±A + B → K	:	Total colectomy
±A + B → L	:	Total proctocolectomy

Operation

Position of patient

For most colectomies, the patient is placed in a modified lithotomy position with the legs supported by Allen stirrups (as described in the chapter on pp. 47–50). Pneumatic compression stockings are used routinely to minimize the risk of thromboembolism and peripheral neuropathy. The supine position is used for right-sided colectomies.

Incision

2   The choice of incision varies widely depending on the particular circumstances of each case.

Knowledge of the underlying pathology, extent of disease, level of the splenic flexure, physical appearance of the patient, previous surgical incisions, and availability of qualified assistants all influence the surgeon's decision. If in doubt, a midline incision is used because it can be extended to expose any area within the abdomen. The midline incision is preferred for patients with inflammatory bowel disease because such patients may require frequent reoperations and may eventually need a stoma. The surgeon usually stands opposite the segment of intestine to be resected, i.e. on the left side of a patient undergoing a right colectomy and vice versa. A first assistant stands across from the surgeon and, when appropriate, a second assistant stands between the legs of the patient who is in a modified lithotomy position. Self-retaining abdominal retractors facilitate exposure and fibreoptic headlights clearly illuminate the operative field, enhancing the safety and ease of the operation.

Exploration

After the incision has been made, the presence of ascites or peritoneal contamination is noted. The surgeon should confirm the preoperative diagnosis and determine resectability of the primary pathology. The uninvolved small and large intestine is assessed to determine the adequacy of the bowel preparation and the presence or absence of obstruction, inflammation, oedema or other factors that might alter the decision to perform a primary anastomosis. All viscera accessible to the surgeon are examined in a standard sequence. Conditions such as an aortic aneurysm, ovarian mass, gallstones or liver metastases may require a change in the operative plan.

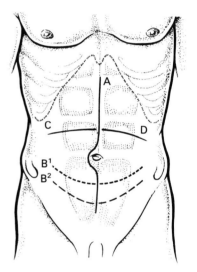

2

A. Midline: versatile
B. Transverse infraumbilical (high and low): primarily for pelvic exposure; if placed near level of umbilicus (B^1), useful for sigmoid colectomy and total colectomy
C. Right trans-supraumbilical: for right colectomy
D. Left trans-supraumbilical: for left colectomy
C + D: used for subtotal colectomy, extended left and right colectomy

Extent of resection

After laparotomy and complete exploration, the surgeon can finalize plans for resection based on knowledge of the patient's primary and secondary pathology.

3 It is useful to think in anatomical terms based on knowledge of colon mesenteric anatomy. For instance, if the goal is to perform a curative resection of a caecal cancer, the planned resection should encompass its field of lymphatic spread. This will require proximal ligation of the ileocolic vessels, including the terminal ileal and right colic vessels and usually the right branch of the middle colic artery. Thus, approximately 15 cm of terminal ileum, the ascending colon, and the right transverse colon to the middle colic artery will be resected. On the other hand, if a cancer of the hepatic flexure is to be resected, the ileocolic and right colic vessels will be resected together with the entire middle colic artery. Thus, less terminal ileum will be removed because the distal ileal vessels will be left intact, but more transverse colon will be resected to ensure removal of the lymphatic bed of the primary lesion along the middle colic vessels. Cancers of the splenic flexure and proximal descending colon may theoretically spread to the lymphatics near the middle colic or the inferior mesenteric arteries. A radical resection with proximal ligation of these two major vessels at their origin would require resection of most of the transverse, descending and sigmoid colon. This would make restoration of continuity difficult. A better alternative, because it does not appear to compromise cancer curability and it eases the technical difficulty of doing a primary anastomosis, is to ligate the left branch of the middle colic artery near its origin from the main trunk, and the left colic artery near its origin from the inferior mesenteric artery. Thus, the right transverse colon and the sigmoid colon can be preserved and a relatively easy colocolic anastomosis achieved.

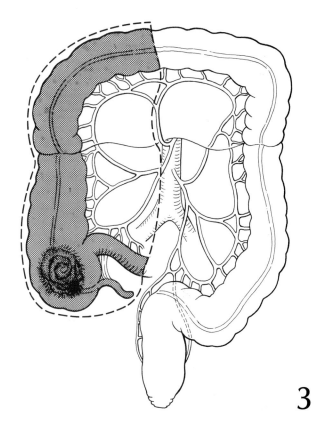

3

Mobilization

The first step is to mobilize the bowel that is to be resected by dividing its peritoneal attachments. The extent of the planned resection determines the type and extent of mobilization of the colon that is necessary. The goals of mobilization are: (1) to expose the mesenteric vessels which need division and ligation; (2) to keep retroperitoneal and other adjacent structures away from the field of resection; and (3) to free sufficient lengths of intestine proximally and distally to allow a tension-free, well vascularized anastomosis to be performed. Thus, for an isolated sigmoid resection, one often has to mobilize the entire left colon including the splenic flexure to conduct a colorectal anastomosis. In general, for a descending colon lesion, it is best to begin

by mobilizing the sigmoid colon, then the descending colon, and finally the left transverse colon. After resection of the descending colon and its mesocolon, a tension-free colocolic anastomosis is performed. Similarly, if an isolated segment of transverse colon is to be resected, it is usually necessary to mobilize both the splenic and hepatic flexures. Usually a mid-transverse colonic resection is incorporated into an extended right, an extended left, or a subtotal or total colectomy. For the last procedures, the author finds it most convenient to begin with mobilization of the entire left colon followed by mobilization of the right side, meeting near the midline in the lesser sac.

Right colectomies

4 The caecum and terminal ileum are gently retracted anteromedially by the surgeon's right hand to expose the lateral and inferior peritoneal attachments. Electrocautery with a blade tip is used to incise through the posterior peritoneum, taking care not to penetrate the mesentery. The surgeon's left index finger is inserted into this plane and easily directed upwards towards the hepatic flexure.

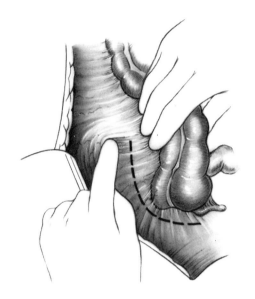

4

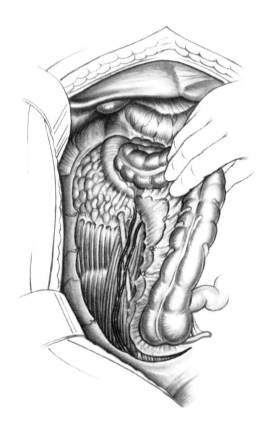

5

5 The assistant incises the exposed, thinned out peritoneum overlying the surgeon's finger with electrocautery. The terminal ileum, caecum including the appendix, and the distal ascending colon is thus mobilized.

6 The underlying right ureter and gonadal vessels are kept posteriorly in the retroperitoneum. By applying gentle anterior retraction on the mobilized right colon the surgeon exposes the duodenum, which is left unharmed in the retroperitoneum by dividing any remaining tissue tethering the colon to the retroperitoneum. Excessive anterior retraction of the colon at the level of the hepatic flexure may result in a tear of one of the fragile veins located in the base of the mesentery near the duodenum. If such a vein is noted to be under tension during the mobilization procedure, it is best to suture ligate and divide it before a troublesome tear occurs. If a tear occurs, packing is used to control the bleeding and to prevent a large haematoma from forming in the base of the mesentery. The packing is slowly removed to reveal the torn vessel, which is suture ligated.

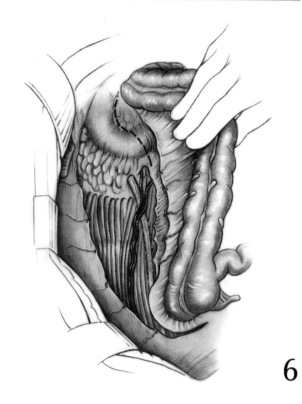

6

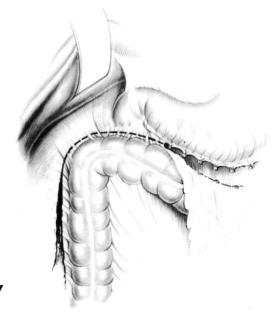

7

7 Adhesions to the gallbladder are divided under direct view. If the omentum is to be resected with the transverse colon, it is divided between clamps with preservation of the gastroepiploic vessels along the greater curvature of the stomach. If the omentum is to be preserved, it is retracted upwards over the stomach, and the relatively avascular attachments between the colon and omentum are divided with electrocautery.

Left colectomies

8 Mobilizations of the sigmoid, descending and left transverse colon are considered together. The sigmoid colon is retracted anteromedially by the surgeon's left hand to expose the lateral peritoneal attachments. Electrocautery dissection along the white line of Toldt is instituted.

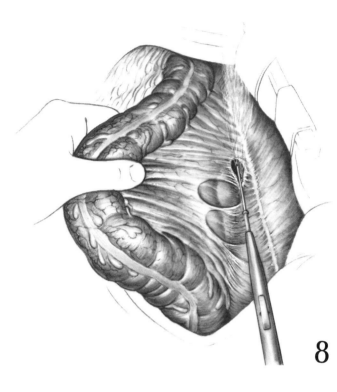

9 The full thickness of the peritoneum is incised but the mesentery itself is not entered. The gonadal vessels and left ureter are gently displaced posteriorly using a stick sponge. The surgeon's right hand is inserted into the plane posterior to the descending colon and used to separate the colon from the retroperitoneal structures. It is important to get into the proper plane of dissection. If too deep, troublesome retroperitoneal bleeding occurs and, if too superficial, the colon will remain fixed to the retroperitoneum. By rolling the right hand out from under the descending colon, the right lateral peritoneal attachments are exposed for division by the assistant positioned between the patient's legs.

It is important not to pull down on the descending colon because this can result in a splenic injury. Instead, the thrust of the dissection is upwards towards the splenic flexure. The surgeon's left hand retracts the now mobilized sigmoid and distal descending colon anteromedially, allowing its mesentery to serve as a fan-like retractor, keeping the small intestine from interfering with the remaining lateral mobilization. At this time, the splenic flexure is visualized, and any peritoneal bands to the spleen or splenic–omental adhesions are divided under direct view by electrocautery. Once that is accomplished, the left transverse colon is gently retracted inferiorly towards the left lower quadrant by an assistant. The surgeon's right hand in the plane posterior to the descending colon is gently passed up to the splenic flexure. By rolling the right hand, the remaining lateral peritoneal attachments are exposed for division by the assistant.

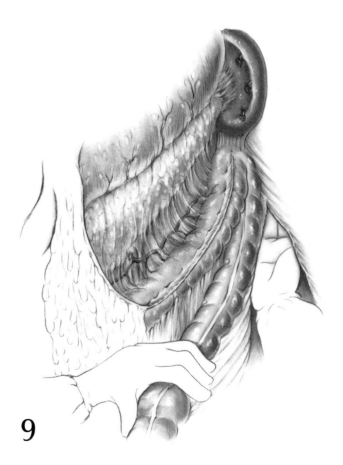

10 At this point, it is important to stay adjacent to the superolateral margin of the colon. The splenocolic ligament is often quite thick and may be best divided between clamps and secured with ties. Omental adhesions may overlie this area and must be clamped and divided initially to expose the deeper attachments. As these attachments are divided, the left colon is held up in a fan-like manoeuvre to enhance exposure of the retroperitoneum. As the splenocolic ligament is divided, the lesser sac is entered and the dissection continues medially. The omentum is handled as noted earlier. If the splenic flexure is difficult to expose, it is sometimes helpful to enter the lesser sac in the midline before completing division of the splenocolic ligament. Thus one can work at the most difficult point of dissection from two sides: along the left transverse colon from within the lesser sac, and along the descending colon in the retroperitoneum.

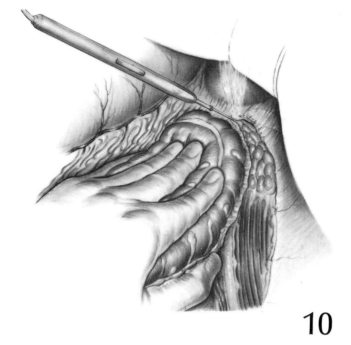

10

Division of mesentery and resection

11 The mobilized colon is retracted so that its mesentery can be exposed and transilluminated. The primary vessels such as the ileocolic, middle colic and inferior mesenteric or their major tributaries are exposed by incising the overlying peritoneum. These major vessels are triply clamped, divided and doubly tied on the proximal end. For cancers, a proximal ligation is standard.

If mobilization was properly performed, this step should be quite safe because the ureters, gonadal vessels, duodenum and other retroperitoneal structures should be out of the field of mesenteric vessel ligation. For benign conditions, ligation is performed where 'comfortable', without risking proximal mesenteric dissection. Once the major vessels are divided, the mesentery supplying the intestine at the sites of the proposed anastomosis is assessed, divided between clamps, and ligated. Inflammatory conditions such as Crohn's disease may thicken the mesentery, making division in the standard fashion quite hazardous. Suture ligation and small bites of tissue can overcome this problem. A short distance of only 1 cm or less is cleared along the mesenteric surface of the intestine to allow accurate suture placement without compromising the vascularity of the anastomosis. The mesenteric flow at the proposed anastomotic sites should be pulsatile. The blood supply to the splenic flexure area is variable and may be tenuous, especially in elderly patients, after ligation of the middle colic artery or the inferior mesenteric artery. If there is doubt about the adequacy of the blood supply, the left colon should be resected.

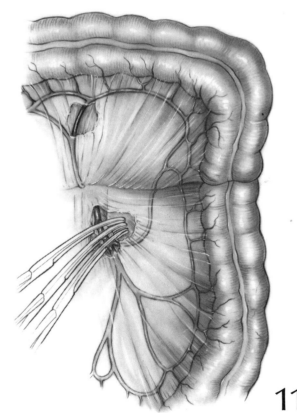

11

If a hand-sewn anastomosis is planned, non-crushing clamps are placed across the intestine at the sites for division, with two crushing clamps being placed in parallel on the 'specimen side' of the non-crushing clamps. The intestine is resected and is sent to the pathology department for review of the adequacy of resection.

Mesenteric closure

12 Mobilization should allow the two ends of intestine to come together without tension. After alignment, the mesocolon is closed with a continuous polyglycolic acid suture from its base near the proximal ligation point to within 5 cm of the site of anastomosis. This is best accomplished at this stage since the base of the mesocolon defect is most easily exposed before the anastomosis is created. Care is taken not to damage any vessels along the cut edges of the mesocolon which might diminish blood flow to the anastomosis. The remaining 5-cm gap in the mesentery is closed after completion of the anastomosis.

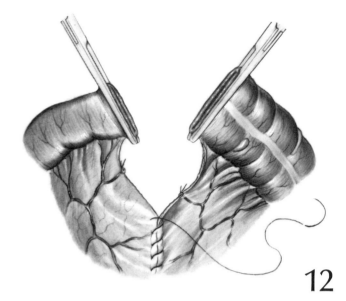

12

Anastomosis

Ideally, a primary anastomosis is performed following a colectomy. The surgeon's sound judgement is essential to assure success. Factors that must be considered include the patient's overall status, the condition of the peritoneal cavity, the condition of the intestine and completeness of its preparation, and the assurance that the necessary technical demands of an anastomosis, i.e. vascularity, lack of tension, and accurate approximation, can be met. We generally prefer a semiclosed, hand-sutured, minimally inverting technique approximating the intestine in an end-to-end fashion (as described in the chapter on pp. 51–73).

13 The site of anastomosis is isolated from the surrounding field with laparotomy pads. The bowel clamps are held parallel, approximately 3 cm apart, by the assistant, who directs the tips towards the surgeon's dominant hand.

The clamps are rotated through 90° to expose the posterior wall, and interrupted 4/0 seromuscular sutures are placed at approximately 1-cm intervals. The sutures at the mesenteric and antimesenteric sides are left untied and tagged.

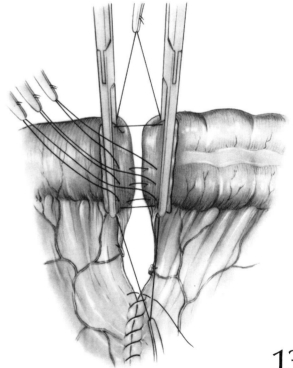

13

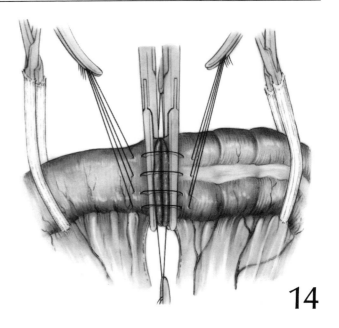

14

14 The other sutures are serially tied and trimmed as the assistant holds the parallel Dennis clamps together. The Dennis clamps are rotated through 180°, thus exposing the anterior wall. A series of 4/0 seromuscular sutures are placed about 1 cm apart and the ends tagged. Occlusion of the intestine 3–4 cm from the ends is achieved by gentle digital compression or by a shod non-crushing clamp gently applied across the intestinal lumen only.

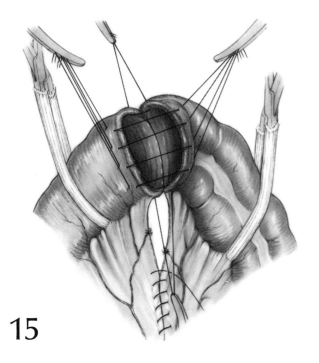

15

15 The non-crushing clamps are removed from first one cut end of intestine and then the other. While the tagged sutures are held up to open the intestinal lumen, an assistant is ready to use suction if any stool begins to leak from the cut end.

16 After ensuring that none of the sutures have inadvertently picked up the opposite wall and that there are no major arterial 'pumpers', the surgeon ties all suture pairs. Proximal occluding pressure or shod clamps are removed. The anastomosis is completed by placing 4/0 interrupted, full-thickness sutures between each of the previously placed sutures. The surgeon must be certain that the anastomosis is well vascularized, widely patent, under no tension, and that the technique was not compromised in any way. The mesocolic suture is completed up to the wall of the intestine.

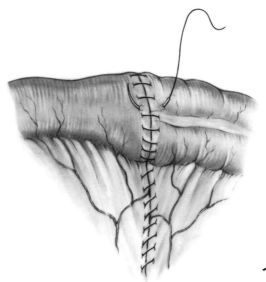

16

Alternative anastomotic techniques

Unique problems demand flexibility on the part of the surgeon, and other anastomotic techniques may be preferred.

Size discrepancy

Major size discrepancy in the two limbs of intestine does not usually pose a problem if the technique described above is used. The technique of continually halving the distance to guide suture placement on each end of cut intestine can be used to easily accommodate a major size discrepancy. An acceptable alternative anastomotic technique is a side-to-side functional end-to-end stapled anastomosis (as described in the chapter on pp. 74–83). A total abdominal colectomy and ileorectal anastomosis may involve two limbs of intestine with major size discrepancy. If the rectum is large and the ileum small, the author's preferred approach is to use a double-staple technique (as described in the chapter on pp. 74–83).

Distal anastomosis

Most colonic anastomoses are easily accessible and lend themselves to suturing. If a distal anastomosis to the upper or middle third of the rectum is required after a segmental or total colectomy, the circular stapled end-to-end anastomosis may be easier (as described in the chapter on pp. 74–83).

Oedematous bowel

Obstruction often results in oedematous bowel which can be hazardous to approximate because sutures or staples may pull out. A two-layer technique or reinforcement of a stapled anastomosis may be preferable in such situations. Alternatively, the oedema may preclude a safe primary anastomosis, and a colostomy or ileostomy may be necessary as a first step (as described in the chapter on pp. 397–415).

Wound closure

After achieving haemostasis, the abdomen is irrigated, fluid is suctioned, and the fascia is closed, usually with a running, heavy, slowly absorbable monofilament suture. The subcutaneous tissue is irrigated, and in most instances the skin is approximated by subcuticular sutures or skin staples.

Postoperative care

Nasogastric aspiration is maintained after the operation if there was evidence of obstruction, but otherwise it is not used unless the patient develops nausea, distension or vomiting. Clear liquids are begun when the patient has a soft abdomen with normal bowel sounds and expels flatus and/or stool without nausea, vomiting or distension. If tolerated, the diet is advanced to a normal intake over the next 2 days. Intravenous fluids are maintained until the patient is taking sufficient fluids orally. The urinary catheter is normally discontinued between the second and fourth day after surgery. If there is evidence of infection or sepsis without an obvious aetiology, the surgeon must suspect a leaked anastomosis (as described in the chapter on pp. 93–104). Patients have generally recovered sufficiently to be discharged 6–8 days after surgery.

Colectomy for malignant disease of the colon: the 'no touch' isolation technique

D. G. Jagelman MD, FRCS, FACS
Chairman, Division of Surgery and Chairman, Department of Colorectal Surgery, Cleveland Clinic Florida, Fort Lauderdale, Florida, USA

History

The majority of patients with metastatic colorectal carcinoma develop liver involvement because of venous invasion with transit of malignant cells through the portal system. Cancers may be disseminated by the trauma of surgical excision, and an initial direct approach to the origin of the artery and vein of the cancer-bearing segment may limit the potential of the venous dissemination and maximize the excision of metastatic lymphatic disease. This method has been termed the 'no touch' isolation technique and was first described by Barnes[1] in 1952 and popularized by Turnbull et al.[2] in 1967.

We recommend that this technique is used in conjunction with the standard operation for the treatment of large bowel tumours.

Principles and justification

Carcinoma of the caecum and the ascending colon should be treated by right hemicolectomy with ileotransverse colonic anastomosis with *en bloc* resection of the lymphatic drainage of the cancer-bearing segment. Carcinoma of the mid-transverse colon is best treated by total colectomy and ileorectal anastomosis. Carcinoma of the splenic flexure and left colon should be treated by total left colectomy with colorectal anastomosis, and carcinoma of the sigmoid colon by sigmoid colectomy with anastomosis of the upper descending colon to the rectum. Colectomy and ileorectal anastomosis should also be considered for young patients with colonic malignancy and patients with synchronous colonic carcinoma and synchronous adenomatous polyps.

Preoperative

Patients who enter hospital for elective resection of cancer of the colon will have undergone either proctosigmoidoscopic or fibreoptic sigmoidoscopic examination, or both. An air contrast barium enema or, preferably, a colonoscopy (when possible) should be performed to exclude synchronous carcinomas that occur in approximately 6% of cases or synchronous adenomatous polyps that occur in as many as 30% of patients. A general physical examination is performed with particular reference to respiratory and cardio-vascular status. Haemoglobin, urea, electrolyte determinations, liver function tests, prothrombin time and urinanalysis are undertaken routinely. A baseline carcino-embryonic antigen (CEA) test should also be performed. Chest radiographs and electrocardiograms are obtained. Anaemia, if present, is corrected by appropriate blood transfusion and blood is grouped and cross-matched for the day of surgery. In recent years the use of autologous blood and/or donor-directed blood has been preferred.

Adequate mechanical bowel preparation is essential to minimize septic complications; this is achieved using a 1-day bowel preparation. The patient is placed on a fluid diet the day before surgery and is given 1 litre of 10% mannitol solution to drink over a 2-h period. This technique is well tolerated by patients, has no significant side effects, and has reduced patient discomfort and nursing time appreciably. Neither laxatives nor enemas are given. An alternative method of preparation, however, is to use GoLytely. An intravenous infusion is started the night before surgery to avoid the dehydration produced either by the bowel preparation and/or the necessary fasting from midnight before the operation. The patient is anaesthetized with endotracheal intubation.

Operation

Position of patient

Patients undergoing left-sided resections are placed in the extended lithotomy position in stirrups (*see* page 48), and the rectum is irrigated with 1 litre of normal saline until the fluid returning is clear. A wide mushroom catheter is used for this purpose and is left in the rectum to drain any residual fluid from the large bowel during the dissection. A urinary catheter is placed to empty the bladder and allow assessment of renal function during and after the procedure.

Incision and abdominal exploration

The abdominal skin is prepared with povidone-iodine (Betadine), 10% solution, and the abdomen is opened by a long midline incision which can be extended upwards or downwards as needed for access to the peritoneal cavity. The cancer-bearing segment of the colon is inspected but not palpated, and a search is undertaken for peritoneal nodules and liver metastases. Needle biopsy specimens are taken from any liver nodules and sent for frozen section. The remainder of the colon is examined for synchronous pathology.

RIGHT COLON RESECTION

1 Carcinoma of the right colon is treated by resection of the terminal few centimetres of ileum, caecum, ascending colon and right side of transverse colon. In addition, the bowel mesentery and lymphatic pathways up to the origins of the ileocolic and right colic arteries, and the right (hepatic) division of the middle colic artery are excised.

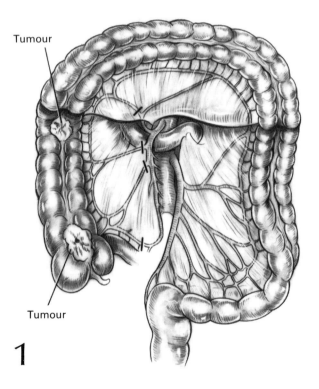

Tumour

Tumour

1

2 With the surgeon standing on the patient's left side a retroperitoneal approach to the lymphovascular pedicles of the right colon is preferred. The small intestine is reflected to the right side of the abdomen and the duodenojejunal flexure is exposed. The peritoneum is incised from this point towards the caecum.

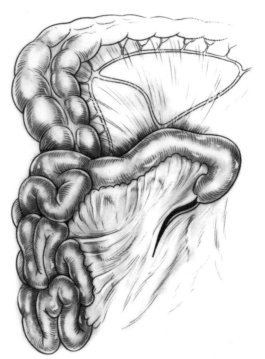

2

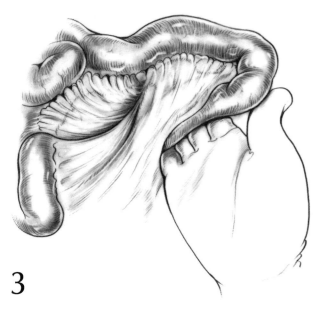

3

3 The index and middle fingers are inserted along the lateral border of the third portion of the duodenum, dissecting the duodenum from the base of the small bowel mesentery. The index finger easily reaches the third part of the duodenum. This allows for the assessment of possible duodenal invasion of a right-sided colonic carcinoma. The fingers should then be beneath the origin of the ileocolic artery. Care should be taken not to dissect under the duodenum to avoid injury to the small vessels around the pancreas.

4 With the fingers of the left hand lying along the lateral border of the duodenum, the small bowel is replaced in the abdomen thus lying over the palm of the left hand which is beneath the root of the mesentery. The superior mesenteric, ileocolic (IC) and right colic (RC) arteries now lie across the left index finger. The tip of the finger can be seen through a window in the mesentery between the ileocolic and the right colic arteries.

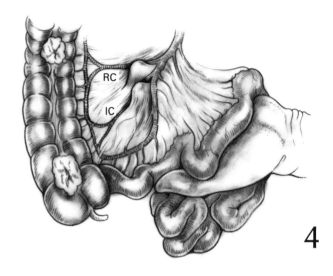

4

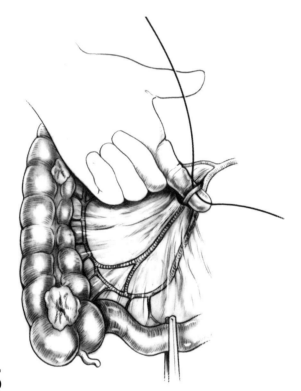

5

5 By palpation, the origin of the ileocolic lympho-vascular bundle is defined, ligated and divided from the superior mesenteric artery where it crosses the third portion of the duodenum.

6 Next, the right colic artery is selected, ligated and divided at its origin.

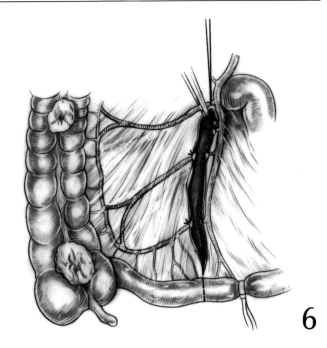

6

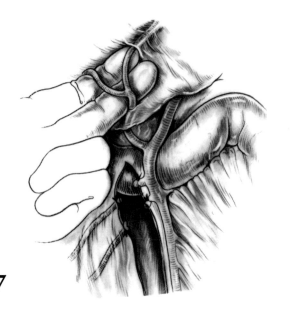

7

7 The hepatic flexure division of the middle colic artery is similarly isolated, clamped and ligated. After the main colonic vessels have been ligated and dissected, the ileocolic mesentery is divided from the duodenum to the ileum approximately 12 cm proximal to the caecum. A broad linen tape is placed around the ileum just proximal to the line of division and is knotted tightly to prevent intestinal spillage during subsequent anastomosis.

8 The lesser sac is entered along the greater curvature of the stomach and the gastrocolic omentum is stripped down from the greater curvature of the distal stomach. This frees the right side of the transverse colon from the stomach and duodenum. If the tumour is near to the hepatic flexure, the gastrocolic omentum is taken down flush with the gastric wall, inside the gastroepiploic arch.

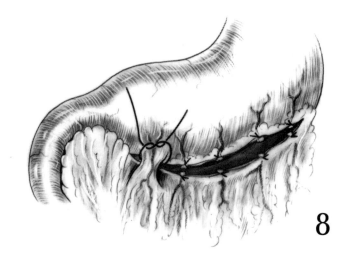

8

9 The remaining mesentery and mesenteric vessels of the transverse colon are then clamped and divided. The point of anastomosis to the mid-transverse colon is then selected, clamped and divided. A linen tape is placed just distal to the line of transection on the transverse colon to prevent retrograde faecal spillage at the time of anastomosis.

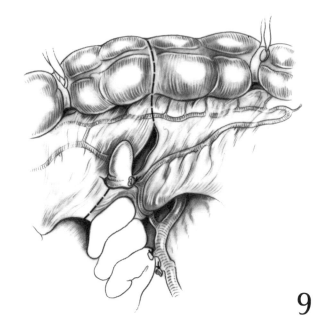

9

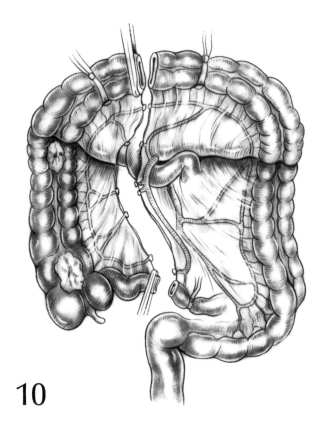

10

10 The isolated cancer-bearing segment is then reflected laterally and removed. The mesentery of the ascending colon is separated from the ureter and gonadal vessels and from the surface of the right kidney. Finally, all of the peritoneum of the right paracolic gutter is removed with the cancer-bearing segment.

Method of anastomosis

An end-to-end sutured anastomosis is preferred (*see* chapter on pp. 51–73). If there is a disparity in the size of bowel lumen, an antimesenteric (Cheatle) slit is used to widen the smaller lumen. This ensures a wide open anastomosis. The bowel is checked for good pulsatile blood supply and the bowel ends are swabbed with 10% povidone-iodine solution as an antiseptic and a tumoricidal agent.

Ileotransverse colonic anastomosis can be achieved using a combination of the TA 55 and the GIA staplers (*see* chapter on pp. 51–73).

There is often a disparity in luminal diameter between the terminal ileum and the transverse colon. An end-to-side anastomosis overcomes this problem and the use of the EEA instrument facilitates the anastomosis (*see* chapter on pp. 74–83).

Wound closure

The mesenteric defect is obliterated by continuous interlocking 3/0 chromic catgut. The abdomen is closed with an interrupted 1 Maxon figure-of-eight mass closure technique through all layers. Finally, the skin is approximated with clips.

CARCINOMA OF DISTAL TRANSVERSE AND LEFT COLON

11 Carcinoma of the distal transverse colon and descending colon is treated by early ligation of the appropriate lymphovascular pedicles; that is, the inferior mesenteric and splenic branches of the middle colic artery and vein. Division of the transverse colon in its mid-portion and of the rectum at the level of the sacral promontory is followed by end-to-end colorectal anastomosis.

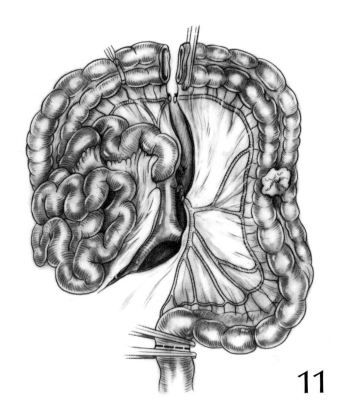

11

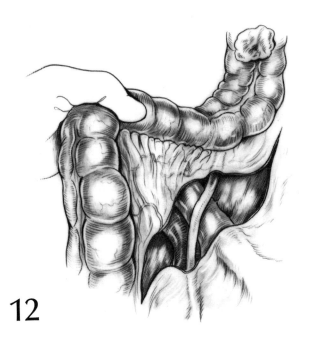

12

12 The sigmoid colon is gently lifted upwards and out of the abdomen and the peritoneum on its lateral border is incised. With combined sharp and blunt dissection the avascular plane anterior to the gonadal vessels and ureter is defined and entered. The sympathetic chain can be seen passing over the bifurcation of the aorta and should be avoided.

It is then possible to pass the left hand under the sigmoid colon and define the origin of the inferior mesenteric lymphovascular pedicle on the aorta.

13 The inferior mesenteric artery and vein are then clamped and divided individually. If the tumour is in close proximity to the site of mobilization of the sigmoid and descending colon, a direct ligation in continuity with the inferior mesenteric artery and vein is performed before mobilization of the sigmoid. The vessels can then be divided after full mobilization of the sigmoid and left colon, vascular dissemination having thus been prevented.

The splenic flexure branch of the middle colic artery is next ligated and divided by lifting up the transverse colon and incising into the mesentery. The left colon is then isolated from a lymphovascular viewpoint. A point of division is selected in the midtransverse colon and the gastrocolic omentum and transverse mesocolon are divided and individual vessels are tied as they are transected. The bowel is divided between clamps. Dissection is continued along the greater curvature of the stomach to remove the gastrocolic omentum as far as the splenic flexure.

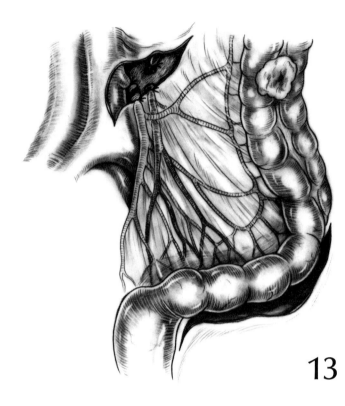

13

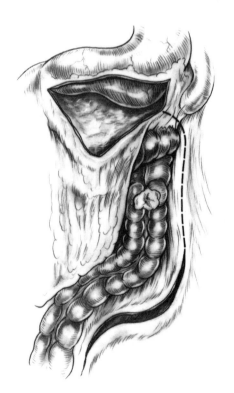

14

14 The incision along the left paracolic gutter is then extended upwards towards the splenic flexure and finally, by gently grasping both limbs of the colon at the splenic flexure, the peritoneum can be divided to allow the colon to be brought down out of its splenic bed. The descending colon and its mesentery can be swept across from the anterior surface of the left kidney as far as the ligament of Treitz.

15 The lateral peritoneal incision is continued down towards the rectum on the left side, and the peritoneum is divided from the origin of the inferior mesenteric artery down to the level of the sacral promontory on the right side. Before transecting the rectum it is irrigated with 10% povidone-iodine solution as an antiseptic and tumoricidal agent through the mushroom catheter previously inserted into the rectum. The rectum is transected at the level of the sacral promontory without entering the presacral space.

The colon can then be removed. A colorectal anastomosis is performed between the transverse colon and the rectum at the level of the sacral promontory.

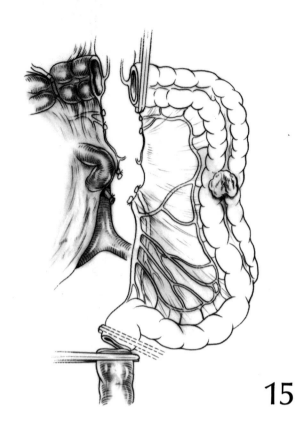

15

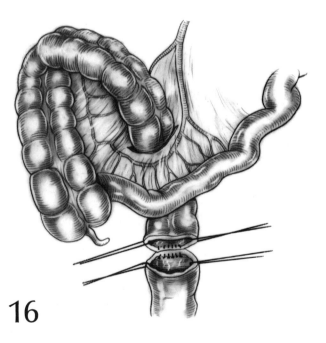

16

16 If there is difficulty in approximation of the bowel ends without tension or if there appears to be undue distortion of the small intestine and its mesentery, the transverse colon should be brought through an opening in the mesenteric vascular window of the terminal ileum between the ileocolic artery and the superior mesenteric artery. The right side of the gastrocolic omentum needs to be divided as far as the duodenum to allow extra mobility of the remaining transverse colon. The opening in the mesentery is sutured to the transverse colon to prevent the possibility of herniation of small bowel through the mesenteric window.

The colorectal anastomosis is performed as previously described, including the use of the Cheatle slit if necessary to achieve equal size of the lumen of the two ends of intestine.

CARCINOMA OF SIGMOID COLON

17 Carcinoma of the sigmoid colon is treated by early vascular ligation of the inferior mesenteric artery and vein, by division of the colon at the mid-descending level, and by division of the rectum just below the sacral promontory. Mobilization and resection is as for the left hemicolectomy previously described.

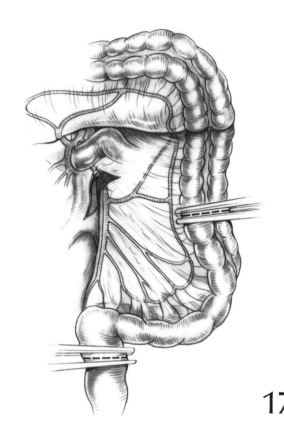

17

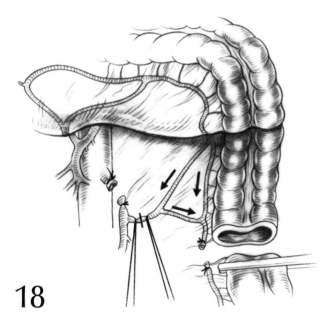

18

18 After division of the inferior mesenteric artery at its origin, the left colic branch is identified. This is divided proximal to its bifurcation. It is hoped that retrograde blood flow will pass down the preserved left colic bifurcation and supplement the marginal artery to supply the colon at the point of transection. The anastomosis is performed in the manner previously described.

An alternative to conventional colorectal anastomosis utilizing suture is by means of the EEA stapling instrument (*see* chapter on pp. 74–83). It is preferable to use the largest (31-mm) cartridge for this type of anastomosis (*see* also chapter on pp. 456–471).

References

1. Barnes JP. Physiologic resection of the right colon. *Surg Gynecol Obstet* 1952; 94: 722–6.

2. Turnbull RB, Kyle K, Watson FR, Spratt J. Cancer of the colon: the influence of the 'no touch isolation technic' on survival rates. *Ann Surg* 1967; 166: 420–7.

Illustrations by Gillian Oliver and the late Robert Lane

Elective surgery for sigmoid diverticular disease

Mark Killingback FRCS, FRCSEd, FRACS
Sydney Adventist Hospital, Sydney, Australia

Principles and justification

Patients may have significant clinical problems attributable to diverticular disease caused by functional colonic muscle abnormalities without local inflammation of the colon being present. This concept has led to a better understanding of the indications for surgical treatment. Furthermore, there may be a discrepancy between the clinical and radiological assessments in these patients – a barium enema may underestimate or exaggerate the apparent significance of the diverticular disease.

In recent years there has been a better appreciation of the response of symptoms to dietary manipulation. The effect of increasing food residue with a high fibre diet has greatly reduced the number of patients requiring surgery for 'failed medical treatment'.

Indications

Caution must be exercised in attributing abdominal and intestinal symptoms to diverticular disease, particularly in those patients whose principal complaint is chronic abdominal pain. Irritable bowel syndrome may be indistinguishable from the symptoms of non-inflammatory functional chronic diverticular disease. The author does not believe that there is any pathological relationship between these two conditions.

Prophylactic resection of sigmoid diverticular disease is not justified in the early stage of the disease in an attempt to prevent complications, such as perforation and fistula formation. Their development is largely unpredictable and is often the first manifestation of the disease. If symptoms have become refractory, however, surgery is indicated because the inflammatory focus has become irreversible and will cause progressive fibrosis of the wall of the colon, the mesentery and the pericolic tissues with or without a concomitant abscess.

Most elective resections are performed for complicated disease such as chronic phlegmonous diverticulitis, chronic pericolic or pelvic abscess and fistulae. Some of these patients will present for a second-stage elective procedure after a previous laparotomy for acute diverticulitis, drainage of an abscess, or frank peritonitis.

Despite conservative management with a high-residue diet and unprocessed bran, persistent symptoms may warrant elective surgery. In this group, patients with irritable bowel syndrome should be diagnosed and excluded.

Repeated attacks of acute diverticulitis of significance may occur with evidence of peritoneal irritation, fever and systemic effects. Such attacks usually settle with antibiotic therapy in a few days, but often leave a focus for subsequent attacks. Such an episode which subsides slowly and leaves a focus of tenderness, with or without a mass on palpation, is better managed by resection in an otherwise fit patient. If the attack is less severe in an elderly patient with accompanying medical problems, it may be preferable to observe the patient for a period and advise surgery on the basis of future episodes.

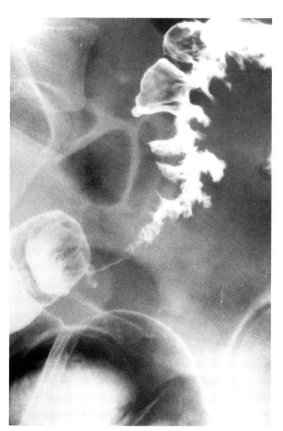

1a

1a, b A persistent inflammatory mass for more than 4–6 weeks is an indication for resection in the fit patient. Invariably it will be associated with a stricture on radiography (*see Illustration 1a*), and this in turn will raise the possibility that a carcinoma is present. Although the inflammatory stricture usually shows mucosal continuity (*see Illustration 1b*) indicating its benign nature, the radiograph can appear indistinguishable from a carcinoma.

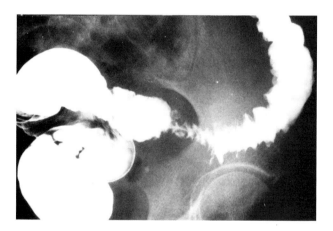

1b

2 A barium enema may show extravasation beyond the wall of the colon, indicating localized perforation. There may or may not be an associated stricture, and it is likely that there is an associated inflammatory mass. While this situation may be tolerated in the unfit patient without symptoms, the colon is best resected.

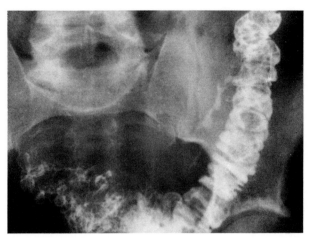

2

Flexible sigmoidoscopy or colonoscopy can differentiate some but not all of these lesions, because stenosis, fibrosis and angulation of the colon may impede the passage of the endoscope. Computed tomography (CT) can be very helpful in acute diverticulitis by demonstrating a related abdominal or pelvic abscess. Its value in patients with chronic or intermittent symptoms, however, is yet to be demonstrated.

Colovesical and colocutaneous fistulae are common and may complicate sigmoid diverticulitis. Less common fistulae are colovaginal, coloenteric and colofallopian, but diverticular disease can form a fistula into any organ and many bizarre fistulae have been described. Such fistulae are usually an absolute indication for surgery, but in frail patients without evidence of an active abscess or ascending renal tract infection (colovesical fistula), the compromise for conservative treatment may be acceptable.

Resection is usually indicated as a secondary procedure if emergency surgery for acute diverticulitis with peritonitis has previously been carried out. Such patients may have an associated fistula, and a proximal stoma may be present. Patients in whom a Hartmann operation has been performed as an emergency will need careful assessment to see if further resection of proximal and/or distal residual disease is needed before an anastomosis is carried out.

Interval elective surgery is indicated very occasionally between recurrent episodes of profuse colonic bleeding. While most bleeding of this type is due to vascular dysplasia (most often from the right colon), bleeding from diverticula may be demonstrated by angiography and histology. If colonoscopy, scintigraphy, or angiography has demonstrated a bleeding site, a segmental resection can be performed. If the episodes of bleeding recur significantly without localization, colectomy and ileorectal anastomosis should be considered as an elective treatment.

Preoperative

Preparation for the patient with diverticular disease is the same as for any major colorectal operation and will include a full blood count, blood biochemistry, chest radiography and electrocardiography. Intravenous pyelography is not mandatory before sigmoid resection for uncomplicated disease, but is important if complications are evidenced by the presence of a palpable mass or radiological stricture, which may be close to the left ureter on the pelvic brim and left wall of the pelvis. It may also reveal an incidental urinary tract abnormality, such as ureteric duplication, deviation of the ureter, non-functioning of one kidney, or obstruction of the ureter by the inflammatory disease in the pelvis.

Mechanical bowel preparation is carried out the day before surgery by the oral administration of 3 litres of polyethylene glycol preparation over a 2-h period. Usually with this preparation no additional aperients or enemas are administered. During the intraoperative and early postoperative period, prophylatic broad-spectrum antibiotics are given parenterally.

Ureteric catheterization

In patients in whom a large pelvic inflammatory mass is evident on rectal examination, considerable extraperitoneal pelvic fibrosis is likely. In such patients, the introduction of ureteric catheters before operation is most helpful. The author has employed ureteric catheters in 9% of patients resected.

Operation

Position of patient

The Lloyd-Davies position (modified lithotomy-Trendelenburg position) with Lloyd-Davies stirrups is preferred. This allows better retraction by the second assistant standing between the patient's legs, vaginal examination which may assist in a difficult anterior dissection (particularly after a hysterectomy) and is necessary for the use of the intraluminal stapling instrument, which is the author's preferred method of anastomosis.

Incision and laparotomy

A midline incision is made from the pubic symphysis to as far above the umbilicus as necessary to gain wide exposure. A thorough laparotomy is performed to assess the diverticular disease, its complications and any other intra-abdominal pathology.

In assessing the diverticular disease, the possibility of carcinoma must be considered. If there is doubt about such a diagnosis, the problem is usually diverticular disease. Any attachment of the diverticular disease to adjacent organs should be noted. The extent of the diverticular disease along the colon proximally must be assessed, as well as any abnormal muscular thickening. A similar examination of the rectosigmoid and upper rectum is important to assess possible inflammatory disease and associated muscle changes with diverticula.

Despite preoperative investigations and careful intra-operative assessment, real doubt may exist that the disease is benign. In this situation a careful examination of a preoperative barium enema may show mucosal continuity along the stricture, indicating that the disease is not malignant. While flexible sigmoidoscopy may not have been useful before operation, its use during the operation, assisted by the abdominal surgeon, may confirm a diagnosis.

If carcinoma cannot be excluded, then the surgeon will need to perform an appropriate cancer operation, resecting adherent organs *en bloc*. Although resecting a segment of bladder wall *en bloc* for diverticulitis (mistaken for carcinoma) may be surgically acceptable, further extension of radical pelvic surgery is not. In such a circumstance, it is preferable to dissect between the bladder and the sigmoid pathology, and extend the operation as appropriate if examination of the lumen of the resected sigmoid has revealed carcinoma. Distending the bladder with saline may lift the pathological segment out of the pelvis and facilitate this part of the operation.

Mobilizing the sigmoid and descending colon

3   After placement of a plastic ring wound protector in the abdominal wound, incision of the parasigmoid peritoneum along the line of the mesenteric and parietal fusion will expose the gonadal vessels and lower part of the ureter. Careful identification of the mesenteric layer of the left colon will ensure the correct anatomical plane.

Gentle digital dissection medially and upwards is used to displace the colon mesentery forwards, and the gonadal vessels, left ureter and perinephric fascia posteriorly. Troublesome bleeding may occur if large ovarian veins are not manipulated with care. This dissection should stop at the mid-point of the left kidney, as further manipulation may cause a traction injury to the splenic capsule which is not under vision during this manoeuvre.

With the upper sigmoid and lower descending colon retracted to the right, further identification of the course of the left ureter to the pelvic brim is made. The inferior mesenteric artery and vein are clearly identified from this left aspect, distinctly enveloped in fascia. Dissecting across the aorta immediately behind these structures will prevent damage to the preaortic nerve plexus, and when followed distally will lead to the correct anatomical plane for presacral dissection.

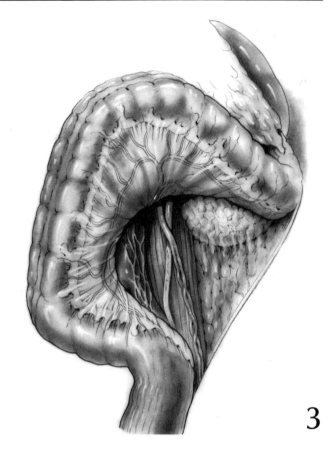

3

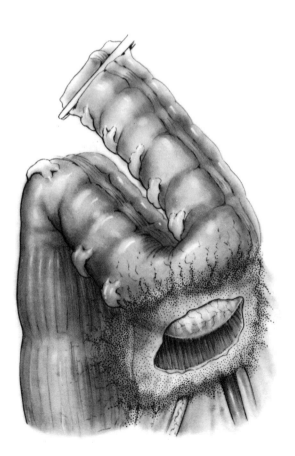

4

Specific difficulties in resecting sigmoid diverticulitis

The apex of the sigmoid colon is often fixed into the pelvis by adhesion to a deep chronic pelvic abscess, and until this is mobilized adequate dissection of the sigmoid colon is not possible. This pelvic dissection can often be achieved by careful 'pinching off' manoeuvres. In other instances, however, sharp scalpel dissection (too tough for scissors) or diathermy is required to cut through the very hard fibrosis that may join the sigmoid colon to the parietal peritoneum or pelvic structures. It is in this circumstance that ureteric catheters, which can be palpated, are most helpful.

4   If the sigmoid colon cannot be mobilized from the pelvis as the first step in the operation, then exposure of the left ureter will be difficult. Dissection in this area, and then to the left pelvic brim, will be facilitated by transecting the colon as an early step in the operation and lifting the sigmoid colon forward to expose the left posterior abdominal wall and the pelvic brim. This latter area can be a potentially hazardous dissection, with thick fibrosis obscuring the left ureter and left common iliac vessels. In such a circumstance, the sigmoid can be mobilized from this site by dissecting the adherent sigmoid in its intramural plane, thus avoiding damage to vital structures.

Splenic flexure mobilization

In most resections for diverticulitis, mobilization of the splenic flexure will be necessary. Up to this point in the operation, care is taken to avoid traction on the left aspect of the greater omentum and the splenic flexure of the colon to avoid capsule injuries to the spleen.

Mobilization of the splenic flexure is best performed by the surgeon operating from the right side of the table with the first assistant standing between the patient's legs, which maximizes his view and ability to assist. A second assistant on the left side of the table retracts the wound and the left costal margin. It is for this part of the operation that the incision in the upper part of the wound should be adequate.

5 The first three steps in mobilization are: (1) release of omental adhesions to the anterior border of the spleen; (2) release of omental adhesions to the left paracolic gutter at the level of the lower pole of the spleen; and (3) division of the peritoneum between the colon and the lower border of the spleen. This peritoneum is over the upper pole of the left kidney, and the incision is continued laterally to complete the incision of the left paracolic gutter.

These three manoeuvres release the spleen and will effectively prevent traction injuries to the splenic capsule.

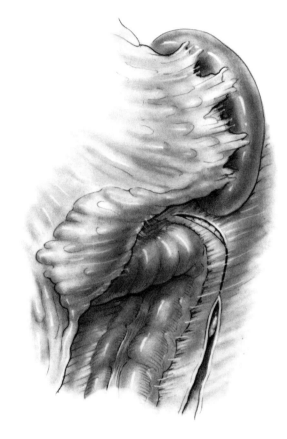

5

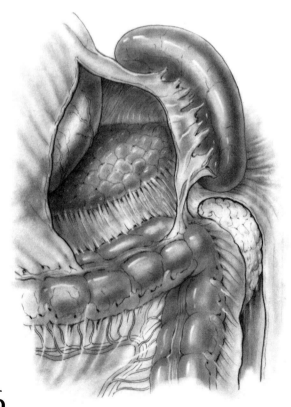

6

6 With the greater omentum retracted upwards and to the right, the lesser sac can be exposed by incising above the left transverse colon and/or opening the left lateral limit of the lesser sac, which is a short distance proximal to the splenic flexure.

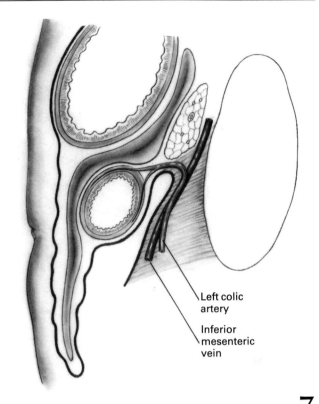

Left colic artery

Inferior mesenteric vein

7

7, 8 With the structures on the posterior wall of the lesser sac exposed, further mobilization (if required) can be achieved by dividing the anterior layer of the transverse mesocolon, which will allow the left colic vessels adjacent to it and the peritoneum posterior to these vessels to be dissected from the left perinephric fascia. Care must be taken medially of the inferior mesenteric vein, if it is to be preserved. The splenic flexure will now be fully mobilized.

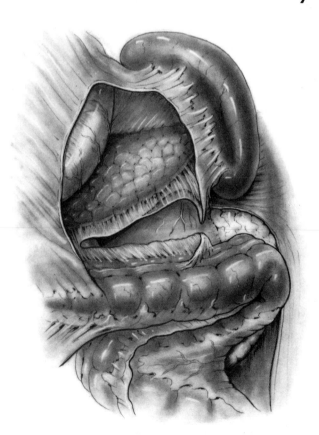

8

9 If necessary, division of the inferior mesenteric vein below the duodenum will give further length to the left colon by allowing the course of the left colic artery to 'unwind', which is thus preserved as an additional source of circulation to the left colon.

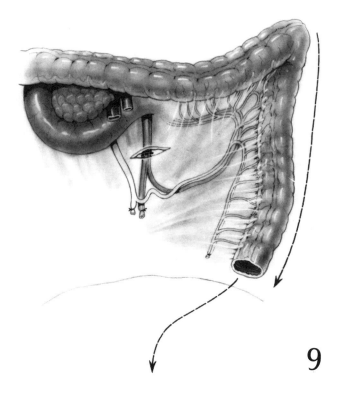

9

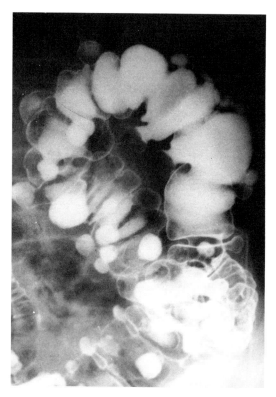

10

Selecting the proximal level of resection

In deciding the proximal extent of resection, several aspects are important. Obviously, active chronic infection in the colon and mesentery must be included. Muscle thickening, which may be proximal to the sigmoid colon, is best removed, and it is preferable to remove colon that contains many diverticula.

10 In the fit patient it may be reasonable to include the descending colon and distal transverse colon in order to remove extensive diverticulosis. More proximal excision of the colon requiring division of the middle colic vessels is not recommended.

11 It may be difficult to detect diverticula if there is much pericolic fat. By 'milking' gas and fluid into the segment in question, the luminal pressure will increase and expand the colon, causing occult diverticula to 'balloon' and be revealed. Although one or two diverticula can be inverted at or near the anastomosis if unavoidable, it is preferable to use normal colon free of diverticula.

In the author's series, the level of proximal resection was near the sigmoid descending junction in 60% of patients, and at varying levels to the distal transverse colon in the remaining 40%.

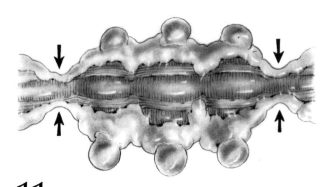

11

Vascular preparation of the colonic mesentery

12 If the proximal level of resection is in the vicinity of the sigmoid–descending colon junction, the left colic artery should be preserved, and the inferior mesenteric vein and artery ligated below the origin from that artery. This ligation is similar to cancer surgery, as there is no advantage in ligating branches and tributaries of the sigmoid vessels closer to the intestinal wall. If more proximal colon is to be removed, then both the inferior mesenteric artery and vein will be divided.

The marginal vessels of the descending colon run close to and parallel to the colon, but in the proximal sigmoid colon these vessels are often further from the intestine and lie in a looped formation, making them more vulnerable to inadvertent surgical interruption.

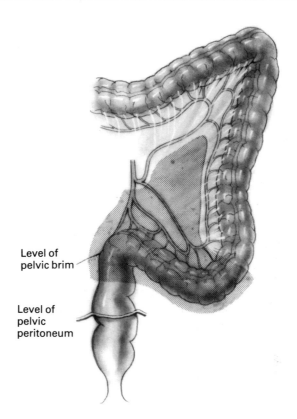

Level of
pelvic brim

Level of
pelvic
peritoneum

12

13 Division of the marginal vessels should be more distal than the level of the colon transection ('overshoot') to provide a safe margin to avoid damage to the vasa breva and vasa longa, which are related to the area for anastomosis. The marginal artery flow should be tested by allowing it to bleed. If flow is poor, and more proximal resection is inadvisable, this may be an indication for a proximal stoma.

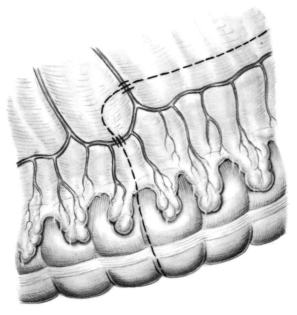

13

Stapled anastomosis in diverticular disease

14 The author's preference is to use circular stapling wherever possible after resecting diverticular disease. The results are satisfactory, but not all patients are suitable, and approximately 5% of patients are best managed with a sutured anastomosis. These are patients with chronic pelvic floor fibrosis, which restricts the safe use of the stapler, patients who exhibit persistent spasm of the upper one-third of the rectum even under anaesthesia, and patients whose left colon is markedly contracted after a period of defunctioning by a proximal stoma.

The stapling technique is a good discipline for the surgeon, because both the proximal and distal ends of intestine must be normal, supple and free of inflammatory changes or muscle thickening for the technique to be satisfactory.

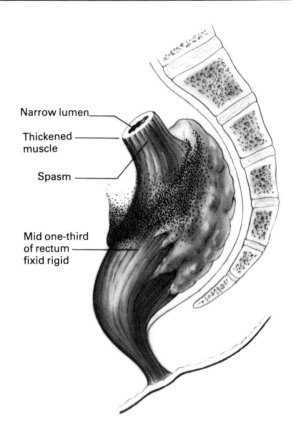

Narrow lumen

Thickened muscle

Spasm

Mid one-third of rectum fixid rigid

14

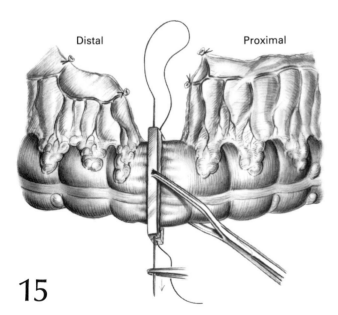

Distal   Proximal

15

Preparation of the colon

Minimal excision of terminal branches of the vasa breva and vasa longa should occur to secure a bare segment of colon for anastomosis. For convenience, one or two obtrusive appendices epiploicae can be excised (preserving the vasa within the base of the appendix).

15 A 1.5-cm segment of colon can be cleared to facilitate the application of an occlusive bowel clamp, and immediately proximal to it a purse-string clamp that is used in all cases to insert a purse-string suture. This clamp should leave no more than 1.0 cm of 'bare' colon between it and the proximal pericolic fat and vessels. A double-ended 0 polypropylene (Prolene) round-bodied malleable needle (3.5 metric) is passed through the purse-string clamp, and the colon is divided between the clamps.

16 Before dividing the colon, a nylon tape is tied around it (being careful not to include the marginal vessels) 10 cm proximal to the area for anastomosis. The edges of the colon are held in a pair of Babcock's forceps and a segment is thoroughly irrigated with water to remove all faecal debris.

If the colon is poorly prepared or loaded with faeces, intraoperative colonic lavage should be performed via the caecum or ileum to cleanse it completely.

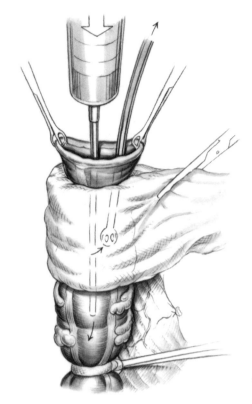

16

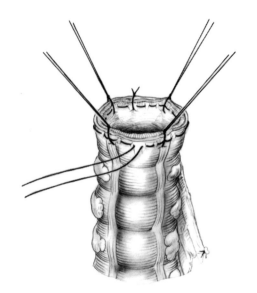

17

17 Four stay sutures are then placed on the margin of the divided colon. Two of these should pass through the antimesenteric taenia. A fifth short suture is used to 'trap' the mesenteric taenia. These five sutures include the purse-string suture to reinforce its function, and the stay sutures facilitate the insertion of the anvil into the colon.

Selecting the distal level of resection

The distal level of excision is also determined by the site of inflammation in the wall and mesentery of the intestine. It is important to remove distal diverticula that may be obscured in the pericolic and perirectal fat just above or below the rectosigmoid junction. Careful examination of the barium enema radiograph may also help to localize the distal limit of diverticula formation. The longitudinal muscle coat is usually thickened in the rectosigmoid region and sometimes in the upper rectum, and it is preferable to remove this abnormality. Therefore, the distal level of dissection is usually below the promontory of the sacrum through the upper third of the rectum.

18 Unusually, extensive diverticular disease may affect the upper one-third of the rectum.

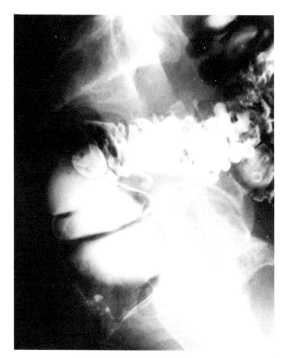

18

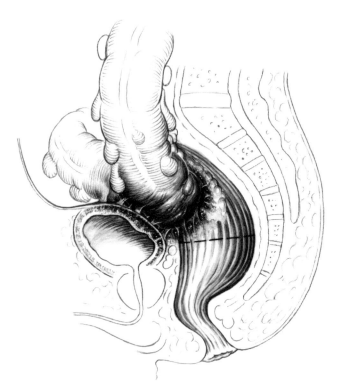

19

19 Secondary involvement of the upper one-third of the rectum is important in determining the distal level of transection. If a pelvic abscess involves the rectovaginal or rectovesical pouch but leaves the upper part of the rectum unaffected, the level of transection can be through healthy intestine in the upper one-third of the rectum. If this part of the rectum is abnormal due to contiguous inflammation, the transection level must be far enough distal to be through healthy rectal wall. In some cases this will mean an extraperitoneal level, and very occasionally through the lower one-third of the rectum.

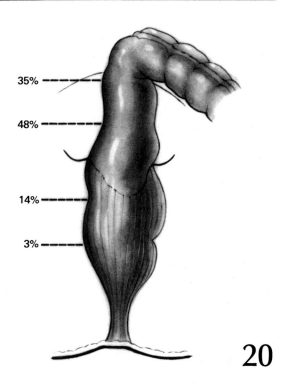

20 The levels of distal resection of 172 consecutive cases are shown.

20

Preparation of the rectum

With the usual level of transection in the upper one-third of the rectum, the presacral space is dissected, but not completely to the tip of the coccyx. The peritoneum lateral to the rectum is usually incised and a variable division of lateral ligaments of the rectum performed. At the selected level the mesorectum is divided transversely between artery forceps. The left forefinger and thumb are used to feel the wall of the rectum and 'pinch' the mesentery safely away from the intestine to allow safe application of the forceps. As this posterolateral clearing of the rectum occurs, the released rectal wall stretches to reveal at least 2 cm of 'bare' rectum suitable for anastomosis.

21 A right-angled rectal clamp is applied to the proximal part of the bare rectal wall (from right to left). The rectum is thoroughly irrigated through the anus with a rectal catheter through a proctoscope. The water is delivered by hand pump or large syringe to allow meticulous cleansing of all faecal debris, which is vital to the technique of circular stapling through the anus.

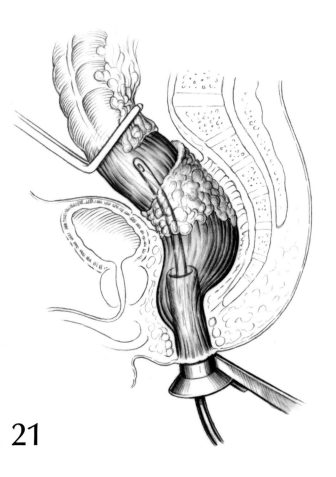

21

22 The purse-string clamp is applied right to left and used in 99% of patients to insert the purse-string in the wall of the rectum.

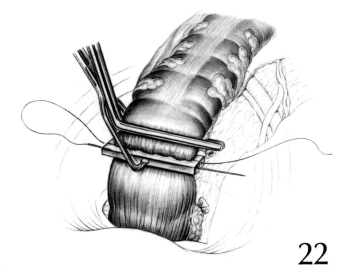

22

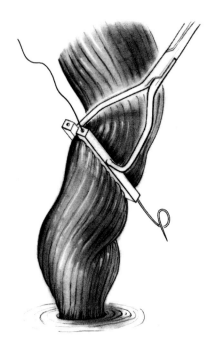

23

23 This manoeuvre is more difficult if the transection level is extraperitoneal, but it is achieved by rotating the rectum anticlockwise and angling the right side of the clamp upwards. Bending the soft needle as it emerges from the clamp on the left side overcomes any further difficulty.

The rectum is divided 3–4 mm above the purse-string clamp, and the specimen is removed. Before the purse-string clamp is removed, a Foss–Eisenberg non-crushing right-angled clamp is placed to control the rectum and stop bleeding from the cut edge. At least eight silk stay sutures are inserted and tied to trap the purse-string suture, to improve its function and to assist in control of the rectal stump.

Specific recommendations on stapling technique

Not all the details of the technique of circular stapling are described here, but certain important points are emphasized, of which some are specifically important in treating diverticular disease. For example, spare anvil heads in various sizes should be available to test the diameter of the colon so that the appropriate stapler will be selected, and hyoscine butylbromide, 20 mg given at least 5 min before the insertion of the stapler, is effective in overcoming spasm in the colon and rectum. The diameter of the stapler is not related to postoperative narrowing of the anastomosis, and there is no need to 'stretch' the intestine excessively to fit a larger size of stapler. In addition, the perineal operator should examine the anal canal and gently dilate it if there is stenosis sufficient to obstruct the stapler.

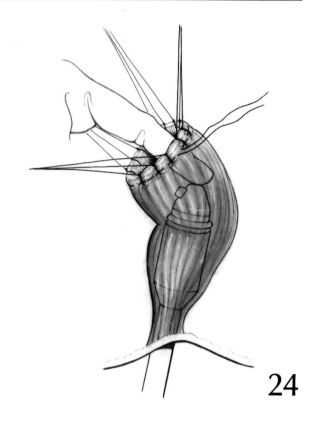

24

24 The abdominal operator should insert the right forefinger into the cleansed rectal stump to guide the stapler through a tight anal canal and to prevent any sudden thrust against the rectal wall.

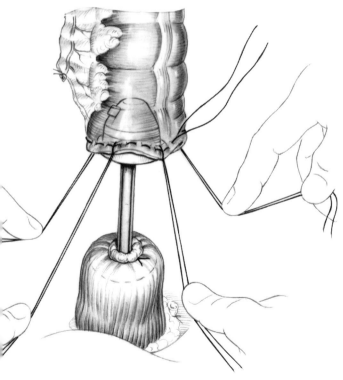

25

25 The detachable anvil head has greatly facilitated safe insertion into the colon, but if not available then the technique shown is recommended, using the stay sutures to 'see-saw' the colon gently over the anvil.

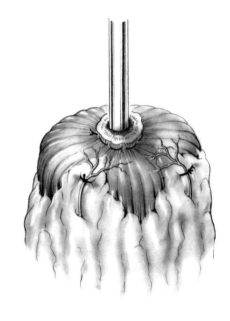

26 Significant arteries that lie over the edge of the anvil or the cartridge should be underrun with a 3/0 polyglactin suture, as they may cause significant postoperative bleeding or haematomas in the anastomosis.

It is specifically important in diverticular disease that, in the final stages of approximation of the cartridge or anvil, two or three pauses in the compression are necessary to allow the fluid to be squeezed from the compressed muscle; muscle damage may otherwise occur and the taenia may evert and escape the line of the staples.

The author has no experience with or enthusiasm for using the 'stab' technique in the closed rectal stump after a Hartmann resection and prefers to dissect out the rectum to obtain healthy and supple rectal wall for anastomosis.

26

Colovesical fistula

The management of a colovesical fistula is principally that of the diseased colon with all its implications. The fistula in the bladder wall is usually not a difficult technical problem and may not be identifiable. The operation is usually performed in the chronic phase of diverticulitis, and a preliminary colostomy followed by a second-stage resection is usually unnecessary. Blunt digital dissection will usually separate the colon from the bladder and if a small defect is noted in the vault of the bladder (usual site) it may, in some instances, be closed with a single layer of 2/0 polyglactin suture. On rare occasions a larger defect in the bladder wall is present with fibrotic margins, and in these circumstances excision of the defect in the wall of the bladder is preferable with a two-layer closure: the inner (mucosal) layer with continuous 2/0 plain catgut and an outer (mucosal) layer with interrupted 2/0 polyglactin sutures. It is important to separate the bladder repair from the colorectal anastomosis, particularly in the presence of chronic residual pelvic granulation tissue which could subsequently suppurate. If omentum is available, it can be placed between the intestinal anastomosis and the bladder. The use of the prolonged pelvic drainage technique (*see Table 1*) will prevent the sequence of sepsis–anastomotic defect and possible anastomotic–vesical fistula.

The indications for a complementary proximal stoma are those referred to when resecting diverticulitis and are not specifically related to the problem of the colovesical fistula (*see* below).

The bladder is drained with a urethral catheter, during which time urinary drainage is checked to ensure blockage of the catheter does not go undetected. It is in this circumstance that use of the new smaller suprapubic catheters may be preferable to drainage with a urethral catheter. Whichever method is used, the bladder should be drained for 10 days.

Drains

Anastomotic drains, as such, are not used. Presacral drains, in a fully dissected presacral space, remain of unproven value, even though they are often used in the belief that they may prevent secondary pelvic sepsis, which may damage the anastomosis. Presacral drains are certainly useful if optimal haemostasis in the pelvis is difficult to achieve.

27 Prolonged drainage at the site of a chronic abscess (the inflammatory 'nest' of Turnbull) is important. It is indicated if the parietal walls/floor of the abscess cannot be excised (even though the granulation tissue may be cleaned by curettage). This focus, if not controlled by drainage, will form a secondary abscess and damage the anastomosis. It may also take a long period to resolve. The principle is to convert the infected site to the dimension of the drain with carefully balanced, continuous irrigation–suction until a well established channel exists around the drains. The regimen is shown in *Table 1*.

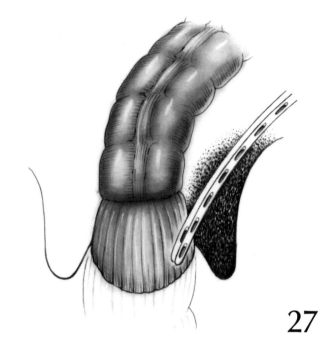

27

Table 1 Prolonged pelvic drainage

Day	Irrigation with saline via 12-Fr Nelaton catheter*	Suction via a 20-Fr Ventrol sump drain†
1	6 l/24 h	−80 mmHg
2–10	1 l/24 h	−80 mmHg
11	Remove	Remove

*Indoplast Pty Ltd, Sydney, Australia; †Mallinckrodt, Athlone, Ireland.

28 On day 11 the two drains are replaced with one Nelaton catheter which is used for the sinogram. This usually shows the optimum size of track, which signifies that the previously infected pelvic space has been 'neutralized'. The drain can be gradually removed over the next 5 days. This technique has enabled anastomoses to be performed in the presence of a chronic pelvic abscess and has practically eliminated the Hartmann operation as an elective procedure.

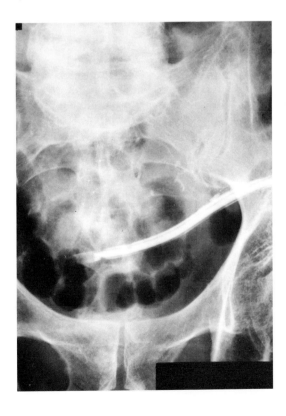

28

Indications for a proximal stoma

If the above criteria are used to select the proximal and distal ends of intestine for anastomosis, the use of a proximal stoma at the time of operation will be minimal. Currently, the author uses a proximal stoma in fewer than 10% of cases. In recent years, preference for a loop ileostomy instead of a loop colostomy has developed in association with higher standards of stomal management. In the event of a long-term stoma being necessary, the loop ileostomy is associated with a lower incidence of prolapse and hernia.

The following indications may each, or in combination, be reasons for performing a proximal stoma:

1. Technical problems with the anastomosis, such as muscle separation, tearing or haematomas, or demonstrated leaks that cannot be overcome satisfactorily by supporting sutures.
2. Poor blood supply to the colon or rectum despite all care having been taken with vascular preparation.
3. Thickened and oedematous wall as a result of pre-existing large intestinal obstruction.
4. Residual inflammatory changes in the rectum near the anastomosis which may not be resectable for some reason.
5. A combination of factors such as poor general health, prolonged and complex operation, and significant blood loss.

Postoperative care

Intravenous therapy usually continues for 7 days. Nasogastric intubation and aspiration are not used routinely, but they are used promptly if indicated by intense nausea, hiccoughs, abdominal distension, or vomiting. This approach is used in 30–40% of patients. Oral feeding is usually not commenced until the seventh day. The urethral catheter is removed on the fourth day. If a loop ileostomy is present, the plastic rod under the loop is removed on the tenth day.

As part of an ongoing study on anastomotic healing, the author routinely has the anastomosis assessed by a limited Gastrografin enema 10–12 days after surgery. A small catheter must be used, and no pressure can be generated in the rectum during the injection of contrast material as anastomotic disruption might occur. Specific instruction must be agreed by the radiologist for this investigation or, alternatively, the surgeon or surgical assistant should conduct the test. Although not necessarily recommended as routine postoperative monitoring it is wise to carry out at least this investigation before an operation to close a proximal stoma.

Complications

Postoperative complications are those that might follow any resection of the left colon and rectum. Secondary sepsis related to the chronic infected focus may occur if prolonged drainage is mismanaged. If a septic focus does occur, it may be possible to drain it by a CT-guided catheter, but in some instances it will still take a long time to resolve.

Outcome

Since the strict insistence on the use of a normal rectal segment for the anastomosis to avoid any inflammatory change in the intestinal wall, the author's anastomotic leakage rate has beome insignificant. On occasion, the upper rectum at the sacral promontory becomes involved in the inflammatory process because of contiguous inflammation in the sigmoid colon, and under these circumstances the extraperitoneal middle one-third of the rectal segment or below may be required for the anastomosis. In 109 consecutive stapled anastomoses for elective resections of diverticular disease, two (1.8%) minor leaks have occurred, which have only been detected on routine postoperative contrast radiography.

Colonic surgery for acute conditions: perforated diverticular disease

J. M. Sackier MB, FRCS
Associate Professor of Surgery, University of California, San Diego, California, USA

History

Colonic diverticula are acquired pulsion herniations consisting of mucosa and submucosa which occur at the small openings for nutrient vessel entry most commonly found on the antimesenteric border of the bowel[1]. The most frequent site for occurrence is the sigmoid colon but, in reducing order of frequency, they are also found in the descending, transverse and ascending colon.

Occasionally a giant diverticulum may be found alongside the sigmoid colon, but this is rare. The disease is extremely common and is found in approximately 10% of adults in the western world by the age of 40 years and in 65% by 80 years of age. Most diverticulosis is asymptomatic and acute perforations may be the first presentation.

Classification

The choice of treatment largely depends upon the extent of the disease at the time of presentation. The classification proposed by Hinchey and colleagues[2] is of value.

1a–d

Stage 1: a pericolic abscess confined by the mesentery.

Stage 2: a pelvic abscess caused by local perforation of a pericolic abscess.

Stage 3: peritonitis resulting from rupture of a pericolic or pelvic abscess into the general peritoneal cavity. There is no communication between the lumen of the bowel and the abscess cavity because of obliteration of the neck of the diverticulum by the inflammatory process. This is also known as acute non-communicating diverticulitis.

Stage 4: faecal peritonitis resulting from free perforation of the diverticulum. This usually develops rapidly and is also known as acute communicating diverticulitis.

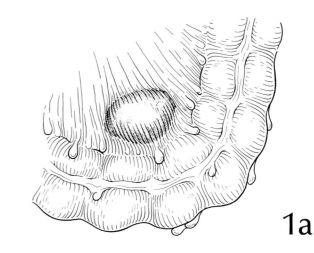

1a

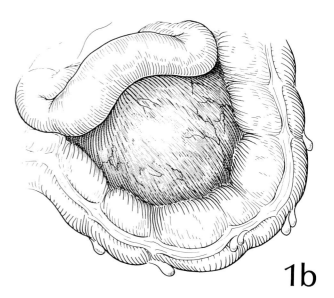

1b

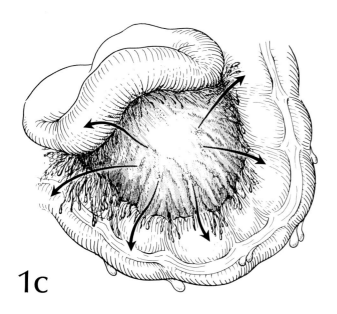

1c

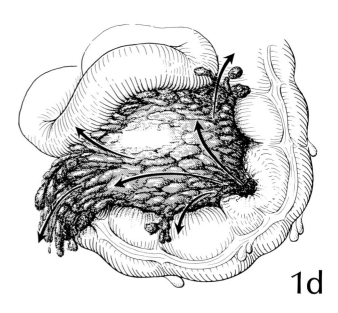

1d

Preoperative

Assessment

Patients who present with acute diverticular disease should be admitted to hospital for resuscitation, conservative treatment and the establishment of a more specific diagnosis.

Initial investigations should include a full blood count, and assessment of the function of the kidneys, heart and lungs. If cardiac disease is present, it may be necessary, if the patient is in an unstable haemodynamic state, to use a Swan-Ganz catheter to help manage cardiopulmonary function. Radiographic films of the chest and abdomen (erect and supine) are required. The most accurate test to stage the disease is the abdominal computed tomography (CT) scan, which can differentiate a bowel phlegmon, local abscess and free perforation.

Barium enema should be avoided because of the risk of perforation, producing a barium peritonitis which may be life-threatening. If a contrast study is thought necessary, a water-soluble medium should be used. Endoscopy is usually unhelpful because it is difficult to negotiate a tortuous and inflamed sigmoid colon. However, it may be of some value to see an unbreached mucosa which can help to differentiate acute perforated diverticulitis from a perforated carcinoma.

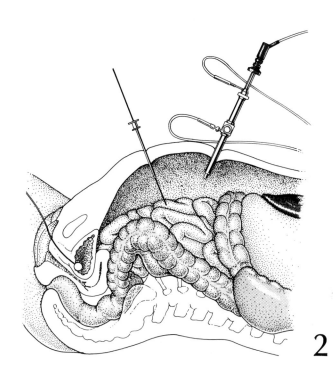

2

2 Occasionally it may be difficult to reach a firm preoperative diagnosis, especially in the elderly or rotund patient. In this circumstance, diagnostic laparoscopy may be useful. If free pus or faeces is seen, then the patient requires immediate laparotomy. Patients who have a localized peridiverticulitis can avoid open surgery. A unilocular abscess can be drained under direct vision as an alternative to drainage under CT control.

Preparation

Preoperative resuscitation and treatment are instituted together in the form of intravenous fluids, antibiotics and no oral intake. Nasogastric intubation is usually unnecessary and merely adds to the patient's discomfort. If, at the time of CT scan a localized abscess with defined walls is identified, it may be treated initially with percutaneous drainage under radiological guidance. This may avoid an emergency operation, although a high percentage of patients will require later elective resection. Although many of these patients are moderately sick, some (particularly the elderly) may need vigorous resuscitation and cardiopulmonary support aided by a Swan-Ganz catheter. Occasionally, perforated diverticulitis may present with fasciitis of the

abdominal wall or the thigh. This complication may be associated with a gas-forming organism and is an indication for early surgery and wide debridement of the area. Occasionally, further early surgery is required for excision of the fasciitis. More usually, and apart from the obvious free perforation or ruptured pericolic abscess, the indication for surgery is failure to improve on maximum medical therapy 24–48 h after admission to hospital.

Anaesthesia

General anaesthesia with endotracheal intubation is required. Regional spinal anaesthesia adds unnecessarily to the time taken for the surgery but can be used.

Position of patient

The patient is positioned supine on the operating table with the legs in stirrups. This position distributes the assistants around the operating table and provides access to the perineum to irrigate the rectum, to use an end-to-end stapling machine, and occasionally to allow for a cystoscopy to place ureteric stents. The abdomen and perineum are prepared and draped.

Selection of operative procedure

The choice of surgical procedure will depend not only on the extent of disease, but on the experience of the surgeon, the clinical condition of the patient before and during the operation, and the severity of coexisting disease. For instance, the surgeon confident and skilled in techniques of primary anastomosis may choose to perform a Hartmann's procedure in a patient who becomes unstable during surgery or for patients who are on steroids because of the high incidence of anastomotic breakdown under these circumstances.

3a–f The full spectrum of surgical choices is as follows.

1. Proximal diverting colostomy and placement of drains (*Illustration 3a*).
2. Bowel exteriorization (von Mikulicz operation, *Illustration 3b*) – of historical interest only.
3. Resection with colostomy and mucous fistula (*Illustration 3c*).
4. Resection with colostomy and Hartmann's pouch (*Illustration 3d*).
5. Resection and primary anastomosis with or without proximal defunctioning stoma (*Illustrations 3e, f*).

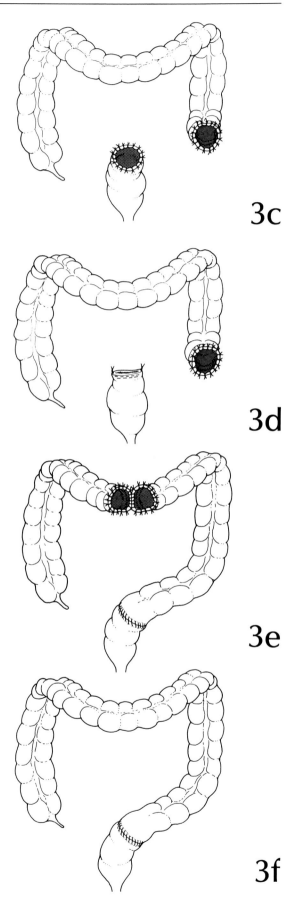

3c

3d

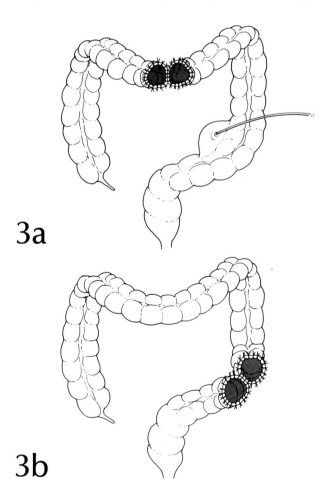

3a

3b

3e

3f

Proximal diverting colostomy and placement of drains

At one time this was standard therapy for the treatment of perforated diverticular disease which was supplemented with local suture plication if a hole was seen in the intestinal wall. However, over the past 20 years it has become accepted that this is inadequate therapy because stool located between the site of the stoma and the intestinal perforation will frequently continue to emerge into the peritoneal cavity resulting in an expected high mortality rate. However if, at the time of abdominal exploration, an acute phlegmonous diverticulitis is found *without* free perforation or abscess formation, local irrigation of the inflamed area (with or without local drains and with or without a defunctioning proximal loop stoma) has been reported to be associated with a good outcome. Under adverse conditions, an inexperienced surgeon might treat free perforation of the intestine with vigorous intraperitoneal irrigation, proximal stoma and local perforation closure using an absorbable synthetic suture material buttressed with omentum. Such a procedure should be seen as a temporary measure until such time as the patient can be transferred for more definitive therapy or the availability of a more experienced surgeon. Preferably, a fully trained surgeon should proceed to one of the excisional techniques described below for the treatment of perforated diverticular disease.

Resection with colostomy and mucous fistula

This procedure results in the removal of the diseased bowel but gives the patient two stomas to manage. The benefit of a mucous fistula is that bowel reconstruction is somewhat easier than after a Hartmann procedure.

Resection with Hartmann's pouch

When there is an insufficient length of distal colon to bring to the abdominal wall, the bowel may be closed as a Hartmann's pouch with either sutures or staples. The stump should then be secured to the sacral promontory with non-absorbable sutures to prevent it from descending into the pelvis and to facilitate subsequent bowel reconstruction. The second operation to reconstruct the bowel is often a difficult procedure because of small intestine adhesions in the pelvis which obscure the Hartmann's pouch. These adhesions tend to resolve with time; therefore a 16–20-week waiting period is recommended before the second operation. The commonly experienced difficulties with intestinal reconstruction after the Hartmann procedure and its associated morbidity and mortality rates should be borne in mind when contemplating the optimum procedure for each individual patient.

Resection with primary anastomosis

Resection of the diseased bowel to include the rectosigmoid junction followed by immediate bowel anastomosis is a controversial recommendation. The belief that an anastomosis in the presence of peritonitis may lead to a higher incidence of anastomotic failure has dissuaded many surgeons from performing this procedure. However, experience has shown that the overall morbidity and mortality rates from 'staged' procedures are as high or even higher than from a carefully planned and executed single-stage operation. Furthermore, if the surgeon is unsure about the security of the anastomosis, a proximal stoma (loop colostomy or loop ileostomy) is an additional safeguard which is relatively simple to reverse at a later date. Two developments have made the operative approach safer: first, 'on-table' orthograde colonic lavage[3, 4], and second, the intraluminal bypass tube[5] (Coloshield).

Operations

COLOSTOMY WITH DRAINAGE

A lower midline incision is made and the diagnosis of a localized abscess is confirmed. If frank peritonitis or faecal soiling is found, bowel resection is then the preferred treatment.

4 The abscess is usually located in the mesentery or between the mesentery and lateral abdominal wall. Gentle blunt dissection with the operating finger placed in a gauze swab, working downwards from the abdominal wall, will allow the cavity to be entered. Soft Penrose drains should be placed and brought out laterally with as straight a tract as possible to facilitate drainage.

The adjacent small bowel may adhere to the mass and should be gently separated away, taking care not to injure the serosa of the bowel.

In placing the colostomy (*see* chapter on pp. 274–283) the surgeon should remember that the greater the distance from the distal limb to the perforation, the more faecal material can leak; however, placing the colostomy close to the perforation may render subsequent resection difficult.

On rare occasions it may be considered safer to close a perforation with interrupted, absorbable synthetic sutures as a temporary measure. Great care is necessary because the tissues are friable and the perforation may be enlarged, which would then mandate intestinal resection.

RESECTION WITH COLOSTOMY AND MUCOUS FISTULA

A lower midline incision is made and extended above the umbilicus as required. The patient is placed in a head-down position and rotated towards the right so that the small intestine drops away from the operative field. Once the small intestine has been carefully dissected free of the mass, it is placed in warm moist packs. The sigmoid colon is gently manually retracted towards the midline to expose the fascial layer of Toldt, which is incised, taking great care to note the gonadal vessels and ureter, which may be palpated and visualized as it lies over the iliac vessels.

The colon should be palpated above until normal bowel is felt. To prevent further faecal soiling, a soft clamp should be placed across the bowel at this point; this will form the proximal line of resection.

The distal dissection should be carried down towards the peritoneal reflection beyond the diseased bowel at the top of the rectum.

If there is any concern about the presence of malignant disease, a cancer operation should be performed. The distal margin is defined and clamps are

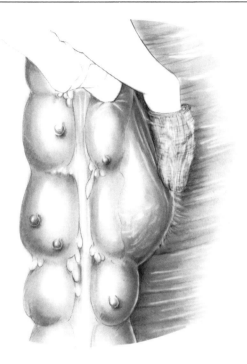

4

placed at the resection margin in the upper rectum. The vessels may be secured and divided close to the intestine when the surgeon is certain that a malignancy is not present. However, in practice this is difficult because the mesentery tends to be oedematous and thickened and it is usually technically easier to locate and divide the vessels towards the base of the mesentery.

It will usually be necessary to mobilize the splenic flexure to provide sufficient length to fashion an anastomosis without tension, but great care should be taken to avoid splenic injury. The intestine may be divided using the GIA stapling device and this renders it easier to draw the proximal colon through the circular incision for the colostomy.

Once the specimen has been resected, the abdomen should be copiously lavaged and the site of the colostomy in the abdominal wall should be chosen. Ideally this should be along a line joining the anterior superior iliac spine with the umbilicus, but the state of the patient's abdomen and previous scars and skin creases may dictate otherwise (*see* chapter on pp. 274–283).

The closed distal intestine is brought out of the lower end of the wound and secured to the skin. The abdomen is then closed in layers. Once the main wound has been covered, the colostomy is sutured with interrupted mucocutaneous sutures of chromic catgut.

If there is gross peritoneal soiling, a delayed primary closure of the skin may be used by inserting a series of interrupted, loosely tied sutures to the skin and interposing this with a ribbon gauze soaked with povidone-iodine. The ribbon gauze is changed twice daily by the nursing staff. If the wound is clean at 3 days, the pack may be removed and the sutures tightened.

HARTMANN'S PROCEDURE

5 The operation is carried out as described in the previous section; however, if the distal bowel is too short to be brought out as a mucous fistula, the upper rectum may be closed as a Hartmann's pouch with a transverse stapling device or by suture. The pouch should then be secured to the sacral promontory with two large silk sutures to prevent the upper rectum from falling into the pelvis, becoming kinked (which may result in a small closed loop bowel obstruction), and to facilitate finding the rectal stump at a subsequent operation. It is unnecessary to place drains into the pelvis.

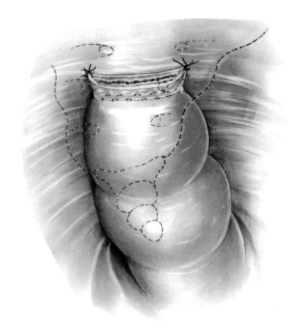

5

RESECTION WITH PRIMARY ANASTOMOSIS AND PROXIMAL COLOSTOMY

During this operation it is necessary to locate healthy intestine with minimally thickened muscle, and splenic flexure mobilization is usually required to achieve this objective. However, splenic flexure mobilization should not be attempted in the unstable patient or by the inexperienced surgeon.

6 The anastomotic technique should be the surgeon's preference. The author uses an interrupted single layer of inverting sutures with absorbable synthetic material (2/0 polyglycolic acid). The usual tenets of colonic anastomosis must be strictly adhered to: there must be no anastomotic tension (by mobilization of the splenic flexure); a good blood supply (pulsatile bleeding) should be present; and careful attention must be paid to the technical details of suture placement (*see* chapter on pp. 51–73). It is useful in this circumstance to place the sutures in guy-rope fashion and run them down in groups once the posterior layer has been completed.

If the pelvis is narrow, the surgeon may choose to use a stapled anastomosis, but the ends of the intestine tend to be sufficiently thickened that concern for staple penetration through the intestinal wall may be justified.

A right-sided proximal transverse colostomy is then raised, which should be reversed at about 6 weeks after operation once a contrast study demonstrates anastomotic integrity. The use of drains should be avoided.

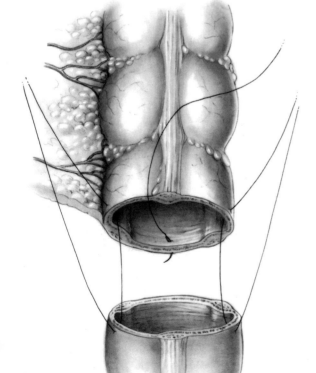

6

RESECTION WITH PRIMARY ANASTOMOSIS WITH NO COLOSTOMY

As mentioned earlier, this is a challenging procedure for an experienced surgeon. Two recent developments may improve success: first, on-table colonic lavage (*see* chapter on pp. 397–415) and second, the intracolonic bypass tube.

Intracolonic bypass tube

This device has been demonstrated experimentally to be of value in reducing faecal soiling of the anastomosis and is associated with improved anastomotic healing. It has been used in colonic perforation[6] as an adjunct to primary anastomosis to avoid the need for a proximal defunctioning stoma.

7a, b After the diseased bowel has been removed, it is necessary to evert a cuff of approximately 4 cm of proximal colon. This is easier when there has been an element of obstruction which leads to proximal colonic dilatation. Four intraluminal stay sutures of silk are placed, and a gentle traction eversion is achieved. Babcock forceps may also be placed on the edge of the intestine and a section of proximal colon induced through this lip. If the intestine is very contracted, Hegar dilators can be used to widen it. The author has not found the administration of glucagon to be of value.

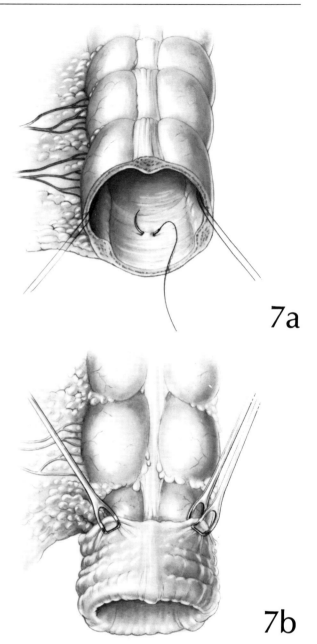

7a

7b

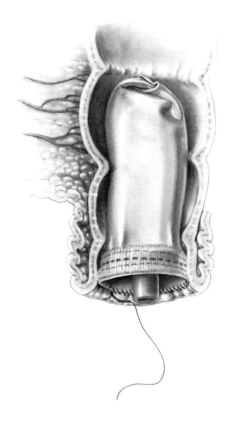

8

8 An appropriately sized intracolonic bypass tube is selected, always trying to use the largest available but without forcing the device into position. The tube is folded in parachute fashion and may be lubricated to ease insertion. If the intestine is very contracted, it is preferable to open the bypass tube so that the proximal polyester reinforcing band can be apposed directly to the inside of the lumen of the proximal bowel. The tube should be sutured to the proximal colon with a locking, running stitch of 2/0 polyglycolic acid, being sure to pick up mucosa and submucosa. There is a very definite feel to incorporating this latter bowel layer and some experience is required to recognize this sensation.

9 Once the tubocolonic anastomosis has been completed, it should be checked by trying to insert a pair of mosquito forceps in between the tube and the colon to look for gaps. If present, they should be closed with interrupted polyglycolic acid sutures.

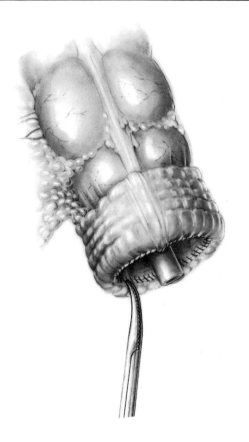

9

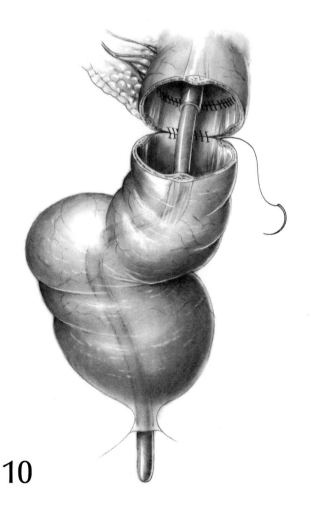

10

10 The everted cuff should now be returned to its previous position and the serosa of the colon checked for perforation of the tubocolonic anastomotic line. If present, a serosal horizontal mattress suture should be placed.

For a sutured anastomosis, the rectal probe is now attached to the intraluminal bypass tube; this is a useful 'handle' to lift up the intestine. The author prefers a single layer of interrupted inverting polyglycolic acid sutures and these are now placed. The rectal probe is then passed distally and retrieved at the anus by an unscrubbed assistant.

The tube can be unravelled at this juncture, but the author prefers to leave it in position because of the risk of perforating the tube with the anterior sutures.

The anterior layer of colorectal anastomotic sutures is now placed.

Traction on the rectal probe will lead the intraluminal bypass tube to unravel and come to lie across the anastomosis while providing for luminal continuity.

If the assistant gently pulls on the rectal probe, the surgeon will be able to feel the tubocolonic anastomosis and ensure that it is patent.

11 Once the mesenteric defect, peritoneal cavity and abdomen have been closed, the surgeon's attention should be directed to the perineum. Gentle traction should be placed on the tube and it should then be incised. A finger should be placed inside the lumen of the tube to ensure that the latex surfaces are not adherent so that faeces may pass. The tube may now be fully cut across and will then retract and come to lie within the rectal ampulla.

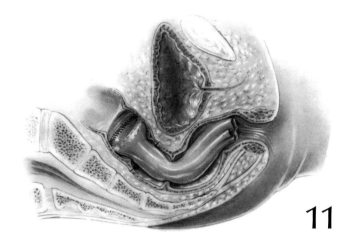

11

Postoperative care

Antibiotics should continue and be adjusted as indicated by the sensitivity of intraoperative cultures. Intravenous fluids should be administered according to metabolic need. The patient should ideally spend the first 24 h in the intensive care unit, as elderly patients are at great risk from the complications of septicaemia. A nasogastric tube is usually necessary and will have been placed during operation. The urinary catheter may be discontinued when the patient has achieved fluid balance and is alert enough to urinate. When the ileus resolves, the nasogastric tube may be spigotted and residual volumes taken. When these decrease, the nasogastric tube is removed, oral fluids are commenced and the patient can progress to a normal diet. For the patient with a colostomy, nursing care should be supplemented with psychological support.

References

1. Painter NS, Burkitt DP. Diverticular disease of the colon: a deficiency disease of Western civilization. *BMJ* 1971; 2: 450–4.

2. Hinchey EJ, Schaal PGH, Richards GK. Treatment of perforated diverticular disease of the colon. *Adv Surg* 1978; 12: 85–109.

3. Munro A, Steele RJC, Logie JRC. Technique for intra-operative colonic irrigation. *Br J Surg* 1987; 74: 1039–40.

4. Radcliffe AG, Dudley HAF. Intraoperative antegrade irrigation of the large intestine. *Surg Gynecol Obstet* 1983; 156: 721–3.

5. Ravo B. Colorectal anastomotic healing and intracolonic bypass procedure. *Surg Clin North Am* 1988; 68: 1267–94.

6. Ravo B, Mishrick A, Addei K, Gastrini G, Pappalardo G, Gross E. The treatment of perforated diverticulitis by one-stage intracolonic bypass procedure. *Surgery* 1987; 102: 771–6.

Illustrations by Gillian Lee

Colonic surgery for acute conditions: obstruction

L. P. Fielding MB, FRCS, FACS
Chief of Surgery, St Mary's Hospital, Waterbury, Connecticut, Clinical Professor of Surgery, Yale University School of Medicine, Connecticut, USA and Visiting Clinical Scientist, St Mary's Hospital, London, UK

Principles and justification

Large bowel obstruction is a relatively common complication of lesions in the colon and rectum, usually caused by a primary tumour. The discussion in this chapter will be centred on this aetiology, although the principles of mangement can be applied to any other cause of large gut obstruction. The two specific disease processes of toxic megacolon and volvulus are discussed in other chapters (*see* pp. 420–435). One of the problems about discussing the relative merits of different methods of treatment of intestinal obstruction is that there is no clear definition of the condition. It seems reasonable, therefore, to divide the subject into three subsections: (1) bowel stenosis resulting in faecal loading but without obstruction to intestinal gas; (2) complete obstruction to the onward flow of faecal matter, fluid and gas, but without major systemic upset; and (3) the addition of major systemic metabolic problems, usually caused by longstanding obstruction with or without bowel perforation.

The implications for therapy of these three subsets of large bowel obstruction will be discussed at the relevant points during the chapter. In a survey[1] which reviewed the clinical practice of 84 surgeons, it was clear that there was a spectrum of methods employed to treat these conditions. However, the overall figures indicated that immediate tumour resection (with or without bowel reconstruction) was practised more frequently at all sites than the method of bowel decompression followed at a later date, by tumour resection (staged resection): right colon 96%; splenic flexure 75%; left colon 55%. Over the last 10 years the trend towards immediate resection, even for left-sided obstructing colonic tumours, appears to have increased. Thus, at each site primary tumour excision will be described first and a staged procedure will be described as an alternative method of treatment.

Preoperative

General assessment of patient on admission

1 The severity of clinical illness suffered by patients with intestinal obstruction is very variable, ranging from the patient with colicky abdominal pain alone to a severely ill person with gross systemic and metabolic derangement associated with multiorgan failure. It is worthwhile, therefore, to review systematically all principal body systems, obtain baseline information on each and be prepared to monitor the function of all. In particular, in haemodynamically unstable patients, a Swan–Ganz catheter is necessary to assess cardiac function and provide fluid resuscitation to establish maximal cardiac output without central overload. Pulmonary and renal function need to be reviewed and supported. This will generate a large volume of information which should be integrated by an experienced surgeon and the most ill patients should be placed in the critical care unit. It seems that the key to good results is the presence and active participation of a senior and interested surgeon at *all* stages of management.

Anaesthesia

It is usual for these patients to have general inhalation anaesthesia with muscle relaxants and positive pressure ventilation. Some anaesthetists will include as part of their technique an epidural or spinal anaesthetic, which will reduce the need for muscle relaxant drugs and their reversal. The latter techniques improve the operative field, reduce blood loss and assist with immediate postoperative pain control.

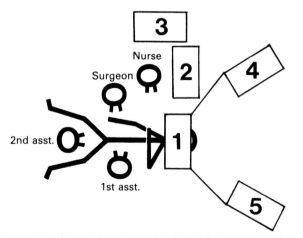

1, overhead table; 2, instrument trolley; 3, instrument trolley; 4, anaesthetic machine; 5, anaesthetic table

2

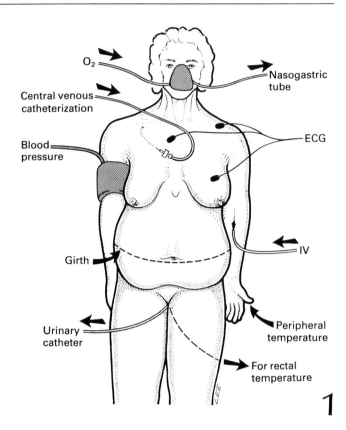

1

Operations

Position of patient

2 It is useful to place the patient in the lithotomy-Trendelenburg position with Allen stirrups, which allows an approach to be made to the anal canal during surgery and places a second surgical assistant in a position to be of greater help than when the patient is in the simple supine position (*see Illustration 3* on page 48). However, this operative set-up does have its disadvantages in that it is somewhat more difficult for the instrument nurse to see the operative field (and therefore to assist the surgeon), and the anaesthetist will need to make special arrangements to maintain access to the patient's head and shoulders.

The essential features of the position are that there should be a small sandbag under the sacrum, which should be sited at the end of the table proper (the bottom leaf of the table should be removed), and that the legs are in the stirrups, which are also level with the end of the table. This allows the legs to be raised, but the hip joint is abducted then flexed to a *minimal* degree. A large neurosurgical type of overtable is placed above the head end of the operating area. Once this position has been achieved, the patient is catheterized, placed in 15° head-down tilt, cleansed and draped.

Abdominal incision

3 Assuming that the object of therapy is to carry out a primary tumour resection, a long midline incision skirting the umbilicus is made at the very start of the procedure. The incision should extend from the pubic skin crease to two-thirds of the way between the umbilicus and xiphisternum. In patients with gross intestinal obstruction and obesity, a full length pubis to xiphisternum incision should be carried out.

Some surgeons may disagree with an immediate tumour resection and wish to fashion a so-called 'decompressive loop transverse colostomy', in which case a modest-sized left paramedian incision or a midline incision is carried out to preserve the upper right quadrant for the stoma.

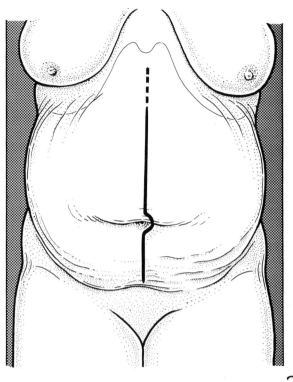

3

Bacteriology

4 Once the abdomen is opened there is always some free fluid present, some of which should be placed in a sterile screw-capped pot and sent for aerobic and anaerobic culture.

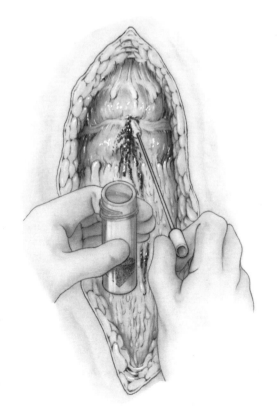

4

Bowel decompression

Once the abdomen has been opened, irrespective of the site of the obstructing lesion, the next procedure is to deflate the distended bowel, which will allow greater access to the abdominal cavity and reduce the risk of intestinal perforation. The caecum is inspected to make sure a perforation has neither taken place nor is imminent. Assuming that the caecum is undamaged three techniques are described that can be used singly or in combination.

Needle aspiration

5   A 14-gauge intravenous needle is attached to the sucker system and passed obliquely through a taenia coli into the lumen of the transverse colon. Care is taken to keep the tip of the needle within the luminal gas rather than the fluid content because if the needle touches fluid faeces it immediately becomes blocked. Gas can be transferred from the remainder of the bowel to the transverse colon by applying pressure in both flanks simultaneously.

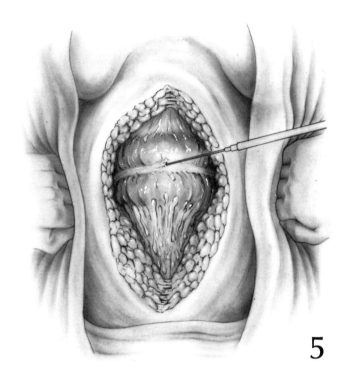

5

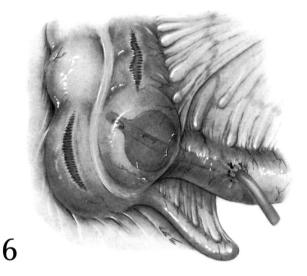

6

Foley catheter decompression

6   It is frequently found that simple needle aspiration alone is not adequate to decompress the right side of the colon. This can be achieved by passing a large Foley catheter through a purse-string placed in the distal ileum, through the ileocaecal valve and then on into the colon. Gentle intermittent suction on the catheter will eventually allow considerable quantities of liquid faeces to be aspirated, thus decompressing the bowel

An alternative site of access to the bowel for the Foley catheter is the appendix stump. However, this site may be more prone to leakage.

Small bowel decompression

7 In patients with an incompetent ileocaecal valve (or as a secondary phenomenon to adherence to a tumour) the small bowel itself is frequently found to be distended. If this occurs in the distal small bowel, fluid may be 'milked' into the caecum and then aspirated through the Foley catheter (*see Illustration 6*). When the upper part of the small intestine is affected, gas and fluid may be 'stripped' back through the pylorus into the stomach and then aspirated through a large nasogastric tube.

It must be noted at this point that if a segment of small bowel is attached to the primary tumour or if a lymph node with secondary tumour is present the small bowel must *not* be 'peeled-off' but must be resected *en bloc* with the tumour and then the bowel reconstructed. This is a basic concept in surgery for tumours and if it is not observed the surgeon can expect to find a cluster of intraperitoneal secondary deposits occurring 9–18 months after tumour resection. Once the bowel has been decompressed, a full laparotomy is possible.

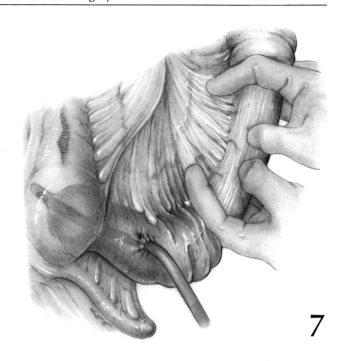

7

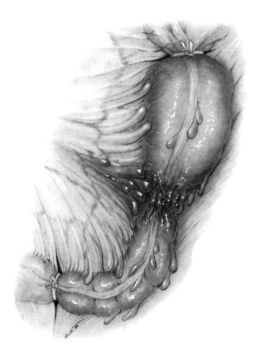

8

Laparotomy findings

8 First, the nature of the obstructing lesion should be sought and, if it is a tumour, some assessment of its mobility should be made gently at this stage of the operation. Sites of secondary spread to the peritoneum or liver are sought and then a systematic laparotomy is carried out.

Assuming that the tumour is considered removable, tapes are tied around the bowel both proximal and distal to the obstructing tumour to prevent intraluminal spread of malignant cells. The remaining small and large bowel are packed away into the abdominal cavity or may be exteriorized into a plastic bag.

Once the large and small bowel have been completely decompressed, resective surgery can continue as for the elective case.

IMMEDIATE TUMOUR RESECTION FOR OBSTRUCTING LEFT-SIDED COLONIC LESIONS

The mobilization of a left-sided tumour may be divided into six basic phases:

Phase 1: division of arterial supply and venous drainage and visualization of the left ureter.
Phase 2: mobilization of the left colon.
Phase 3: mobilization of the splenic flexure.
Phase 4: complete distal mobilization.
Phase 5: division of the bowel.
Phase 6: consideration of immediate anastomosis.

Phase 1: securing vascular supply

Depending on the bulk of the transverse colon and small bowel, it may be possible to pack these organs into the upper abdomen, or it may be necessary to place the small bowel in a plastic bag which can then be exteriorized on the abdominal wall.

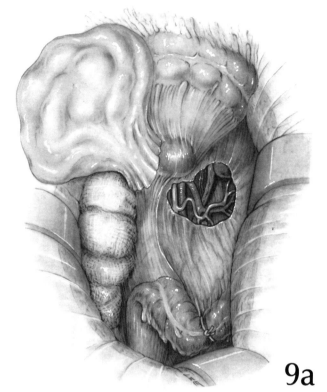

9a

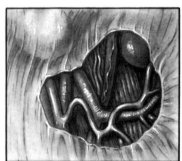

9b

9a, b The aorta is displayed below the fourth part of the duodenum and, assuming that a radical resection is possible, the inferior mesenteric artery is divided at its origin from the aorta (for distal lesions, this vessel may be divided just distal to the ascending branch of the left colic). The mobilization of this part of the mesentery requires the control of small arteries and veins by electrocoagulation.

The dissection then moves 1.5–2 cm left and laterally where the inferior mesenteric vein is found running due 'north' to join the splenic vessel. This structure is divided according to the level of division of its sister artery.

10 As the mesentery is mobilized and lifted forward, the central portion of the left ureter must be identified and protected. The dissection is then carried laterally in front of the plane containing the ureter, continuing the mobilization of the bowel mesentery. The mesentery is divided at the site of bowel division. There should be at least 5 cm of normal-looking bowel between the tumour and the resection margins. There is usually more at the proximal resection site because this site is determined by the colour of the bowel after the required vessels have been divided – at least 5 cm must be removed proximal to the site at which the bowel colour changes from pink to blue.

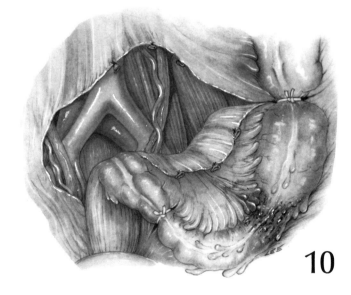

10

Phase 2: mobilization of the tumour

11 The colon is then lifted forward and to the patient's right; and the congenital adhesion of the sigmoid colon is divided revealing the ureter and iliac vessels. The peritoneum overlying the left paracolic gutter is similarly divided. There is usually a tendency for the gonadal vessels to be taken forward on to the specimen. If these structures are well away from any tumour and are not fixed or tethered, they may be swept posteriorly and preserved. If the tumour is at the rectosigmoid junction or in the upper rectum itself, the rectum will require mobilization (*see* chapter on pp. 456–471).

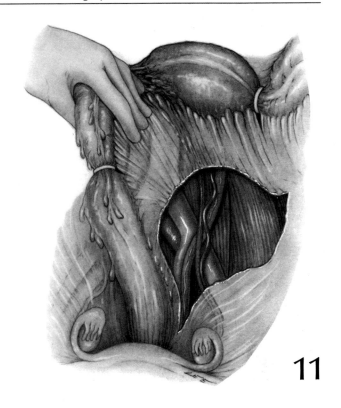

11

Phase 3: mobilization of the splenic flexure

In almost all radical left-sided resections it is necessary to mobilize the splenic flexure and this procedure is carried out in three separate stages. The surgeon should stand to the patient's right.

Posterior dissection

12 Having started to divide the peritoneal reflexion in the left paracolic gutter, the surgeon carries this incision in the peritoneum upwards towards the spleen. The colon itself is pulled across to the patient's right and with blunt dissection the mesentery to the colon is separated from perirenal fat. At this stage of the procedure it is very easy to go too far posteriorly and lift the kidney forward. This must be avoided because it leads into the wrong plane and also opens up, unnecessarily, a false plane.

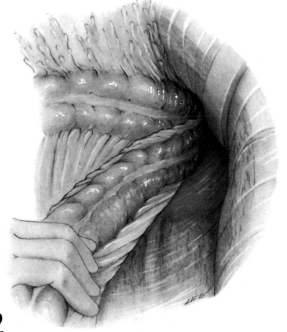

12

13 Once the correct plane is achieved this tissue line is developed by blunt finger and gauze dissection until the surgeon's hand comes to lie behind the splenic flexure.

No attempt is made at this time to pull the colon down towards the pelvis because this may rupture small adhesions on the spleen itself.

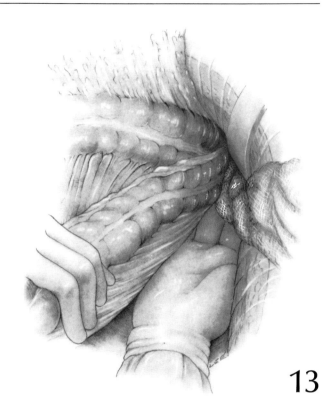

13

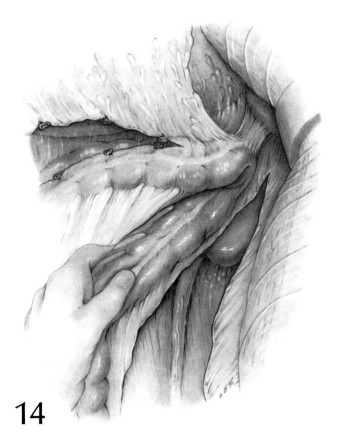

14

Anterior dissection: mobilization of the great omentum

14 If the lesion is distal the omentum may be dissected free from the 'bloodless plane' of the colon, gradually working towards the apex of the splenic flexure. Here again the transverse colon should not be pulled forcibly towards the midline for fear of splenic damage.

15 For more proximal lesions, when the left part of the omentum needs to be taken *en bloc* in a specimen, the great omentum is mobilized from the stomach by dividing the short vessels leading from the epiploic arch to the greater curve. When the short vessels from the splenic hilum are encountered, the left gastroepiploic vessel is divided and the dissection directed to the apex of the splenic flexure.

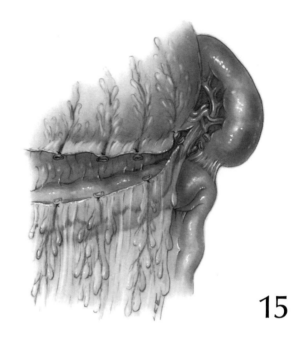

15

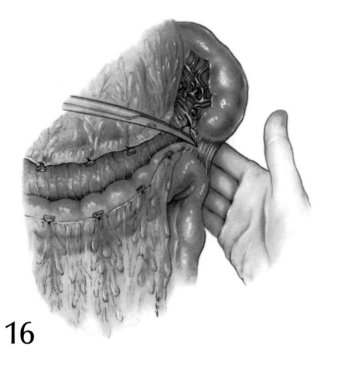

16

Release of splenic flexure

16 Having established the posterior and anterior parts of the dissection, the operator's right hand is placed behind the splenic flexure and, using long dissecting scissors with the left hand, the remaining attachment of the splenic flexure to the spleen is divided under direct vision. Sometimes vessels at this point need to be formally ligated.

For tumours near the splenic flexure, when direct invasion of the spleen or the tail of the pancreas may have occurred, the dissection follows the line between the left gastroepiploic vessels and the stomach but continues up, dividing the short gastric vessels. The peritoneum around the spleen is divided, mobilizing this structure, which can then be brought down with the tail of the pancreas to be taken *en bloc* with the resected specimen. The splenic vessels are divided. The pancreas is divided by traversing the gland with a knife and three structures will then need to be ligated separately – the superior and inferior pancreatic vessels and the pancreatic duct. It is usually possible then to suture the tail of the pancreas by interrupted sutures to complete its closure.

Phases 4 and 5

The mobilization of the distal colon is then completed to a point at least 5 cm distal to the tumour. The proximal and distal points of bowel transection are now ready to be divided before discarding the specimen.

Phase 6: immediate *versus* delayed anastomosis

At this point in the operation the surgeon must decide either to prepare for an immediate anastomosis or to delay this procedure to a second operation. If the patient is relatively fit, if the bowel is judged to be suitable to take sutures securely and if the surgeon is confident of achieving primary anastomotic union, the anastomosis is performed. If not, the anastomosis is delayed. The techniques involved in these two procedures will be discussed in turn.

'On-table' orthograde bowel lavage[2]

Before an anastomosis can be constructed safely the proximal bowel needs to be mechanically empty, which can be achieved by 'on-table' bowel lavage. A Foley catheter is inserted into the distal ileum as described for bowel decompression (*see Illustration 6*).

17, 18 A long length of presterilized anaesthetic scavenging tubing is attached very firmly, with a watertight fit, to a 10-cm long metal connector, which is inserted into the bowel, having discarded the specimen some 8 cm distal to the site of the eventual anastomosis. Packs need to be placed carefully around the area to catch any spillage and three tissue-holding (Babcock) forceps are placed on the edge of the bowel to aid the introduction of the anaesthetic tubing. Once the metal connector is in place, two strong nylon tapes are secured around the bowel, tying the colon to the metal tube.

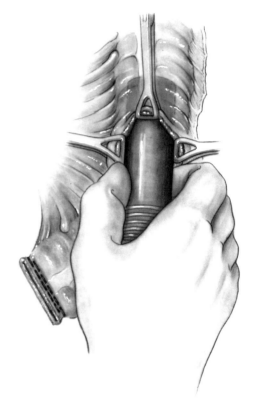

17

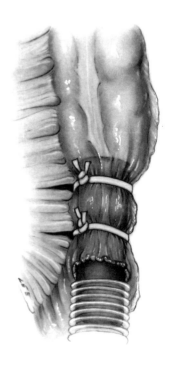

18

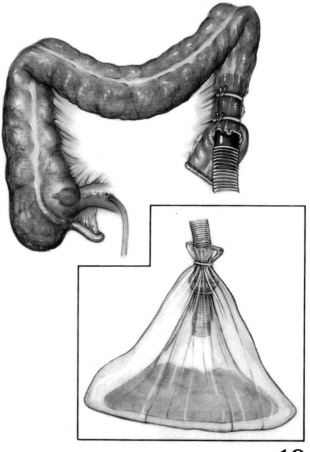

19 The distal end of the anaesthetic tubing is placed over the table and into two plastic bags, one inside the other, and tied on to the tubing to form a closed system. Physiological saline or Hartmann's solution, which must be warmed to body temperature to avoid cooling the patient, is then instilled into the proximal colon through the Foley catheter.

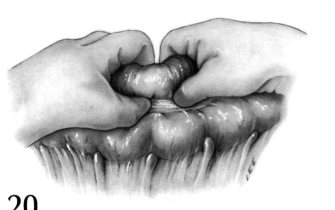

20 While this fluid is progressing through the colon, any faecal matter is broken down by finger pressure into pellets of not more than half the diameter of the anaesthetic scavenging tubing.

21a, b Blockage of the tubing by faeces will eventually cause extreme technical difficulty and result in faecal contamination of the peritoneal cavity. The irrigant fluid is helped around the colon by intermittent pressure on the ascending and transverse and (possibly) descending colon, so that no segment becomes over-distended.

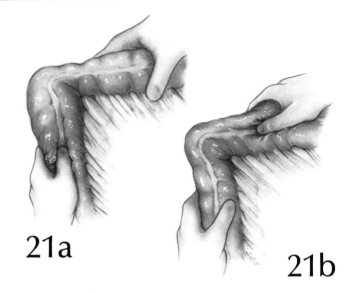

21a

21b

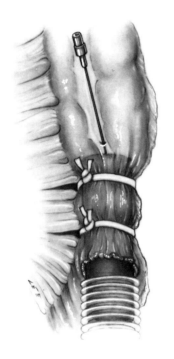

22

22 As fluid flows down the anaesthetic tubing, a negative pressure is produced, sucking the colon into the tubing. This can be avoided by placing a large intravenous hypodermic needle, which acts as a vent, through the proximal colon.

23 The procedure is continued until all faecal residue has been manipulated out of the colon and the effluent is running clear.

The distal (usually somewhat damaged) colon is then discarded, along with the anaesthetic tubing, at the site of anastomosis.

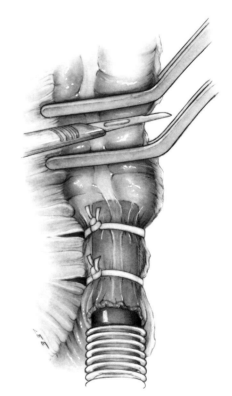

23

Cleansing of the distal segment

24 A proctoscope is passed into the anal canal and through it a large calibre (28 Fr) Foley catheter is inserted. Through the catheter physiological saline is introduced to wash the rectum and low sigmoid colon below the occluding clamp. At the end of this procedure the irrigant fluid is changed to mercury perchloride 1:500, which will prevent seeding of any residual malignant cells at the anastomotic site.

A second crushing clamp is placed distal to the first and the intervening short segment of colon is discarded. The anastomosis then proceeds and the author uses an open technique of one-layer, interrupted, musculosub-mucosal sutures, 3–4 mm apart (*see* chapter on pp. 456–471). After the anastomosis, this area and the whole peritoneal cavity are extensively lavaged with warmed physiological saline containing tetracycline (1 g/l). If the anastomosis is below the peritoneal reflexion suction drains are placed anteriorly and posteriorly. These are removed on the second day postoperatively. The author does not use drains after an intra-abdominal anastomosis.

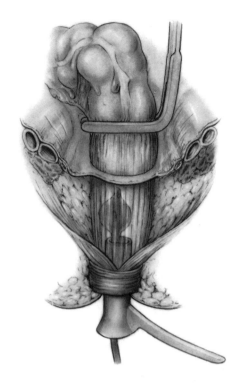

24

Techniques for delayed anastomosis

If the conditions to consider a primary anastomosis do not apply, the proximal colon should be brought out as an end-colostomy using the techniques described in the chapter on pp. 488–496. One modification of this technique which has been found useful after adequate bowel decompression is to bring the bowel out through the abdominal wall leaving the bowel closed for some 2–3 days to allow the bowel to adhere to its surroundings before being contaminated by faeces.

If the distal end of the bowel is not long enough to reach the anterior abdominal wall the rectum is irrigated as described above. The second crushing clamp is placed across the bowel after this irrigation and the intervening short segment of gut is gradually excised at the same time that the rectal stump is oversewn using the 'cut and stitch' method to prevent any rectal contents spilling into the pelvis. Alternatively, the rectal stump may be stapled closed with a TA 55 stapler.

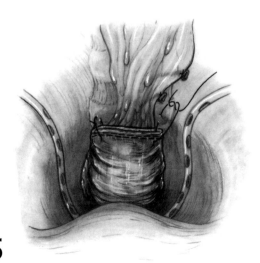

25

25 In order to avoid the rectum falling into the pelvis and becoming kinked, the apex of the rectal stump is sutured to the presacral fascia. This will assist in a subsequent operation if reconstruction is undertaken (*see* chapter on pp. 488–496).

Two suction drains are placed into the pelvis and removed when no further serosanguineous fluid is obtained.

26a, b If the distal bowel is long enough to reach the anterior abdominal wall, the distal bowel may be divided between crushing clamps of the Zachery–Cope design – the distal crushing element is not removed from the bowel, which is brought out through the lower end of the laparotomy incision. Sufficient length of bowel needs to be left so that a gauze dressing may be placed underneath this crushing clamp to raise it above the closed abdominal wound surface by about 2–3 cm.

The length of 'proud' bowel may be excised once it has become fixed into the wound (8–10 days) thus forming an open mucous fistula. The rectum itself should not be mobilized in order to make adequate length to bring to the abdominal wall as this opens up planes in the pelvis which may give rise to troublesome, and occasionally severe, pelvic sepsis. If there is not adequate length, it is better to close the distal bowel as a Hartmann's procedure (*see* above).

Before closing the abdomen, any site of tumour attachment or any possible peritoneal or liver secondary tumours should be biopsied so that adequate tumour staging can be obtained in consultation with the histopathologist.

An alternative method of handling the distal bowel is to divide it using the GIA machine, leaving sufficient length for the bowel to rest easily 0.5–1.0 cm above the abdominal wall skin once closed. At the end of the closing sequence, the bowel is *not* opened but sutured to the skin. Depending on the patient's further management, the site may remain closed, be opened as a stoma or, if there are no plans to reconstruct the bowel and if there is no distal obstruction in the rectum, the bowel above the level of the skin can be trimmed under local anaesthesia and a simple running absorbable suture used to close the stoma. Eventually the skin will heal over the area, leaving the closed bowel end in the subcutaneous tissue where it can be opened with ease should the need arise.

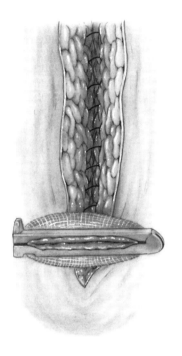

26a

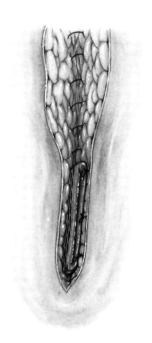

26b

Closing sequence

After all these procedures, extensive lavage is carried out with warmed physiological saline containing tetracycline 1 g/l to remove blood and debris, to prevent possible contamination of faecal matter and also to reduce the *concentration* of organisms within the abdominal cavity and on the wound. All these patients run the risk of intra-abdominal complications of sepsis or adhesive obstruction and therefore it is important to have the most efficient technique of gastric decompression. For this reason the author performs a gastrostomy in all these patients, except those who have been on long-term steroids.

27a, b Abdominal wall closure is achieved with a mass suture technique, using a continuous 1 polydioxanone suture; each bite should be 1 cm from the incision line and each loop of the suture placed 1 cm apart. In the obese patient, care should be taken to include as little fat as possible because the tension in the suture line will rapidly diminish as the fat gives way.

Deep tension sutures should never be used. If there is any significant tension on the abdominal wall because of bowel distension or increased oedema of the bowel caused by the resuscitation fluids, forcing the bowel closed merely increases intra-abdominal tension and reduces the vascular supply to the gut. Furthermore, the increased tension in the abdominal wall may give rise to disruption or a serious fasciitis with tissue breakdown.

To avoid closing the abdominal wall under great tension, a mesh insert should be sutured in place to the fascia to maintain the gut *in situ*. One edge of the mesh is trimmed in a curve to fit the abdominal wall opening. The edge itself is then folded over so that there is a double layer of mesh being attached to the fascial edge. Once the first side of the mesh is in place, the abdominal wall is placed into a position where the second edge of the mesh can be trimmed, and once sutured will lie as 'snug' fit, but without tension.

When the patient's general condition has improved and the abdomen has become soft and less distended, the mesh may be divided in the midline, the omentum and bowel beneath gently lifted away from it. The mesh is then sutured, taking 2-cm bites of mesh on either side of the midline to gradually approximate the fascial edges. With a large mesh insert, this may need to be performed more than once. Subsequently, under general anaesthesia the mesh is removed and a routine mass closure of the fascial layer carried out. Although this process of mesh insert and 'graduated removal' appears laborious, it is important to remember that gut blood flow and venous return must not be compromised in these already very ill patients.

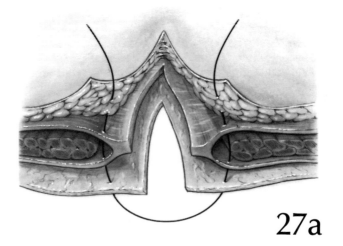

27a

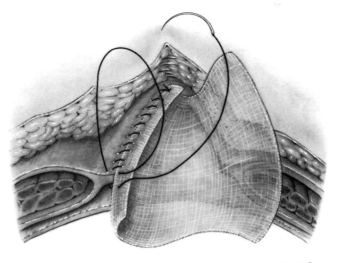

27b

28 Finally, after a further irrigation, the skin and subcutaneous tissues are lightly packed with dry gauze in preparation for delayed primary closure 48–72 h later.

Protection of anastomosis after immediate bowel reconstruction

This is a controversial subject in elective surgery and more so in patients undergoing immediate tumour resection and anastomosis in the face of bowel obstruction. The author's preference is to decide before starting the anastomosis whether undue difficulty will be encountered. If difficulty is likely, the author prefers not to proceed to anastomosis, but to construct an end colostomy and to either close the distal rectum as a Hartmann's procedure or to bring it out as a mucous fistula. The occurrence of a clinically significant anastomotic leak, especially in these patients (who are frequently elderly and ill) is, in the author's view a greater risk than that associated with the second operation when the patient has fully recovered. Furthermore, some patients may wish not to undergo a second procedure, having successfully survived the first.

Some surgeons advocate anastomotic 'protection' in all potentially compromised anastomoses (in the setting of obstruction, after irradiation, and even after ultra-low

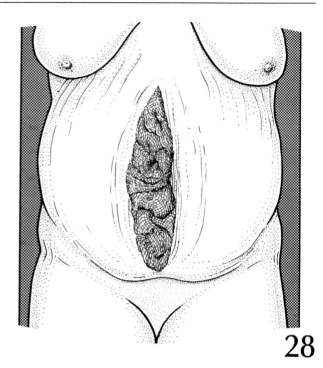

28

anterior resection of the rectum), by loop ileostomy (*see* pp. 243–269), transverse loop colostomy (*see* pp. 274–283), or the insertion of a Coloshield apparatus. The author has not used an anastomosis-protecting stoma or Coloshield in the setting of obstruction but recognizes that this represents a reasonable approach to anastomotic protection.

IMMEDIATE TUMOUR RESECTION FOR OBSTRUCTING RIGHT COLONIC LESIONS

The principles of management for these lesions are the same as those for obstructing left-sided tumours, but the detailed anatomy is different.

Securing vascular supply

29 The mesentery to the distal part of the small bowel is spread out towards the patient's right iliac fossa, so that the vascular supply may be studied.

Nylon tapes are passed around the small bowel and large bowel proximal and distal to the lesion to occlude the lumen. The ileocolic, right colic (and for transverse colon tumours the middle colic) vessels are divided at their origins.

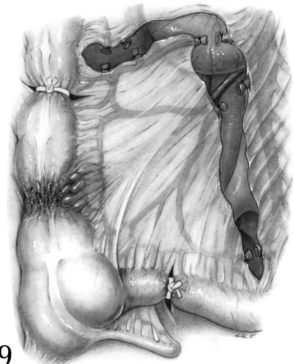

29

30 The dissection is then taken to the deep side of the mesentery supplying the bowel which is lifted forward, and the ureter, vena cava and aorta are identified.

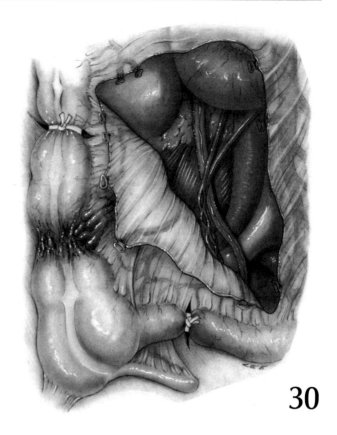

30

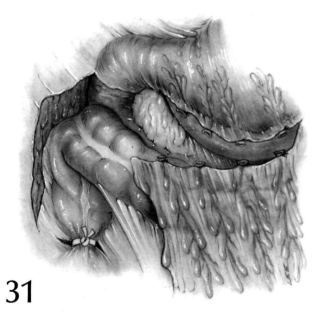

31

31 The hepatic flexure is then mobilized: either the greater omentum is dissected free in the 'bloodless plane' or, for lesions near the hepatic flexure, the omentum is mobilized between the right gastroepiploic vessels and the greater curve of the stomach. In the latter case the dissection is taken down over the inferior part of the first and second parts of the duodenum, dividing the right gastroepiploic vessel at its origin. The dissection is then taken laterally, dividing the top end of the peritoneum overlying the right paracolic gutter. The plane of the dissection at this point is the duodenum and great care must be taken not to damage this structure.

32 Before these two dissections are joined, it is useful to return to the pelvic brim and divide the peritoneum demonstrating the ureter and iliac vessels. Once these structures have been identified, the peritoneum under the caecum is mobilized and the remaining portion of the right paracolic gutter is mobilized.

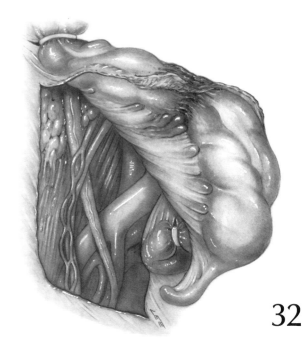

32

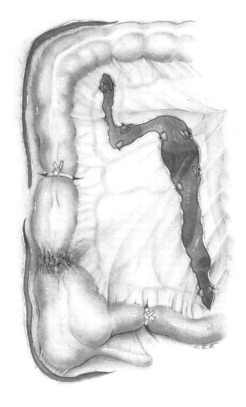

33

33 The parts of the dissection are then joined by lifting the tumour forward: the medial part, where the principal vessels have been ligated; the superior part, bordered by the duodenum; the inferior part, in which the ureter and iliac vessels have been identified; and the lateral part of the paracolic gutter.

As the tumour is lifted forward, the gonadal vessels tend to adhere to the underside of the dissection. They may frequently be left *in situ*, being mobilized by blunt dissection; however, if adherent to the tumour, they are divided.

Finally, the proximal small bowel and distal colon are divided between crushing clamps.

Immediate *versus* delayed anastomosis

It is usual for an immediate anastomosis to be carried out but if there is 'peritonitis' of the bowel surface or the bowel wall itself is very friable, the bowel ends should be brought out. However, in most patients a very carefully performed end-to-end anastomosis can be constructed.

If there is heavy distal colonic faecal loading, a retrograde on-table gut irrigation may be carried out, using a similar technique to that described above.

Closing sequence

The procedures are the same as those described above: lavage with warmed physiological saline containing tetracycline 1 g/l; no drains; gastrostomy; mass closure of abdominal wall; delayed primary closure of skin and subcutaneous tissues.

All these patients should, at the end of the procedure, continue to have positive pressure ventilation and be managed, where possible, in an intensive therapy unit. There is strong evidence that even short periods of hypotension or hypoxia will prejudice the long-term outcome, and the risks of respiratory/cardiac failure will be mitigated by accepting this advice on every occasion. Furthermore, an intensive therapy unit gives an opportunity for careful measurement of urinary output, good pain control, adequate physiotherapy and detailed clinical observation by staff experienced in the care of the seriously ill.

EXTENDED RIGHT HEMICOLECTOMY

For obstructing lesions of the distal part of the transverse colon, splenic flexure and proximal descending colon, an extended right hemicolectomy is a useful procedure. The anatomical dissection will be a combination of the techniques described above and will allow, in most patients, immediate anastomosis.

DELAYED RESECTION POLICY (STAGED RESECTION)

Some surgeons remain of the opinion that immediate tumour resection for left-sided obstructing lesions is not to be undertaken and that a 'defunctioning' transverse colostomy should be carried out as the only primary procedure. The author does not advocate this method.

PAUL–MIKULICZ OPERATION: DOUBLE-BARRELLED COLOSTOMY

Some surgeons, after a radical resection, have brought the ends of the colon out through a single opening in the abdominal wall, so that a full laparotomy to reconstruct bowel continuity may be avoided. If this procedure is carried out, the bowel ends can be mobilized, trimmed, sutured or stapled and returned to the abdominal cavity without further bowel mobiliza-tion. However, the operation is difficult to get 'just right' and perhaps the safest procedure is a simple end colostomy and mucous fistula, as described above. One of the dangers of the Paul–Mikulicz procedure is that the small bowel is always at risk by attachment to the underside of the two limbs of the colostomy; because of the local nature of the mobilization, this adherence of small bowel may not be appreciated and fistula formation may occur. The author does not favour the use of this procedure.

MANAGEMENT OF FIXED TUMOUR

If the tumour is found to be fixed or adherent to vital structures, no attempt should be made to resect it at the first operation. In particular, surgeons should refrain from trying to develop a plane of cleavage directly between the tumour and the attached organ. Under these circumstances, the following sequence is suggested:

1. For right-sided lesions, an ileocolonic anastomosis is fashioned to establish an internal bypass. For more distal lesions, a transverse colostomy is necessary.
2. Before undertaking the bypass or transverse colostomy, decompression of the bowel should be undertaken using the techniques described above. Before an ileocolonic anastomosis, the segment of the small bowel to be used should be chosen as the site for Foley catheter decompression; for more distal lesions, the site of the transverse colostomy is used for needle decompression.
3. Radiopaque 'clips' are placed around the tumour area (it may be possible to irradiate the lesion and render it operable).
4. Closing sequence as described above.

Once the patient has recovered from the acute illness and after the consideration of radiotherapy, the patient should undergo a second laparotomy by an experienced colorectal surgeon in an attempt to excise the primary tumour.

References

1. Fielding LP, Stuart-Brown S, Blesovsky L. Large bowel obstruction caused by cancer: a prospective study. *BMJ* 1979; ii: 515–17.

2. Dudley HAF, Radcliffe AG, McGeehan D. Intraoperative irrigation of the colon to permit primary anastomosis. *Br J Surg* 1980; 67: 80–1.

Colonic surgery for acute conditions: massive haemorrhage

E. L. Bokey MS, FRACS
University of Sydney, Department of Colon and Rectal Surgery, Concord Hospital, Concord, New South Wales, Australia

P. H. Chapuis DS, FRACS
University of Sydney, Department of Colon and Rectal Surgery, Concord Hospital, Concord, New South Wales, Australia

Principles and justification

The most common causes of massive haemorrhage of the large intestine are angiodysplasia and diverticulosis of the colon. Other causes include inflammatory bowel disease (notably Crohn's disease), ischaemic colitis, and radiation injury to the colon. Haemangiomas, leiomyomas, lipomas and colonic varices are rare causes, and secondary haemorrhage after endoscopic polypectomy may occur very occasionally. The presence of telangiectasias on the lips and buccal mucosa suggests the Osler–Rendu–Weber syndrome (hereditary haemorrhagic telangiectasia) as the cause for bleeding. Some patients with angiodysplasia are more likely to bleed if they have associated aortic valve disease[1].

Preoperative

Initial assessment

Most patients with massive haemorrhage ideally should be cared for in a high-dependency area and their management is largely influenced by the rate of bleeding. Initial resuscitation is often necessary before an accurate history can be obtained or a complete physical examination performed. Resuscitation includes the insertion of an adequate peripheral line, a urinary catheter and a nasogastric tube and preferably a central venous line. A careful history, including details of drug usage, may provide a clue to the source of haemorrhage, but often the history and physical examination are not helpful.

If the patient's condition improves and the bleeding stops spontaneously there is time to select appropriate investigations. However, should bleeding persist, urgent investigations become necessary. Early upper endoscopy may exclude gastric and duodenal lesions. Proctoscopy to exclude bleeding haemorrhoids is useful and simple to perform. Sigmoidoscopy (preferably with a flexible instrument) may identify distal pathology.

Colonoscopy

1   Emergency colonoscopy is possible at the time of bleeding, but must be carried out by an experienced endoscopist. Generally, it is best performed once the patient is stabilized and following an adequate bowel preparation. Excessive air insufflation should be avoided as this will efface the mucosa and collapse small arteriovenous malformations. Typically, angiodysplasias seen at colonoscopy are multiple, bright red in colour with a central vessel and a peripheral flare. They occur throughout the colon but are usually found in the right side.

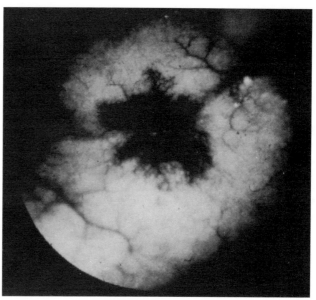

1

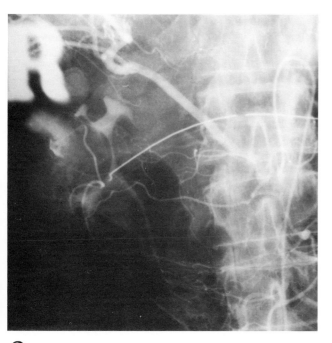

2

Angiography

2   Selective angiography is sometimes helpful, but its success is proportional to the rate of bleeding and the experience of the radiologist. Diagnostic features of angiodysplasia include a vascular blush, early draining vein, and large submucosal veins. Extravasation of contrast material into the lumen confirms the bleeding site. If an active site is identified, selective injection of vasopressin may be successful as an interim measure to stop bleeding. Occasionally, if the bleeding site has not been identified, the catheter may be left *in situ* for further emergency angiographic studies should bleeding recommence.

The illustration shows the late arterial phase with the catheter in the superior mesenteric artery, from which the right hepatic artery is arising. There is moderate extravasation of contrast into the bowel lumen from the right colic artery, adjacent to the pyelogram. Also note gallstone near 'R' marker.

Nuclear scanning

Nuclear scanning generally lacks the accuracy of angiography. This investigation may take up to 4 h to complete and is recommended only in a relatively stable patient. Occasionally, a technetium-labelled sulphur colloid scan will demonstrate the bleeding site, if bleeding is occurring at the time of injection, usually at the same rate as that required for angiography (minimum 1 ml/min). A ^{99m}Tc scan may demonstrate bleeding from ectopic gastric mucosa in a Meckel's diverticulum.

Endoscopic management

Coagulation

If diagnosed, angiodysplasia may be treated successfully by endoscopic coagulation. Hot biopsy forceps or laser may be used, according to personal preference. Coagulation using the hot biopsy forceps requires a setting of 2–3 V. The mucosa is touched or lightly grasped by the forceps and the current is applied until blanching occurs. Treatment for lesions larger than 5 mm diameter should begin around the periphery of the lesion and be directed to its centre. It is advisable not to overdistend the colon to avoid perforation.

Laser

Coagulation with a neodymium yttrium aluminium garnet (NdYAG) laser can be performed using a similar technique with the laser enabled at a power setting adjusted to deliver 40 W for 0.5 s at a working distance of 1 cm. This low setting is chosen to avoid perforation of the thin-walled right colon. At the completion of colonoscopy, the colon must be deflated to avoid delayed perforation.

Operation

The details of surgical treatment depend on whether the cause and source of haemorrhage have been identified and whether the operation is urgent or elective.

Whenever possible the patient should be counselled by a stomal therapist, and all patients (even those who are bleeding profusely) should be sited for an ileostomy and sigmoid colostomy.

Unknown source of haemorrhage

The procedure of choice is total colectomy with ileostomy, rectal mucous fistula or oversewing of rectal stump.

Patients are catheterized and placed in stirrups. A long midline incision is made. A full laparotomy is performed (with careful palpation of the small bowel); this usually confirms blood in the colon but rarely discloses the cause. Blood in the small intestine may be present when the source of bleeding is in the colon. Arteriovenous malformations cannot be identified by inspection or by palpation. The presence of diverticula does not imply that they are the cause of haemorrhage. It is best to avoid intraoperative endoscopic manoeuvres. They are time consuming, potentially hazardous, and rarely helpful.

If the patient's condition permits, an immediate ileorectal anastomosis may be performed.

Known source of haemorrhage

The procedure will depend on the cause and site of the haemorrhage.

If angiodysplasia has been identified in the right colon, then right hemicolectomy with immediate ileotransverse anastomosis is performed.

In the rare event that a sigmoid diverticulum in the left colon has been identified as the source of bleeding, a Hartmann's procedure is advised.

Profuse bleeding is rare in patients with inflammatory bowel disease. Where it occurs it is usually associated with Crohn's disease. When bleeding becomes life-threatening despite intensive medical treatment, emergency total colectomy with ileostomy and rectal mucous fistula may become necessary. It is important to ensure that the rectum can be exteriorized without tension. It should not be oversewn or stapled and returned to the pelvis as these patients are at significant risk of anastomotic disruption. On very rare occasions, if the rectum as well as the rest of the colon is bleeding profusely, an emergency proctocolectomy may be necessary.

The surgical specimen

3 The cause of bleeding is often not identified before or during surgery, because angiodysplasias are difficult to see with the naked eye. Arterial injection of barium into the resected specimen may help the pathologist to confirm the diagnosis[2].

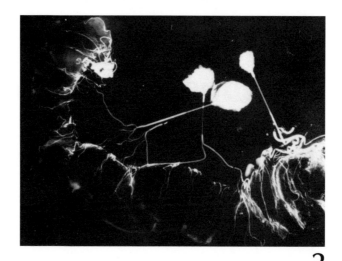

3

4 Examination of the open specimen after barium injection will show areas of barium pooling in the mucosa and will direct the pathologist as to where tissue should be sampled for sectioning.

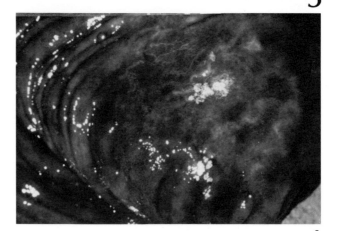

4

5 Histological examination will show barium-filled vascular spaces in the mucosa, continuous with ectatic submucosal vessels typical of angiodysplasia[3].

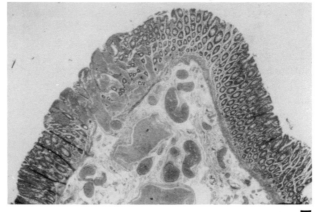

5

Acknowledgements

Illustration 2 is reproduced by courtesy of Dr G. R. Faithful.

References

1. Price AB. Angiodysplasia of the colon. *Int J Colorectal Dis* 1986; 1: 121–8.

2. Alfidi RJ, Caldwell D, Riaz T *et al*. Recognition and angio-surgical detection of arteriovenous malformations of the bowel. *Ann Surg* 1971; 174: 573–82.

3. Hayward PG, Bokey EL, Chapuis PH, Kneale KL, Faithful GR. The use of barium injection studies to confirm the diagnosis of colonic angiodysplasia. *Coloproctology* 1984; 6: 156–7.

Colonic surgery for acute conditions: volvulus of the colon

David N. Armstrong MD, FRCSEd
Clinical Instructor, Department of Surgery, Yale University School of Medicine, New Haven, Connecticut, USA

G. H. Ballantyne MD, FACS, FASCRS
Associate Professor of Surgery, Department of Surgery, Yale University School of Medicine, New Haven, Connecticut, USA

History

Torsions of the colon have plagued mankind throughout history. The Greeks called this condition 'ileus', the Romans 'volvulus'. The natural history of sigmoid volvulus was detailed in the Papyrus Ebers from dynastic Egypt – the twist of colon either 'rotted in the belly' or it untwisted and the patient rapidly recovered. Asclepiades defines 'ileus' as 'a severe and prolonged twisting of the intestine'. The method of treatment advocated by Hippocrates suggests that he was treating sigmoid volvulus. He advised insertion of a ten-digit long (about 22 cm) suppository into the rectum, and this manoeuvre often relieved the obstruction. Indeed, this technique heralded the modern derotation of sigmoid volvulus with a rigid sigmoidoscope 25 cm in length.

Treatment of all forms of intestinal obstruction remained primarily non-operative until late in the 19th century. Although Praxogaras, in ancient Greece, had advocated 'making an incision in the pubic region, then cutting open the rectum, removing the excrement, and sewing up the rectum and abdomen', few physicians had entrusted their patients to surgeons for these heroic measures. Occasional descriptions of operative treatment of intestinal obstruction crept into the surgical literature after the Renaissance. In 1692, for example, Nuck reported the successful reduction of a volvulus by 'gastrostomy'.

Satisfactory techniques for enteric suturing and anaesthesia did not evolve until the 19th century. Successful operative treatment of colonic obstruction and sigmoid volvulus became more common in the 1880s. Atherton reported the first successful operative detorsion of a sigmoid volvulus in Boston in 1883. Treves, in his monograph on intestinal obstruction published in 1884, recommended colectomy when a gangrenous colon was encountered. In 1889, Senn sought to apply the principles advocated by Travers for the treatment of obstruction. He advised enterotomy for decompression of the intestine proximal to the volvulus. Because of the high likelihood of recurrence, Senn also suggested 'shortening of the mesentery' of the sigmoid colon (sigmoidopexy). Thus, by the close of the 1890s, operative treatment of sigmoid volvulus rapidly became, for many, the standard therapy.

Operative detorsion or obstructive resection of the Paul–Mikulicz type remained the recommended treatment of colonic volvulus for the first half of the 20th century. In the second half, however, primary therapy of sigmoid volvulus has returned to non-operative techniques. In 1859, Gay had observed during an autopsy of a patient who had died from a sigmoid volvulus that 'with a tube, per rectum, the bowel could be relieved of its contents; and then, by rolling the body over, the bowel (would) right itself'. This form of therapy, of course, brings to mind the ten-digit suppository used by Hippocrates for decompression of patients with volvulus. Unfortunately, the value of non-operative decompression of sigmoid volvulus with a rigid sigmoidoscope and rectal tube was not widely recognized until 1947, when Bruusgaard reported his results in the treatment of 168 episodes of sigmoid volvulus. His data demonstrated that whenever possible, patients with sigmoid volvulus should undergo non-operative techniques for decompression and derotation of the twisted sigmoid colon.

Caecal volvulus occurs less commonly than sigmoid volvulus. Classical physicians were silent on this condition. In 1646, Fabricius Hildanus described the autopsy of a young boy who had succumbed to a caecal volvulus and Treves accumulated only five cases of caecal volvulus. The first major treatise on caecal volvulus was published in 1900 by Von Manteuffel and the first major series in English in 1905 by Smith and Perry. Throughout the 20th century, three different operations have been advocated for this condition: caecopexy, caecostomy and right hemicolectomy. Because of the great success of non-operative decompression for the treatment of sigmoid volvulus, similar attempts have been made for the non-operative reduction of caecal volvulus but with intermittent success.

In English-speaking countries, sigmoid rather than caecal volvulus is more commonly encountered. Non-operative decompression and derotation of a sigmoid volvulus followed by elective sigmoid resection has become the standard therapy. In contrast, caecal volvulus generally requires urgent operative treatment after resuscitation.

Principles and justification

Aetiology

Large intestinal volvulus accounts for 3–5% of large intestinal obstruction in Western populations, and for over 50% of obstruction in the 'volvulus belt' of Africa and the Middle East.

Volvulus of the sigmoid colon occurs in the presence of three conditions:

1. Elongation of the sigmoid colon.
2. Narrowing of the base of the sigmoid mesocolon (mesosigmoiditis).
3. A torque force applied to the sigmoid colon.

In the West, the sigmoid colon elongates as a result of neurological disease, laxative abuse, or chronic constipation, most often seen in occupants of chronic care facilities. The base of the sigmoid mesocolon becomes foreshortened as the scar tissue generated by the chronic mesosigmoiditis contracts. This occurs because of repeated episodes of torsion.

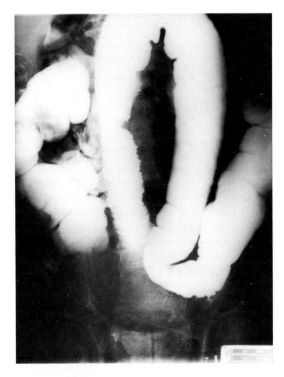

1

1   Barium enemas in these patients reveal the close apposition of the descending colon–sigmoid colon junction to the rectosigmoid junction. As a result, the narrow base acts as a fulcrum, about which the sigmoid colon twists.

In African and Middle Eastern societies, a high-fibre diet results in an overloaded sigmoid colon whose weight provides the rotational force to initiate torsion. A shift in the relative positions of the intra-abdominal organs, as seen in pregnancy or tumours, may also precipitate an episode of sigmoid volvulus.

Barium enema showing close apposition of descending colon junction and rectosigmoid junction in a patient who has had recurrent episodes of sigmoid volvulus.

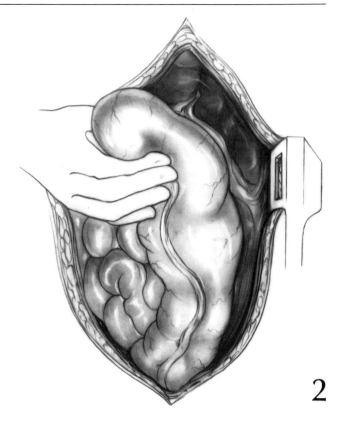

2

2 Caecal volvulus occurs in patients with incomplete peritoneal fixation of the caecum. In a series of post mortems in the USA, the caecum retains a complete mesenterium ileocolicum commune without any retroperitoneal fixation in about 11% of patients. Axial torsion of the caecum can produce a caecal volvulus when the right colon retains this degree of mobility.

In another 25% of patients, the ascending colon is fixed to the retroperitoneum, but the caecum remains unattached. In these patients the caecum can fold anteriorly, producing a caecal bascule. Thus, the caecum of about one-third of the American population has sufficient mobility that it can twist and generate a caecal volvulus.

Indications

Large intestinal volvulus is a life-threatening condition. Non-operative reduction of the volvulus provides excellent initial therapy for the majority of patients with sigmoid volvulus and an occasional patient with caecal volvulus. Unfortunately, following non-operative reduction, there is a high probability of recurrence with a high concomitant mortality. Consequently, almost all patients in whom a colonic volvulus is discovered should undergo definitive operative treatment during the same hospitalization.

Choice of operation

Sigmoid volvulus

When non-operative reduction of sigmoid volvulus is achieved, the patient can receive a standard mechanical and antibiotic bowel preparation. This allows construction of a primary anastomosis after resection of the twisted segment. When non-operative detorsion can not be achieved, the patient must undergo emergency sigmoid resection. Under these circumstances, a temporary stoma may be required. Simple sigmoidopexy is followed by too high a recurrence rate to be recommended.

Caecal volvulus

Non-operative derotation of a caecal volvulus is seldom achieved. As a result, almost all patients afflicted by caecal volvulus require emergency surgical intervention after a rapid period of resuscitation and stabilization. Necessarily, the patients undergo operation without a bowel preparation. Excellent results have been reported after three operations: caecopexy, caecostomy and right hemicolectomy.

Caecopexy

Caecopexy prevents future torsion of the right colon by fixation of the ascending colon to the abdominal wall near the right gutter. The major advantage of this procedure is that the colon is not opened, and thus no contamination of the abdominal cavity occurs. The great disadvantage of the procedure, however, is that decompression is not achieved and the right colon remains distended. Hence, closure of the abdomen is difficult. In addition, large quantities of 'toxins' remain within the colon, and bacterial translocation may continue to plague the patient in the postoperative period.

Caecostomy

In this operation, the caecum is intubated with a large catheter, decompressed and drained of its faecal contents. In addition, the right colon is secured in place both by sutures, as in caecopexy, and by the caecostomy tube. Consequently, the right colon is decompressed and drained. Recurrence rates of caecal volvulus after caecostomy are very low. None the less, the greatest disadvantage of a caecostomy is the risk of contamination of the abdomen during decompression of the caecum and placement of the catheter. In addition, abdominal wall infections can occur around the caecostomy site. This may lead to separation of the caecum from the abdominal wall and drainage of caecal contents into the free abdominal cavity. Finally, persistent drainage through the caecocutaneous fistula requires prolonged wound care and lengthens the period of disability after operation.

Right hemicolectomy

Right hemicolectomy offers a definitive treatment for caecal volvulus and avoids the problems of caecopexy and caecostomy. Resection of the right colon eliminates any chance of recurrence of caecal volvulus. Transection of the ileum and transverse colon with stapling instruments, which simultaneously seal both the specimen side and the patient's side of the intestine eradicates any significant abdominal contamination. The obstructed segment and its contents of 'toxins' are removed, and the risk of persistent sepsis is minimized. As the distended segment is removed, closure of the abdominal wound is also facilitated. In most patients a primary anastomosis can be safely constructed.

Preoperative

Clinical presentation

The average age of patients with volvulus is 60–66 years. Caecal volvulus occurs more commonly in patients who have undergone operations that partially or completely mobilize the right colon. Sigmoid volvulus is more commonly reported in blacks than other ethnic groups and more commonly in men than in women. Patients generally have a sedentary lifestyle and may be inhabitants of chronic care facilities, such as nursing homes or psychiatric hospitals. Many report a prolonged history of constipation.

Patients develop the signs and symptoms of colonic obstruction with abdominal distension, abdominal pain and obstipation evolved over 3–5 days. Some become nauseated or begin to vomit. Physical examination typically reveals abdominal distension, increased tympany and perhaps some abdominal tenderness. On digital examination, the rectal vault is often empty.

Diagnosis

3–5 The characteristic appearance of a caecal or sigmoid volvulus on a plain abdominal radiograph will confirm the diagnosis in the majority of patients. The distended intestine assumes two characteristic silhouettes in caecal volvulus: the appearance of a 'coffee bean' in axial torsion of the caecum and ascending colon and a solitary inverted tear-drop in caecal bascule. In sigmoid volvulus, the colon often appears like a 'bent inner tube'.

In doubtful cases, a limited Gastrografin enema will reveal the characteristic 'bird's beak' appearance of the apex of the sigmoid volvulus in the proximal rectum. During rigid or flexible sigmoidoscopy, spiralling folds of mucosa at the rectosigmoid junction establish the diagnosis.

Occasionally the sigmoid volvulus spontaneously derotates before the diagnosis is documented by abdominal radiography. Under these circumstances, colonoscopy can often confirm that the sigmoid colon was recently twisted. Colonoscopic examination in these patients reveals discrete segments of inflammation at the rectosigmoid junction and at the descending colon–sigmoid junction. Each segment of inflammation is about 5 cm in length and is characterized by loss of the vascular markings, thickening of the intestinal wall, erythema and sometimes granularity or friability. These findings strongly support the diagnosis.

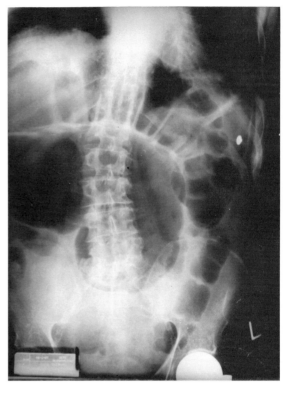

3

Abdominal radiograph of caecal volvulus produced by axial torsion of the caecum and ascending colon showing 'coffee bean' appearance of obstructed right colon.

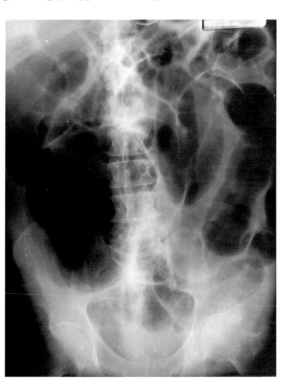

4

Abdominal radiograph of caecal volvulus produced by a caecal bascule showing 'inverted tear-drop' appearance of obstructed caecum.

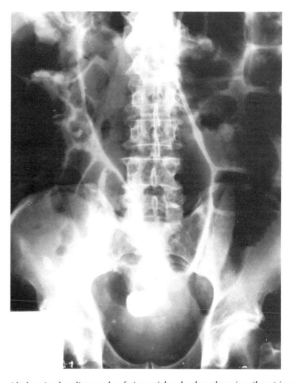

5

Abdominal radiograph of sigmoid volvulus showing 'bent inner tube' appearance of obstructed sigmoid colon.

Resuscitation

The first priority is resuscitation of the patient, although these patients generally appear reasonably stable. Colonic obstruction carries a very high mortality rate, however, because it precipitates large volume shifts and often generates cardiovascular complications because of endotoxin and bacterial translocation.

All patients are admitted to a surgical intensive therapy unit. Oxygen saturation is monitored by pulse oximetry. Pulse, blood pressure and central venous pressure are continuously monitored. A Swan–Ganz catheter is required when the patient has significant associated cardiac disease. The patient is laid in the left lateral position to improve venous return, which may be compromised as a result of massive abdominal distension. Oxygen is given because splinting of the diaphragm impedes respiratory efforts and results in shunting of blood through the pulmonary circulation. A Foley catheter is inserted to help assess fluid balance. All patients should be intubated with a nasogastric tube because of the high mortality rate from aspiration of gastric contents. Parenteral antibiotics to cover aerobic and anaerobic organisms must be given to all patients to treat potential sepsis and as prophylaxis against inadvertent perforation during sigmoidoscopic intubation.

The rate of fluid resuscitation is determined by the success of non-operative attempts at derotation of the volvulus. If an emergency operation proves necessary, the patient is rapidly resuscitated over a 4–8-h period with a balanced electrolyte solution. If the volvulus is successfully reduced, the patient is rehydrated more cautiously over a 48-h period.

Non-operative decompression and derotation of sigmoid volvulus

The patient is placed in the left lateral position. A 25-cm rigid sigmoidoscope is advanced into the rectum under direct vision. Air insufflation is not generally required. Spiralling folds of rectal mucosa are traversed at the rectosigmoid junction. Intubation of the obstructed loop of sigmoid colon is heralded by the almost explosive propulsion of gas and liquid stool through the sigmoidoscope. The tip of a well-lubricated no. 32 rubber rectal tube is pushed gently into the sigmoid colon through the sigmoidoscope. This serves to maintain decompression of the sigmoid colon during the few days before elective resection of the sigmoid colon.

On occasion, initial attempts at detorsion of the volvulus are unsuccessful. The patient is placed in the knee–elbow position; this may allow the colon to fall away and open up the angle of the volvulus. The temptation to push a narrow, rigid probe into the apex should be resisted, as this may perforate the already compromised intestinal wall. If visibility is poor, the end of the sigmoidoscope is placed directly on the twist at the rectosigmoid junction. Without moving the sigmoidoscope, the tube is pushed up the sigmoidoscope, so that the tip lies at the apex. Undue force should never be used, nor attempts to poke blindly. There will be no doubt when decompression has been achieved. A polythene-lined bucket should be on hand to avoid unnecessary spillage from the sudden, forceful rush of gas and liquid stool.

In some patients the rigid sigmoidoscope is not long enough to reach into the obstructed segment of sigmoid colon, but a flexible sigmoidoscope or colonoscope can be advanced into the twisted segment. There is no sudden rush of gas and fluid, as the endoscope works with a closed system. The obstructed sigmoid colon is slowly decompressed with suction. The flexible instruments are not as effective for drainage of the faecal contents of the sigmoid colon because of the narrow calibre of the suction channel. None the less, decompression of the sigmoid colon with flexible instruments will generally result in detorsion of the volvulus.

Successful non-operative reduction of volvulus

Sigmoidoscopic decompression is successful in over 90% of patients in whom the sigmoid colon remains viable at the time of presentation. When successful, decompression should be confirmed radiologically, and the rectal tube taped securely to the buttocks. The patient is stabilized and assessed for surgery, undergoes a standard mechanical and antibiotic bowel preparation, and elective surgery is scheduled 5–7 days later.

Unsuccessful non-operative reduction of volvulus

When endoscopic attempts at detorsion of the volvulus fail, the patient should receive operative therapy immediately following adequate resuscitation because the sigmoid colon is strangulated and usually necrotic.

Operations for sigmoid volvulus

Position of patient

For operations to correct sigmoid volvulus, the patient is placed in the Lloyd-Davies position (as described in the chapter on pp. 47–50).

Incision

A lower abdominal midline incision extending to the umbilicus allows adequate exposure for correction of sigmoid volvulus. Care must be taken when entering the peritoneum not to inadvertently cut the distended colon.

COLOPEXY

Several techniques of colopexy have been described. The simplest involves suturing the sigmoid colon to the lateral abdominal wall using interrupted sutures. More elaborate methods include enclosing the sigmoid in a lateral retroperitoneal 'pouch', plicating the mesentery (mesenteropexy), Gore-tex banding of the sigmoid colon to the abdominal wall, and sigmoid colostomy. All of these techniques have recurrence rates similar to those in unoperated patients and, furthermore, are often more time-consuming than a simple resection.

RESECTION: SIGMOID COLECTOMY

Sigmoid resection provides the simplest approach and has the lowest rate of recurrence. The small intestine is packed into the right upper quadrant with warm, moist packs. The sigmoid colon is mobilized on its primitive mesentery by dividing the 'white line' laterally. As a result of repeated torsions, the mesocolon is foreshortened and the peritoneal reflection shifted laterally. This often facilitates the dissection. The left ureter is identified and preserved.

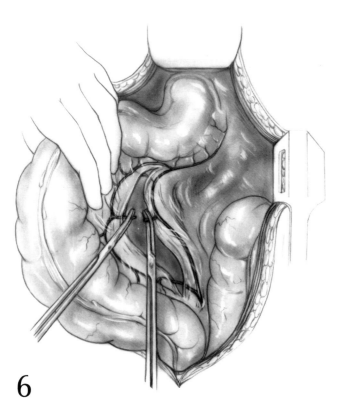

6

Extent of resection

6   As a result of foreshortening of the mesentery, the peritoneal reflection of the rectum and the descending colon are brought into close proximity. Recurrence rates are lowest after simple resection of the omega loop of the sigmoid colon. More extensive resection is unnecessary. The inferior mesenteric artery is preserved, as this is a benign disease process, and this will ensure an adequate blood supply to the proximal rectum. The sigmoid branches are divided near their origin on the inferior mesenteric vessels. The remaining mesentery is divided between clamps and tied with 3/0 silk. The sites of transection are chosen to allow a well-perfused, tension-free anastomosis.

Side-to-side (functional end-to-end) colorectal anastomosis

7a, b The intestinal wall is not cleared of mesenteric tissue. The descending colon is transected near its junction with the sigmoid colon with a GIA 60 stapler. This closes both the descending colon and the specimen with double rows of titanium staples. Even in unprepared colon, faecal soiling seldom occurs. The rectum is divided just distally to the rectosigmoid junction, also with a GIA 60 stapler. The distal descending colon and the proximal rectum are usually contiguous because of scarring of the mesentery from chronic mesosigmoiditis.

The antimesenteric sides of the rectum and descending colon are aligned with two silk sutures. One is placed 1 cm from the end of the two staple lines near the mesentery. The second suture is placed 6 cm from the staple lines. The corners of the two staple lines are excised with curved Mayo scissors. A third GIA 60 stapler is introduced through the two colotomies. The third staple line should run along the taenia on the descending colon. After firing the stapler, the staple line is inspected for haemostasis. The edges of the remaining enterotomy are approximated with four Allis' clamps. The silk suture near the enterotomy is removed. The previous staple lines at the end of the rectum and descending colon can be aligned so that they either form an X or one continuous everted closure. The enterotomy is closed using a TA 55 stapler with 3.5-mm staples. A third silk suture is placed in the 'crotch' at the end of the third GIA staple line.

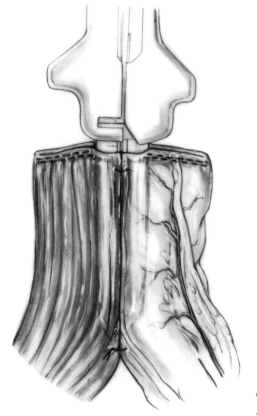

7a

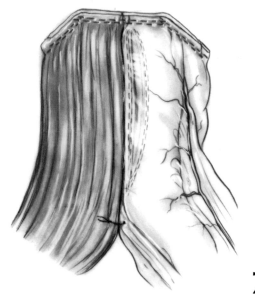

7b

End-to-end colorectal anastomosis (double stapling technique)

8 The points of resection are identified at the descending colon–sigmoid colon junction and the rectosigmoid junction. The proximal rectum is divided with the GIA 60 stapler. In some patients it may be necessary to use the Roticulator-55 stapling device to close the rectum, because the shape of the pelvis does not allow access with the more bulky GIA device. The specimen side of the rectum is secured with a right-angled bowel clamp, such as a Foss–Pemberton clamp. The intestine is divided and the specimen removed.

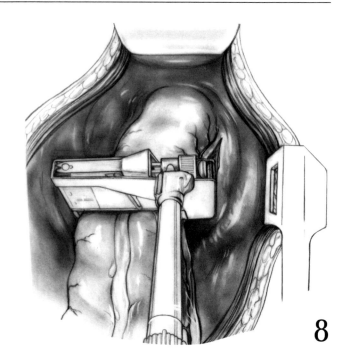

8

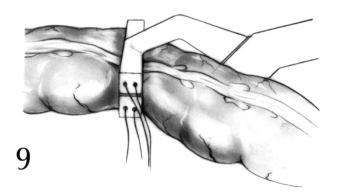

9

9 Mesenteric attachments and epiploic fat tags are cleared from 2.5 cm of intestinal wall. An automatic purse-string device is applied at the distal limit of the cleared colonic wall. A crushing bowel clamp is placed across the specimen side of the intestine near the purse-string. The intestine is divided with a scalpel or pair of heavy scissors. The purse-string device is left attached to the intestine and acts as a clamp until the specimen is removed. The wound is inspected for haemostasis.

10 The purse-string device on the descending colon is opened. The edges of the colon are grasped with three Babcock's clamps. The colon is usually dilated from the recent obstruction and does not require dilatation. The diameter of the colon is measured with sizers. Whenever possible, the 31-mm Premium CEEA should be used. When necessary, the descending colon can be dilated with the surgeon's thumb, or alternatively by slow distension with water in a Foley catheter with a 30-ml balloon. The anvil shaft assembly of the Premium CEEA is detached from the central rod and positioned within the descending colon. The purse-string is tightly tied within the groove on the shaft.

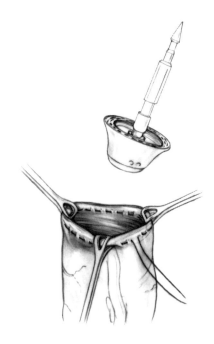

10

11a–c

The anus is dilated to admit four fingers. The trocar is positioned in the centre rod of the Premium CEEA and withdrawn below the level of the staples. The head of the stapler is introduced into the rectum and advanced to the stapled closure of the proximal rectum. The trocar is advanced through the centre of the staple line by turning the wing nut at the base of the stapler. Once the tip of the trocar becomes visible, scissors are used to open the overlying intestinal wall. This facilitates passage of the trocar and prevents tearing of the rectum.

The centre rod is advanced until its orange neck is visible. The trocar is removed. The shaft of the anvil is inserted into the centre rod. The wing nut is turned until the green area becomes visible in the tissue thickness gauge. The stapler is fired. One Lembert suture of 3/0 silk is placed anteriorly on the staple line. This is used to provide counter traction as the stapler is withdrawn. The anvil is opened three and a half turns, twisted left and right and removed. The 'doughnuts' of tissue should be complete circles.

A rigid sigmoidoscope is introduced into the rectum and the staple line is inspected for haemostasis. The pelvis is filled with water. The rectum is insufflated until air escapes through the anus around the sigmoidoscope. The anastomosis should be air-tight; no air bubbles should float to the surface of the water in the pelvis.

Wound closure

The fascia is closed with a continuous monofilament suture (1 polydioxanone). The skin edges are approximated with a continuous subcuticular absorbable suture (4/0 coated polyglycolic acid). A sterile dressing is applied to the wound.

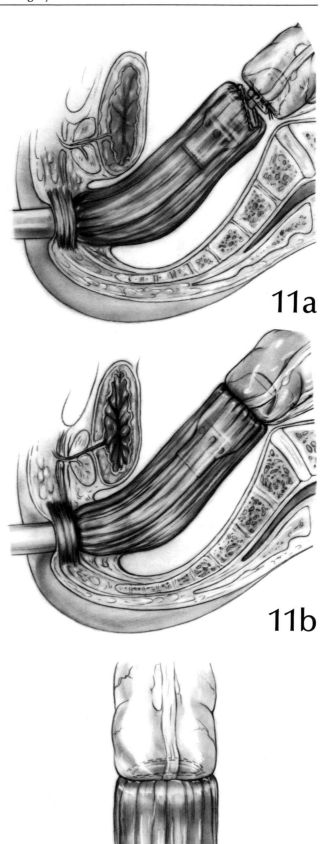

FAILED NON-OPERATIVE REDUCTION OR SUSPECTED ISCHAEMIC GUT

Failed sigmoidoscopic reduction or the presence of local peritonitis require urgent operative reduction and resection of the twisted sigmoid loop. A low midline incision is mandatory to provide the necessary exposure of an often enormously dilated sigmoid loop. Where possible, the surgeon should not untwist the colon because this manoeuvre may 'release' the contained stagnant venous blood into the circulation, which might cause septic shock. Similarly, the obstructed succus entericus would gain access to an absorptive surface in the intestine, both proximal and distal to the volvulus, with a similar outcome. Therefore, the colon should be clamped in the twisted position, and the mesentery clamped to occlude the vessels. Once control has been obtained, the colon can then be untwisted and removed.

The sigmoid colon generally twists anticlockwise, the caecum clockwise. When the base of the mesocolon is inspected, the direction in which to reduce it will be obvious. Several options for resection are available:

1. Paul–Mikulicz exteriorization and resection.
2. Hartmann's procedure.
3. Resection and primary anastomosis.

Paul–Mikulicz resection

The abdomen is entered through a lateral flank incision and the strangulated segment of sigmoid colon is exteriorized through the incision. The sigmoid loop is amputated at skin level distal to crushing clamps. A double-barrelled colostomy is fashioned using interrupted all-coats intestine to subdermal sutures and a few interrupted sutures are placed between the two adjacent limbs of the colostomy. This procedure is of largely historical interest.

Hartmann's procedure

Colorectal anastomoses constructed when the patient has not received a mechanical and antibiotic bowel preparation carry a high risk of leakage. Perforation of the sigmoid colon and significant peritoneal soiling also increase the risk of primary anastomosis. The incision, mobilization and resection of the sigmoid colon are the same as described above. Additional mobilization of the descending colon may be required, so that its divided end will reach the anterior abdominal wall. When the colon is unprepared, transection of the gut with a GIA 60 stapler minimizes the risk of spillage of stool. The apex of the rectal pouch is sutured to the sacral promontory with two or three non-absorbable sutures. This prevents retraction and allows easy identification of the pouch when the time comes for closure of the colostomy (as described in the chapter on pp. 488–496).

Resection and primary anastomosis

In selected patients with colonic obstruction, primary anastomoses have been constructed with a satisfactory outcome and with low leakage rates. Absence of peritoneal soiling and viable intestinal ends are prerequisites. Intraoperative cleansing of the colon is required (as described in chapter on pp. 397–415). The procedure is as described for sigmoid colectomy.

Operations for caecal volvulus

Position of patient

The patient is placed in a supine position. Access to the anus is not required.

Incision

The abdomen is entered through a midline incision for caecal volvulus. It should extend from the mid-epigastrium to below the umbilicus. Other incisions are possible but may interfere with the positioning of a stoma if a primary anastomosis proves unwise.

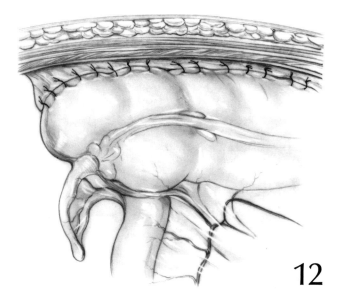

CAECOPEXY

12 The volvulus is derotated. Interrupted seromuscular sutures of 3/0 silk are placed along the antimesenteric border of the ascending colon. These are used to secure the right colon to the abdominal wall near the right gutter. Low rates of recurrence of volvulus after this simple technique have been reported, but additional fixation of the ascending colon with an elevated flap of parietal peritoneum or polyvinyl alcohol sponge has been advocated.

CAECOSTOMY

The caecal volvulus is untwisted. A colotomy is made through the anterior taenia coli of the caecum. The caecum and ascending colon are decompressed and drained of as much faecal material as possible with a large-core suction catheter. Irrigation of the caecum with warmed saline may be necessary to obtain satisfactory drainage of the right colon. Alternatively, the appendix can be excised and the caecum cannulated through the appendiceal orifice.

13 Two concentric purse-string sutures of a strong non-absorbable suture, such as 2/0 silk, are placed around the colotomy. The caecum is intubated with the largest available Mallincrot or Foley catheter. The catheter is secured in place with the purse-string sutures.

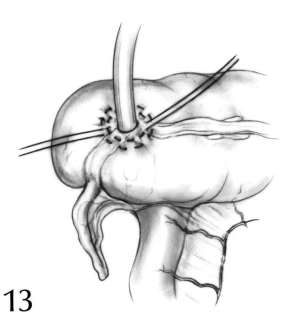

14 Interrupted seromuscular sutures of 3/0 silk are used to secure the antimesenteric border of the right colon within the right gutter, as with a caecopexy. A small stab wound is made approximately at McBurney's point in the right lower quadrant. A curved clamp is passed through the abdominal wall and used to withdraw the end of the catheter through the stab incision. Interrupted seromuscular sutures of 3/0 silk placed around the catheter seal the caecum to the anterior abdominal wall. Two heavy sutures, such as 1 silk, bind the catheter to the skin and prevent migration of the catheter.

After closure of the abdominal incision, a bulky dressing is placed around the catheter. This dressing maintains the first few centimetres of the catheter in a position perpendicular to the abdominal wall, which prevents kinking at the level of the fascia. The catheter is placed on continuous suction.

After the operation, the caecostomy catheter requires frequent attention. It must be cautiously irrigated with water several times a day. Abdominal radiographs should be obtained to confirm continued satisfactory decompression of the caecum. The catheter is removed approximately 3 weeks after the operation. In the majority of patients, the caecocutaneous fistula will spontaneously close. Occasionally, operative closure is required.

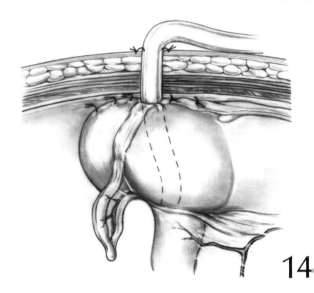

14

RESECTION: RIGHT HEMICOLECTOMY

Mobilization of the caecum is facilitated by the presence of a long mesentery. The retroperitoneal attachment of the caecum is opened near the common iliac vessels and the ureter is identified. A hand is passed palm-up behind the ascending colon and anterior to the ureter up to the hilum of the kidney. With the ascending colon retracted anteriorly, the lateral attachments of the colon are incised up to the hepatic flexure. The attachments of the mesocolon to the duodenum are sharply divided. The right colon is mobilized medially to the vena cava and the mesentery of the terminal ileum is freed of its retroperitoneal fixation. This allows sufficient mobility for the terminal ileum to be rotated up to the transverse colon for the anastomosis.

The lesser sac is entered through the avascular plane between the omentum and transverse colon. The omentum is freed from the proximal half of the transverse colon and preserved. The remaining points of fixation of the hepatic flexure are divided with cautery.

15 The right colon is elevated. The terminal ileum is divided with a GIA 60 stapler near the end of the ligament of Treves. The ileal arcades in the mesentery are divided between curved clamps. The ileocolic, right colic and right branch of the middle colic vessels are identified and divided near their origin and doubly ligated with 2/0 silk sutures.

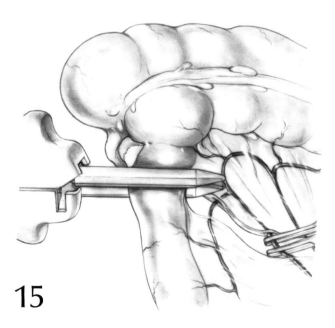

15

16 The transverse colon is divided with a GIA 60 or GIA 80 stapler near the preserved arcades of the left branch of the middle colic artery. The remaining mesentery near the chosen points of resection are divided between clamps and tied with 3/0 silk sutures. The specimen is held off the field and opened to ensure that no unsuspected neoplasms are found near the margins of resection.

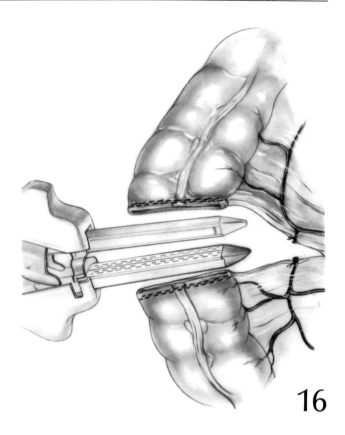

16

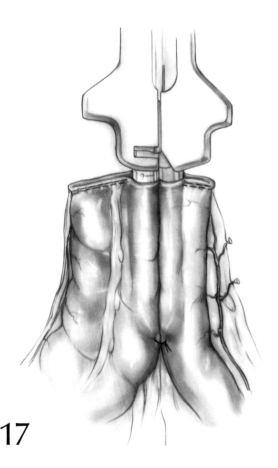

17

Side-to-side (functional end-to-end) ileocolic anastomosis

17 If the operation has proceeded smoothly without significant contamination of the abdomen with faecal material, a primary anastomosis can be constructed. The caudad surface of the transverse colon and the cephalad surface of the terminal ileum are approximated and fixed with two sutures of 3/0 silk. The mesentery of the terminal ileum is inspected to ensure that it is not twisted. The corners of the two staple lines are opened with a pair of heavy Mayo scissors. A large-bore suction catheter is passed into both the transverse colon and terminal ileum. The anastomosis is constructed along the antimesenteric border of the transverse colon with a GIA 60 stapler and the staple line inspected for haemostasis.

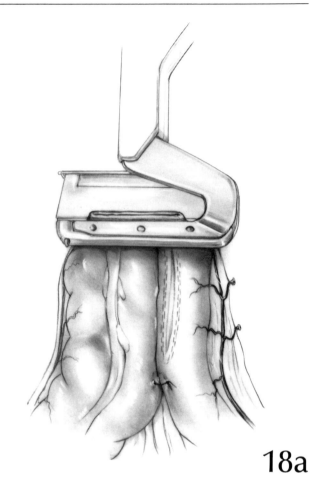

18a

18a, b
The silk suture near the enterotomy is removed. Four Allis' clamps are used to approximate the intestinal wall of the remaining enterotomy. This is closed with a TA 55 stapler using 4.8-mm staples. A 3/0 silk suture is placed in the 'crotch' of the anastomosis and the abdomen is liberally irrigated with warmed saline.

BROOKE ILEOSTOMY

If the caecum has ruptured or there is gross spillage of stool into the abdominal cavity, a primary anastomosis should not be constructed. An end (Brooke) ileostomy and mucous fistula are fashioned (as described in the chapter on pp. 243–269). The closed end of the transverse colon is tacked to the cephalad end of the incision. It is not opened. The abdominal incision is closed, and the wound protected. The stapled closure of the terminal ileum is excised with a pair of curved Mayo scissors and the stoma constructed.

Closure

The fascia is closed with a continuous monofilament suture (1 polydioxanone). The wound is irrigated with an antibiotic-containing solution and the skin edges are left open. The wound is packed with gauze soaked in povidone-iodine. The skin wound can be closed 3–4 days after operation with Steri-strips.

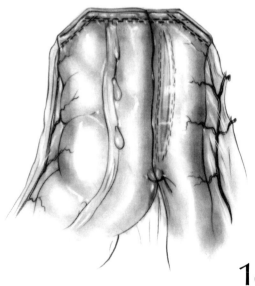

18b

Postoperative care

The management of patients after operation for large intestinal volvulus is the same as after resection of the colon for other diseases. The patient receives one additional dose of antibiotics after surgery. The nasogastric tube is removed on the first day after operation and the Foley catheter is removed when the patient is ambulatory. The patient begins eating when postoperative ileus resolves and is observed for signs and symptoms of abdominal sepsis and wound infection. If an intra-abdominal abscess is suspected, computed tomography of the abdomen with both intravenous and oral contrast media is performed. Abdominal abscesses can often be treated with percutaneous drainage.

Preliminary assessment of the integrity of a stapled anastomosis can be made on the basis of a plain abdominal radiograph. The staples of an intact anastomosis will form one of several different continuous patterns depending on the type of stapling technique that was used. A break in the continuity of the staple line strongly suggests anastomotic dehiscence. If an anastomotic leak is suspected, a Gastrografin enema is given to confirm its presence. Clinically significant dehiscence of the anastomosis is generally treated by removing it and constructing an ileostomy or colostomy. If no complications evolve during the postoperative course, the patient is discharged 7–10 days after operation.

Outcome

The results of treatment for large intestinal volvulus are largely determined by the condition of the twisted segment of colon at the time of operation. When the colon is viable, hospital mortality rates below 10% can be achieved in patients with either sigmoid or caecal volvulus. Unfortunately, the mortality rate of necrotic sigmoid colon is extremely high. Thus, early treatment either by non-operative or operative means is the primary determinant of outcome.

Caecopexy is followed by a 5–10% recurrence rate of volvulus. Recurrence after caecostomy is rare. Right colectomy obviously precludes recurrence. None the less, hospital mortality rates for patients afflicted with caecal volvulus are primarily determined by the condition of the intestine at the time of operation; mortality rates of 12% have been reported for patients with viable intestine at the time of operation and 32% for those with a necrotic right colon. As Lord Moynihan stated in 1905: 'Anything over a 10% mortality is the mortality of delay.'

Further reading

Ballantyne GH. Review of sigmoid volvulus: history and results of treatment. *Dis Colon Rectum* 1982; 25: 494–501.

Ballantyne GH. Review of sigmoid volvulus: clinical patterns and pathogenesis. *Dis Colon Rectum* 1982; 25: 823–30.

Ballantyne GH. The meaning of ileus: its changing definition over three millenia. *Am J Surg* 1984; 148: 252–6.

Ballantyne GH, Brander MD, Beart RW Jnr, Ilstrup DM. Volvulus of the colon: incidence and mortality. *Ann Surg* 1985; 202: 83–92.

Burke JB, Ballantyne GH. Cecal volvulus: low mortality at a city hospital. *Dis Colon Rectum* 1984; 27: 737–40.

Colonic surgery for acute conditions: injuries to the intra-abdominal colon

L. W. Baker FRCSEd, FRCS, MSc, FNU
Professor Emeritus, Department of Surgery, University of Natal, Durban, South Africa

S. R. Thomson ChM, FRCS
Senior Lecturer, Department of Surgery, University of Natal, Durban, South Africa

History

Colon injuries result from a variety of mechanisms. Blunt and iatrogenic trauma are relatively uncommon, whereas penetrating trauma is responsible for the majority of injuries. The rising tide of civilian violence and urban terrorism, and the increasing use of firearms, demands that the practising surgeon familiarizes himself with the prinicples of surgical treatment of these injuries. Traditional wartime management was that of exteriorizing the wound as a colostomy[1]. Although this proved safe and effective, it had a high morbidity rate and involved two operations and prolonged hospitalization[2,3]. Nevertheless, it is probably the best option for those who treat such injuries only occasional-ly. It is, however, being increasingly realized that it is the pathophysiological events set in motion by the injury – faecal contamination and shock – that determine the outcome rather than the method of surgical repair of the colonic wound, provided that this is performed with technical competence[2-5]. The authors' prospective evaluation of more than 1000 colonic injuries confirms these views and indicates that intraperitoneal primary closure should be employed in the majority of colon injuries[2]. Methods involving exteriorization should be reserved for patients with complex injuries.

Principles and justification

Mechanisms of injury

Penetrating injuries

The vast majority of colonic injuries are due to penetrating trauma.

Knives, stilettos, screwdrivers and spokes penetrating the anterior aspect of the torso from nipple to pubis often penetrate the abdominal cavity. The colon (particularly the transverse and sigmoid) ranks third after small intestine and stomach in frequency of injury. Most injuries are through-and-through, and serious suspicion should be aroused by an odd number of holes. Penetration is less likely, but more difficult to diagnose, with posterior abdominal wounds.

Firearm injuries are classified according to the muzzle velocity[6,7]. High-velocity injuries are defined as those caused by a muzzle velocity of greater than 600 m/s. This is an artificial classification in civilian practice, because the firearm is often unidentified and the speed at impact unknown. The destructive force of an individual missile depends on two factors: first, its wounding energy, which is the difference in the kinetic energy of the bullet on impact and on leaving the body; and second, with missiles travelling at greater than 600 m/s, the creation of temporary cavitation which may cause tissue damage up to 30 times the diameter of the missile track and suck in debris from outside. Both cavitation and wounding energy depend on missile shape, and each component contributes a variable amount to the severity of an individual injury. Many hand guns deliver missiles with muzzle velocities in excess of 600 m/s, and shotgun injuries at close range may produce high-velocity damage. A large exit wound and gross tissue or bone destruction are highly suggestive of a high-velocity injury, but it may be extremely difficult to determine the velocity of an injury from the nature of the entry and exit wounds. Low-velocity missiles, which dissipate all their energy in the body, can be equally as destructive as high-velocity missiles, and both may produce a complicated intra-abdominal tract involving multiple organs.

Uncommon modes of injury

Colonic injury occurs in fewer than 5% of patients having a laparotomy for blunt trauma. This mechanism is often associated with extensive serosal bruising and mesenteric haematoma with delayed perforation. Iatrogenic colonic perforation after polypectomy at colonoscopy is well described. Perforation may occasionally follow sigmoidoscopy, barium enema, laparoscopy, culposcopy, or percutaneous pyelolithotomy. Foreign bodies swallowed or inserted into the anus may also cause occult injury to the colon. The relative rarity of these types of injuries dictates that their management has to be individualized.

Principles

The best results will be attained in patients in whom the effects of peritoneal contamination and hypovolaemic shock are reduced to a minimum. This can be achieved by rapid transport to hospital, vigorous adequate resuscitation, early administration of antibiotics followed by prompt repair of their injuries.

Indications

The approach to the diagnosis and the indications for laparotomy in the traumatized patient are controversial, particularly with respect to stab wounds. Refractory shock and peritonitis remain absolute indications to explore the abdomen. Institutions that receive many trauma victims have evolved management algorithms to reduce the number of negative explorations. All algorithms include frequent reassessment, preferably by the same experienced surgeon. Surgeons who manage penetrating injuries sporadically, however, should open the abdomen if penetration is suspected. After blunt trauma, diagnostic peritoneal lavage is often invaluable in determining the need for laparotomy.

Choice of colonic wound management

The trauma victim has had an acute pathophysiological insult, and it is the severity of this insult that dictates whether circumstances are favourable to effect primary repair in the individual patient or whether an exteriorization procedure should be performed.

Unfavourable circumstances for primary repair

Unfavourable circumstances for performing primary repair are most likely to occur in the severely injured patient, caused by high-velocity missiles, close-range, low-velocity firearms whose missiles arrest in the torso, or blunt trauma. These patients may require a lengthy operation to repair multiple intra-abdominal and extra-abdominal injuries, and they are often acidotic and hypothermic at the end of the procedure. In addition, a major vascular injury and persistent haemodynamic instability are not uncommonly present. Massive transfusion may precipitate a dilutional coagulopathy. These factors give rise to poorly perfused oedematous intestine with the consistency of wet blotting paper, which holds sutures poorly and mitigates against primary repair. Primary repair should probably also be avoided when delay with contamination has resulted in generalized peritonitis.

It is the presence of these factors, usually in combination, that suggests that these patients may be better served by exteriorization of the injury rather than primary repair. There remain, however, three situations which mandate such a procedure:

1. Complex pancreaticoduodenal injuries.
2. Vascular injury with a prosthetic repair.
3. Associated rectal injury.

Indications for exteriorization

Although primary repair is being used more often, exteriorization procedures still have a place in the management of certain injuries. It has particular merit in two situations: first, when repair is effected in the presence of generalized peritonitis; and secondly, when there is extensive associated subserosal bruising or a large mesenteric haematoma, even if the large intestinal wall appears viable. Whenever exteriorization is deemed necessary, the method with the lower morbidity is that of exteriorization of the primarily sutured wound, rather than exteriorization of the wound as a colostomy, because in up to 75% of patients the repaired colon can be returned to the abdomen between 5 and 7 days. Thus, prolonged colostomy care and subsequent readmission for closure with its attendant morbidity is avoided in the majority of patients.

Preoperative

Resuscitation

On admission, the patient is resuscitated and a full clinical examination, including the back and the rectum,

is carried out to assess the extent of the injuries. Blood must be taken for cross-matching, and a wide-bore (12-gauge) intravenous cannula is inserted in a forearm vein. A urinary catheter and a central venous line should be placed in all shocked patients and adequate oxygenation should be ensured. An erect (preferably posteroanterior) chest radiograph should be obtained to exclude concomitant thoracic injury. Abdominal radiography is not essential, but may be helpful in locating bullet fragments remaining in the body. Other investigations may be indicated depending on the nature and extent of the associated injuries.

Antibiotics

The optimal dose schedule has not been determined, but the trend for prophylaxis is towards a single intravenous dose of a second-generation or third-generation cephalosporin before operation, supplemented by one or two doses during or after operation, depending on the pharmacokinetics of the drug and the length of operation. The authors believe that therapeutic antibiotics continued for 5 days are seldom necessary and are best reserved for patients with established peritonitis or gross faecal soiling. In such cases, the addition of metronidazole provides the most effective anaerobic cover.

Operations

Position of patient

The lithotomy-Trendelenburg (Lloyd-Davies) position must be used when rectal injuries are suspected. This position has merit for surgery of all abdominal trauma, although the supine position is also satisfactory.

Incision

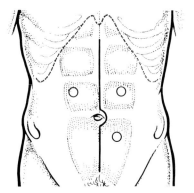

1   A long midline incision is the most suitable. This access ensures that the entire lateral abdominal wall remains available for exteriorization of the colon. In the shocked patient who responds poorly to preoperative resuscitation, it should be made initially from xiphisternum to pubic symphysis. On opening the abdomen, blood and contents should be removed using large abdominal packs to cope with, and control, massive ongoing haemorrhage for which suction is inadequate. The surgeon's first priority is to obtain haemostasis, whereupon systematic laparotomy can be carried out and all injuries identified and repaired. Colonic wounds should be next for repair after the control of haemorrhage.

INTRAPERITONEAL PRIMARY CLOSURE

The vast majority of colonic injuries may be managed by primary repair. This can be performed safely in stable patients even if it involves resection and anastomosis. Associated diaphragm or renal injuries are not contraindications to primary repair. A possible leak of urine should be drained retroperitoneally. Faecal contamination without peritonitis does not negate primary repair. Good peritoneal and wound toilet will minimize the risk of septic complications.

2 Gross faecal contamination, if present, is removed first. After milking the contents proximally and distally away from the wound, non-crushing intestinal clamps are applied to the transverse or sigmoid colon to prevent further spillage. The edges need to be debrided only if they are contused or devitalized. A small wound of less than 2 cm can be closed in the line of the wound. Large or complex adjacent through-and-through wounds should be closed transversely, to avoid stricture formation, or resected with primary anastomosis.

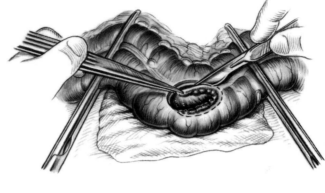

2

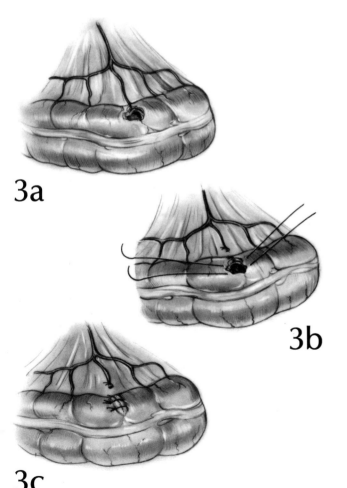

3a

3b

3c

3a–c It is imperative to assume that the posterior colonic wall has also been penetrated. After closing the anterior laceration, the colon is inspected to find the paired wound. It may be concealed by subserosal or mesentric haematomas, which must be explored to find the exit wound. Small wounds on the mesenteric border can be easily closed by serosubmucosal sutures. After ligating one of the small feeding vessels obscuring the wound, enough muscle is exposed to allow the placement of two or three interrupted sutures. These are tied after they have all been inserted. The placement of a second layer in this situation only serves to jeopardize the blood supply to the area and is not recommended.

Inspecting the retroperitoneal colon

The colon is mobilized in the area adjacent to the injury by dividing the parietal peritoneum of the paracolic gutter sufficiently to allow careful inspection of the posterior surface. In the case of injury to the flexures, wider mobilization is required.

4 Particular care should be exercised in mobilizing the splenic flexure. The left side of the lesser sac is entered by dividing the gastrocolic omentum below the gastroepiploic arch vessels. The lateral peritoneum of the descending colon should then be divided. Simultaneous gentle traction on the distal transverse colon and proximal descending colon in an inferomedial direction facilitates division between clamps of the condensation of peritoneum running from the apex of the splenic flexure to the tail of the spleen, thus avoiding the risk of a capsular tear of the spleen.

Retrocolic structures (ureter and gonadal vessels) are inspected for injury, and if a posterior colonic laceration is confirmed, it is debrided and sutured. On the right side, inferior vena caval injury becomes all too obvious when the retroperitoneal haematoma is disturbed and requires control and immediate repair. Duodenal injury may be more occult and is associated with a pancreatic injury. Both organs must be mobilized for careful inspection because they carry a very high mortality if injury to them is missed.

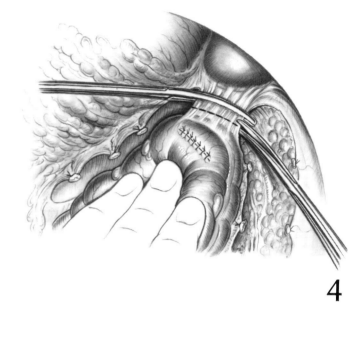

4

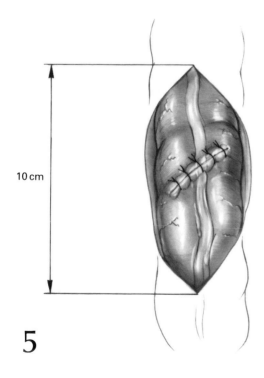

10 cm

5

EXTERIORIZATION OF THE PRIMARILY SUTURED COLON

A detailed description of this valuable method is merited because attention to technical detail determines its success or failure.

5 The abdominal wall is incised in the same direction as that taken by the part of the colon to be exteriorized. The length of the incision should be 10 cm (four finger widths). This will appear excessive when made in the paralysed anaesthetized patient. Too short an incision leads to oedema of the colon from compression by the abdominal wall and is a cause of early breakdown of the suture line, leading to the necessity for a colostomy. Too long an incision may allow small intestinal herniation alongside the exteriorized loop.

The injured colon must be mobilized so that the portion to be exteriorized will be clear of the skin, thus avoiding the possibility of necrotizing fasciitis should dehiscence of the colon wound occur with release of colonic contents into the subcutaneous fat.

Exteriorization fixation

6, 7 The exteriorized loop should be easily retained in position without tension by an 8-mm soft latex rubber tube. The tube is sutured to each edge of the wound and should be of sufficient length and rigidity to hold the subcutaneous tissue and skin open. It is then cut close to the sutures to allow a colostomy bag to be applied in which the colon is completely enclosed. Dressings of any description are avoided because they rapidly produce serositis of the colon wall. The warm, moist environment inside the sealed colostomy bag appears to favour wound healing.

If the incision in the abdominal wall is adequate, gas that collects in the exteriorized loop is easily emptied both proximally and distally into the intra-abdominal colon. This manoeuvre also confirms an adequate lumen for passage of intestinal contents through the loop.

Failure of the suture line to heal often has a technical basis. The loop may have been mobilized inadequately or the incision for exteriorization may be too small. Ileus with gaseous distension is transmitted to the exteriorized loop and the resulting tension on the suture line may cause dehiscence.

Return of healing loop

8 After it is clear that intraperitoneal sepsis has been avoided or has resolved, the healing exteriorized loop may be returned to the peritoneal cavity under general anaesthesia. This should not be performed if the suture line is unhealthy or if there is evidence of breakdown. Under no circumstances should a small hole in the suture line be repaired immediately before reduction. Replacement will normally be indicated between the fifth and tenth day and is usually accomplished by blunt digital dissection of the intestine from the wound edge.

If the intestine has been exteriorized for more than 10 days, sharp dissection is necessary to mobilize the colon loop. To promote a colocutaneous fistula should a leak subsequently occur, a soft latex rubber drain is placed to the site of the returned intestine. The abdominal wall is loosely approximated around the drain. A leak is uncommon if the policy described is followed.

Breakdown of the repair is more likely the longer the colon is out of its normal intraperitoneal environment. It occurs most commonly at about the seventh day, but exteriorization has been successfully used for up to 26 days without colonic breakdown.

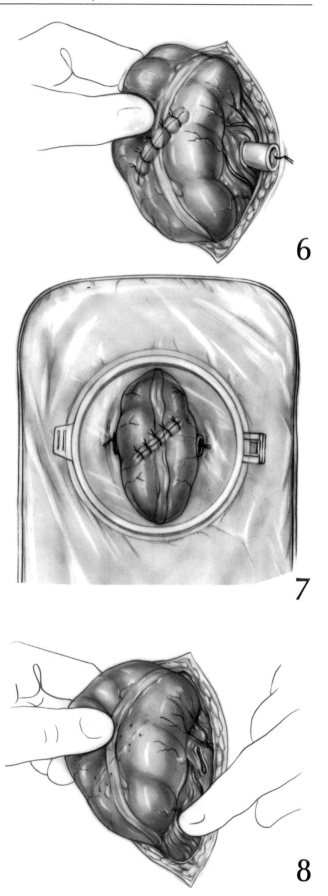

6

7

8

INJURIES REQUIRING RESECTION

9, 10 High-velocity bullet wounds produce an explosive 'bursting'-type injury of the colon, with diffuse vascular and tissue injury, extending several centimetres on either side of the laceration. The single most important therapeutic objective is wide debridement of all damaged tissue, which in the case of the colon demands resection back to healthy intestine. Except where there has been mesenteric injury with an expanding haematoma to the mesocolon, resection for trauma follows the technique used for total colectomy in inflammatory bowel disease. Vascular ligation is undertaken as close to the intestinal wall as is convenient. If conditions are favourable, continuity can safely be restored at the same time. The anastomosis must be performed without tension in the presence of a good blood supply to both ends. The authors perform the anastomosis using an interrupted serosubmucosal appositional technique with 2/0 polyglactin sutures. A two-layer sutured or a stapled anastomosis may also be safely employed.

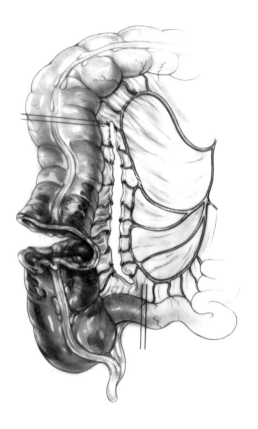

9

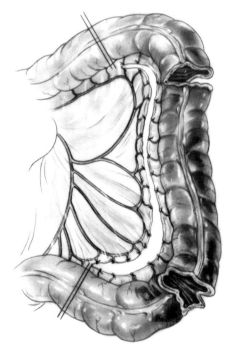

10

Formation of an end colostomy

11 If it is deemed unsafe to restore continuity after resection, an end colostomy should be constructed. The damaged intestine is resected using de Martel clamps. Adequate mobilization to allow the end of the colon to sit comfortably on the skin at the selected site without tension is essential. A disc of skin is excised at the selected site. The muscles are divided obliquely, and the peritoneum is entered. The knife is then turned at right angles, and a cruciate musculoperitoneal incision is made to allow three fingers to be passed into the peritoneal cavity. The colon end occluded by the de Martel clamp is passed through the defect created with the correct orientation of the mesentery.

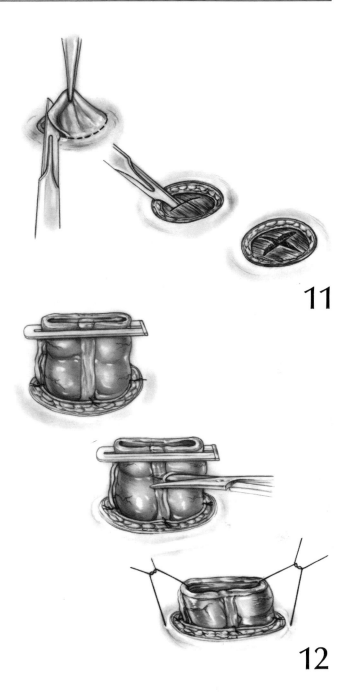

11

12 After the midline wound has been closed, the colon is fixed with three 2/0 polyglactin seromuscular sutures to the external oblique aponeurosis on both lateral aspects and its antimesenteric border. Mucocutaneous apposition is obtained using interrupted 3/0 polyglactin on a cutting needle.

The authors favour closing the distal end with a linear stapler with oversewing of the staple line using a 2/0 polypropylene suture which can be left long and used to hitch the colon to the peritoneum of the lateral aspect of the anterior abdominal wall. The distal end can be readily identified when restoration of continuity is undertaken. The distal end may be brought out as a mucous fistula. This requires careful placement to avoid its site impinging on the stoma appliance for the functioning colostomy. In addition, creation of the mucous fistula does not obviate the need for laparotomy to restore continuity.

Whenever possible the end colostomy should be sited to accept a well-fitting colostomy appliance, usually midway between the anterior superior iliac spine and the umbilicus.

12

Conclusion of operative procedures

Peritoneal toilet

When the intra-abdominal procedures have been completed, and before the removal of the colonic clamp, the peritoneal cavity should be irrigated with large quantities of warmed isotonic saline until the effluent is clean and free from all particulate matter. There is still controversy regarding the instillation of antibiotics into the peritoneal lavage fluid, but the authors favour the addition of tetracycline to the lavage solution.

Closure of the abdominal incision

Mass closure of the abdominal wall is performed with an 0 loop nylon or 1 polypropylene suture. The subcutaneous tissues should be closed unless there has been gross contamination or established peritonitis. Under these circumstances, they should be left open for either delayed primary closure or spontaneous healing.

The entry and exit wounds into the peritoneal cavity should be closed from the inside with 1 polyglactin suture incorporating transversus abdominis muscle to prevent herniation. The external traumatic wounds should be debrided and left open. High-velocity injuries should be debrided of all doubtfully viable muscle and the skin incised to allow good open drainage of the wound.

Postoperative care

Those patients with minimally to moderately severe injuries should be managed in a high-dependency nursing area for 12–24h. If they remain stable, the nasogastric tube and the Foley catheter should be removed by 48h. Oral fluids are commenced when postoperative ileus has resolved. Severely injured patients with colonic injuries require intensive care support, which will often entail rewarming, correction of acidosis, administration of blood products and ventilatory support. Those treated by primary repair will have the shortest stay.

Control of infection

The precise interrelationship between shock, sepsis and the development of multiple organ failure remains unclear. What is clear, however, is that the majority of deaths occur from multiple organ failure, that intraperitoneal sepsis is often present, but that the repaired colonic wound seldom breaks down. Therefore, alertness to the development of sepsis at various sites is imperative. Soft tissue sepsis related to the traumatic and surgical abdominal wounds may take several days to evolve. Although rare, extensive necrotizing fascitis or clostridial myonecrosis are life threatening and must be treated by wide drainage and debridement. The management of suspected intraperitoneal sepsis is controversial. The authors favour early 'second look' laparotomy to exclude signficant intra-abdominal collections and also advocate its use in high-velocity injuries where cavitation effects can produce delayed perforations in intestine that looked normal at the original operation. There is no clear indication when 'second-look' surgery should be performed, but after 48–72h it is reasonable to re-explore.

Later in the recovery period, ultrasonography or computed tomography may allow percutaneous drainage of well-localized abscesses in certain sites. Reoperative approaches often necessitate management of the open abdomen, which is messy and requires attention to detail over a prolonged intensive care course while organ failures are supported. The authors favour the use of a mesh or membrane to maintain closure after repeated operations. The operative treatment of colonic wounds is only one facet of the complex management of these patients.

Enterocutaneous fistula

Enterocutaneous fistulae may occur at any stage. Those that occur early may be related to missed injuries or anastomotic failure. Late fistulae occur in those patients with septic wound dehiscence or when an abdominal wound is managed by the open method. The establishment of a controlled fistula, with appropriate drainage of associated abscesses, and adequate nutritional support are the mainstays of management. The majority of fistulae, particularly those with a high output, are from small intestine and require intravenous nutritional support. Low-output colocutaneous fistulae can usually be effectively managed by enteral nutritional support until they heal. Unless there is mucocutaneous continuity or distal obstruction, these fistulae are likely to close spontaneously, and the healing process can be accelerated by the use of somatostatin. Operative closure should only be performed when the patient is in an optimal nutritional state.

Stoma management

Those patients in whom a stoma has been created do not have the advantage of preoperative siting or counselling, and the stoma may not be optimally placed. Hence, a stoma care nurse forms an integral part of the management team and must be involved early. It is also wise for the surgeon to allay fears regarding the colostomy. He must reassure the patient that the stoma is temporary and that continuity will be restored, usually 6–8 weeks after the initial operation.

References

1. Imes PR. War surgery of the abdomen. *Surg Gynecol Obstet* 1945; 81: 608–16.

2. Baker LW, Thomson SR. The current status of the management of civilian colon injuries. In: Nyhus L, ed. *Surgery Annual*. Connecticut: Appleton and Lange, 1990: 203–23.

3. Stone HH, Fabian TC. Management of perforating colon trauma: randomisation between primary closure and exteriorisation. *Ann Surg* 1979; 190: 430–6.

4. George SM, Fabian TC, Voeller GR et al. Primary repair of colon wounds. *Ann Surg* 1989; 209: 728–34.

5. Chappuis CW, Frey DJ, Dietzen CD et al. Management of penetrating colon injuries. *Ann Surg* 1991; 213: 492–8.

6. Owen-Smith MS. *High Velocity Missile Wounds*. London: Edward Arnold, 1981.

7. Cooper GJ, Ryan JM. Interaction of penetrating missiles with tissues: some common misapprehensions and implications for wound management. *Br J Surg* 1990; 77: 606–10.

Illustrations by Angela Christie

Colonic surgery for acute conditions: amoebiasis

Frederick M. Luvuno FRCS(Ed), FRCS(Glas)
Senior Consultant Surgeon, King Edward VIII Hospital and Senior Lecturer, Department of Surgery, University of Natal, Congella, Durban, South Africa

Background

Amoebiasis is common in the tropics and subtropics, but with the ease of air travel it can be found anywhere. Invasive amoebiasis begins when trophozoites of *Entamoeba histolytica* invade the colonic mucosa and ingest red blood cells; this indicates their invasive potential. Complicated amoebic colitis (transmural amoebic colitis) has a high mortality rate whether treated conservatively or by major colonic resection[1]. Resectional surgery, which necessitates that the protective adhesions be undone to assess the extent of transmural ischaemic necrosis of the colon, is associated with considerable mortality rates. Experience of resectional surgery in this hospital reveals a mortality rate of 24%[2]. However, the mortality rate for non-resectional surgery was less than 12%[3] initially, and currently it has decreased to 9%. Non-resectional surgery evolved from the fact that a clean peritoneal cavity found at laparotomy in the presence of advanced transmural amoebic colitis suggested that the results of surgery might be improved if the protective adhesions attracted by the ischaemic colon with transmural amoebic colitis were not disturbed. In fact, these adhesions protect the peritoneal cavity mechanically should the necrotic colon perforate. Further bacterial contamination from the colon is minimized by perileotomy on-table antegrade colonic lavage with removal of colon contents through the anus[4]. The lavaged colon is defunctioned by an ileostomy (phase 1 surgery) which is maintained for 6 weeks before closure (phase 2 surgery). The operation performed for complicated amoebic colitis treated by laparotomy, colonic lavage and ileostomy decompression (phase 1 surgery) is described here. Restoring continuity of the bowel after 6 weeks (phase 2 surgery) will be only briefly described as it is an elective procedure.

Mucosal amoebic colitis

1 Mucosal amoebic colitis is defined as patchy necrotic ulceration confined to the mucosa of the colon. The colon muscle and serosa are normal. This is a medical condition and responds well to oral metronidazole, 800 mg 8-hourly for 7–10 days if possible, or 500 mg intravenously 8-hourly. Mucosal disease will be excluded from this discussion. However, extensive mucosal disease, usually extending from the rectum to the caecum, is clinically indistinguishable from, and can merge imperceptibly into, complicated transmural amoebic colitis, the surgical management and treatment of which is described here.

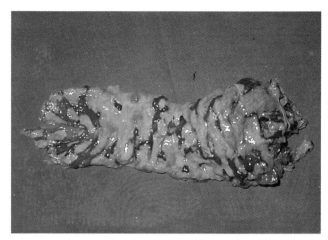

1

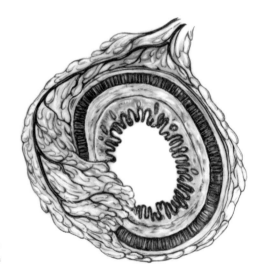

2

Transmural amoebic colitis

2 Progress of amoebic colitis from mucosal disease to transmural amoebic colitis[1] is due to thrombotic occlusion of vessels supplying a segment of colon. Transmural amoebic colitis is defined as progressive, segmental, ischaemic necrosis of the entire thickness of the colon wall, including the serosa, and has two elements: (1) necrosing colon at the centre, surrounded by (2) viable vascular adhesions on the outside called the 'adhesive wraps'.

Adhesive wraps[5] are defined as adhesions attracted by ischaemic colon caused by transmural amoebic colitis. The adhesive wraps protect the peritoneal cavity mechanically from faecal soiling should perforation of the colon occur. Hence the laparotomy finding of a clean peritoneal cavity in the presence of advanced transmural necrosis of the colon is the rule. Furthermore, these adhesive wraps act as vascular grafts to the ischaemic colon.

Postamoebic syndromes

These are symptom complexes resulting from treated severe amoebic colitis associated with postamoebic strictures and postamoebic dysentery. Strictures may require elective surgery.

Preoperative preparation (phase 1 surgery)

The preoperative principles in transmural amoebic colitis are to minimize the risk of misdiagnosis by having a high index of suspicion of amoebiasis in all patients with an acute abdomen, diarrhoea or proctitis. In all patients with an acute abdomen or diarrhoeal illness the following must be performed: inspection of the diarrhoeal stool for slough; digital rectal examination feeling for rugged ulceration; and proctosigmoidoscopy to confirm the ulceration and to allow biopsy of the edge of the ulcers. Patients requiring a laparotomy should be placed in the Lloyd-Davies position in anticipation of misdiagnosis because transmural amoebic colitis may mimic many surgical conditions[2].

Diagnosis of amoebic colitis

Although diagnosis is difficult, it is helpful to note the following:

1. Ulceration felt by finger on rectal examination and seen on sigmoidoscopy.
2. Identification of haematophous amoebae in the stool or tissue biopsies.
3. Finding of characteristic adhesive wraps at laparotomy.

Resuscitation

Resuscitation includes correction of fluids and electrolytes with a trial of oral metronidazole, 800 mg 8-hourly if possible, or 500 mg 8-hourly intravenously for 24–48 h. A Foley catheter should be placed to monitor urine output and the central venous pressure should be measured to allow adequate volume and colloid replacement without the risk of overhydration, which these hypoalbuminaemic patients tolerate poorly. Serial plain abdominal radiographs are useful as they will indicate extraluminal gas or obstruction[3], previously referred to as the toxic megacolon of amoebic colitis.

Indications for surgery[6]

Indications for surgery are failure to respond to, or deterioration during, medical treatment; extraluminal gas such as air under the diaphragm or retroperitoneal mottling; intestinal obstruction indicated by persistent abdominal distension associated with radiological evidence of megacolon; and rectal bleeding.

Operation

The operative strategies in transmural amoebic colitis are as follows:

1. To establish the diagnosis very soon after entering the abdomen by finding a clean peritoneal cavity and a colon buried in omental wraps in a patient with an 'acute abdomen'.
2. Minimal disturbance of adhesive wraps.
3. Avoidance of resectional surgery with its accompanying massive peritoneal faecal soiling and marked blood loss, both of which greatly compromise the patient.
4. Prograde colonic lavage to decrease bacterial contamination by the colon of the peritoneal cavity, and protection of the lavaged colon by a defunctioning ileostomy maintained for 6 weeks (phase 1 surgery).

PHASE 1 TECHNIQUE

At operation all patients are placed in the Lloyd-Davies position (*see Illustration 3* on page 48) with facilities for carrying out on-table prograde colonic lavage with discharge of the effluent through an anal tube[4].

3   The anal tube is a transparent corrugated anaesthetic elephant tube which is held in place with a purse-string at the anus with 2/0 black silk on a cutting Colt needle. The suture is tied firmly at the anus and is not cut, but a knot is made about 4–5 cm from the anal purse-string and tied again to the elephant tube to prevent the tube from disconnecting from the weight of the irrigation fluid. The distal end of the elephant tube is tied to a transparent waste plastic bag to produce a closed system through which the irrigation fluid can be inspected to judge its clarity during lavage. The refuse bag is placed in a bucket with wheels so that it is mobile and can be pushed back and forth for inspection of the lavage fluid.

The bottom draping towel is placed astride both legs from the pubic symphysis to hang over the toes, leaving the anus exposed. This is particularly important to allow access in cases where amoebiasis was not suspected in an acute abdomen and is diagnosed by finding a clean peritoneal cavity with adhesive wraps. The anus is accessible to an assistant who can place the corrugated anaesthetic tube by getting under the leg towels without disturbing or contaminating the abdominal exposure. The scrub nurse stands on the left with the tray over the leg towels. The irrigation fluid stand should be placed away from the tray, preferably behind the upper drapes to allow a constant supply of irrigation fluid. A big Y-shaped connector facilitates the change over of the irrigation fluid reservoirs which prevents delays during the change of empty bottles. Isotonic saline is preferable because its physiological nature is less damaging to the ulcerated colonic mucosa than water.

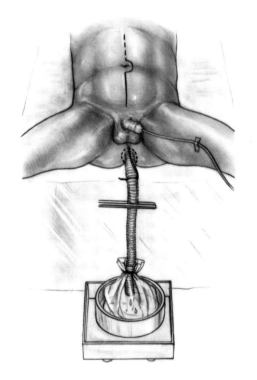

3

Incision

4   If a diagnosis of amoebiasis has been made before operation, a short midline incision is made from the umbilicus to the pubic symphysis. If diagnosis was missed, no rectal tube is *in situ* and a long abdominal incision has been made, the upper part of the incision is closed up to the umbilicus to restore the tamponading effect of the abdominal wall and the assistant is requested to insert an anal tube.

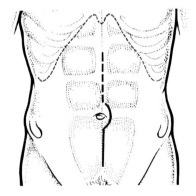

4

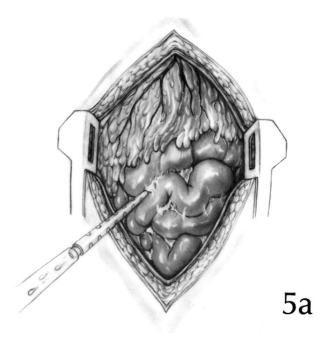

5a

Identification of terminal ileum

5a, b With minimal disturbance of the wraps, the terminal ileum is isolated and brought out as a loop. A peritoneal fold on the antimesenteric border of the terminal ileum is a useful marker to identify the terminal ileum among loops of small bowel. This peritoneal fold is constant and triangular in shape, with its base extending from the caecum to the caecoileal junction. The fold may rise more than 1 cm above the oedematous bowel and terminates in an apex, which is usually only 4–6 cm from the ileocaecal junction. This marker is easily seen in oedematous bowel and thus helps to avoid delivering the wrong small bowel loop from the incision.

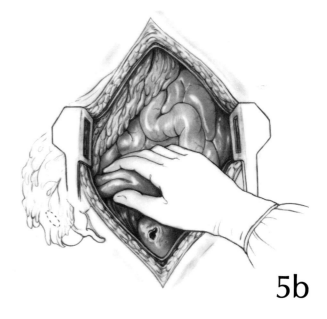

5b

6 When an ileal loop long enough to reach the skin surface of the abdomen without tension has been delivered, an ileotomy is performed, a 28-Fr Foley catheter is passed through the ileotomy as far distally as is possible, and a purse-string is tied around the catheter after distending the catheter bulb to prevent it from slipping out. A soft bowel clamp is applied just proximal to the ileotomy to prevent retrograde flow of irrigation fluid. The Foley catheter is then connected to the irrigation system and 10–12 litres of warmed fluid are used during irrigation. The endpoint of irrigation is clear fluid seen through the transparent closed collecting system.

If the abdominal incision is long, the tamponading effect of the abdominal wall is lost and colonic distension by irrigation fluid is common. This can be frightening but merely indicates that in amoebic transmural disease of the large bowel there is usually an element of obstruction which may present clinically as the so-called toxic megacolon. Warm packs for compression over the short subumbilical incision minimize the distension of the colon. Abdominal agitation is necessary to hasten the lavage procedure and minimal leaks of irrigating fluid, which merely trickle through the compressive packs at the abdominal incision, are ignored.

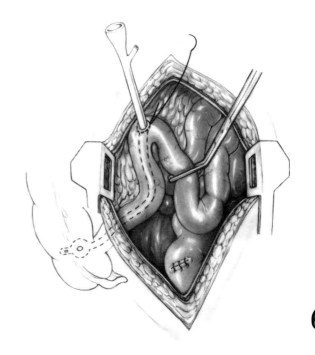

6

7

Massive leaks

7 Massive leakage of irrigating fluid, making lavage inefficient, is usually caused by inadvertent disturbance of caecal or sigmoid wraps on initial ileal mobilization. The perforation is closed watertight by a simple suture with an absorbable material or patched with omentum, usually after extending the laparotomy incision. The incision is then again partially closed to the umbilicus to restore the tamponade effect to the upper abdomen. Suture patching of the perforations can be frustrating as the bowel easily cuts through and is friable. Gentle traction just to approximate the edges (with tension being taken up by the patching omentum or small bowel) is crucial to success. Insignificant leaks often persist but they do not interfere with effective lavaging.

Once the effluent is clear when viewed through the transparent bag (usually after 10–12 litres of saline), a defunctioning ileostomy is performed.

Defunctioning ileostomy

8 A pair of artery forceps is pushed through the mesentery of the ileum very close to the intestine directly opposite the previous ileotomy. A Jacques catheter is pulled through and its two limbs clamped with a pair of artery forceps. The irrigation Foley catheter is also clamped and disconnected from the lavage system.

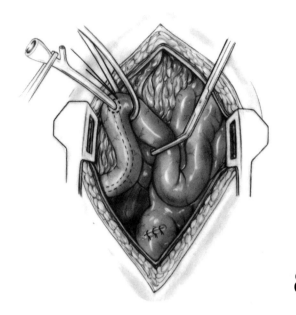

8

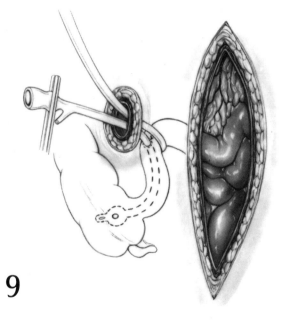

9

Delivery of ileostomy with intubation of distal and proximal limbs

9 The occluding soft bowel clamp on the proximal ileal limb of the ileostomy is removed. An adequate ileostomy incision is made at the right iliac fossa, usually admitting three or four of the operating surgeon's fingers. A tight wound around the ileostomy is the major cause of small bowel fistulae at that site. A big artery forceps (e.g. a Robert's) is passed through the abdominal ileostomy wound and the Jacques and the Foley catheters are serially delivered, taking care not to tear the bowel during traction. The distal limb is easily recognized because it is intubated with a Foley catheter.

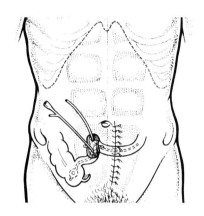

10a

10a, b

The proximal limb is then intubated with a latex tube under vision before closing the abdominal wound. The intubation of the proximal and distal ileostomy limbs allows postoperative egress of fluid and gas, thereby preventing the build-up of intracolonic pressure which could disrupt the wraps.

Drainage of associated amoebic abscess

The liver is always palpated for the presence of an associated amoebic liver abscess in those patients who have not had liver ultrasonography which might exclude it. At operation, the hand is inserted between the undisturbed adhesive wraps and the abdominal wall to palpate the liver to exclude an amoebic liver abscess. Whereas small abscesses are not important even when missed, large abscesses are intubated blindly percutaneously and led into a sterile closed system.

Lavage of abdominal cavity

This is important only when there has been soiling and should be done with great care so that adhesive wraps are not disturbed.

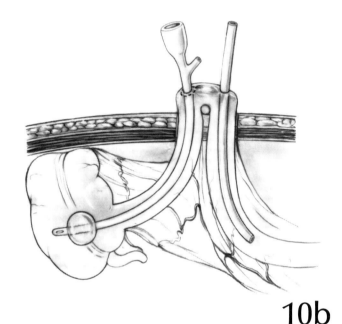

10b

Abdominal wound closure

The abdominal cavity is closed in mass fashion with nylon. If there has been no gross contamination, the skin is closed. Finally the corrugated anaesthetic elephant tube which was fixed at the anus is removed. The ileostomy is left *in situ* for 6 weeks.

PHASE 2 SURGERY

Before ileostomy closure, usually at 6 weeks, the colon is assessed by barium enema for strictures as these may require resection and anastomosis or stricturoplasty depending on the calibre of the lumen. If barium flows freely, even in the presence of radiological narrowing, the ileostomy is closed while the healed diseased bowel is left alone.

Postoperative care

Complications

Fluid overload

Fluid overload with consequent pulmonary oedema and respiratory failure is the major cause of death. Fluids should be given with absolute caution because these patients will not tolerate even the standard postoperative fluid requirements.

Intestinal fistulae

Compression of the ileostomy by the abdominal wall and even strangulation of ileostomy limbs are the main causes of small bowel fistulae.

Wound infection

Infection occurs only if there has been gross contamination of the wound and there is usually partial disruption not requiring resuture.

Other complications

These include colovesical or colosplenic arterial fistulae, which usually occur during the second week of recovery when ischaemic necrosis is removed by the healing process, thereby exposing the adhesive wraps to the lumen of the colon. Erosion of vessels of the adhesive wraps may cause a life-threatening bleed requiring surgery. Arterial embolization should be attempted; if this fails, laparotomy is performed to ligate the bleeding vessel. However, localization of the source of bleeding may be very difficult.

After lavage, patients are anorectic; they may refuse to eat and die from metabolic derangement.

Establishment of bowel continuity (phase 2 surgery)

Approximately 6 weeks after prograde colonic lavage and ileostomy decompression, bowel continuity is established after radiological assessment which is performed through the anus and the ileostomy. Gentle pressure is used during barium examination to avoid barium leaking into the peritoneal cavity. Most patients will require only closure of the ileostomy, although some may require resection or stricturoplasty.

References

1. Luvuno FM, Mtshali Z, Baker LW. Vascular occlusion in the pathogenesis of complicated amoebic colitis: evidence for an hypothesis. *Br J Surg* 1985; 72: 123–7.

2. Luvuno FM. Role of intraoperative prograde colonic lavage and a decompressive loop ileostomy in the management of transmural amoebic colitis. *Br J Surg* 1990; 77: 156–9.

3. Luvuno FM. Letters to the Editor. *Am J Surg* 1987; 155: 451–8.

4. Dudley HAF, Racliffe AG, McGeehan D. Intraoperative irrigation of the colon to permit primary anastomosis. *Br J Surg* 1980; 67: 80–1.

5. Luvuno FM. The role of adhesive wraps in the pathogenesis of complicated amoebic colitis: evidence for auto-tissue graft and revascularization of ischaemic colon. *Br J Surg* 1988; 75: 713–16.

6. Luvuno FM. Surgery for complicated amoebiasis. In: Watters DAK, ed. *Baillière's Clin Trop Med Commun Dis* 1988; 3: 349–65.

Pelvic and rectal surgery: introductory comment

Keith A. Kelly MD, FACS, FRCSEd
Professor and Chair, Department of Surgery, Mayo Clinic and Mayo Medical School, Rochester, Minnesota, USA

The operative approach to pelvic and rectal diseases has taken a quantum leap forward, as outlined in the chapters in this section. These advances in surgery have been possible because of concurrent advances in basic sciences pertinent to the field, improved surgical techniques, and better preoperative, operative and postoperative care.

Advances in basic sciences

The anatomical course of the nervi erigentes is now known more accurately. Today these nerves can be preserved at operation, even though wide excision of the rectum is performed. A clearer understanding of pararectal, presacral and perianal anatomy has allowed direct repair and better drainage of rectal and anal injuries.

Recent advances in physiology have taught us the importance of a compliant, adequately sized rectal reservoir and an intact anal sphincter for the maintenance of faecal continence. With these points in mind, surgeons writing here describe the preservation or reconstruction of the reservoir and the protection of the sphincter in more patients than previously when treating benign or malignant conditions of the proctodeum.

Careful studies in pathology have given us a better understanding of the spread of malignant tumours. Extensive excisions (>3 cm) distal to rectal cancers are now recognized to be necessary only infrequently, allowing the distal rectal wall and the anal canal to be preserved for restoration of enteric continuity and transanal defaecation. The spread of malignant cells, not only superiorly along the superior rectal lymphatic chain but also laterally along the middle haemorrhoidal chain, has supported the resection of the lateral nodes and the superior nodes when operating for malignancy.

The use of molecular biology techniques, such as recognizing the diploid chromosomal pattern of more benign, less invasive rectal malignancies, has allowed an increased use of local resection or fulguration when treating these tumours.

Improved surgical techniques

The surgeons writing these chapters have also used new transanal, laparoscopic and stapling techniques to make their pelvic and rectal operations better tolerated, less costly and followed by a quicker recovery. Current transanal procedures are described for benign tumours and enterocoeles of the rectum, and for certain small, low grade, mobile, minimally invasive, non-ulcerated, less aggressive malignant tumours. In these operations, no cutaneous incision is required. Colonic resections via the laparoscope, with less postoperative disability, a shorter hospital stay, and a more rapid return to good health and to the workplace, are described. The proximal colon or even the small intestine can be stapled to the anal canal to restore transanal faecal flow and reasonable faecal continence after colorectal resections. These stapling techniques are often faster and safer than the conventional, hand sewn anastomoses.

Better patient care

The recognition of the importance of an adequate bowel preparation, attention to nutrition and resolution of concomitant medical problems before operation has meant safer conduct of the procedures described, fewer complications and a more rapid return to good health. Invasive and non-invasive monitoring during the procedures has prevented perioperative complications or allowed such complications to be recognized promptly and treated early, before they progress. Pain after operation is controlled with epidural anaesthesia. Patient-controlled, intravenous analgesia has decreased postoperative discomfort and has speeded recovery.

Better antibiotics have prevented, or treated more effectively, infections related to the disease or to the operation.

Future directions

In summary, these features and others outlined in this section have greatly improved patient care, restored patients to a better quality of life after operation, and probably reduced the costs of care. Continued application of these advances will bring excellent results to our patients in the future.

Anterior resection of the rectum

R. J. Heald MA, MChir, FRCS, FRCSEd
Consultant Surgeon, Colorectal Research Unit, Basingstoke District Hospital, Basingstoke, Hampshire, UK

Prepared with the advice and collaboration of the former author of this chapter:

J. C. Goligher FRCS
Emeritus Professor of Surgery, University of Leeds, Leeds, UK

History

Until 20 years ago, anterior resection of the rectum, although a well established procedure, was considered appropriate for only the 30–50% of patients in whom the tumour was in the upper part of the rectum: it is now the accepted operation for 80–90% of all patients with rectal cancer. However, some of the lower lesions so treated impose special difficulties and carry a greater risk of complications.

Three important changes in surgical technique have led to the increased usage of this operation: (1) the recognition that a margin of clearance of 2.0 cm of apparently uninvolved intestinal wall beyond the palpable distal edge of the growth (or possibly less) is adequate, instead of the 5-cm margin previously considered necessary; (2) the availability of stapling devices that enable a colorectal anastomosis to be constructed with good results as low as the top of the anal canal; and (3) the appreciation that a thorough dissection and complete mobilization of the rectum and the cancer by the abdominal operator is necessary before deciding whether a sphincter-saving resection is possible.

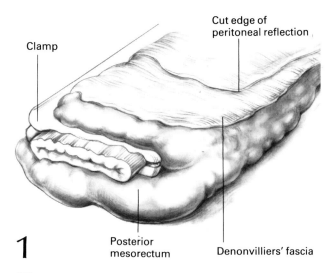

Clamp

Cut edge of peritoneal reflection

Posterior mesorectum

Denonvilliers' fascia

1

1 Good results can be attained by rectal mobilization in which the avascular plane between the visceral and parietal structures is identified under direct vision as a delicate filamentous latticework of areolar tissue. This encapsulation of the rectum and its mesorectum within a surgically definable plane provides one of the finest opportunities in surgery for a clear monobloc resection of a cancer-bearing organ and its principal field of direct, lymphatic and vascular spread. The precise development of the plane in the depths of the pelvis does, however, present special difficulties, and failure to excise this monobloc of tissue completely may explain the considerable differences in the incidence of local tumour recurrence recorded by different surgeons[1, 2].

Principles and justification

Several procedures are appropriate, depending on the circumstances. Each should be considered carefully.

Abdominoperineal excision (*see* also pp. 472–487)

This procedure is appropriate only for carcinomas that invade the anal sphincter or for those tumours which, after full mobilization in the visceroparietal plane, are so close to the sphincter that a clamp cannot be placed safely below the palpable edge of the tumour with an adequate margin of clearance. Thus, an abdominoperineal excision is more frequently necessary in an obese man with a narrow pelvis than in a woman. It may also be preferred to a very low anterior resection when anal sphincter tone and function are impaired, although some surgeons may prefer to undertake a Hartmann's procedure (*see* chapter on pp. 488–496) in this situation.

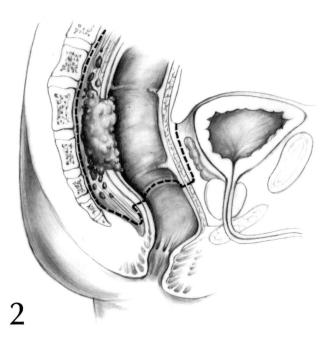

2

Low anterior resection with total mesorectal excision

2   The authors believe that the complete mesorectum should be removed as part of the proper clearance of all mid and low rectal tumours[3]. After full mobilization, the distal 'tail' of the mesorectum may be trimmed posteriorly and removed with the specimen to leave a 3–4-cm reservoir of rectal muscle tube above the anal canal. The precise site of the tumour will determine the length of distal rectum that can remain. The anastomosis (for which most surgeons will find the stapled technique easier) may thus lie up to 5 cm from the dentate line.

Usually, mobilization of the splenic flexure will be necessary to achieve an adequate length of colon for an anastomosis at this level. In addition, the large cavity created in the pelvis must be 'filled' with viable tissue and effectively drained with suction for the first 48 h after surgery. The large size of this cavity and the small size of the rectal reservoir distal to the anastomosis are important factors contributing to the risk of anastomotic leakage (*see* also chapter on pp. 93–104).

Many surgeons regard temporary defunctioning of the anastomosis by a proximal loop transverse colostomy or loop ileostomy as a wise precaution in these cases of very low anastomosis.

High anterior resection and mesorectal division

3   In this procedure the mesorectum is transected 5 cm below the tumour and the anastomosis is constructed in the middle third of the rectum, giving a rectal stump 8–10 cm long above the dentate line. Thus the size of the cavity remaining in the pelvis is smaller, and the higher and relatively easier anastomosis can be made manually or stapled according to the surgeon's preference. It is appropriate for patients with tumours above the peritoneal reflection in whom mobilization achieves sufficient length for the mesorectum to be divided 5 cm below the lower edge of the cancer. Full mobilization of the splenic flexure is usually unnecessary, suction drainage can often be omitted, and defunctioning is almost never required. The procedure is less of an undertaking than a low anterior resection with complete mesorectal excision and is associated with a much lesser incidence of anastomotic dehiscence and other complications.

Surgeons vary in the frequency with which they use high anterior resection. One of the authors (RJH) feels it appropriate in only about 15% of true rectal cancers because of the fear of local tumour recurrence arising from lymphatic and other satellite deposits of growth in the mesorectal tissues which are not excised. High anterior resection is used rather more frequently by JCG, particularly in patients whose rectal lesions lie 10 cm (or more) above the anal verge when measured at the preoperative sigmoidoscopy.

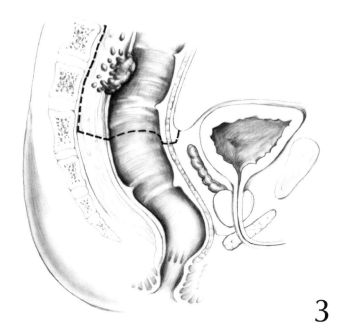

3

Abdominoanal, abdominosacral and abdominotransanal resections

These operations were popular with some surgeons when anterior resection was confined to growths of the upper rectum. The development of low anterior resection techniques and the advent of staplers have made these methods less useful alternatives (*see* chapter on pp. 546–556 for further details).

Extended Hartmann procedure

The extent and technique of excision of tissue in this operation is identical to that of a low anterior resection, but no anastomosis is performed. Instead the patient is left with an iliac colostomy, an intact anal canal, and a small (open or closed) distal rectal stump, extending just above the pelvic floor (*see* chapter on pp. 488–496). It is appropriate for patients in whom an anastomosis is undesirable or likely to be unduly risky, a colostomy is acceptable, and in whom the tumour can be mobilized sufficiently for the bowel to be divided below it with an adequate margin of clearance. It may be particularly applicable if irremovable extensions of growth in the pelvis make local recurrence inevitable, or if the reason for avoiding an anastomosis is a patulous anal sphincter.

Local excision

This is appropriate for small mobile cancers in the lower half of the rectum that have not invaded the muscle coat of the intestinal wall, particularly those so close to the anal sphincter that only an abdominoperineal excision would provide adequate clearance. The indication is considerably strengthened if the patient is deemed to be an especially poor risk for abdominoperineal excision.

Preoperative

Clinical assessment

Frail patients may be judged unsuitable for the major surgery involved, and thus assessment of the general and cardiopulmonary condition of the patient is of great importance. Cardiac function tests may be useful, and assessment of peripheral vascular supply to the legs is always necessary because acute (and possibly fatal) postoperative leg ischaemia can occur when visceral collaterals, which have maintained a tenuous arterial supply to the legs, are interrupted by surgery[4].

The quality of the anal sphincter and its tone on rectal examination are also important: a patient prone to leakage or incontinence with a patulous sphincter would be unsuitable for very low colorectal or coloanal anastomosis. Previous intestinal resections and/or coexisting gastrointestinal disease causing diarrhoea or urgency might also influence the decision as to the most appropriate operation. The patient's own desire to avoid a stoma needs to be balanced against any of these relative contraindications.

Biopsy

A biopsy to confirm the diagnosis is essential before proceeding to surgery of this magnitude. However, the presence of a high-grade (poorly differentiated) tumour is no longer regarded as a contraindication to the performance of a sphincter-conserving operation.

Imaging

Both computed tomography (CT) and ultrasonography have enabled identification of local tumour spread and nodal metastasis. Substantial extrarectal spread more than 5 mm in diameter, or obvious nodal spread, apparent on a CT scan may also provide a guide towards the use of full-dose preoperative radiotherapy. Improved CT, ultrasonography and magnetic resonance imaging techniques will give the surgeon more precise information concerning the extent of tumour spread.

An intravenous pyelogram is of value with lesions which are close to the ureter (e.g. rectosigmoid, sigmoid and caecal tumours) and in the few large fixed rectal tumours which occupy the whole pelvis. However, it has little relevance to the routine mid-rectal carcinoma because the ureter is anterior to such lesions.

The entire large intestine should be examined using either double-contrast radiology or colonoscopy to exclude the presence of synchronous tumours (which occur in 3.5–4.0% of cases) and polyps. When the obstructive nature of the primary rectal tumour makes this impossible, careful palpation at operation should be combined with colonoscopy during the first 6–12 months after surgery to establish that the patient has a truly 'clear colon' (see chapter on pp. 142–150).

Examination under anaesthesia

Patients should be examined rectally under general anaesthesia, and bimanual abdominovaginal examination in a woman should always be performed. In selected cases, cystoscopy may be necessary for bladder inspection and to insert ureteric stents. The assessment of tumour mobility and the extent of invasion of local structures will help the selection of locally advanced tumours for preoperative radiotherapy. Assuming that the surgeon decides to proceed with an operation, a urethral catheter is then inserted.

Bowel preparation

An empty large intestine is desirable, and can be achieved satisfactorily by combining clear fluids by mouth for 48 h before surgery with oral laxatives. During surgery, if more than minimal residual faeces are found in the colon, an on-table lavage can be performed (see chapter on pp. 397–415). Systemic antibacterial agents, including those effective against anaerobes (such as metronidazole) are commenced 1–2 h before surgery and administered every 6 h thereafter for 24 h.

Operations

LOW ANTERIOR RESECTION WITH TOTAL MESORECTAL EXCISION

Position of patient

The lithotomy-Trendelenburg position is used (see chapter on pp. 47–50) which ensures a choice of operation in the light of the operative findings (sphincter-saving resection or abdominoperineal excision). In the event of a restorative resection, this position permits the anal insertion of a staple gun. The patient is kept horizontal during the initial abdominal phase of the operation and only tilted 15–20° head down when the pelvic dissection commences.

Good lighting of the operative field is extremely important. It can be obtained by readjusting the readily moved and focused operating room lights to meet the needs of different phases of the dissection, a headlight (which some surgeons find rather irksome) and by incorporating lights into retractors.

Incision and abdominal exploration

4 The best access to the abdomen and pelvis is provided by a long vertical median or left paramedian incision extending from the pubic symphysis to well above the umbilicus. In obese male patients, anything short of an incision from the pubic symphysis to the xiphoid is unlikely to be satisfactory. Some surgeons advocate a long transverse incision, but in the authors' experience this is less satisfactory for the pelvic dissection than a conventional vertical approach.

The next step is a thorough exploration of the abdominal cavity to determine the presence of any extensions of the growth, special attention being directed to the liver, the greater omentum and peritoneal surfaces, the small intestine, the entire large intestine, and finally the rectum and the primary lesion itself. If no contraindication to excision is found, a self-retaining retractor is inserted. Loops of small intestine must be displaced away from the intended dissection in the left lower abdomen by enclosing it in a plastic bag which is then placed to the patient's right in front of the abdominal wall, into the right upper peritoneal compartment, or by packing the individual coils of intestine into the right upper compartment with a 20-cm wide roll of gauze, tightly rolled and held in place by an assistant's hand or a Finnochetto retractor.

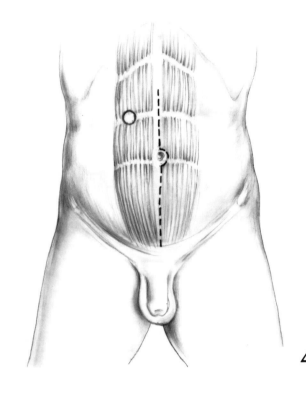

4

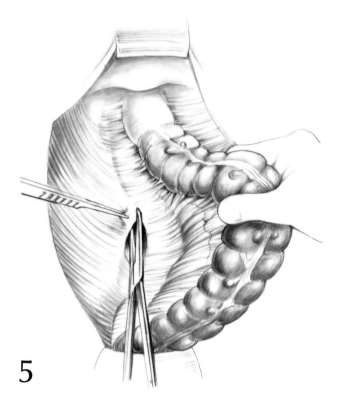

5

Initial incision of the visceral peritoneum

5 This will generally begin to the left or to the right of the pelvic brim. The left side is customary, the white lines of congenital adhesions between the left leaf of the mesosigmoid and the posterior parietal peritoneum providing a convenient starting point. It is important to gain access to the avascular plane between the mesentery and the surrounding parietal structures: a valuable clue to this is the mobility of the tissues which can be readily seen through the transparent peritoneum. A perfectly avascular plane can be developed in front of the bifurcation of the presacral nerve as it crosses the aortic bifurcation.

The process of lifting forward the superior rectal vessels and mesorectum is thus initiated. If a perfect avascular plane is not readily found to the left of the mesocolon, the operator should make a corresponding incision on the right side where vision and lighting are often better. The orientation provided by this plane is important for the satisfactory dissection of the more distal parts of the dissection.

6 Further dissection is divided into three stages.

1. Extension of the peritoneal cut around the left side of the splenic flexure, fully mobilizing the left colon and exposing the termination of the inferior mesenteric vein.
2. Extension of the right cut to encircle and facilitate the ligation of the inferior mesenteric artery and vein.
3. Extension of both planes downwards into the pelvis around the fully mobilized mesorectum, rectum, and the cancer.

The order in which these procedures are performed will vary according to circumstances: for example mobilization of the splenic flexure is not needed if an abdominoperineal excision becomes necessary, if the tumour can be resected with mesorectal division and a relatively high anastomosis, or if a trial dissection leads to the decision to refer the patient for radiotherapy; in some low cases an exceptionally long and well vascularized sigmoid may be safely used for the anastomosis. In all these situations the early mobilization of the splenic flexure would be inappropriate.

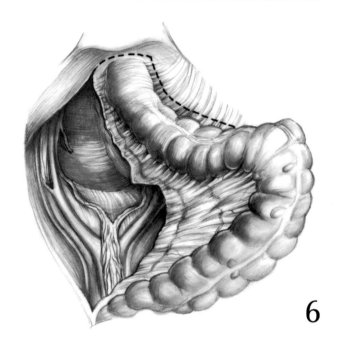

6

Mobilization of the splenic flexure

7 The wound is retracted superolaterally to the left while the peritoneum is divided and the subperitoneal fascia divided as a separate layer. The gonadal vessels, the ureter and the autonomic nerve plexuses are carefully preserved. The omentum is lifted forwards and upwards and the colon dissected from its posterior leaf and down from the adhesions to the hilar region and lower pole of the spleen. If the correct planes are followed, it will become apparent that the entire blood supply of the omentum comes from the gastric leaves so that the mobilization of the left colon should be virtually bloodless. Various adhesions can, however, make this part of the operation tedious. Once near the midline, the omentum becomes so mobile that later it can be brought down into the pelvis to wrap around the anastomosis.

7

Ligation and division of the inferior mesenteric vessels

8 In most cases the inferior mesenteric artery will be ligated and divided about 2 cm from the aorta in order to preserve those autonomic nerves which split around its origin. Some distance away, above and to the left, the inferior mesenteric vein disappears behind the lower border of the pancreas to the left of the duodenojejunal flexure. For a low anastomosis, the vein is best divided here because this gives the greatest amount of mobility to the splenic flexure so that the colon can lie easily in the bottom of the pelvis. In approximately 10% of patients a substantial branch from the superior mesenteric artery lies near the inferior mesenteric vein and supplies the descending colon. Judgement is required to determine if this vessel should be preserved or if it must be divided to provide sufficient intestine to reach the pelvic floor.

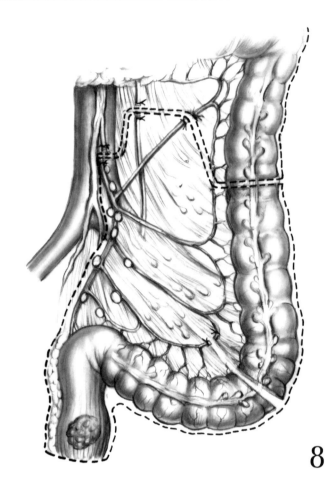

8

Mobilization of the mesorectum, rectum and cancer

This is the most important stage of the operation. The surgeon must develop a mental picture of the exact position of the tumour and its local spread based on the initial investigation and the preoperative assessment. To cut across or to leave satellites of tumour in the pelvis is to expose the patient to a very high risk of local recurrence.

Many surgeons prefer to divide the colon at this stage to facilitate the posterior and lateral dissections. The GIA stapler is ideal for this, but the colonic end will need to be revised and washed out later before the anastomosis is undertaken.

Posterior dissection

9 The avascular areolar tissue plane which surrounds the mesorectum must now be identified. The posterior surface of the mesorectum is similar to a bilobed lipoma. As the rectum is lifted gently forwards from the bifurcation of the presacral nerves, the areolar plane is opened under direct vision by sharp dissection and is extended downwards around the curve of the sacrum in the midline, past the coccyx, and forwards in front of the anococcygeal raphe. A St Mark's retractor (with integral illumination) greatly helps this process, particularly during the distal parts of the dissection which require the mesorectum to be drawn forwards so that the lowest part of the dissection can be seen.

Lateral dissections

10 The lateral attachments are mobilized by extending the plane of dissection forwards from the posterior midline around the side walls of the pelvis. It is important to appreciate that the inferior hypogastric plexuses curve forwards tangentially around the surface of the mesorectum in close proximity to it. The slender nervi erigentes (on which erection depends) lie more posteriorly in the same plane as the presacral nerves, which should be seen and preserved, although it is all too easy to 'tent-up' the nerves and cut them.

The nervi erigentes curve forwards from the sacral foramina; they converge like a fan to join the presacral nerves and form the neurovascular bundles of Walsh[5]. Thus the nerves lie at the outer edges of Denonvilliers' fascia and are in great danger at 10 o'clock and 2 o'clock in the anterolateral position just behind the lateral edges of the seminal vesicles. More distally they curve forwards out of danger.

As the dissection moves deeper into the pelvis, one or two middle rectal vessels may be divided: occasionally one is of sufficient size to demand diathermy or ligation after occlusion by carefully placed slender curved artery forceps. If the areolar plane surrounding the mesorectum has been faithfully followed, it is unlikely that there will be enough lateral pedicle to divide between clamps as has often been recommended.

If bleeding is encountered, a small adrenaline-soaked swab should be placed on to the bleeding point and attention moved to another part of the dissection. Any bleeding will be more easily controlled after the tumour has been removed.

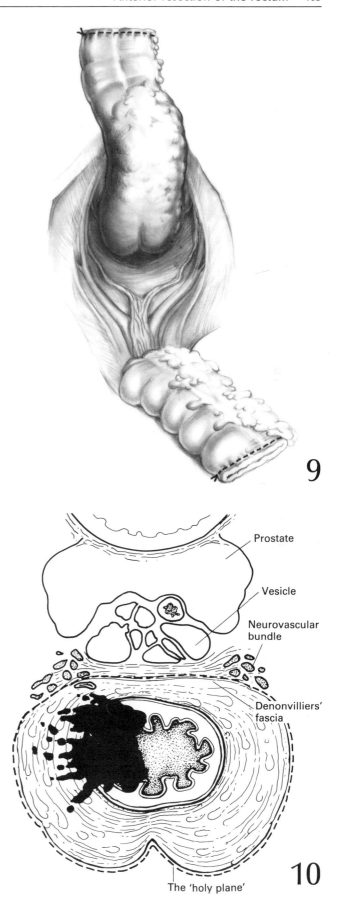

9

Prostate

Vesicle

Neurovascular bundle

Denonvilliers' fascia

The 'holy plane'

10

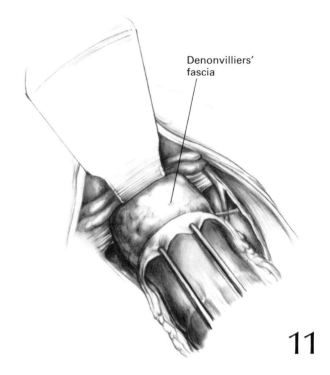

Denonvilliers' fascia

11

Anterior dissection

11, 12 In the male, a transverse incision is made through the peritoneum anterior to the peritoneal reflection in the pelvis, to descend straight to the superior aspect of the seminal vesicles. In drawing the tumour upwards it is important not to pull directly on the intestinal wall and tumour for fear of rupturing the tumour, and increasing the risk of local recurrence by malignant cell spillage. After the peritoneum at the rectovesical pouch has been divided, the posterior cut edge of the peritoneum should be grasped by long haemostats and gentle upward traction applied. This manoeuvre lessens the chance of the tumour being pulled apart.

A swab is laid on the anterior surface of the rectum, and the plane of dissection downwards immediately in front of Denonvilliers' fascia may now be developed, with great care, in the midline. Even greater care is required as this plane is extended laterally to meet the lateral dissection, because it is at the outer edge of Denonvilliers' fascia that the autonomic nerve fibres converge to form the neurovascular bundles that control both potency and bladder function. Denonvilliers' fascia marks the anterior limit of the dissection plane and the anterior surface of the 'tumour package'. It lies like a bib in front of the anterior mesorectum behind the vesicles, and below it fuses with the posterior fascia of the prostate. Therefore the fascia must be divided with scissors to 'cone-down' onto the anterior wall of the lowest few centimetres of the rectum, but this should not occur until well beyond the lower edge of the cancer.

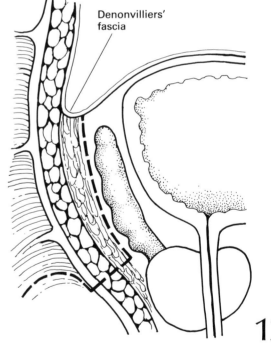

Denonvilliers' fascia

12

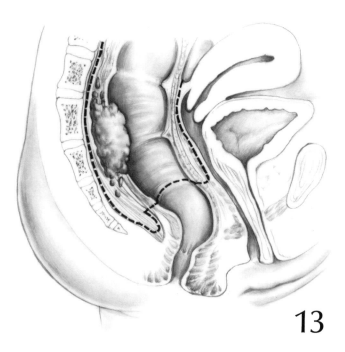

13 In the female, anterior dissection is generally straightforward provided that the uterus is lifted well forward. A common difficulty is to find a clean avascular plane behind the cervix and posterior fornix without encountering bleeding from the venous plexus. The peritoneal reflection itself may adhere to the posterior fornix; in this case (and the cancer permitting), the anterior peritoneal cut may be placed at the level of the posterior fornix to enter the dry plane just behind the posterior vaginal wall. Denonvilliers' fascia, often less well developed than in the male, is excised as the anterior surface of the specimen.

Anterolateral dissections

The joining of the anterior and lateral dissection planes is critical in the preservation of the pelvic autonomic nerves. It is particularly important in the male, but placement of the cuts requires careful judgement in both sexes. The anterior plane in the midline is clear of the nerves while the front of the lateral plane is marked by the presacral nerves and neurovascular bundles which have already been identified. The peritoneal and subperitoneal cuts are 'coned' medially to preserve these bundles as they curve inwards, and the lateral mesorectal edge is developed forwards to Denonvilliers' fascia and the circle is thus completed.

Extended resections in special cases

Adherent adjacent organs should be excised *en bloc* with the primary tumour without splitting open a malignant adhesion. Although about half the adhesions to a cancerous segment are not caused by tumour invasion, it is safer to resect attached organs rather than to peel them away.

Uterus and vagina

It is practical to enter the vaginal vault at this stage and to excise a segment of vaginal wall with the cancer if the tumour is tethered or fixed at this point. However, if the cancer is large or fixed it is wise to clear all the anterior tissue medial to the nerves and the ureters and to perform a hysterectomy with excision of the vaginal vault and posterior vaginal wall before completing the anterior resection. If there is a large vaginal defect which cannot be closed, a low colorectal anastomosis should be wrapped around with the mobilized omentum and a loop stoma should be fashioned to defunction

the anastomosis. These patients should not have sexual intercourse for several months after the operation until the area has healed.

Seminal vesicles

If these are very close to the tumour, the plane anterior to the seminal vesicles may be safely entered, allowing their excision *en bloc* with the rectum, carefully preserving the ureters. The neurovascular bundles will be in particular danger in such a dissection.

Prostate

It is occasionally appropriate, although difficult, to cut away an adherent part of the prostate or, when the prostate is greatly enlarged, to precede the rectal excision with a prostatectomy. The authors have encountered cases where transvesical or retropubic prostatectomy was necessary simply for access. The modern nerve-preserving 'radical prostatectomy' may be used as a part of extended *en bloc* anterior resection in a very small number of selected patients. The operation requires that the neurovascular bundles are carefully dissected distally, dividing the vessels emerging from them, ligating the troublesome penile dorsal venous complex, and removing the whole prostate with its capsule[5]. The distal prostatic urethra must be carefully divided above the triangular ligament.

Ureters

The ureters may be involved in rectosigmoid or colonic cancer but are seldom in danger in dissection for mid or low rectal cancer. However, it is always safe to divide the tissues anterior to the ureteric tunnels in both sexes because they pass in front of the nerve plexuses and are crossed only by the vasa, which may be sacrificed. If one ureter is invaded or obstructed, the adherent portion should be resected. Depending on the size of the resulting defect and height of the ureteric resection, it may be possible to effect a scalloped end-to-end anastomosis of the ureter or to implant the proximal end into the bladder or the opposite ureter[6]. The authors favour ureteroureterostomy as the most useful option and a pigtail stent across the interureteric anastomosis is a desirable safety measure if urological back-up is not readily available.

Bladder

The bladder may be involved in high (intraperitoneal) rectal cancers and the segment can be resected as a disc followed by reconstruction. The management of a mid-rectal tumour with anterior invasion of the bladder base is more difficult: it may be best approached by opening the bladder, catheterizing the ureters and resecting the bladder base at the point of adherence. A course of preoperative irradiation may facilitate such an operation. If firm attachment to the base of the bladder is encountered, the surgeon may be advised to close the abdomen without a resection, arrange a full course of radiotherapy, and then carry out a full laparotomy 8–12 weeks later, when conditions for curative resection may be more favourable.

Inferior hypogastric nerve plexuses and presacral nerves

Much of this chapter has emphasized the exploration of the plane within these nerves so that they may be preserved. If, however, a large tumour is invading the area, these must be resected with the cancer and the prevascular plane outside the nerves along the aorta and major vessels developed (a 'peri-adventitial strip'). If only one side is affected, the nerves on the other side may be preserved. There may, particularly in a female patient, be no serious functional consequences to nerve section, but stripping away of nerves not involved by the cancer is unnecessary.

Internal iliac nodes and the pelvic side wall

There is a wide variation in the reported incidence of internal iliac node involvement. Some surgeons regard lateral lymph node clearance as an essential part of radical surgery[7], but most limit extended resections to cases where there is either direct invasion and fixation of the region of the internal iliac vessels or a palpable or visible abnormal node within the chain concerned. If

the tumour is found on preoperative evaluation to be bulky or fixed, a full course of preoperative irradiation will improve local cancer control and avoid the morbidity of extended lateral pelvic wall clearance. However, in the presence of direct invasion surgery may be modified to include ligation of the anterior division of the internal iliac artery and vein, and clearance of the pelvic side wall in the plane lateral to these vessels. Venous bleeding may be troublesome and this step should not be undertaken lightly. The nerve plexuses on the relevant side will be sacrificed; therefore they should be carefully preserved on the other side if possible.

Synchronous primary tumours

Arguments have been advanced for subtotal colectomy and ileorectal anastomosis for multiple cancers, and occasionally proctocolectomy with an ileal pouch and ileoanal anastomosis may be justified. However, ultra-low resection is more likely to be followed by good functional results when proximal large intestine is preserved. There is no evidence that a synchronous tumour may not be treated as effectively by a separate conventional resection without sacrificing the entire large bowel. This approach is preferred when the rectal cancer necessitates a low or ultra-low anastomosis. However, the remaining parts of the large intestine will need to be reviewed at regular intervals.

Liver metastases

This has become a highly specialized subject and is fully covered in the chapter on pp. 105–115. Small superficial and accessible deposits should be excised with a margin of normal liver of at least 1 cm whenever possible. However, the surgeon should be certain that there are no other metastases before undertaking synchronous resection of liver metastases. Intraoperative ultrasonography is used to determine the full status of the liver with regard to metastasis: when more deeply seated deposits are detected, it is better to complete the rectal excision and to document the full extent of the disease. In the postoperative period, CT scanning may give a clear picture of the extent of hepatic involvement, possibly avoiding fruitless re-exploration. Liver metastases should not normally be biopsied as implantation may occur.

Anastomosis

The most challenging part of the operation is now complete and the specimen is attached to the pelvic floor by a clean tube of anorectal muscle. The objectives remaining are to produce a perfect low anastomosis and to avoid implanting malignant cells into the soft tissues of the pelvis or the anastomosis itself.

14 The last remnants of the mesorectal 'tail' are drawn upwards with a swab and trimmed off the back of the rectum to create a clean muscle tube. The operator must carefully judge the position of the lower edge of the tumour. The intestinal wall is compressed with a finger and thumb distal to the tumour, and a right-angled clamp is placed below these with a 'safe' margin of intestinal wall between. Most rectal cancers may safely be given a clearance of 2 cm or less. Microscopic mural spread beyond the palpable lower edge is very rare and the compromise of mural margins does not appear to be a significant cause of local recurrence[8].

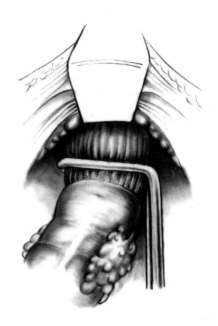

14

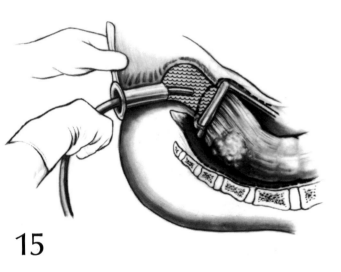

15

15 A proctoscope is introduced anally and fluid is delivered by a 50-ml syringe or through a catheter. Plain water is more cytocidal than saline; aqueous cetrimide or povidone-iodine solutions are probably best for this purpose.

Once the intraluminal washout is complete, and with the pelvis itself still awash with aqueous cetrimide, the anorectum is divided, preferably with a pair of large Goligher scissors. A few millimetres of intestinal wall should be left beyond the clamp so that it does not slip off. Upward traction must be applied only to the clamp; traction on the intestine itself may pull the cut edges through the clamp, with consequent spillage of malignant cells.

It may be difficult to achieve complete haemostasis, particularly in a long, narrow male pelvis. The middle rectal arteries themselves seldom bleed significantly and may usually be left until the pelvic side wall can be more readily inspected after the tumour has been removed. Gentle diathermy or a few ligatures are generally all that is required, although haemostatic gauze with local pressure may be helpful if a wide area of pelvic wall persists in oozing. Excessive use of diathermy may damage the hypogastric plexuses and should be avoided.

16 Insertion of the distal purse-string suture is important for a good stapled anastomosis. Upward pressure in the perineum is essential to bring the rectal stump into view. The principal operator's left hand should be inserted through the anus, or an assistant should apply direct pressure on a large swab. Countertraction with a St Mark's or wide-lipped pelvic retractor draws the bladder and vesicles forwards away from the anorectum which is thus made accessible for the suture. A 0 nylon or polypropylene (Prolene) suture (2/0 is rather easily broken) is mounted on a small half-circle atraumatic needle. A simple over-and-over continuous suture is appropriate, taking bites 5 mm from the cut edge of bowel and 5 mm apart.

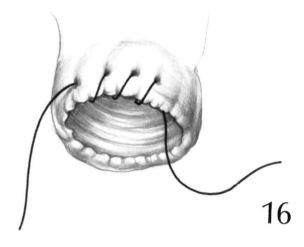

16

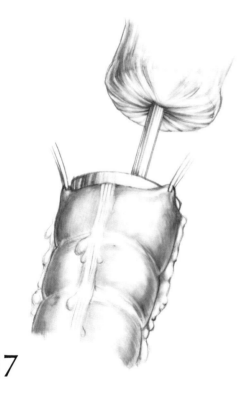

17

17 A pulsatile blood supply is essential so that the marginal artery is divided at a more distal point than the bowel itself. Usually, after full splenic flexure mobilization and double high ligations, the wide, well vascularized bowel which was formerly in the region of the spleen will be ready to lie comfortably in the sacral hollow without tension. However, great care is necessary in planning good vascular divisions that will preserve both adequate length and excellent blood supply for the crucial colonic component of the anastomosis. The proximal purse-string suture generally poses no problem and is performed with a simple over-and-over continuous stitch with 0 polypropylene.

The colonic end should be sucked out and washed clean with a cytocidal solution before being prepared for the anastomosis. This can be accomplished through the open bowel end using a 50-ml syringe and the sucker. The colonic end is eased over the anvil with the aid of three Babcock forceps. The intestinal wall drawn down onto the shaft should be cleaned of any mesenteric fat that may otherwise become interposed between the inverted opposed rims of colon and rectum. There is little good, and some harm, however, in cutting back the mesentery beyond the exact outer point of the inverted rim.

18 If the anvil has been disconnected from the body of the stapler, the introduction of the latter into the anus must be aided with lubricant and the assistant's fingers. The abdominal operator may pass a finger down through the lumen from above to meet the stapler, ease aside the mucosa and facilitate its upward passage. With the spindle fully advanced the lower purse-string suture is tightened and the upward-facing disc of rectal wall cleaned of any excess mesenteric fat.

The two halves of the stapler are now fixed together and the instrument is closed, taking great care not to catch adjacent structures such as vaginal wall or vesicles. When the gap is just within the recommendations (i.e. the widest permissible to avoid crushing the inturned rims), the gun is fired.

To remove the stapler, the gap between the shaft and the anvil must be opened while the gun is tilted, rotated and gently manipulated down through the anastomosis. The perineum may be steadied by the abdominal operator's left hand and the fingers used to help ease the instrument through the anal canal.

19 The purse-string sutures and a complete ring of intestinal end should be identified from both the rectal and the colonic sides in order to check the gun rings. Cutting and withdrawing the purse-string will avoid errors with a very slender ring. The anastomosis may be further checked by filling the pelvis with water and injecting air into the rectum through the anus.

20 If anastomotic integrity is in doubt it is common practice to add reinforcing sutures, and formation of a defunctioning loop stoma is wise in such a case. Only the distal (anorectal) ring should be sent for histology to confirm that tumour has not spread distally.

A double-stapling technique has many advocates, although it has not been proved superior to the use of a single-stapling approach. The TA55 or RL60 staplers may be used to divide the rectum about 5 cm from the dentate line or the TA35 or RL30 may be used to divide the anorectum in a very low anastomosis. To accommodate the thickness of the intestinal wall, the longer staple length is required. These staplers must be used only after the right-angled clamp has been applied and cytocidal washout completed. This means that the double-stapling method is inappropriate in the case of a very low-lying tumour because there is not enough room to place both the occlusive right-angled clamp and the stapler below the tumour. The technique does, however, save time if there is sufficient length of rectal stump to apply the stapler and clamp simultaneously.

With an ultra-low anastomosis, a J pouch may be created in the end of the proximal colon and stapled to the anus (*see* chapter on pp. 689–697).

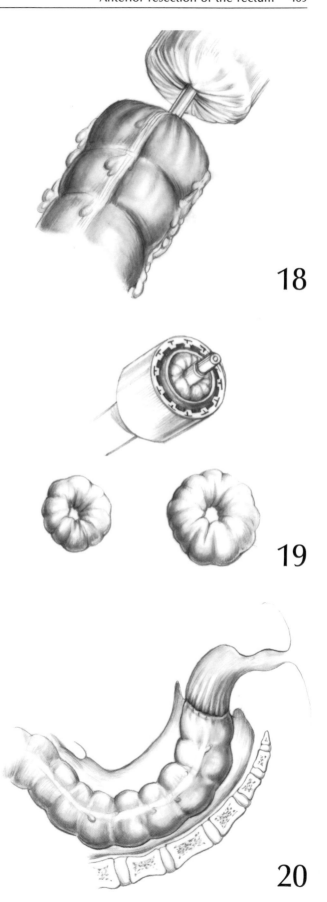

18

19

20

Defunctioning stomas

The question of whether to defunction a low or ultra-low anastomosis with a stoma remains controversial. With few exceptions, anastomotic leakage is reported in 10–15% of patients with anastomoses below 5 cm. The authors have adopted a cautious approach to intestinal defunction in such cases and use a loop right transverse colostomy. This stoma must be placed well to the right in the transverse colon because damage to the blood supply of the left transverse colon would be disastrous. We prefer to avoid a defunctioning ileostomy in the belief that episodes of band obstruction are more likely to occur after formation of a distal ileal stoma and its subsequent closure than after a loop transverse colostomy, which is performed entirely in the supracolic compartment. The stoma is closed 6–8 weeks after surgery, after a water-soluble contrast study has shown satisfactory healing of the colorectal anastomosis.

HIGH ANTERIOR RESECTION AND MESORECTAL DIVISION

Tumours above the peritoneal reflection, with a sigmoidoscopic height of about 10–15 cm from the anal verge, would not usually be considered by most surgeons to require an operation of the magnitude of a low anterior resection with total mesorectal excision. Treatment in these cases is by high anterior resection of the rectum, the initial stages of which are identical to those described for low resection except that mobilization of the splenic flexure may not be necessary.

After posterior mobilization of the rectum and the upper part of the lateral dissection have been performed, the tumour is lifted well out of the pelvis so that the mesorectum may be divided 5 cm below the lower edge of the cancer to ensure that any tumorous lymphatic invasion close to the primary lesion is removed. The superior rectal vessels are clamped and ligated, and the rectal wall is carefully cleaned and clamped as previously described.

The wall is then divided immediately below the clamp. Normally there is no problem in bringing down the upper sigmoid or descending colon for either a stapled anastomosis, using the technique described for low anterior resection (see also chapter on pp. 74–83), or manually inserted sutures (see chapter on pp. 84–92). Anastomoses at this level should not require defunctioning and, because the pelvic cavity is largely filled by the remaining rectum and mesorectum, there is usually no need for suction drainage.

Postoperative management

Pelvic drains

Sump drains require continuous suction by extrinsic pumps. Interruption of suction during the transfer of the patient from the operating room to the ward may allow blood clots to form and block the air channel. Therefore, the authors prefer to use two medium-sized suction drains which are connected to the operating room pump as soon as they are inserted and to a closed suction bottle as soon as the abdominal closure is commenced. The suction bottle can be transported with the patient to the ward without further attention.

Anastomotic leakage

The large cavity created by rectal and mesorectal excision does not readily drain despite suction, and may become the site of an infected presacral haematoma which can become a presacral abscess. In the second or third week after surgery, this abscess may discharge through or near the anastomosis into the bowel lumen and may occasionally require further opening of the abscess into the rectum to give adequate drainage. The closer the anastomosis is to the anus, the greater the risk of a chronic abscess and possible anastomotic failure.

Anastomotic leakage of a different kind may sometimes occur during an apparently good recovery[9]. This problem may be caused by 'faecal extrusion': peristalsis driving the faeces downwards against a closed sphincter and forcing faecal material through the anastomosis into the pelvic tissues, leading to pelvic sepsis and septicaemia. Thus, despite the apparent initiation of normal bowel function, such patients sometimes become unwell, develop abdominal pain and peritonitis or simply deteriorate in a way that leads to suspicions of pulmonary embolus or cardiac event. In such patients an urgent radio-opaque enema should be undertaken to identify the leakage as the cause of septicaemia.

Anastomotic leakage is managed as in the chapter on pp. 420–435.

Loop stoma

Once the patient has progressed satisfactorily and the likelihood of anastomotic leakage is small, the supporting bar under the loop stoma can be removed, usually 10–14 days after surgery. If there are signs of an anastomotic leakage, then the supporting bar should be retained for a few extra days. About 4–5 weeks after surgery, a water-soluble contrast enema is carried out as a prelude to closure of the colostomy to make sure that the anastomosis is intact. If a leak is observed, the stoma should be left in place for a further few weeks and the contrast study repeated.

Anastomotic stricture

All low stapled anastomoses may be readily palpated during follow-up visits. A narrowing to 1–2 cm is very common in the early months and gentle dilatation may be appropriate at the time of colostomy closure, and occasionally in the ensuing months. Persistent symptomatic stricture is rare unless there has been colonic ischaemia, inadequate colonic length or gross pelvic sepsis. It cannot be overemphasized that the colon proximal to a low anastomosis must lie without tension in the hollow of the sacrum to avoid ischaemic complications. Very occasionally, reoperation may be required to achieve sufficient length of colon.

Postoperative anorectal function

If the sphincters were effective before surgery, it is rare for incontinence or stool seepage to be a problem with even the lowest anastomosis. Urgency and frequency of defaecation (the 'absent reservoir' syndrome) improves gradually over the initial 12–18 months. Very occasionally, reversion to a permanent colostomy may be requested by the patient and should be considered if symptoms are severe.

Local recurrence

This chapter is dedicated to techniques designed to prevent the dismal complication of local tumour recurrence, which is seldom amenable to curative treatment. If pelvic recurrence occurs, the patient should be considered for a full course of irradiation therapy, and further surgery can be contemplated 8–12 weeks after the end of this treatment. A repeat anterior resection may, very occasionally, be possible, or an abdominoperineal resection (*see* chapter on pp. 472–487) or a pelvic exenteration (*see* chapter on pp. 523–537) may be indicated.

Adjuvant therapy

Most surgeons believe that full-dose radiotherapy confers some benefit in selected cases, particularly for the locally advanced bulky lesion. Preoperative radiotherapy has the advantage that much of the fully irradiated tissue is removed by subsequent surgery. This treatment also has the theoretical attraction that it may shrink the tumour sufficiently to render the surgical dissection planes less likely to be transgressed by viable cancer cells. The role of chemotherapy is somewhat more controversial, although its use is undoubtedly on the increase.

References

1. Philips RKS, Hittinger R, Blesovsky L, Fry JS, Fielding LP. Local recurrence after curative surgery for large bowel cancer. The overall picture. *Br J Surg* 1983; 71: 12–16.

2. Hermanek P, Friedl P. Locoregional recurrence in rectal carcinoma. Experience from a German multicentre study (SGCRC). *Abstr Acta Chirurg Austr* 1991; (Suppl. 93): 9–10.

3. Heald RJ, Husband EM, Ryall RDH. The mesorectum in rectal cancer surgery – the clue to pelvic recurrence? *Br J Surg* 1982; 69: 613–16.

4. Ward AS, Heald RJ. Leg ischaemia complicating colorectal surgery. (In press).

5. Walsh PC, Schlegel PN. Radical pelvic surgery with preservation of sexual function. *Ann Surg* 1988, 208: 391–400.

6. Cranston D. Ureteroureterostomy. In: Whitfield HN, ed. *Operative Surgery: Genitourinary Surgery*, 5th edn, Volume 1, Oxford: Butterworth-Heinemann, 1993: 180–2.

7. Hojo K, Sawada T, Moriya Y. An analysis of survival and voiding, sexual function after wide iliopelvic lymphadenectomy in patients with carcinoma of the rectum, compared with conventional lymphadenectomy. *Dis Colon Rectum* 1989; 32: 128–33.

8. Karanjia ND, Schache DJ, North WRS, Heald RJ. 'Close shave' in anterior resection. *Br J Surg* 1990; 77: 510–12.

9. Karanjia ND, Corder AP, Holdsworth PJ, Heald RJ. Risk of peritonitis and fatal septicaemia and the need to defunction the low anastomosis. *Br J Surg* 1991; 78: 196–8.

Abdominoperineal excision of rectum

John J. Murray MD
Staff Surgeon, Department of Colon and Rectal Surgery, Lahey Clinic Medical Center, Burlington, Massachusetts, USA

Malcolm C. Veidenheimer MD
Staff Surgeon, Department of Colon and Rectal Surgery, Lahey Clinic Medical Center, Burlington, Massachusetts, USA

Principles and justification

Indications

Abdominoperineal resection for the treatment of patients with distal rectal carcinoma remains the standard against which all other options of treatment must be compared. As described by Miles in 1908, the operation involves abdominal exploration with ligation and division of the proximal lymphovascular pedicle and mobilization of the rectum. The perineal dissection permits subsequent removal of the rectum. Although the two phases of the operation can be performed as sequential steps that involve repositioning the patient from the supine to the lateral decubitus position, the operation is most commonly performed as a synchronous combined procedure with two teams operating simultaneously when the lesion has been judged to be resectable. Although small carcinomas in the distal rectum may be treated with curative intent by local measures such as electrocoagulation or full-thickness excision, abdominoperineal excision is the customary treatment for most tumours involving the distal third of the rectum and for selected bulky tumours of the mid-rectum. Abdominoperineal excision of the rectum is also performed for inflammatory bowel disease. When undertaken for this diagnosis, the abdominal dissection differs from the technique described in this chapter so that the autonomic innervation to the bladder and sexual organs is preserved. The perineal dissection in patients with inflammatory bowel disease can be confined to the intersphincteric plane to reduce the size of the perineal wound.

Preoperative

Preoperative preparation begins with endoscopic and digital examination of the rectum to assess the size and location of the tumour. For carcinomas located in the anterior quadrant of the distal rectum, this evaluation includes an assessment for possible involvement of the prostate and bladder in men and the rectovaginal septum in women. A full course of preoperative radiation therapy may facilitate subsequent abdominoperineal excision of large tumours or tumours that appear fixed because of extension to other pelvic structures. Computed tomography, magnetic resonance imaging and transrectal ultrasonography may further delineate the extent of the pelvic tumour, but this information is unlikely to alter the plan of treatment. A definitive assessment regarding the resectability of a rectal carcinoma can only be made at laparotomy.

All patients require mechanical cleansing of the colon before operation. A lavage preparation using a balanced electrolyte solution with polyethylene glycol is employed in this department at present. Patients receive oral antibiotics before operation to reduce bacterial colonization of the large intestine. Parenteral antibiotics are provided during the operative period. Patients are seen before operation by an enterostomal nurse who begins instruction in stomal care. The enterostomal nurse also selects the most appropriate site on the abdominal wall for the colostomy. Prophylactic measures to reduce the risk of deep vein thrombophlebitis are mandatory in patients undergoing abdominoperineal excision of the rectum.

Operation

Position of patient

1 The patient is placed in the lithotomy Trendelenburg position with a pad beneath the sacrum to provide simultaneous access to the abdomen and perineum. The legs are positioned in stirrups that provide support to the knees and feet while avoiding compression of the perineal nerve. A Foley catheter is inserted into the bladder using sterile technique. We have not found the routine use of ureteric catheters to be helpful. Their use is restricted to patients who have previously undergone extensive pelvic surgery or who have received radiation to the pelvis. A 2/0 purse-string suture of silk is used to occlude the anal orifice.

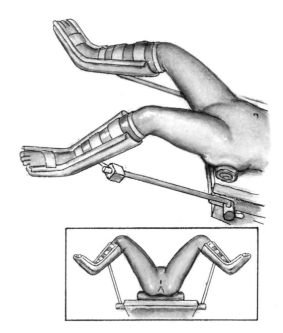

Incision

2 A midline incision extending cephalad from the superior margin of the pubic symphysis and passing to the right of the umbilicus provides access to the abdominal cavity without encroaching on potential sites for placement of the abdominal stoma. The colostomy should be situated over the body of the rectus muscle to reduce the risk of paracolostomy herniation. The site should be chosen to avoid deformities of the abdominal wall and bony contours. Most commonly, the best site for the stoma is in the left lower quadrant at the apex of the infraumbilical skin fold. In this location the stoma is easy for the patient to see, enabling correct placement of the colostomy appliance.

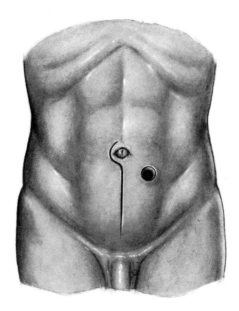

Technique

3 The extent of colonic resection necessary to accomplish abdominoperineal excision of the rectum is determined by the blood supply to the rectum and the level at which the proximal vascular pedicle is ligated. The left colic and superior rectal arteries, as well as a variable number of sigmoid branches, originate from the inferior mesenteric artery. The middle rectal arteries are derived from the internal iliac arteries and pass across the superior aspect of the levator ani muscles. The inferior rectal arteries originate from the pudendal arteries and have anterior and posterior branches that pass through the ischiorectal fossae. Ligation of the superior rectal trunk adjacent to the bifurcation of the aorta preserves the left colic artery. This approach improves perfusion to the proximal sigmoid colon and permits the apex of the sigmoid loop to serve as the site for proximal transection of the colon. Ligation of the inferior mesenteric artery at its origin from the aorta to encompass the para-aortic lymphatic tissue in the operative specimen has not been demonstrated to improve the chance for cure after abdominoperineal excision of the rectum. High ligation of the vascular pedicle impairs the blood supply to the proximal sigmoid colon, however, and usually requires more extensive resection of the colon.

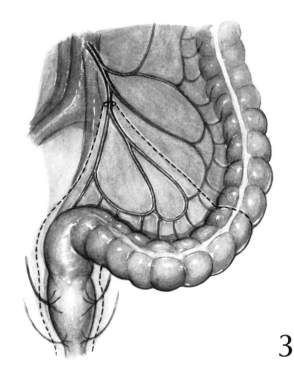

3

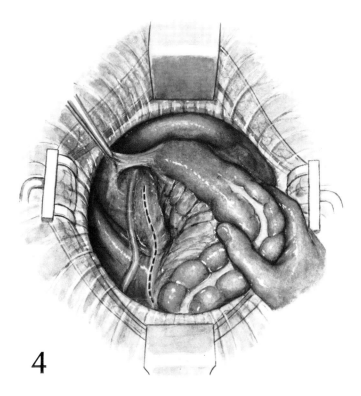

4

4 After exploration of the abdomen to assess the full extent of the tumour, a plastic drape is placed around the margins of the wound to minimize contamination of the skin. Exposure is maintained with a self-retaining retractor. Congenital adhesions in the left paracolic gutter are divided to begin mobilization of the sigmoid and rectosigmoid colon.

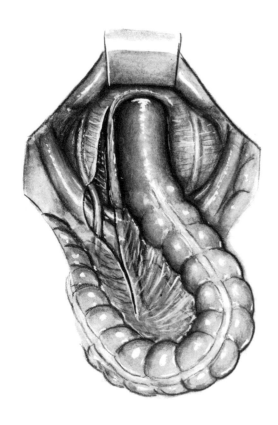

5 The peritoneum along the base of the rectosigmoid mesentery in the left gutter is incised with scissors. The incision is extended proximally across the sigmoid mesentery to the planned site for transection of the colon. The incision is carried distally across the brim of the pelvis and extends to the base of the bladder. During the course of this dissection, the left ureter is identified and protected.

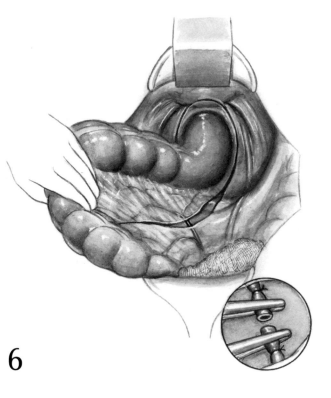

6 The sigmoid colon is retracted to the left. In a similar fashion, the peritoneum on the right side of the sigmoid mesentery is incised. The incision begins adjacent to the planned site for proximal transection of the colon. The dissection proceeds across the sigmoid mesentery to a point adjacent to the aortic bifurcation. From this point, the incision is extended along the root of the rectosigmoid mesentery and across the pelvis to the base of the bladder. The peritoneal incisions are joined across the base of the bladder just above the floor of the rectovesical pouch. Before the peritoneum is incised, the right ureter can usually be identified as it crosses the brim of the pelvis. The branches of the inferior mesenteric vessels are isolated, divided between clamps and ligated.

7 After the vascular pedicle has been divided, the remaining sigmoid mesentery is dissected from the posterior abdominal wall with scissors. Dissection progresses in a caudad direction, exposing the sacral promontory. While maintaining anterior traction on the rectosigmoid, the presacral space is entered by inserting dissecting scissors into the loose areolar tissue just anterior to the sacral promontory.

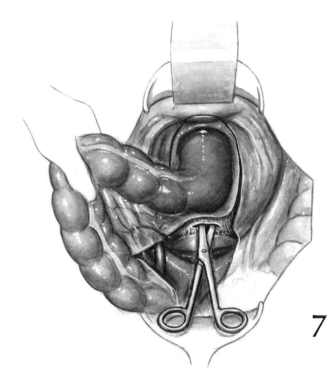

7

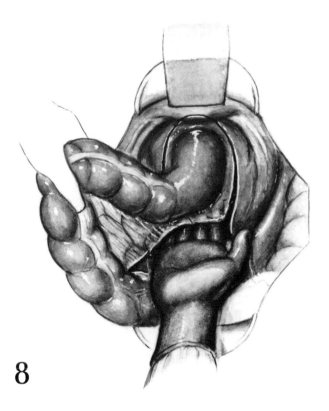

8

8 When the plane of dissection has been demonstrated, the right hand is inserted, and the rest of the presacral dissection is accomplished by blunt finger dissection and gentle anterior displacement of the rectum.

9 Blunt dissection in the presacral space is carried distally to the level of the tip of the coccyx, which can be appreciated on the back of the middle finger. Care is taken to ensure that the dissection is performed in a plane anterior to the presacral fascia to avoid injury to the presacral venous plexus. As the dissecting hand is swept laterally in the presacral space, the lateral attachments proximal to the lateral ligaments are thinned. These proximal lateral attachments are avascular and can be divided with sharp dissection.

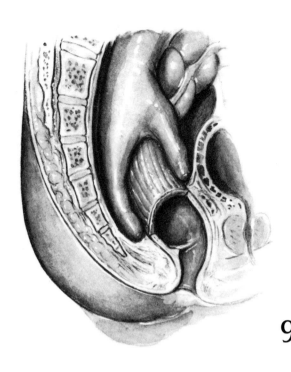

9

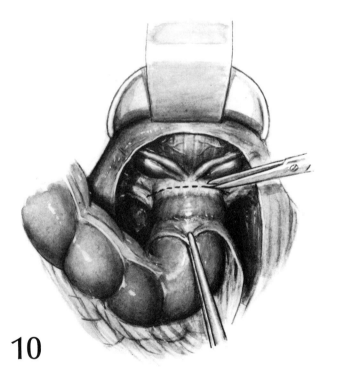

10

10 The anterior dissection, aided by retraction on the posterior edge of the peritoneal incision, is now carried to a deeper plane. The posterior wall of the bladder and the seminal vesicles are demonstrated by a combination of sharp and blunt dissection. Denonvilliers' fascia is exposed and incised by sharp dissection. In women, the anterior dissection commences at the base of the pouch of Douglas and exposes the cervix and the posterior fornix of the vagina.

11 Incision of Denonvilliers' fascia exposes the longitudinal muscle of the rectal wall. While countertraction on the rectum is maintained, the bladder and prostate are swept away from the anterior rectal wall by blunt finger dissection. Dissection in this plane is carried distally until the indwelling Foley catheter can be palpated within the membranous urethra when the examining finger is pressed against the undersurface of the pubic symphysis. In women, the posterior vaginal wall is swept from the rectum by finger dissection. This dissection should be carried into the distal third of the rectovaginal septum.

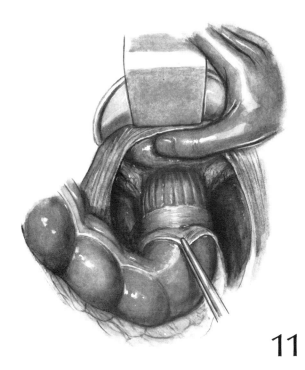

11

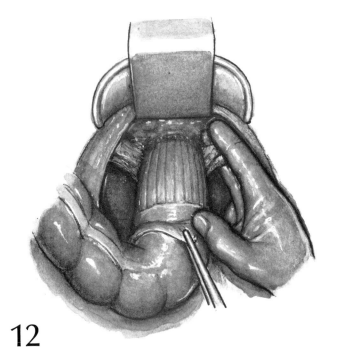

12

12 Lateral mobilization of the rectum is completed. The lateral ligaments may contain branches of the middle rectal vessels. While the rectum is displaced to the opposite side of the pelvis, the lateral ligament is thinned by placing the index finger in the anterior plane of the rectal mobilization and the middle finger in the posterior plane. The fingers are moved back and forth to thin the intervening band of tissue.

13 By means of a corkscrew movement of the index finger passed along the lateral border of the rectum, the lateral ligament on each side of the rectum is hooked on the finger, clamped and divided. Division of the lateral ligaments should be accomplished as close to the pelvic side wall as possible to encompass adjacent lymphatic tissue in the operative specimen. After division of the lateral ligaments, abdominal mobilization of the rectum is completed.

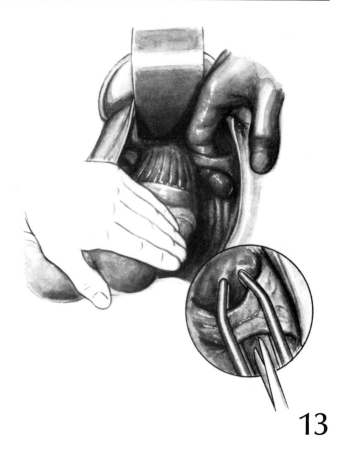

13

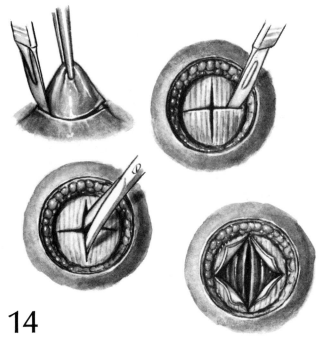

14

14 While midline traction on the lower abdominal wall is maintained by means of a Kocher clamp, the previously marked skin site for the colostomy is grasped in a Kocher clamp. A circle of skin approximating the diameter of the colon is excised. In obese patients, a plug of subcutaneous tissue and fat is removed with the overlying circle of skin. A cruciate incision is made in the exposed anterior sheath of the rectus muscle. The fibres of the rectus abdominis muscle are split using Mayo scissors and the peritoneum is incised. The defect in the abdominal wall should be of sufficient size to accommodate two fingerbreadths.

15 The colon is divided with a linear intestinal stapling instrument. The proximal end of the colon is drawn through the defect in the abdominal wall using Babcock clamps.

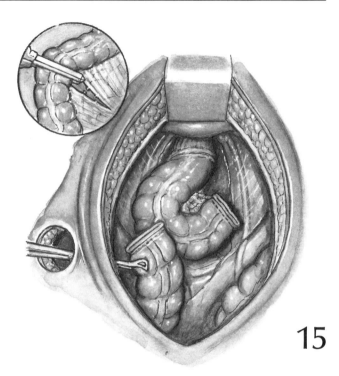

15

16 After the surgical specimen has been removed, the pelvic cavity is irrigated. The peritoneum along the pelvic side walls is mobilized to a degree that will permit closure with a continuous suture of absorbable material. Alternatively, the pelvic peritoneum can be left unapproximated. In this instance, closed suction drainage catheters are placed in the depths of the pelvis and brought through abdominal stab wounds.

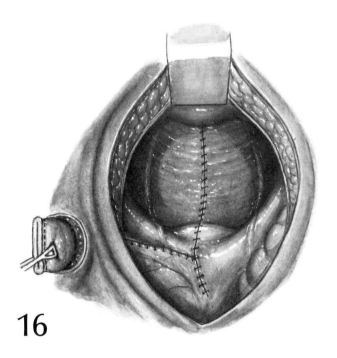

16

17 Adjuvant radiation therapy to reduce the risk of local recurrence of the tumour has become standard practice in the management of patients with advanced carcinoma of the rectum. Operative measures to exclude the small intestine from the pelvis may reduce the risk of radiation injury. A pedicled flap of omentum based on the left gastroepiploic vessels can be used to obliterate the pelvic dead space and displace the small intestine. The omentum is dissected from the transverse colon, permitting entry into the lesser peritoneal sac. The right half of the omentum is separated from the greater curvature of the stomach. Care is taken to preserve the gastroepiploic vessels as well as the omental blood supply arising from the left gastroepiploic artery.

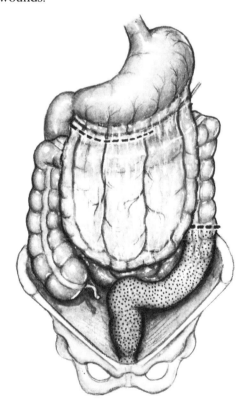

17

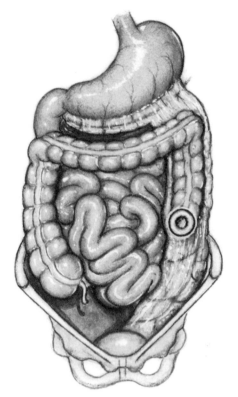

18 The pedicle of omentum is brought lateral to the afferent limb of the colostomy in the left paracolic gutter to fill the pelvic cavity and displace the small intestine.

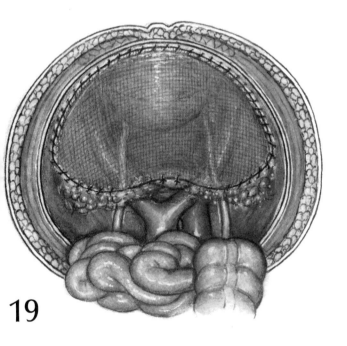

19 If the omentum is attenuated or unavailable, absorbable polyglycolic acid mesh can be used to create a temporary intestinal sling that will exclude the small intestine from the radiation portals during the period of treatment. The sling is anchored to the posterior abdominal wall below the aortic bifurcation with two 2/0 polyglycolic acid sutures. The sutures are run laterally in opposite directions, with care taken to avoid the ureters and iliac vessels. The sutures are continued across the lateral paracolic gutters and along the posterior aspect of the anterior abdominal wall.

20 Fixation of the mesh to the abdominal wall advances in a cephalad direction as the sutures are run from the posterior abdominal wall to the anterior abdominal wall. The sutures are approximated in the anterior midline above the level of the umbilicus as the midline fascial incision is closed. Closed suction catheters are placed in the pelvis below the sling to evacuate any fluid collections.

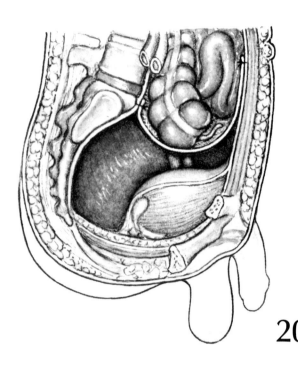

20

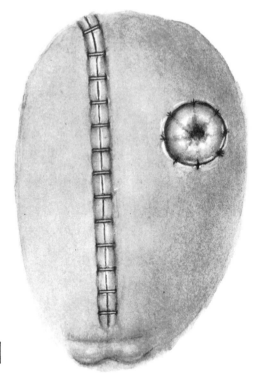

21

21 Copious irrigation of the wound before closure of the skin diminishes the incidence of wound infection. The colostomy is completed by immediate mucocutaneous anastomosis using sutures of 4/0 chromic catgut. A disposable colostomy appliance is secured to the abdominal wall in the operating room.

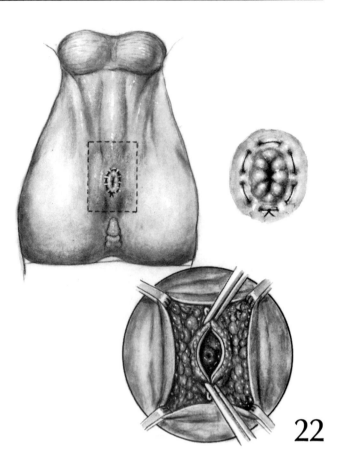

22 When abdominoperineal excision of the rectum is to be performed synchronously by two operating teams, the perineal dissection is started when the resectability of the lesion has been confirmed by the abdominal surgeon. When two operating teams are not available, the abdominal dissection is performed first and the perineal excision of the specimen performed after the colostomy has been fashioned and the abdominal incision has been closed. A rectangular or elliptical incision is outlined using electrocautery. The anterior margin of the dissection overlies the deep transverse perineal muscle. The incision extends posteriorly to the tip of the coccyx. To provide countertraction, the edges of the skin are grasped with Lahey double-hook clamps and the perianal skin is grasped with Kocher clamps.

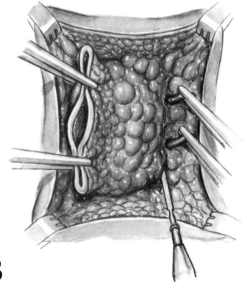

23 The dissection begins laterally. The perianal fat is divided with electrocautery or blunt scissors, providing entry to the ischiorectal fossa. The anterior and posterior branches of the inferior rectal arteries are isolated, divided and ligated.

24 A self-retaining retractor facilitates exposure in the ischiorectal fossa. The anterior dissection is deepened along a plane at the posterior border of the deep transverse perineal muscle.

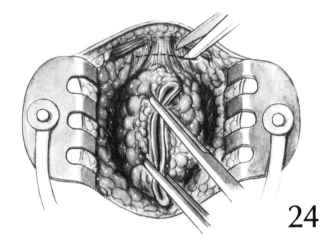

24

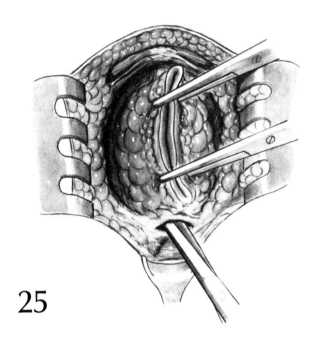

25

25 The anococcygeal ligament is divided by scissors dissection. The presacral pelvic space is entered along a plane anterior to the tip of the coccyx by dividing the levator muscles in the posterior midline. The perineal surgeon is guided by the fingers of the abdominal surgeon, which have been placed in the presacral space. The point of the scissors should be directed anteriorly, aiming at the umbilicus, to avoid inadvertent stripping of the presacral fascia. At this juncture, the abdominal and perineal dissections meet. The rectum and anus will be free in the midline posteriorly.

26 An index finger inserted through the precoccygeal incision is swept across the superior aspect of the levator muscles on each side of the pelvis, and the muscles are divided with scissors or electrocautery. The levator muscles should be divided as close to the pelvic side wall as possible to include a liberal portion of muscle and perirectal fat with the operative specimen. Dissection through the levator muscles is usually avascular.

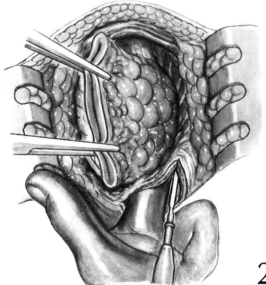

26

27 The abdominal surgeon passes the rectum through the open posterolateral perineal wound. After careful palpation to avoid injury to the urethra, the remaining attachments of the rectum to the recto-urethral muscle are divided.

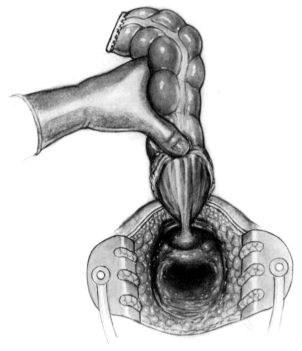

27

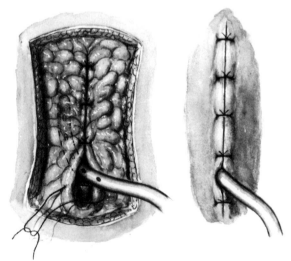

28

28 The perineal wound is copiously irrigated. When the pelvic peritoneum has been closed, a sump suction drain is placed into the pelvic cavity and brought through the posterior aspect of the perineal wound. When the pelvic cavity is to be drained from above, no drains are necessary in the perineal field. No attempt is made to approximate the levator muscles. The ischiorectal fat and subcutaneous tissues are approximated in two layers with interrupted sutures of 2/0 absorbable material. The skin incision is closed with interrupted sutures of nylon.

29 Because of the proximity of the rectum and vagina, and the presence of lymphatic channels within the rectovaginal septum, excision of carcinoma involving the anterior or lateral quadrants of the distal rectum in women should include posterior vaginectomy to ensure adequate clearance of the tumour and to reduce the potential for local recurrence.

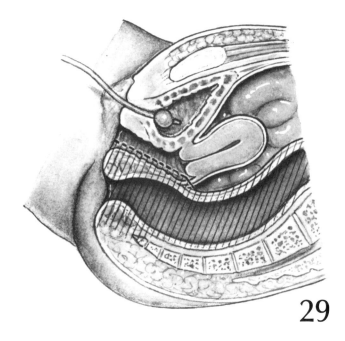

29

30

30 When the perineal dissection is started in women, the lateral margins of the perianal incision are carried anteriorly to the posterolateral aspects of the labia. After the levator muscles are divided and the specimen is delivered posteriorly, the incisions at the base of the labia are extended proximally as full-thickness incisions along the lateral walls of the vagina. A full-thickness transverse incision across the posterior fornix completes the dissection, and the specimen is removed.

31 Reconstruction of the vagina is unnecessary. Bleeding from the transected vaginal wall is controlled with electrocautery or with a continuous running suture of absorbable material. The ischiorectal fat and subcutaneous tissues are approximated in two layers with interrupted absorbable sutures.

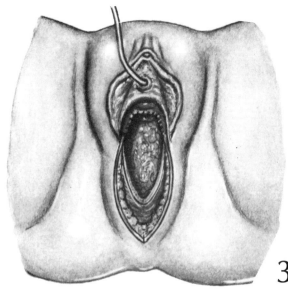

31

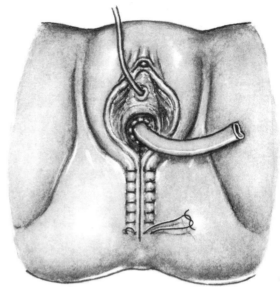

32 Closure of the skin incision is carried anteriorly to the base of the labia to reconstruct the posterior fourchette. The vaginal orifice should accommodate three fingerbreadths. A soft suction catheter is placed through the defect in the posterior vaginal wall to drain the pelvic cavity.

32

Postoperative care

Routine postoperative nasogastric decompression is unnecessary. Ambulation with assistance starts on the first postoperative day. Intake is restricted to intravenous fluids until spontaneous passage of flatus through the colostomy occurs. At this time, a liquid diet is prescribed. The diet is subsequently advanced to an unrestricted diet over the ensuing 24–48 h. When suction catheters are used in the perineal wound, they are removed on the fourth postoperative day. Subsequent care of the perineal wound requires sitz baths and irrigation of the perineal sinus with normal saline solution three times a day. These measures are unnecessary when drains have not been placed in the perineal wound. In this instance, abdominal drains are removed when their daily output has decreased to 20 ml or less. The Foley urethral catheter is left indwelling for 5–7 days after abdominoperineal resection. For patients with symptomatic prostatic enlargement, transurethral resection of the prostate may be necessary after abdominoperineal resection because of compromised bladder function after excision of the rectum. Before discharge from the hospital, patients are instructed in the specifics of managing the stoma, including the option of irrigation of the colostomy.

Acknowledgements

The illustrations in this chapter are reprinted with kind permission of the Lahey Clinic.

Hartmann's operation

Pascal Frileux MD
Professor of Surgery, Hôpital Laennec, Paris, France

Anne Berger MD
Consultant Surgeon, Hôpital Laennec, Paris, France

History

1 In 1923 Henri Hartmann[1] described an operation which is now defined as a resection of the sigmoid colon with construction of a terminal colostomy and closure of the rectal stump. A variable length of rectum may also be resected. The indication was initially cancer of the upper or middle third of the rectum, at a time when anterior resection had not been developed. Today Hartmann's operation is usually performed as an emergency procedure to treat the complications of various colorectal diseases.

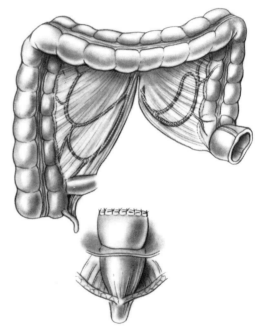

1

Principles and justification

Indications and contraindications

Hartmann's operation is indicated when it is necessary to perform an emergency resection of the sigmoid and/or rectum, when it is unsafe to perform a primary anastomosis, and when it is impossible to raise a mucous fistula owing to an insufficient length of bowel distal to the resection. The advantage of Hartmann's operation over simple diversion is that resection of the lesion is carried out at the primary stage.

Benign diseases

Hartmann's operation represents the 'gold standard' in patients with perforated diverticulitis with generalized peritonitis. There is, however, now a tendency towards primary anastomosis in selected cases[2].

Hartmann's operation is indicated in patients with ischaemic colitis requiring resection when the sigmoid colon is involved[3].

Acute colitis, in the form of toxic megacolon or fulminant colitis, may require an emergency colectomy but it is generally agreed that primary coloproctectomy should be avoided in this situation, and total abdominal colectomy is favoured. Some choose to close the rectal stump, while others (including the authors) prefer a sigmoid mucous fistula to avoid the possible complications caused by leakage from the suture line in the rectum. If Hartmann's procedure is selected, it is necessary to place a tube in the rectal remnant to drain the secretions produced by the inflamed mucosa.

Other indications include: trauma with extensive destruction of the sigmoid or rectum, including iatrogenic perforation; volvulus of the sigmoid colon (*see* chapter on pp. 420–435) with peritonitis and necrosis of the sigmoid colon; and postoperative sepsis after anterior resection in cases where the anastomosis cannot be conserved because of necrosis of the bowel or major disruption of the anastomosis[4].

Malignant diseases

While there was a place for Hartmann's operation in 1921 in the elective therapy of rectal cancer, this is no longer the case because re-establishment of continuity is often not carried out and the patient is left with a permanent colostomy. Malignant obstruction is now better treated by reconstruction after resection (*see* chapter on pp. 436–444). The main indications for Hartmann's operation are in poor risk patients and in some palliative cases associated with perforation of a rectal carcinoma[5].

Operation

The following description applies to cases of perforated diverticulitis.

Position of patient

The patient is placed in the lithotomy position with stirrups (*see* page 48).

Incision

2 While some surgeons favour a left paramedian incision, most perform a midline incision from the pubis to midway between the umbilicus and xiphoid. The edges of the incision are protected with surgical drapes.

The peritoneal fluid is first sampled for bacterial analysis and is then aspirated. Full exploration of the peritoneal cavity is undertaken to identify the primary lesion and occasional associated diseases. In cases of perforated diverticulitis, the origin of the peritonitis is easily recognized.

2

Resection

3 The vessels in the mesocolon are ligated close to the colon, as in any benign disease. The first step is to mobilize the colon, starting from the descending colon where inflammation is minimal. The ureter is identified and the mobilization proceeds distally, using either sharp or blunt dissection according to the type of the inflammatory lesions. There is usually an easy plane of dissection between the sigmoid and the posterior elements (ureter and gonadal vessels), but adhesions may be dense at the level of the pelvic brim. The vessels and mesentery are ligated and divided.

The site of proximal division of the colon varies with the extent of the inflammation; usually it is the limit between the descending and sigmoid colon. A GIA stapler or crushing clamps are used to divide the colon to avoid contamination.

The site of distal division is usually at the level of the sacral promontory because: gross inflammatory lesions rarely extend beyond this point, and if this is the case, they are confined to the mesocolon and do not involve the bowel itself; a sigmoid resection extending down onto the rectum, at the level of the peritoneal reflection, would make the re-establishment of continuity significantly more difficult.

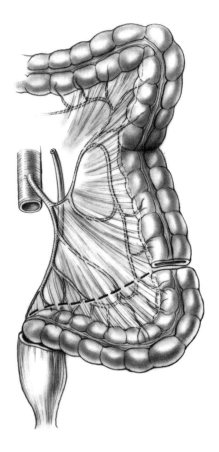

3

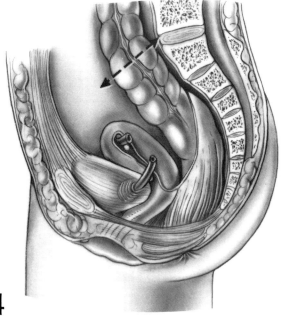

4

4 After the posterior aspect of the rectum at the level of the sacral promontory has been cleared, the rectum is closed using a TA 55 stapler. A clamp is placed above the staple line and the rectum is divided. A suture line over the staples is not necessary, but the rectal stump may be sutured to the sacral promontory to keep it from folding over into the pelvis.

Peritoneal lavage

In the case of peritonitis, thorough peritoneal lavage using saline is indicated to remove fibrinous exudate and pus.

Construction of left iliac colostomy

A separate incision is made in the left iliac fossa at a point equidistant from the anterior iliac spine and the umbilicus. A circle of skin 3 cm in diameter is excised, followed by a cross-shaped incision in the fascia and peritoneal layer. The passage for the colostomy should admit two fingers. If possible, the site of the colostomy should be chosen before the operation, but in emergencies this is not always possible. This colostomy is temporary; therefore, it is not necessary to make a subperitoneal tunnel as for a permanent colostomy (*see* chapter on pp. 472–487). The colon must be well vascularized and brought out without traction; this may require mobilization of the descending colon. The colostomy remains clamped until the abdominal wall has been closed.

Drainage

5 The main postoperative complication of Hartmann's operation is leakage from the rectal suture line. To minimize the consequences of a leak, effective drainage of the pelvis is necessary. The use of tubes, corrugated drains or Penrose drains has been suggested[6], but capillary drainage as described by Mikulicz[7] is used in this department. Large gauze packing is placed in the pouch of Douglas and is exteriorized through the inferior end of the midline incision. The Mikulicz packing is left in place for 12 days and removed under mild analgesia[7]. In addition to efficient drainage, we believe that this technique provides good healing of the peritoneum in the pelvis, thus facilitating reoperation for restoration of continuity.

In the case of generalized peritonitis, some surgeons advocate drainage of the right subphrenic, left subphrenic and subhepatic spaces.

Closure of the abdominal wall

A conventional technique may suffice, but if the patient is old or fragile or there are factors which might lead to abdominal dehiscence in the postoperative period, it is recommended that polyglactin (Vicryl) or polyglycolic acid (Dexon) mesh is placed beneath the abdominal wall.

Evacuation and drainage of the rectum

Gentle dilatation of the anus followed by evacuation and irrigation of the rectal contents is a useful precaution.

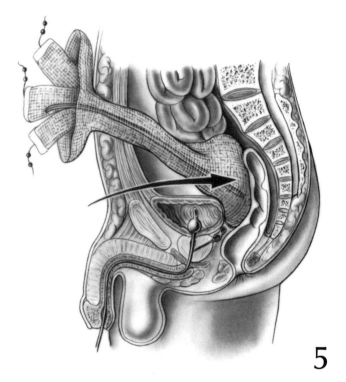

5

Postoperative care

Some patients will require monitoring in an intensive care unit for the management of cardiopulmonary problems. Otherwise, routine postoperative care is required, including inspection of the colostomy and drains. The Mikulicz packing is irrigated from the seventh day to facilitate its removal. Rectal examination can help the diagnosis of pelvic sepsis and sometimes allows the evacuation of a purulent collection.

Outcome

Complications

The incidence of complications is high, approximately 30%, because of the presence of coexistent morbid conditions in elderly, malnourished and septic patients with urinary and pulmonary problems being common.

Sepsis and wound disruption

This occurs in about 25% of patients and in as many as 60% after emergency surgery. Intra-abdominal abscesses requiring percutaneous or surgical drainage occur in 5% of patients[6].

Colostomy complications

These types of complications should be rare, but necrosis may occur: if this is extensive, reoperation may be required[8]; if limited to 1–2 cm of the more distal gut, conservative treatment will suffice. Necrosis is particularly frequent in cases of ischaemic colitis. Most peristomal abscesses can be managed conservatively in the absence of stomal necrosis.

Rectal stump leakage

This occurs in approximately 10% of patients, but results of studies have ranged from zero[9] to 30%[10]. When the pelvis has been drained by a Mikulicz pack, leakage is signalled by a persistent discharge of pus and leakage of water-soluble contrast media seen during diagnostic radiography. Effective drainage may be required to prevent progressive pelvic sepsis and this can usually be achieved through the rectal stump.

Haemorrhage and retention of pus

This may occur in the rectal stump in acute colitis[11]. Conservative treatment with irrigation and packing may be ineffective and emergency proctectomy may very occasionally be required.

Small bowel obstruction

Small bowel obstruction may occur in the early postoperative period because of inflammatory adhesions or recurrent foci sepsis. Guidelines for management are the same as after any major abdominal operation.

Mortality rate

The mortality rate after Hartmann's operation is about 11%, but ranges from 4% to 30%. The mortality rate increases after emergency surgery and in malignant disease. However, most recent series report a lower mortality rate of about 3% for this operation[6].

RESTORATION OF CONTINUITY

The overall rate of restoration of 66%[12] is greater in cases of diverticular disease than in those of cancer, and is increasing with the use of circular staplers[9]. Because the mortality rate of this second procedure is low (0–5%), it is justifiable to propose bowel reconstruction in all cases. However, careful preoperative evaluation is necessary and the timing of surgery is important.

Preoperative

Assessment

Colonoscopy should be carried out to detect neoplasia, diverticular disease or other focal abnormalities in the proximal colon. The rectal stump should be assessed by digital examination and radiography to detect any leak from the suture line and to evaluate the length, volume and compliance of the remaining rectum. Endoscopy and biopsies may be useful, especially in cases of inflammatory bowel disease. Ultrasonography, computed tomography scanning, chest radiography and tumour marker assessment may be useful in patients with malignant disease to detect metastasis, which greatly reduces the indications for further surgery.

The time taken to re-establish bowel continuity is of great importance and depends on the nature of the initial disease and the severity of infection at the time of the first operation. In patients with malignant disease, the delay should be approximately 6 months[3]. In cases of diverticular disease when the procedure is performed in the absence of diffuse sepsis, the delay for reoperation can be quite short (3 months), while delay of 4–12 months is recommended if diffuse sepsis has occurred[13].

Approximately 10% of patients refuse reoperation. These patients are usually elderly and have become used to their colostomy and fear the pain and complications of further surgery. Others have severe or multiple comorbid conditions or an advanced stage of neoplasia, and should be spared the risk of an additional procedure.

Preparation

Bowel preparation is the same as for any colonic surgery. Rectal contents are evacuated and irrigations of the rectal stump are carried out. In 'easy' cases (long rectal stump with normal rectal wall), a conventional colorectal anastomosis may be considered; however, in more 'difficult' cases (short rectal stump or prior operations on the pelvis), the surgeon must be prepared to use either a circular stapler or special techniques, such as the pull-through operations.

Operation

The 'easy' case

The patient is placed in the lithotomy position (*see* page 48). A long midline incision is made, reaching the xiphoid process to give good exposure to the splenic flexure. The operation starts with the dissection of adhesions and a complete exploration of the abdominal cavity. The rectal stump is identified on the sacral promontory where it may be found to be tightly adherent to loops of small bowel, to the uterus in women, and to the posterior aspect of the bladder in men. The aim is to free these adhesions without damage and then find the presacral space so that the limits of the rectal remnant can be identified. This may be difficult because the top of the rectal stump can be adherent posteriorly and the ureters may be pulled towards the midline by the pelvic inflammation. It is useful to localize the ureters before proceeding to dissection of the rectum, and some surgeons pass ureteral catheters at the start of the operation. The dissection may be facilitated by using a sigmoidoscope or inflating the rectum through a Foley catheter to find the apex of the rectum[14]. Others use a large calibre bougie or Hegar dilator. The presacral space is opened and the dissection proceeds downwards posteriorly and laterally. Once a sufficient length of rectum is mobilized (2–3 cm), the level for bowel section is selected where the rectum is supple and large.

The colostomy is dissected from the abdominal wall using instruments which will be discarded because they become contaminated. The left colon and splenic flexure are mobilized, and the end is resected, taking care to prepare a healthy segment of bowel which can reach the level of anastomosis without tension. The anastomosis is then performed as described in the chapters on pp. 51–73 and 74–83. Thorough haemostasis of the operative field and irrigation of the peritoneal cavity terminate the procedure.

The 'difficult' case

Sutured anastomosis

If there has been a leak from the rectal suture line, the top of the rectal stump, including the site of leakage, must be resected, whatever the technique of anastomosis. In the presence of a short rectal stump, the top being below the peritoneal reflection, the operation is often difficult and should be undertaken by a highly experienced surgeon. Despite the use of a sigmoidoscope or a Hegar dilator, localization of the rectal stump is difficult because the bladder (in men) or the uterus/vagina (in women) may be adherent posteriorly to the sacrum, burying the rectal stump. It may only be possible to find a small passage to the rectum from above. If access to the rectum is found posteriorly, then a retrorectal pull-through is indicated (Duhamel operation), provided that the superior part of the rectal stump has not been injured.

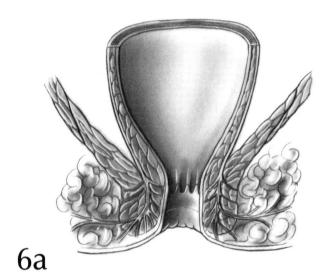

6a

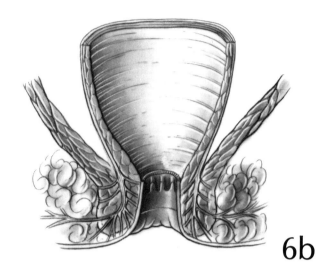

6b

6a–c If the rectal stump is really very short, or has sustained injury during mobilization, it is possible to carry out a mucosal proctectomy from below and to fashion a coloanal anastomosis, which results in a combination of a Soave and Parks operation.

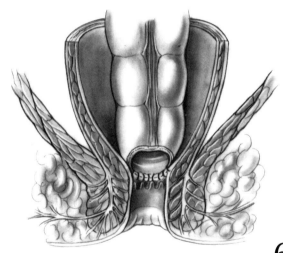

6c

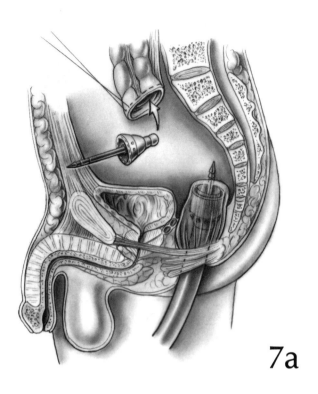

7a

Stapled anastomosis

7a, b The circular stapler is well adapted to this operation[15]; the instrument with the central stem alone is passed through the anus and perforates the rectal stump after minimal dissection, either at the top or at the anterior aspect. However, dissection should be sufficient to avoid taking another organ (bladder, ureter or vagina) between the shaft and the anvil. If the top of the rectum needs to be resected, a double-stapling technique may be used (*see* chapter on pp. 74–83).

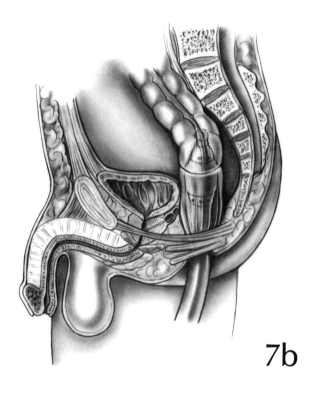

7b

Restoration of continuity in inflammatory bowel disease

The technique in this case is either ileorectostomy (*see* chapter on pp. 347–358) or ileoanal pouch anastomosis (*see* chapter on pp. 604–614), depending on the specific diagnosis: Crohn's disease or mucosal ulcerative colitis.

Postoperative care

When a protective colostomy has been constructed, it should be closed 2 months later after digital and radiological examination of the anastomosis. Anastomotic stenosis is a late complication, and is more prevalent with the use of a small diameter staple machine and after pelvic sepsis associated with anastomotic leakage.

Outcome

The mortality rate is low, ranging from 0% to 5% and complications include wound sepsis, anastomotic leakage and urinary problems.

In conclusion while the indications for Hartmann's operation have changed since 1923, it remains a useful technique in emergency colorectal surgery. It is a safe operation, provided that pelvic drainage is efficient. Restoration of continuity is reasonably easy if the rectal stump is long enough; otherwise it may be challenging.

References

1. Hartmann H. Nouveau procédé d'ablation des cancers de la partie terminale du colon pelvien. *Congrès Français de Chirurgie* 1923; 30: 22–41.

2. Hackford AW, Schoetz DJ, Coller JA, Veidenheimer MC. Surgical management of complicated diverticulitis. The Lahey Clinic experience, 1967 to 1982. *Dis Colon Rectum* 1985; 28: 317–21.

3. Gallot D, Jauffret B, Goujard F, Deslandes M, Sezeur A, Malafosse M. L'intervention de Hartmann. Etude rétrospective de 86 cas. *Ann Chir* 1992; 46: 491–6.

4. Frileux P, Quilichini MA, Cugnenc PH, Parc R, Levy E, Loygue J. Péritonites post opératoires d'origine colique. A propos de 155 cas. *Ann Chir* 1985; 39: 649–59.

5. Doci R, Audisio R, Bozzetti F, Gennari L. Actual role of Hartmann's resection in elective surgical treatment for carcinoma of rectum and sigmoid colon. *Surg Gynecol Obstet* 1986; 163: 49–53.

6. Bell GA, Panton ON. Hartmann resection for perforated sigmoid diverticulitis. A retrospective study of the Vancouver General Hospital experience. *Dis Colon Rectum* 1984; 27: 253–6.

7. Orsoni JL, Mongredien PH, Anfroy JP, Charleux H. Le drainage selon Mikulicz dans les abdomens infectés. Etude critique, technique et résultats à propos de 93 malades. *Chirurgie* 1982; 108: 234–42.

8. Schein M, Decker G. The Hartmann procedure. Extended indications in severe intra-abdominal infection. *Dis Colon Rectum* 1988; 31: 126–9.

9. Cuilleret J, Espalieu PH, Balique JG, Berger JL, Youvarliakis P, Charret P. La place actuelle de l'opération de Hartmann: à propos de 50 cas. *J Chir* 1983; 120: 173–8.

10. Hulkko OA, Laitinen ST, Haukipuro KA, Stahlberg MJ, Juvonen TS, Kairaluoma MI. The Hartmann procedure for the treatment of colorectal emergencies. *Acta Chir Scand* 1986; 152: 531–5.

11. Ona FV, Boger JN. Rectal bleeding due to diversion colitis. *Am J Gastroenterol* 1985; 80: 40–1.

12. Haas PA, Haas GP. A critical evaluation of the Hartmann's procedure. *Am Surg* 1988; 54: 380–5.

13. Lubbers EJ, De Boer HM. Inherent complications of Hartmann's operation. *Surg Gynecol Obstet* 1982; 155: 717–21.

14. Gervin AS, Fisher RP. Identification of the rectal pouch of Hartmann. *Surg Gynecol Obstet* 1987; 164: 176–8.

15. Ramirez OM, Hernandez-Pombo J, Marupidi SR. New technique for anastomosis of the intestine after the Hartmann's procedure with the end-to-end anastomosis stapler. *Surg Gynecol Obstet* 1983; 156: 367–8.

Endoabdominal pull-through resection with colorectal–anal anastomosis

Daher E. Cutait MD, FACS, FRCS
Associate Professor of Surgery, Medical School of the University of São Paulo and Clinical Director, Hospital Sírio-Libanês, São Paulo, Brazil

Felipe José Figliolini MD, TCBC, FACS
São Paulo, Brazil

Raul Cutait MD, TCBC
Associate Professor of Surgery, Department of Surgery, Medical School of the University of São Paulo, São Paulo, Brazil

Principles and justification

Pull-through resections are sphincter-saving operations used to treat malignant and benign lesions of the rectosigmoid region, mostly for tumours of the rectum, particularly in cases where an anterior resection is difficult or technically impossible to perform.

In the abdominal phase of these procedures, the dissection and mobilization of the colon and rectum are identical to those of Miles' operation. Re-establishment of intestinal continuity, which is performed in the perineal phase of the operation, may be executed in two different ways: (1) an anastomosis is constructed between the colon and a segment of retained rectum, as proposed by Maunsell[1] and Weir[2] and later modified by several surgeons such as Black[3] (for cancer), Swenson and Bill[4] (for Hirschsprung's disease), Cutait[5] (for cancer and chagasic megacolon), and Turnbull[6] (for cancer and Hirschsprung's disease). Preservation of a segment of rectum maintains the rectocorticoanal reflex, which is important for preserving continence; (2) the anastomosis may be formed between the colon and the anal canal, as proposed by Hochenegg[7], and subsequently modified and popularized by Babcock[8], Bacon[9] and Waugh[10].

There are a number of ways of performing a pull-through resection. The three procedures used most commonly for cancer and megacolon cases are as follows:

1. Endoabdominal pull-through resection with delayed colorectal anastomosis.
2. Endoabdominal pull-through resection with immediate colorectal anastomosis.
3. Endoabdominal pull-through resection with coloanal anastomosis.

Indications

These procedures may be used in several circumstances.

1. Tumours in the upper (chiefly middle) rectum, when technical difficulties do not permit safe manual or stapled anterior resection.
2. Hirschsprung's disease and chagasic megacolon, in which the dilated sigmoid colon and most of the rectum must be removed.
3. Some benign lesions of the rectum, such as large villous adenomas occupying an extensive part of the wall.
4. Some congenital anorectal anomalies, particularly rectal atresia, when a pouch of normal rectum is present.

Preoperative

The patient should be submitted to a thorough physical examination and admitted to the hospital usually 24 h before the operation. Iced mannitol solution (10%, total volume 1 litre) is given in doses of 150 ml every 10 min in the afternoon, or high colonic washouts are carried out in the morning, afternoon, and night until complete gastrointestinal clearance is achieved. Supplementary washouts are recommended whenever there is evidence of residual faeces in the rectum. Neomycin sulphate, 1 g, and metronidazole 400 mg, are given 18, 12 and 6 h before the operation and prophylactic intravenous cefoxitin, 1 g, is administered 1 h before surgery. This scheme provides a very effective reduction of aerobic and anaerobic flora.

Anaesthesia

The procedure is undertaken under general anaesthesia. As soon as the patient is anaesthetized, the abdomen and perineum are scrubbed with povidone-iodine (Betadine) solution, a Levine tube is introduced into the stomach and a Foley catheter passed into the bladder. In men the penis and scrotum are strapped to the right thigh.

Operation

ENDOABDOMINAL PULL-THROUGH RESECTION WITH DELAYED COLORECTAL ANASTOMOSIS

This technique[5, 11–14] is devised to prevent or minimize disruption of the anastomosis, which is a common complication after using the immediate suture. It is executed in two stages, based on the principle of adhesion by contact between the muscular coat of the rectum and the serosal surface of the pulled-through colon in the first stage, and approximation of the mucosa of the rectum to the mucosa of the colon in the second stage.

Stage 1

Abdominal phase

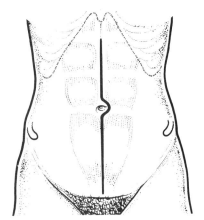

1   The patient is placed in the lithotomy position with moderate flexion of the legs. A midline incision is made, extending from the pubic symphysis to above the umbilicus. The abdominal cavity is explored thoroughly for any intraperitoneal spread and hepatic metastases; the patient is tipped into the Trendelenburg position and the small intestine packed into the upper abdomen. The length of the colon and mesocolon, as well as the vascular arrangement of the segment of the intestine to be used for the pull-through are carefully studied. The procedure should be considered only when the colon and mesocolon are sufficiently long and the marginal arcade adequate.

2   The peritoneum on either side of the mesocolon is incised at its base down to the bladder in the male or to the uterus in the female. The left ureter is exposed and gently swept away from the base of the mesosigmoid. The inferior mesenteric vein is clamped, divided and ligated as high as possible, usually close to the duodenum below the pancreas. The inferior mesenteric artery is ligated close to its origin from the aorta, or just below the left colic branch. The marginal arcade is ligated, and an occlusive ligature of heavy silk applied to the bowel at the same level. The length of colon necessary to extend beyond the anus should be carefully estimated. To facilitate the pull-through, additional length may be obtained by dividing and ligating some vessels in the secondary arcades.

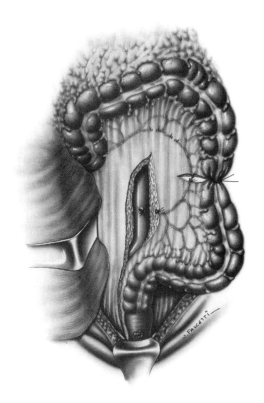

2

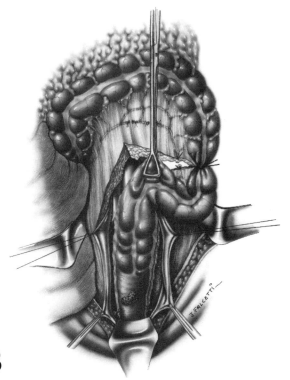

3

3   The rectum is dissected as in Miles' operation: posteriorly to the level of the levator ani muscles, anteriorly through the Denonvilliers' space in males and the rectovaginal space in females, and laterally to a corresponding level. The middle haemorrhoidal vessels are clamped, severed, and tied. Once the rectum is mobilized, the colon above the occlusive ligature must be checked carefully for colour and pulsation of the smaller vessels: pull-through of the colon can be performed with safety only when they are normal. If the viability of this segment is doubtful, additional proximal mobilization must be carried out.

Perineal phase

4 After gentle dilatation of the anal sphincter, an obturator of a sigmoidoscope is introduced through the anus up to the rectosigmoid junction and fixed at this level to the intestinal wall with a heavy silk ligature.

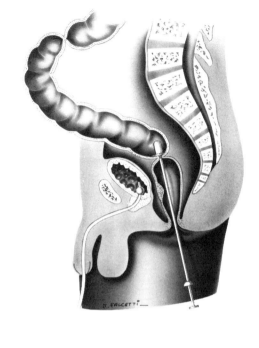

4

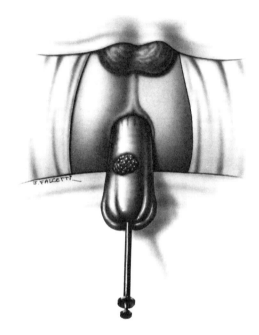

5

5 Gentle downward traction on the obturator promotes eversion of the entire rectum and the pull-through of the lower portion of the sigmoid.

6 The rectal wall is grasped with forceps and incised with scissors approximately 3–4 cm from the pectinate line.

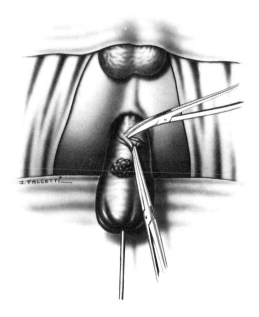

6

7 The incision is completed around the circumference of the rectum, and care is taken not to incise the pulled-through colon.

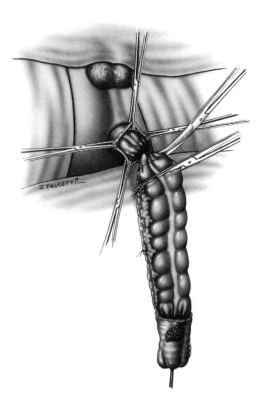

7

8 Haemostasis of bleeding vessels of the proximal cut edge of the rectum is made by ligatures and electrocoagulation.

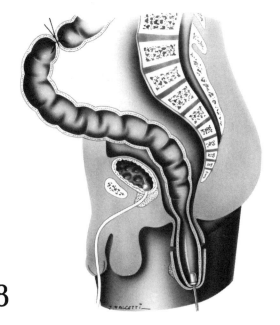

8

9 The bowel is drawn downwards and out through the anus so that the occlusive ligature applied at the abdominal phase of the operation is more than 3 cm from the edge of the everted rectum. The colon is then clamped and divided distal to the ligature.

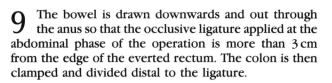

9

10 Four cotton stitches are inserted through the seromuscular coat of the pulled-through colon and the edge of the everted rectum and tied.

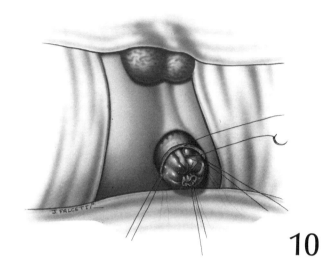

10

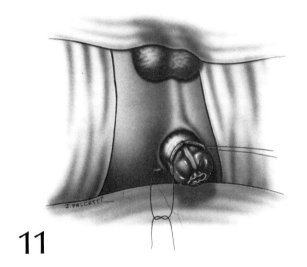

11

11 The two lateral sutures are transfixed and attached to the perineal skin about 2 cm from the pectinate line. This prevents retraction of the colorectal stump. Finally, the stump is covered with petrolatum (Vaseline) gauze.

Closure of the abdomen

While the perineal phase is being performed, assistants working in the abdomen proceed to reconstruct the pelvic peritoneal floor and close the abdomen. The pelvic cavity is drained through a stab wound at the left or right lower quadrant of the abdomen.

The occlusive ligature of the pulled-through colon is removed the day after the operation, after which the pulled-through segment begins to act as a temporary perineal colostomy. The sutures fixing the bowel to the skin are removed 2–3 days after the operation.

Stage 2

This stage is performed about 10 days after stage 1, without anaesthesia.

12 The 10-day period is sufficient to promote firm adhesion of the muscular coat of the everted rectum to the serosal surface of the pulled-through segment of the colon. The adhesion prevents or minimizes the incidence of leakage of the anastomosis.

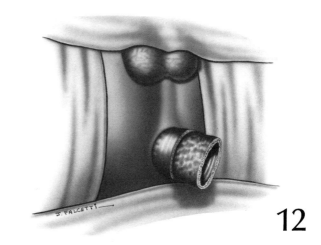

12

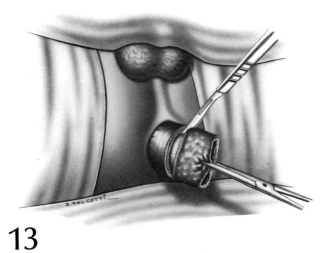

13

13 The colon is grasped with a pair of forceps, and the entire circumference of the seromuscular coat around the border of the everted rectum is incised.

14 The mucosa is then dissected downwards for about 0.5 cm and divided with scissors around the circumference. This dissection permits approximation of the colonic and rectal mucosa without tension.

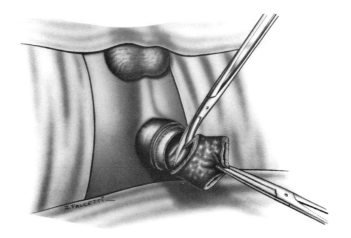

14

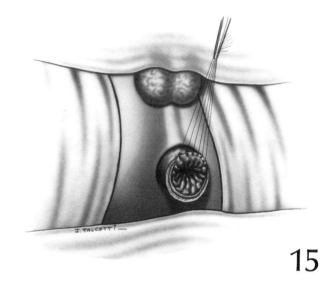

15

15, 16 The rectal mucosa is sutured to the colonic mucosa with interrupted fine cotton stitches.

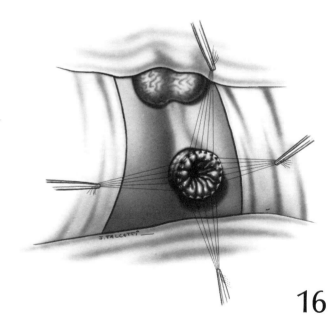

16

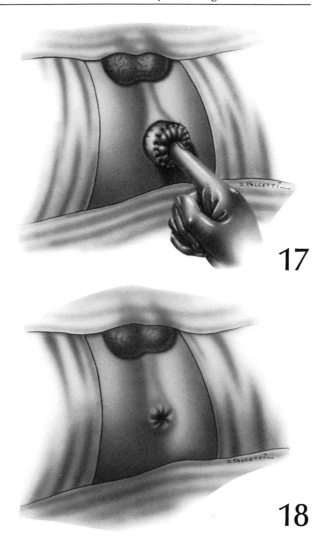

17

18

17,18 Upon completion of the suture, the colorectal stump is forced inside the pelvic cavity with the index finger. In some cases the use of a gauze facilitates this manoeuvre. The patient leaves the hospital after 2–3 days.

Large tumours

In large tumours it is difficult or impossible to evert the rectum by the technique just described, and the colorectal segment is excised in the abdominal phase of the operation.

19 After completion of the colorectal mobilization, the rectum is clamped with a modified Wertheim clamp applied about 5 cm above the levator ani and incised, and the colon is clamped and divided distal to the occlusive ligature.

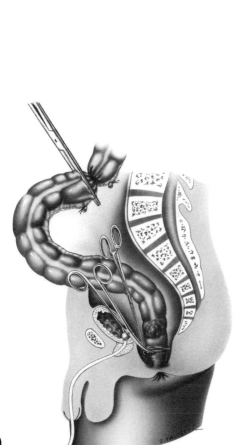

19

20 The surgical specimen is excised and a pair of forceps is introduced through the anal canal to grasp the cut edge of the rectum.

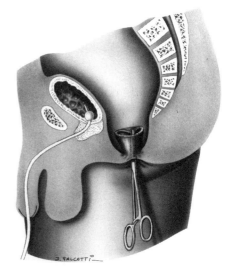

20

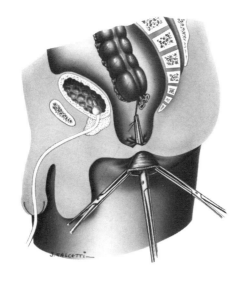

21

21, 22 Gentle traction of the forceps promotes eversion of the rectum. Following this, a clamp is introduced through the anus into the abdominal cavity to grasp the occlusive silk ligature and to pull the colon through and out, so that it protrudes 3 cm beyond the edge of the everted rectum. The operation is then completed as described above.

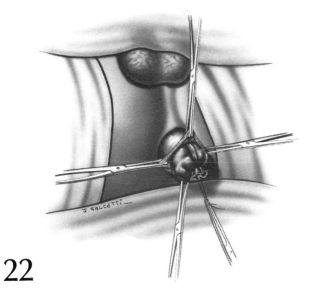

22

ENDOABDOMINAL PULL-THROUGH RESECTION WITH IMMEDIATE COLORECTAL ANASTOMOSIS

This procedure has the disadvantage of being followed by leakage of the anastomosis due to disruption of the suture in more than 20% of cases[14], even after routine transverse colostomy.

The abdominal steps are the same as those described above. The perineal phase is similar, but the colorectal anastomosis is performed and completed in one stage.

23 After intussusception and division of the everted rectum, the colon is pulled down to the level where the occlusive ligature protrudes about 3 cm beyond the edge of the everted rectum.

A two-layer colorectal anastomosis with interrupted cotton stitches is then performed.

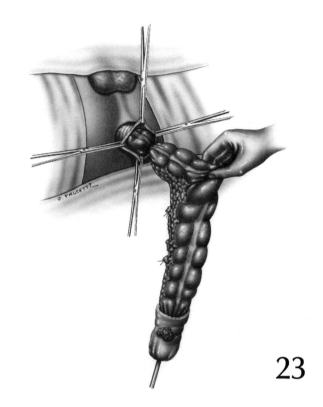

23

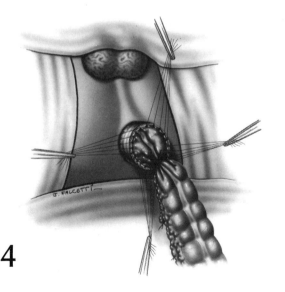

24

24 In the first layer the stitches are applied through the muscular coat of the everted rectum and the seromuscular coat of the pulled-through colon.

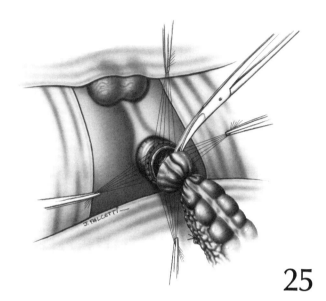

25

25, 26 In the second layer, which is made after division of the colon just distal to the first row of sutures, the stitches penetrate all coats of the rectum and colon. Upon completion of the anastomosis, the rectum is pushed up through the anus with the finger.

A protective transverse colostomy is recommended with this method in order to minimize harmful effects of anastomotic leakage.

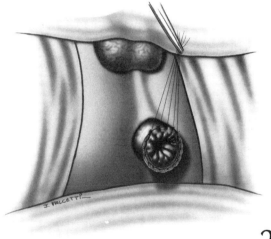

26

ENDOABDOMINAL PULL-THROUGH RESECTION WITH COLOANAL ANASTOMOSIS

The procedure may be used for tumours of the middle rectum[15, 16], but its main indication is cancer of the lower rectum.

The abdominal steps are identical to those described previously. Coloanal anastomosis, which is executed in the perineal phase of the operation, may be carried out using manual or stapled sutures.

Manual anastomosis

27 After mobilization of the colon and dissection of the rectum down to the level of the levator ani muscles, a Wertheim clamp is placed across the rectum below the lesion and the intestine is divided distally with scissors, usually at the level of, or a little above, the anorectal junction.

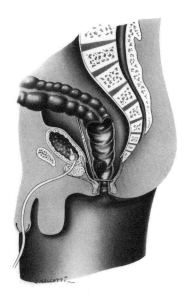

27

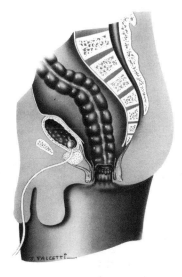

28

28 After careful haemostasis of the cut anal edge, a retractor is placed into the anal canal. The submucosa is infiltrated with a saline adrenaline solution, from the dentate line up to the level of division of the anorectal stump, and the exceeding rectal mucosa is excised with scissors. The colon is then pulled down, and a coloanal anastomosis is performed with interrupted fine cotton sutures. Each stitch transfixes the anal mucosa, a segment of the internal sphincter, and the full thickness of the colon.

A colonic J pouch reservoir[17] may eventually be constructed. In this case, a lateroterminal anastomosis is performed in the same way.

Stapled anastomosis

29 The colorectal segment is dissected and mobilized down to the level of the levator ani muscles, a purse-string suture is applied to the colon and the intestine is divided. A Wertheim's clamp is placed across the rectum distal to the lesion and the gut is divided. At the perineal phase of the operation a purse-string suture is placed in the rectoanal stump. A circular stapler is introduced into the abdomen through the anus, the colonic stump slipped over the anvil and the purse-string suture tied around the centre rod of the instrument. The purse-string suture of the anorectum is then tied around the centre rod, above the cartridge. Straight approximation of both stumps by turning the wing nut clockwise and activating the firing handle complete the anastomosis. This procedure becomes easier with the use of CEEA Premium or DHC staplers.

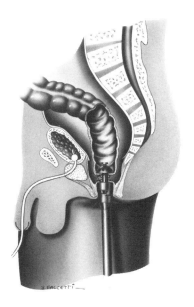

29

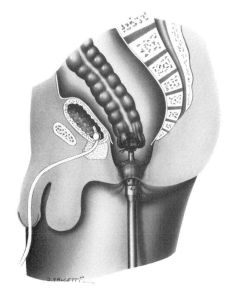

30

Double stapling anastomosis

30 The coloanal anastomosis is performed with the combined use of a Roticulator 55 or RL 60 stapler and a CEEA Premium or DHC stapler, respectively. The linear stapler is applied in the distal rectum at the abdominal phase of the operation. It promotes transection of the gut and closure of the anorectum by a double-line staple suture. The CEEA Premium or DHC stapler is then introduced through the anus without the anvil or anvil shaft. The recessed trocar tip is advanced through the closing stapled line and the tip is removed. The anvil and anvil shaft are introduced into the lumen of the proximal colon, and the previously prepared purse-string suture is tied up. The anvil shaft is then engaged in the instrument shaft of the cartridge. Approximation of both stumps by closing and activating the firing handle promotes a double staggered row of stainless steel staples.

A proximal colostomy is recommended in patients submitted to pull-through resection with coloanal anastomosis, independent of the technique employed.

Postoperative care

Fluid is given intravenously as required. Two additional doses of intravenous cefoxitin (1 g) are administered 6 and 12 h after the preoperative doses. The nasogastric tube is removed as soon as flatus is passed. The urinary catheter is removed about the fifth day after surgery.

Complications

Necrosis of the colon

Sloughing may occur occasionally after pull-through operations with delayed anastomosis: in the distal end of the exteriorized colon, it should not cause alarm. However, when sloughing involves intrapelvic colon, it causes an extensive pelvic abscess and, occasionally, peritonitis. This complication is caused by an inadequate blood supply or undue tension of the colon pulled down through the anus.

It is not always easy to estimate correctly the adequacy of the blood supply of the colon proposed to be used for the pull-through operation. A simple trick may be helpful: after ligation of the inferior mesenteric or sigmoid vessels and marginal arcade, an occlusive heavy silk ligature is applied at the level of the colon to be pulled down to the perineum. This ligature is made before the rectum is dissected. Complete dissection of this segment usually takes 30 min or longer, a sufficient time to evaluate the status of the blood supply of the colon above the occlusive ligature. The blood supply is considered adequate when the colon shows a normal uniform colour and presents pulsation of the vessels or brisk arterial bleeding on incision, contrasting with the cyanosis observed in the colon distal to the ligature. The supply is considered inadequate when the proximal colon has cyanotic colour of variable extent. In the first event, pull-through may be performed with confidence and safety, without danger of necrosis; in the second, additional resection of the colon is necessary.

Extensive sloughing necessitates immediate reoperation to pull down normal proximal colon. However, when unfavourable anatomical conditions or severe infection are present, the only alternative is to resect the necrosed gut and establish a permanent colostomy.

It is important always to have a sufficient length of colon to pull through the anus without tension. This is evaluated by grasping the colon at the level of the occlusive ligature with a Duval clamp and pulling it down towards the pubic area: when it loosely reaches this area, the pull-through procedure may be completed with confidence. Further mobilization of the colon may be needed in some cases. When anatomical conditions are unfavourable, the procedure should be abandoned in favour of another type of operation.

Leakage of the anastomosis

This complication occurs in over 20% of pull-through resections with immediate colorectal anastomosis, even in those with a covering colostomy. Leakage is very rare after delayed anastomosis (about 2%) and is observed in 10–30% of coloanal anastomoses. The incidence is lower when stapled sutures are used (5–10%).

Leakage is usually followed by colorectal or coloanal perineal fistulae, infection and stenosis, but in the majority of cases these subside with proper treatment. However, if these troubles persist, a colostomy may be necessary.

Retraction of the colorectal stump

This is a very rare complication of delayed colorectal anastomosis, and may occur if the rectum is not dissected down to the levator ani floor. In this case, much of the everted rectum lies inside the pelvic cavity. The colorectal stump may thus be affected by the negative pressure of the abdominal cavity during inspiration and be aspirated to the pelvis. Immediately this complication occurs, the colorectal stump should be grasped with an Allis' forceps through a proctoscope and pulled down again. The stump should be closely monitored and covered with a thick petrolatum (Vaseline) gauze dressing until the second stage of the anastomosis can be undertaken.

Pelvic infection

Infection of the presacral space may follow leakage of the anastomosis, necrosis of the intrapelvic colon, retraction of the rectal stump, or even when a large amount of serosanguineous fluid collects in the pelvic cavity. Conservative treatment is indicated for most cases except for necrosis, which usually requires emergency surgical treatment.

Stricture

A slight stricture may be observed in the early postoperative days. It usually subsides spontaneously in a few weeks, but may persist if anastomotic leakage has occurred. Dilatation will usually remedy this complication, but if the narrowing is severe, an internal rectotomy is advised. Colostomy is necessary only in extreme cases of almost complete stenosis.

Anal incontinence

Postoperative diarrhoea and incontinence usually occur in all patients for several weeks following colorectal anastomosis, but subsides spontaneously in the majority of cases. In some patients, however, normal continence is slow to return, but permanent impairment of continence is extremely rare. These complications are more severe in patients who have undergone coloanal anastomosis, and in a significant number of patients incontinence may persist for several months and even become permanent.

Urinary complications

Cystitis commonly occurs following catheterization and should be treated with antibiotics. Urinary retention may occur in some patients and probably results from partial destruction of vesical nerve pathways. It subsides in practically all cases with prolonged catheterization. In some cases, however, retention is secondary to an enlarged prostate gland which may require surgical treatment.

Sexual dysfunction

Sexual dysfunction may occur as a result of damaged nervi erigentes or emotional factors. It must be pointed out that many patients with rectal cancer are old, with little or no sexual activity before surgery. Postoperative sexual neurological disturbances seldom improve, and psychotherapy is usually of little value.

References

1. Maunsell HW. A new method of excising the two upper portions of the rectum and the lower segment of the sigmoid flexure of the colon. *Lancet* 1892; ii: 473–6.

2. Weir RF. An improved method of treating high seated cancers of the rectum. *JAMA* 1901; 37: 801–3.

3. Black BM. Combined abdomino-endorectal resection: surgical procedure preserving continuity of bowel, for management of certain types of carcinoma of midrectum and upper part of rectum. *Proc Staff Meet Mayo Clin* 1948; 23: 545–54.

4. Swenson O, Bill AH. Resection of rectum and rectosigmoid with preservation of the sphincter for benign spastic lesions producing megacolon. *Surgery* 1948; 24: 212–20.

5. Cutait DE, Figliolini FJ. A new method of colorectal anastomosis in abdominoperineal resection. *Dis Colon Rectum* 1961; 4: 335–42.

6. Turnbull RB, Cuthbertson A. Abdominal pull-through resection for cancer and for Hirschsprung disease. *Cleve Clin Q* 1961; 28: 109–15.

7. Hochenegg J. Aus der chirurgischen Klinik des Hofrathes Prof. Albert. Die sacrale Methode der Exstirpation von Mastdarmkrebsen nach Prof. Kraske. *Wien Klin Wochenschr* 1888; 1: 254–7, 272–4, 290–2, 309–11, 324–6, 348–52.

8. Babock W. Experiences with resection of the colon and the elimination of colostomy. *Am J Surg* 1939; 46: 186–203.

9. Bacon HE. Evolution of sphincter muscle preservation and re-establishment of continuity in the operative treatment of rectal and sigmoidal cancer. *Surg Gynecol Obstet* 1945; 81: 113–27.

10. Waugh JM, Turner JC. A study of 268 patients with carcinoma of the mid rectum treated by abdominoperineal resection with sphincter preservation. *Surg Gynecol Obstet* 1958; 107: 777–83.

11. Cutait DE. Technique of rectosigmoidectomy for megacolon; report of 425 resections. *Dis Colon Rectum* 1965; 8: 107–14.

12. Cutait DE. Prevention of pelvic complications in pull-through operations for cancer and benign lesions. *Proc R Soc Med* 1970; 63(suppl.): 121–8.

13. Cutait DE. Abdominoperineale Durchzvgsresektion In: Reifferscheid M., ed. *Rectumkarzinom-Sphinkterehaltende operationsverfahren*. Stuttgart: George Thieme, 1983: 63–71.

14. Cutait DE, Cutait R, Ioshimoto M, Silva JH, Manzione A. Abdominoperineal endoanal pull-through resection: a comparative study between immediate and delayed colorectal anastomosis. *Dis Colon Rectum* 1985; 28: 294–9.

15. Cohen AM, Enker WE, Minsky BD. Proctectomy and coloanal reconstruction for rectal cancer. *Dis Colon Rectum* 1990; 33: 40–3.

16. Gabriele F. Double stapling technique in low anterior resection of the rectum. *Coloproctology* 1991; 13: 218–23.

17. Parc R, Tiret E, Frileux P, Moszkowski E, Loygue J. Resection and colon-anal anastomosis with colonic reservoir for rectal cancer. *Br J Surg* 1986; 73: 139–41.

Illustrations by Gillian Lee Illustrations and the late Robert Lane

Panproctocolectomy and ileostomy

Zane Cohen MD, FRCS(C), FACS
Professor of Surgery, University of Toronto, Surgeon-in-Chief, Mount Sinai Hospital, Toronto, Ontario, Canada

Principles and justification

Panproctocolectomy with end ileostomy was once the standard operative procedure for ulcerative colitis and certain other diseases of the large intestine. However, in the last decade other options have become established: there has been increasing enthusiasm for sphincter-saving operations and, in particular, restorative procto-colectomy with an ileal pouch—anal anastomosis. Other procedures such as colectomy with ileorectal anastomosis and Kock ileostomy (*see* pp. 604–614) are alternatives to an end ileostomy. However, surgeons should not advocate a sphincter-saving operation if it might compromise, in any way, an oncological procedure.

Indications

Panproctocolectomy with end ileostomy is generally accepted as a curative procedure for patients who require surgical treatment for ulcerative colitis, familial adenomatous polyposis and multiple colorectal carcinomas. It is also the operation of choice in certain instances of Crohn's disease involving the large intestine, rectum and anus.

Panproctocolectomy with end ileostomy is also an option for patients with inflammatory and neoplastic diseases of the large intestine and the great majority of such patients manage the end ileostomy extremely well. However, the psychosocial, sexual, and mechanical problems related to an end ileostomy must be discussed with the patient before undertaking the procedure.

Contraindications

Panproctocolectomy should not be offered to patients with toxic megacolon, but colectomy, ileostomy and exteriorization of the sigmoid colon (either closed or open) should be carried out so that all of the above mentioned options remain open for consideration once the patient has made a full recovery.

Preoperative

The patient must be fit enough for this major procedure. If not, the procedure should be staged, with subtotal colectomy and end ileostomy as the initial procedure. The patient should be counselled by an enterostomal therapist to help the patient understand an ileostomy and to alleviate their fear of the unknown. The site of the stoma should be marked on the abdomen (usually in the right lower quadrant), taking into account the patient's shape, occupation and usual clothing habits (*see* chapter on pp. 243–269), and should be within the rectus muscle in order to minimize the chance of paraileostomy herniation. The siting of the stoma is an extremely important part of the preoperative preparation because a well functioning stoma will minimize management difficulties. The surgeon should avoid siting the stoma over a previous scar; however, with the appliances now available this is not as important as in the past.

Mechanical bowel preparation with oral polyethylene glycol (1 litre/h for 3–4h) is undertaken; a prokinetic agent may be given before the lavage to reduce nausea and vomiting. Intravenous metronidazole, 500 mg, and gentamicin, 80 mg, are administered just before the patient is anaesthetized, and continued 8-hourly for three doses.

Operation

Position of patient

The patient is positioned in the lithotomy-Trendelenburg position under general anaesthesia (*see* chapter on pp. 47–50). A nasogastric tube is not routinely used. The perineum is sprayed with tincture of benzoin and in male patients the genitalia are strapped to one thigh with adhesive tape. If necessary, the buttocks are splayed to the side with tape. The entire abdominal wall, from nipples to mid-thigh, and the perineum are prepared with povidone-iodine solution. The anus is then occluded with a purse-string suture of 0 silk inserted through the skin around the anal margin. The patient is then draped. In women it is important to leave the vagina exposed for the operating perineal surgeon.

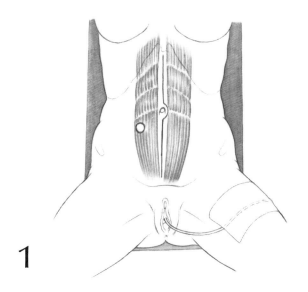

1

Abdominal incision

1 A long midline incision around the left side of the umbilicus will give access to all the abdominal contents. The incision should be carried down to the pubic symphysis in order to maximize exposure of the pelvis. The abdominal contents are then inspected to assess the state of the large intestine and to ascertain whether any other disease is present.

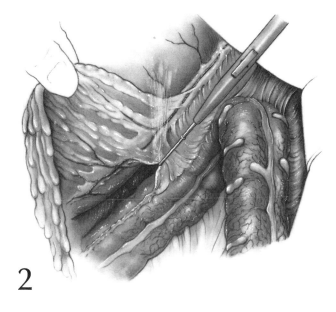

2

Mobilization of the colon

2 The author prefers to mobilize the entire colon before doing the pelvic dissection. This part of the operation may be approached in several ways, but it is preferentially carried out from the right side towards the left side. In inflammatory disease the author's practice is not to preserve the greater omentum; however, for malignant disease the greater omentum is dissected from the transverse colon, leaving it attached to the greater curve of the stomach, so that it can be used as an omental pedicle to fill the pelvis.

In cases where the colon has been perforated and has been sealed off by omentum or peritoneum, the involved area should be mobilized last. The omentum and peritoneum sealing the perforation should be divided in a manner that avoids breaking the seal.

3 The dissection is begun by lifting the right colon to demonstrate the congenital peritoneal reflection visible as a white line (white line of Toldt). Cautery dissection along this line is preferred, but scissor dissection is acceptable. The dissection begins at the caecal portion and extends towards the hepatic flexure. The caecum, terminal ileum and ascending colon are swept forward and lifted above the abdominal wound. The dissection is carried in the plane above the level of the duodenum, and the retroperitoneum is never directly entered. The ureter is identified through the peritoneum.

Mobilization of the right colon is usually quite easy, but care is needed in mobilizing the hepatic flexure because of the underlying duodenum. The dissection of the greater omentum is initiated near to the hepatic flexure, but is not continued at this stage in the procedure. The lesser sac is entered on the left side of the transverse colon, and the omentum is taken down serially between clamps, cut and tied with 0 silk sutures. The fusion plane between the greater omentum and transverse mesocolon is usually quite easily identified, and the dissection is continued from the mid-point of the transverse colon towards the hepatic flexure, thus freeing the entire right colon.

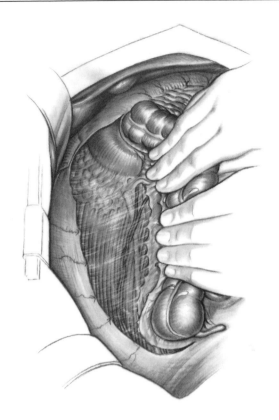

3

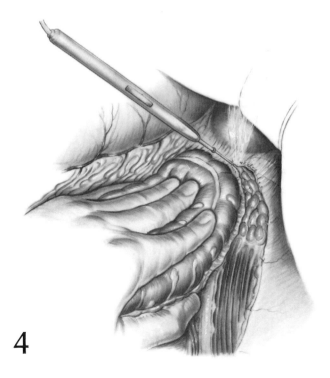

4 The omentum between the stomach and the left portion of the transverse colon is then taken down in a similar fashion, staying quite close to the transverse colon. Blunt dissection in the area of the splenic flexure, or tension on the splenic flexure, should be assiduously avoided so as not to injure the spleen itself.

4

5 The sigmoid colon is mobilized by dividing the congenital peritoneal adhesions as on the right side. Again, by staying just above the white line, the retroperitoneum is not entered. The sigmoid colon (and subsequently the left colon) are held at some tension towards the patient's right side, and the dissection is carried along the left gutter. The entire dissection of the colon and subsequently the rectum is performed with cautery, and vessels encountered in the peritoneal gutter can be coagulated with diathermy before transection. The left ureter is easily identified, but the retroperitoneum should not be breached.

Dissection is then carried up towards the splenic flexure. As it is approached gentle traction should be put on both the left half of the transverse colon and the descending colon, so that the splenic flexure becomes V shaped. This will reveal the lower pole of the spleen, which should be carefully avoided. Staying in the relatively avascular plane the entire left colon, including the splenic flexure, can be mobilized, and the entire colon exteriorized around the abdominal incision.

If the capsule of the spleen is torn during dissection of the splenic flexure, the surgeon should not remove the spleen but should complete the mobilization of the splenic flexure, cover the torn capsule with an absorbable haemostatic gauze, and leave a pack on it until the end of the operation. Re-inspection at this stage will almost invariably show that the bleeding has stopped.

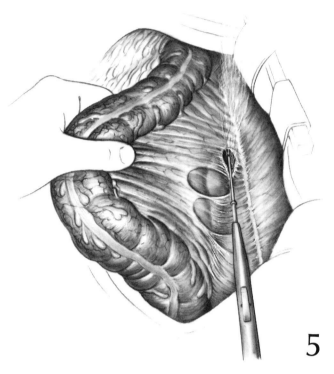

5

In most cases of chronic colitis, mobilization of the splenic flexure is not difficult because of the relative contraction of the colon from the colitis. However, in acute disease there may be microperforations along the left colon and particularly in the splenic flexure region, and in these cases mobilization of the flexure area must be performed very gently. If perforation is suspected, the area of the splenic flexure should be mobilized last, after the abdominal contents have been covered by large abdominal packs.

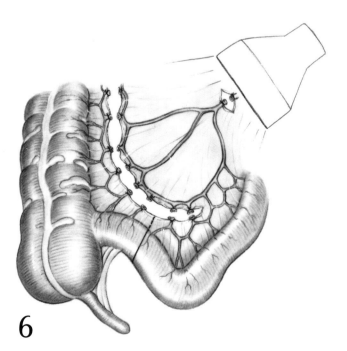

6

6 The mesentery is divided relatively close to the intestinal wall to avoid damaging retroperitoneal structures. However, in cases of neoplastic disease a wider, full oncological procedure should be undertaken. Elevating the bowel will allow the mesentery to be transilluminated in order to demonstrate the colonic vessels and ensure their accurate isolation and division. It is the author's preference to divide the ileocolic artery: this allows the terminal ileum (and subsequently the ileostomy) to be constructed in a straight manner. Even if the mesentery is quite thickened, this manoeuvre will allow a much better functioning stoma.

7 Once the mesentery to the entire colon and terminal ileum have been divided, the terminal ileum itself can be transected. In inflammatory disease this is usually performed as close as possible to the caecum. It is the author's preference to use a linear cutting stapling instrument to divide the terminal ileum which minimizes contamination.

Once the mesenteric dissection is complete the entire colon can be wrapped in a large swab so that it can be moved from side to side when performing the rectal mobilization.

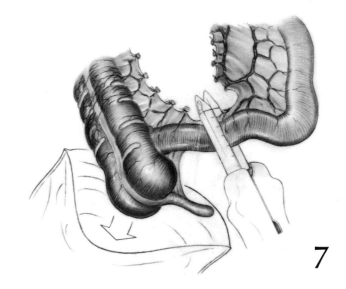

7

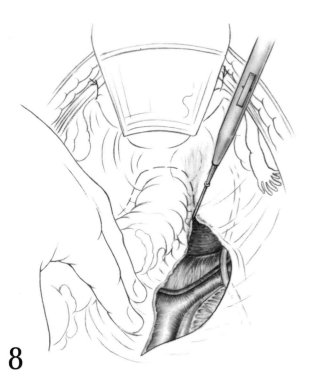

8

Mobilization of the rectum

8 Attention is then turned to the pelvis. A deep-lipped retractor is placed in the rectovesical or rectouterine pouch. If the uterus is bulky, it can be pulled out of the way by inserting sutures around the fallopian tubes and round ligaments on each side, and tying them up to the lower end of the abdominal incision. Incisions in the peritoneum are commenced at the lower ends of the right and left colon dissections and carried down on either side of the rectum using cautery dissection. These incisions are joined anteriorly just at or above the point of the peritoneal reflection in benign disease, and 1 cm distal to the peritoneum in malignant disease.

9 The objectives of the rectal mobilization are to achieve a clean and dry dissection avoiding damage to the pelvic nerves. The hypogastric nerves in the region of the sacral promontory can be easily identified, and careful dissection can be carried out between these nerves and the superior haemorrhoidal vessel. The vascular plane is found and the dissection carried behind the mesorectum, preserving the nerves and the presacral fascia, using cautery or sharp dissection: there is *no* blunt dissection. Once the posterior dissection is almost complete, the right and left side of the rectum are mobilized, cauterizing small vessels (where found) before division. A dissection plane closer to the rectum is maintained for benign disease. In the pelvis no clips are applied and no ties are utilized when the cautery technique is used.

In benign disease, the anterior dissection is carried down through the peritoneum on the intestinal wall. The seminal vesicles in men are usually identified anteriorly through the peritoneum, the fascia of Denonvilliers is divided and the dissection is carried down to the apex of the prostate gland.

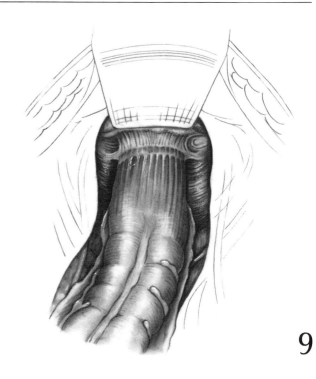

9

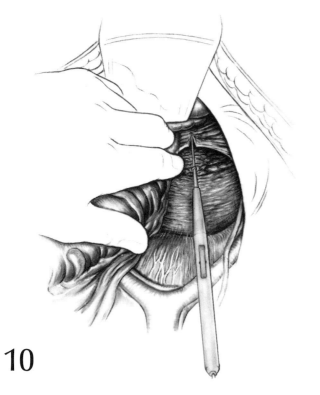

10

10 The rectum may now be pulled up and the lateral attachments cauterized and divided. The posterior dissection has been taken down to below the level of the coccyx, and the lateral dissections will meet this area. Simultaneous dissection by the perineal operator will enable both surgeons to meet posteriorly below the level of the coccyx.

When the perineal dissection is complete (*see* below), the entire colon and rectum are usually removed through the perineal opening. In cases where an extremely bulky colon makes extraction difficult, the perineal operator should place a glove over the anus and tie it onto the rectum. The rectum and anus can then be delivered into the pelvis, and the specimen removed by the abdominal operator. Contamination of the abdominal or pelvic area should be avoided. Using cautery dissection the operative field should be dry but, following pelvic irrigation, a dry pack should be placed in the pelvis and then removed to allow any bleeding points to be coagulated or clipped. It is wise to take the patient out of the Trendelenburg position to allow any venous bleeding to be identified. The pelvis is then irrigated with 1–2 litres of warm saline solution or aqueous chlorhexidine (in malignant cases) to remove clot and debris.

11 The pelvic peritoneum is not closed routinely in the author's proctocolectomy procedures. However, when proctocolectomy is performed for malignant disease and postoperative adjuvant radiation therapy is likely to be performed, a mesh sling (Dexon) is used from the pubic symphysis to the posterior abdominal wall to exclude the small intestine from entering the pelvis. This helps to reduce the incidence of small intestinal complications resulting from irradiation.

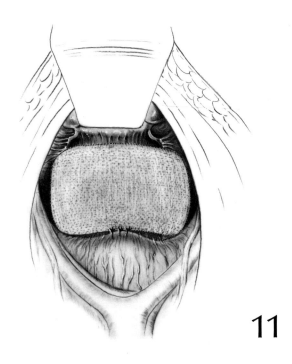

11

Perineal dissection

12 The aim of the perineal dissection for colitis and polyposis coli is to remove only the intestinal wall, not the perirectal tissues. This dissection leaves the pelvic nerves intact and ensures, by maintaining the levator ani, a strong pelvic floor. In both men and women this is achieved by an intersphincteric dissection which commences between the internal and external sphincters. Although this can usually be accomplished without difficulty, it can be technically difficult in patients with Crohn's disease with fistulous communications.

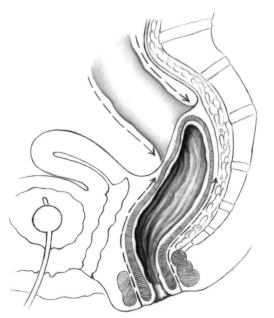

12

13 The perineal dissection can begin when the abdominal surgeon is starting the rectal dissection. The operation should be achieved with anatomical accuracy and with minimal blood loss. The dissection commences with the circumferential incision over the intersphincteric groove. Before making the skin incision, injection of a solution of 1:200 000 adrenaline and saline into the intersphincteric groove helps to separate the internal and external sphincters, making the dissection much easier.

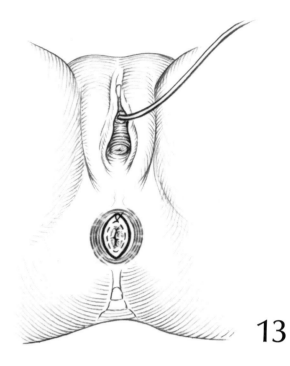

13

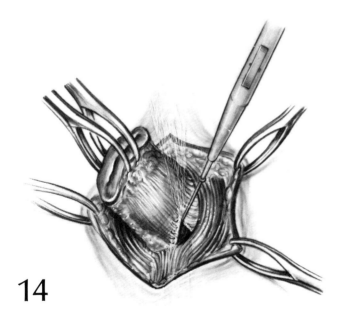

14

14 The dissection is usually started posteriorly and laterally where the intersphincteric groove is most prominent. This plane is usually relatively easy to develop, and with cautery or sharp dissection it can be carried up towards the pelvis.

The dissection is then completed anteriorly. Retraction is accomplished by either a perineal retractor or small self-retaining Gelpi retractors.

15 All of the perirectal tissues should have been mobilized in the abdominal procedure, making the perineal dissection simpler. It is useful for the abdominal operator to have a hand deep in the pelvis both posteriorly and anteriorly to guide the perineal operator. Posteriorly, the abdominal operator can protect the rectum by retracting it anteriorly. The anterior dissection is often the most difficult because the external sphincter decussates in the midline and becomes attached to the fibres of the rectourethralis muscle, making it necessary to cut through some of the fibres of the external sphincter in this plane in order to expose the posterior surface of the prostate. The dissection proceeds higher and, with guidance from the abdominal operator, forwards until the two procedures meet. Continuing the dissection circumferentially will free the entire rectum. It must be remembered that the internal sphincter is the continuation of the inner circular muscle layer of the rectum and, provided that the perineal dissector stays in the correct plane, the operation is simplified.

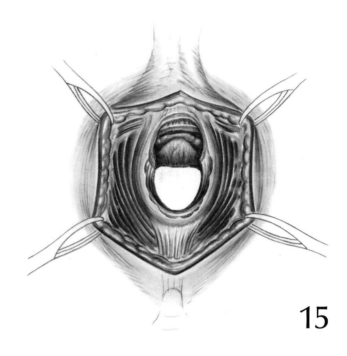

15

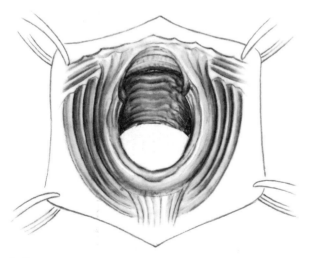

16

16 In women the vagina is dissected forwards, off the anal canal and lower rectum, until the plane opens from above and the rectouterine pouch is reached. The bowel is then free and can be removed.

Wound closure

Perineal wound

17 The pelvis is drained by the abdominal route, because a perineal drain causes discomfort in the postoperative period. A No. 10 Jackson–Pratt drain is inserted through a left lower quadrant stab incision and led down into the pelvis to the perineal region. The drain is placed by the perineal operator and attached to a closed suction system.

The perineal wound is closed using 2/0 polyglactin skin sutures. The musculature is not approximated: this will prevent a potential late-onset supralevator abscess, which can be extremely difficult to detect and treat if the muscle layers have been closed. A simple gauze dressing is then applied to the perineum, and the adhesive tapes holding the buttocks apart are removed; if any tension is encountered when attempting to close the skin, these tapes can be removed before skin closure.

On the rare occasions when bleeding in the perineum is excessive, the area is packed with gauze which is removed gradually over several days. If there is general bacterial contamination of the perineum because of Crohn's disease, it is reasonable to pack the pelvic cavity rather than close the perineal wound primarily.

A conventional end ileostomy is constructed following the removal of the colon and rectum. There is no significant advantage to an extraperitoneal tunnelled ileostomy (*see* chapter on pp. 243–269).

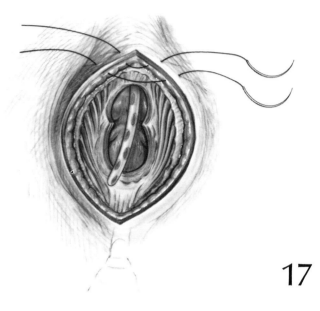

17

Abdominal wall closure

The abdominal wall is closed in layers using continuous and interrupted 1 polyglycolic acid or polyglactin sutures to the linea alba. No abdominal drainage is required, and skin clips are used to close the skin incision.

Postoperative care

The stoma can be inspected easily through the transparent bag, and the skin incision is inspected after 24 h.

Intravenous electrolyte solutions are maintained until the stoma is functioning well. Nasogastric tubes are not used routinely, but may be necessary if abdominal distension, nausea and/or vomiting occur. Initially ileostomy output can be copious, particularly if there have been previous episodes of intestinal obstruction. Ileostomy fluid loss in excess of 800 ml/24 h should be replaced with physiological solutions. The exact elec-

trolyte composition of the ileostomy fluid for replacement can be measured by sending an aliquot of the ileostomy effluent for electrolyte determination.

The urinary catheter is usually removed on the fourth postoperative day, and the skin clips at 7 days. The Jackson–Pratt drain is removed when only serous fluid emanates from the pelvis, and when the volume of drainage is quite low.

Complications

When correctly carried out, this operation is rarely associated with complications in the early postoperative period. However, abdominal distension, high output or an empty ileostomy bag after 72–96 h, even in the absence of colicky abdominal pain, is often an indication of mechanical obstruction rather than continuing ileus. In this case a nasogastric tube should be inserted and maintained on suction to decompress the gut. Once decompression is achieved, the ileostomy will often begin to function. On very rare occasions the patient may require re-exploration in the early postoperative period because of obstruction of the small intestine.

The perineal wound will heal primarily in more than 80% of cases. If perineal infection develops, sutures should be removed to allow adequate drainage of the perineum. The cavity is irrigated twice daily and packed with dry gauze dressings. This cavity will usually heal, but it may take several months or even a year for healing to be complete.

Pelvic exenteration and other extended operations

Alfred M. Cohen MD
Chief, Colorectal Service, Department of Surgery, Memorial Sloan–Kettering Cancer Center and Professor of Surgery, Cornell University Medical College, New York, USA

History

Ultraradical operative procedures for patients with locally advanced primary or recurrent rectal/rectosigmoid adenocarcinoma have traditionally been referred to as exenterations. This term usually meant removal of multiple viscera in the pelvis with a permanent colostomy, frequently a permanent urostomy, and in women the removal of the vagina. These extended operative procedures represent a spectrum of operative resections as well as reconstructive options. The distinctions between the various exenterative procedures will be elucidated below.

Principles and justification

A number of extended operative procedures are performed for sigmoid, rectosigmoid or rectal cancer that are quite routine and will not be described here. Sigmoid or rectosigmoid cancers adherent to the dome or cephalad portion of the bladder are treated by incontinuity colectomy and partial cystectomy. Despite only 50% of such cases showing direct invasion of the bladder, separation of adherent contiguous organs to distinguish inflammatory from malignant invasion may lead to dissemination of malignant cells and is to be avoided. In women, adherence of a rectosigmoid or sigmoid cancer to the uterus requires an incontinuity hysterectomy. Also adherence of an anteriorly based cancer to the rectovaginal septum is an indication for a concomitant total abdominal hysterectomy with posterior vaginectomy. If this is performed as part of an abdominoperineal resection then the posterior vaginal defect may be left open, the small bowel excluded from the pelvis and the defect allowed to heal secondarily. In patients in whom hysterectomy/posterior vaginectomy is performed as part of a sphincter-saving approach, the vaginal defect must either be directly surgically closed (rarely feasible) or covered with an omental, muscle or myocutaneous flap: gracilis or rectus flaps are most suitable.

Patients with primary 'unresectable' rectal cancer with adherence or fixation to the posterior or lateral pelvis or the prostate base of bladder (in males) should be considered for a preoperative radiation therapy strategy. About 4–6 weeks after 4500–6000 cGy of radiation therapy, approximately 75% of these lesions are removable with negative surgical margins.

Definitions of extended operative procedures

Total pelvic exenteration

Traditionally this has meant removal of all pelvic viscera with the formation of a permanent colostomy and urinary diversion, usually by ileal conduit with urostomy. Selected patients may now undergo ileal neobladder formation and avoid a urostomy. All men suffer erectile impotence with this procedure.

1 The coronal planes of importance associated with each type of operation in females are: (A) anterior plane for total exenteration; (B) anterior plane for posterior exenteration with total vaginectomy; (C) anterior plane for post-exenteration with posterior vaginectomy; (D) posterior plane for total exenteration or posterior exenteration; (E) posterior plane for abdominosacral exenteration. Line F shows the optional rectal reconstruction level in posterior exenteration.

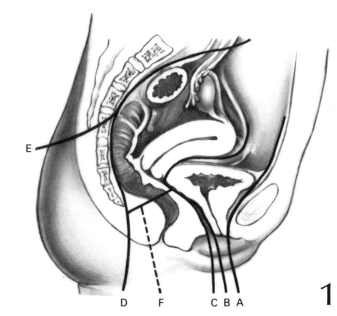

Posterior pelvic exenteration

Posterior pelvic exenteration involves an incontinuity 'radical hysterectomy' with radical rectal resection. The rectal resection may be an abdominoperineal resection or a sphincter-saving reconstruction.

Sacral resection

With tumours adhering to or invading the sacrum all of the above radical operations may be combined with an incontinuity resection of the sacrum. If the bladder is to remain, only a partial sacrectomy is feasible with retention of the S3 nerve roots. However, if the exenterative procedure involves the removal of the bladder as well as the rectum, a high subtotal sacrectomy may be performed. These operative procedures are referred to as abdominosacral, sacropelvic or composite pelvic exenterations.

2 The coronal planes of importance associated with each type of operation in males are: (A) anterior plane for total exenteration; (B) anterior plane for extended abdominoperineal or abdominosacral resection; (C) anterior plane for standard abdominoperineal or abdominosacral resection; (D) posterior plane for standard total exenteration; (E) posterior plane for abdominosacral exenteration.

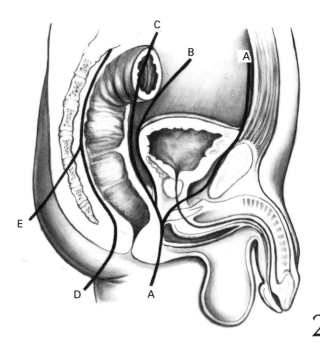

Lateral dissection

The above comments have described various operative procedures as a function of the level of anterior or posterior dissection (coronal plane). An additional consideration is the extent of the lateral dissection (sagittal plane)[1]. The exenterative procedures may be performed at the level of the endopelvic fascia, may involve a lateral pelvic lymphadenectomy with the plane of the dissection on the hypogastric vessels or, in selected patients, a dissection performed lateral to the plane of the hypogastric vessels. This latter plane of dissection is particularly useful in exenterative procedures for recurrent rectal cancer, since it provides not only an additional lateral margin but a virginal plane for dissection.

3 The saggital planes of importance are: (A) the plane on the endopelvic fascia; (B) the plane lateral to the endopelvic fascia, dissecting the hypogastric vessels; and (C) the plane lateral to the hypogastric vessels distal to the superior haemorrhoidal artery.

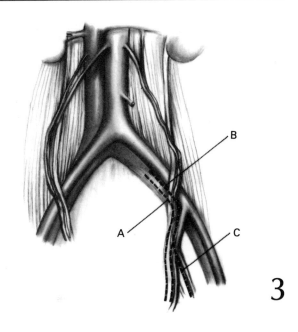

3

Preoperative

These extended operative procedures are associated with considerable morbidity and some mortality. Palliative exenteration is not appropriate. A negative chest radiograph and abdominal computed tomography (CT) scan are imperative. Pelvic CT scans and magnetic resonance imaging evaluations of the pelvis are complementary in terms of determining the extent of disease and the distinction of scar from tumour. Patients with pain in the sciatic distribution are rarely helped by exenterative procedures.

Anaesthesia

These operative procedures are usually performed under general anaesthesia, perhaps combined with regional anaesthesia through an epidural catheter.

In addition to the risk of intraoperative haemorrhage, a major problem in the intraoperative and perioperative period is hypothermia. The patient should be placed on some type of a warming blanket, any exposed skin (particularly the head) covered in plastic and the operating theatre temperature kept higher than many surgeons would prefer.

Operation

Position of the patient

The modified lithotomy steep Trendelenburg position is required, with thighs moderately abducted and slightly flexed with the sacrum supported on a foam pillow. The ischial tuberosities should be kept well away from the edge of the mattress and the sacral support must be above the coccyx. This will allow synchronous dissection which is particularly important with bulky tumours or with reoperations. Occasionally extensive haemorrhage during the transabdominal approach occurs which can only be controlled once the specimen is removed. In extreme circumstances, even major venous bleeding in the pelvis can be controlled with aortic cross-clamping and rapid sharp dissection to remove the tumour by a combined abdominal/perineal approach, after which oversewing of lateral pelvic sidewall bleeding is straightforward.

In order to avoid slippage during a lengthy operative procedure performed in the steep Trendelenburg position, shoulder braces must be used. Bracing is most simply and safely accomplished by taping a pillow underneath the head and nape of the neck which pushes up against the shoulders to keep the patient in position (*see Illustration 2* on page 48).

Management of the anus

The rectum is first cleared of any residual fluid then the anus is sutured closed. If operative findings ultimately dictate a sphincter-saving approach the suture can be removed.

Intraoperative aids

A fibreoptic headlight, adequate long instruments and deep retractors are essential.

Intraoperative evaluation

A meticulous rectal/pelvic examination under anaesthesia and cystoscopy are important in determining clinical resectability of the tumour. At laparotomy the liver and abdomen should be examined to rule out extrapelvic disease: extrapelvic lymph node metastases or peritoneal seeding should preclude ultraradical surgery. Lateral pelvic sidewall involvement also precludes a potentially curative operation. Bimanual examination with the abdomen open is also very useful.

Unfortunately, despite the latest imaging techniques and intraoperative assessment, in many patients undergoing exenterative procedures it is apparent only at the completion of the operation that gross tumour is being left behind. Intraoperative radiation therapy may salvage some of these patients. In patients with recurrent cancer the placement of ureteral stents may be helpful but is not routinely applied.

TOTAL PELVIC EXENTERATION

4 Once extrapelvic disease is ruled out, the peritoneum is incised over both iliac vessels.

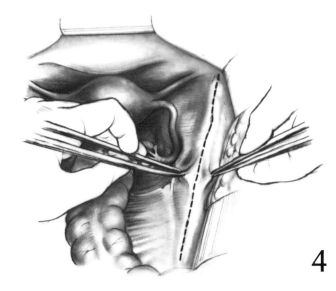

5 The ureters are identified, and in women the ovarian vessels within the infundibulopelvic ligament are ligated and divided on both sides.

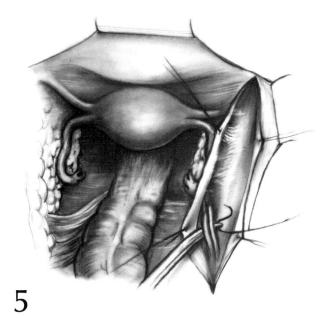

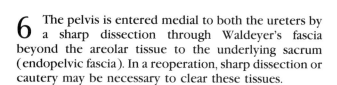

6 The pelvis is entered medial to both the ureters by a sharp dissection through Waldeyer's fascia beyond the areolar tissue to the underlying sacrum (endopelvic fascia). In a reoperation, sharp dissection or cautery may be necessary to clear these tissues.

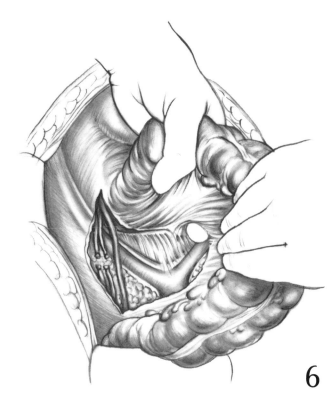

7 The superior haemorrhoidal vessels are ligated and divided. Depending on the amount of sigmoid colon to be removed, this ligation may be performed at the origin of the inferior mesenteric artery.

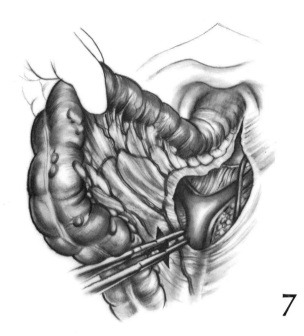

7

8 The mesentery to the proximal sigmoid is divided and the bowel is divided with a linear stapler. The proximal bowel is packed inside the abdomen and scissor or cautery dissection proceeds on the endopelvic fascia in the midline. Care must be taken not to damage the presacral venous plexus.

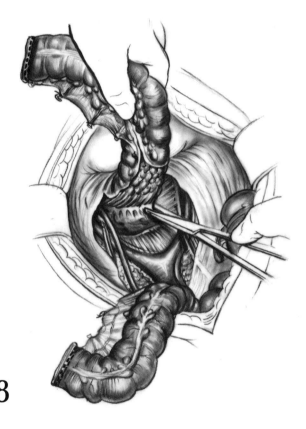

8

9 The paravesical rectal space is more completely exposed and resectability can be determined more conclusively at this time.

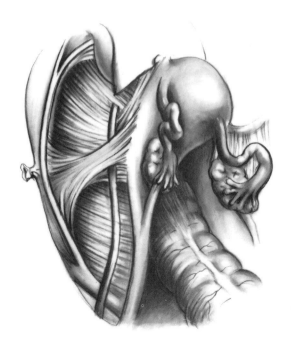

9

10 The ureters are divided, usually at the level of the mid-pelvis. The distal ureter is ligated, but the proximal ureter should not be ligated because in a lengthy procedure this can lead to hyperkalaemia. Ureteric catheters are inserted through the cut ends of the ureters to drain the operative field.

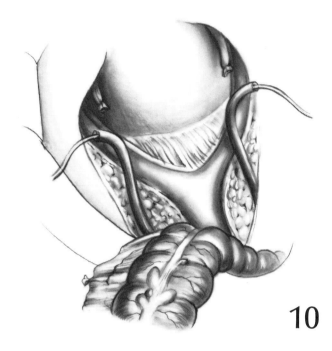

10

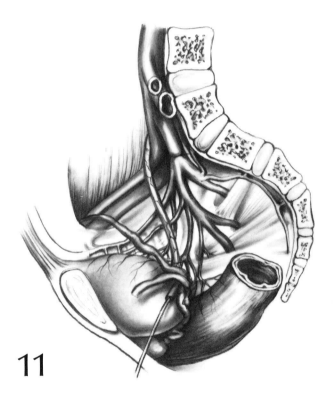

11

11 For total pelvic exenteration, ligation of the hypogastric arteries is usually performed distal to the origin of the superior gluteal artery.

12 Following ligation and division of the hypogastric artery, the pelvic sidewall is dissected along the level of the hypogastric vein.

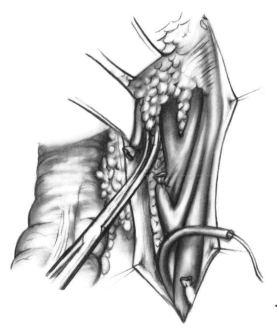

12

13 Scissor and cautery dissection is used to clear the posterior and lateral attachments in a plane that is now deep to the endopelvic fascia, lateral to the hypogastric artery.

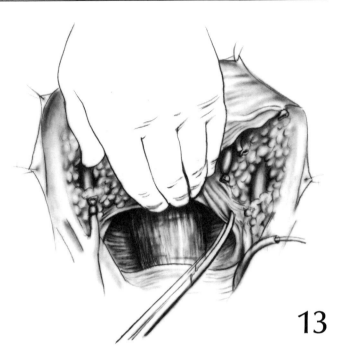

13

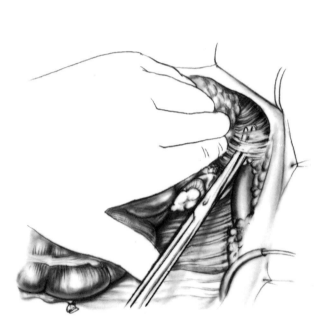

14

14 Attention is now focused more anteriorly, and tissues posterior to the obturator nerve are cleared. As the dissection extends more distally the pelvic floor may be identified in the lateral and posterolateral positions.

15 The endopelvic fascia along the levator ani is sharply incised.

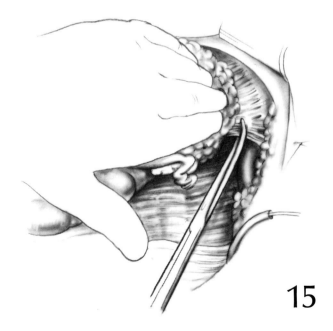

15

16 The posterior dissection is completed using cautery dissection by sharply dividing the rectosacral fascia that binds the posterior rectum to the sacral hollow. Exposure during all of the later stages of the operation is facilitated using a St Mark's retractor.

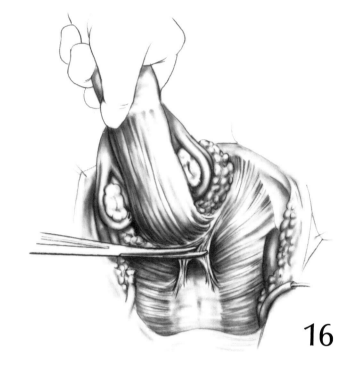

16

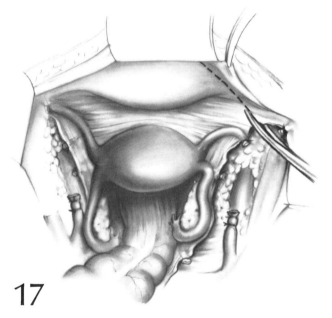

17

17 In women, the round ligaments are ligated and divided and the visceral peritoneum over the periuterine and perivesical spaces divided.

18 By pressing firmly posteriorly on the bladder the periurethral tissues may be identified. The endopelvic fascia along the anterior surface of the levator ani should be incised to separate all attachments except the urethra.

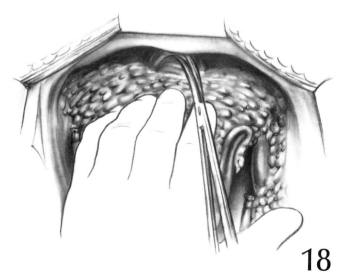

18

19 At this stage, troublesome bleeding from the venous plexus at the junction of the membranous urethra and the prostate can occur in men. The urethra should be identified by palpation of the Foley catheter, and the venous plexus oversewn. Following this the bladder catheter is removed and the urethra is divided and oversewn. Heavy suture ligatures may be necessary to control bleeding from this venous plexus: if they prove inadequate, a Foley catheter is inserted with 30–50 ml in the balloon and placed on traction to tamponade the bleeding.

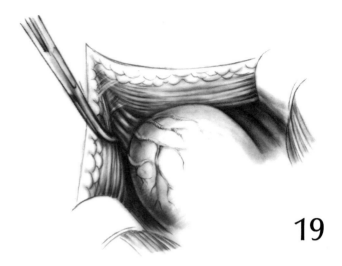

19

At this stage in the procedure the remainder of the resection is performed through the perineum. This is little different from the perineal portion of an abdominoperineal resection. In women, the perianal incision is extended along the labia minora to encompass the urethra and the entire vagina and cautery dissection is used. In both men and women, clamps should be used along the levator muscles laterally and the puborectalis muscles anterolaterally to avoid unnecessary haemorrhage. Once the specimen is removed, these are suture ligated.

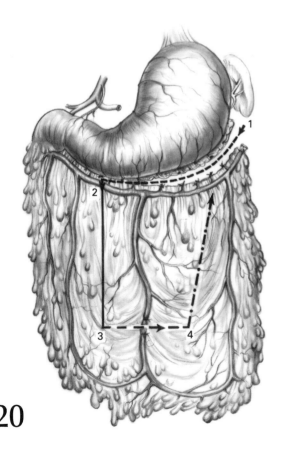

20

20 Following removal of the specimen the small bowel should be excluded from the pelvis, ideally using an omental flap which can be based on either the left or right gastroepiploic artery. With appropriate lengthening the omentum is sewn as a diaphragm to exclude all bowel from the pelvis.

21 If omentum is not available, an absorbable mesh may be used to perform the same function for the first 60–90 days. Absorbable mesh may be combined with the omentum as a double layer. The pelvic space is drained with multiple closed suction drains.

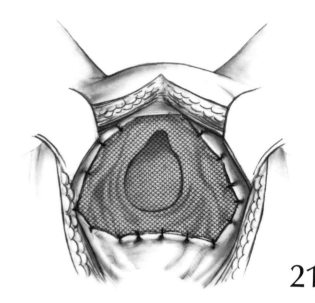

21

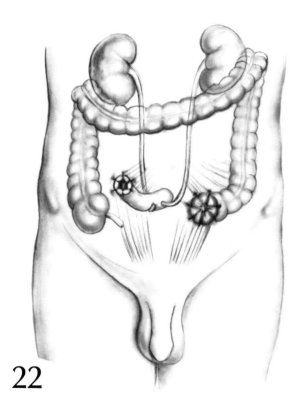

22

22 An ileal conduit is then formed with a urostomy in the right lower quadrant and a colostomy in the left lower quadrant. Both should pass through the rectus muscle to reduce the risk of peristomal hernia.

23 In selected patients, an ileal neobladder may be utilized to avoid a urostomy.

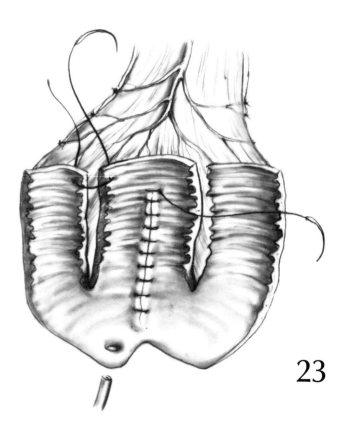

23

TOTAL PELVIC EXENTERATION WITH INCONTINUITY SACRECTOMY

24 The plane of dissection is posterior, through the S3 mid-sacrum.

Position of patient

Except for minor distal sacral/coccygeal resections, it is not possible to perform this procedure with the patient in a single position. The transabdominal component of the operation is performed with the patient supine. The entire mobilization is performed from the transabdominal approach as described for total pelvic exenteration. Both hypogastric arteries should be ligated just distal to the origin of the superior gluteal artery. The lateral and posterolateral dissection is performed to the level of the sciatic nerve. The posterior dissection stops at the level of the mid-sacrum. The decision as to the level of bone division will be based on preoperative scans, operative findings and biopsies. Packs are placed in the pelvis and the wound temporarily closed with through-and-through retention sutures. A sterile dressing is placed on the abdomen. The patient is then placed in the jack-knife position and the perineum prepared and draped.

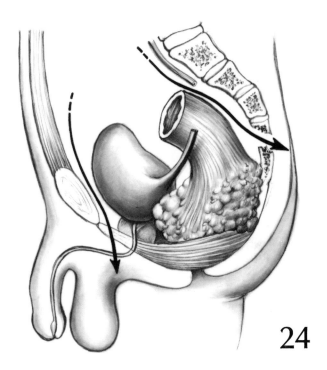

24

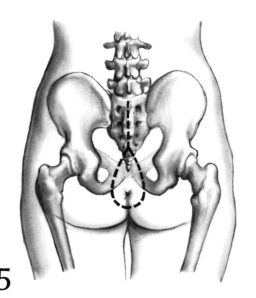

25

25 The incision is outlined and after an initial skin incision using a scalpel the rest of the dissection is performed with cautery. Reversing the direction of dissection, as with an abdominoperineal resection or routine exenteration, the pelvis is entered anteriorly and the levators divided far laterally. All the ligamentous attachments are taken off the sacrum, staying directly on the bone with cautery. Care should be taken not to injure the sciatic nerves.

The pelvis is then entered at the sacroiliac joint and a power saw or Gigli saw used to divide the sacrum. The specimen is removed. The dural sac usually ends at the S1 or S2 level: if it is opened, it *must* be closed. A formal laminectomy to preserve the upper sacral nerve roots is performed if the bladder is to be retained. Careful haemostasis is obtained through the perineal defect using suture ligatures. A meticulous midline closure in layers involving muscle, subcutaneous tissue and skin is performed. Vertical nylon mattress sutures are necessary on the skin.

The patient is then repositioned supine on the operating table, the abdomen re-prepared and draped and the abdominal incision is opened. Additional haemostasis is then obtained from the abdominal approach and the urinary conduit is fashioned. The colostomy is then completed and the small bowel is excluded from the pelvis with an omental pedicle and/or absorbable mesh. Suction drains are used in the pelvis.

EXTENDED ABDOMINOPERINEAL RESECTION IN MEN

26 In an abdominoperineal resection in men the anterior plane of dissection is directly posterior to the dense Denonvilliers' fascia (A). However, if the rectal cancer extends anteriorly or a recurrence abuts the base of the bladder, an additional margin can be obtained by dissection anterior to Denonvilliers' fascia (B) including the seminal vesicles.

The vasa deferentia are ligated and divided, following which the seminal vesicles are completely exposed and may be amputated at the level of the prostate. Dissection then proceeds directly on the prostatic capsule. It is important to transect Denonvilliers' fascia once again as it wraps around the most caudad portion of the prostate.

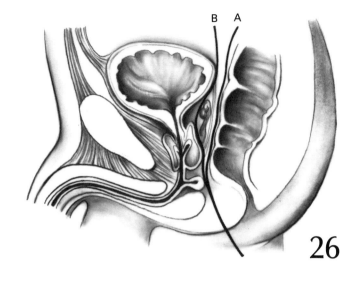

POSTERIOR EXENTERATION IN WOMEN

In this procedure an abdominoperineal resection or a low anterior resection of the rectum is combined with a radical hysterectomy.

27 The visceral peritoneum over the broad ligaments is excised, exposing the base of the bladder.

28 The round ligaments are ligated and divided, the ovarian vessels are similarly ligated and divided and all of the peritoneum overlying the lateral anterior portions of the uterus and broad ligaments is incised.

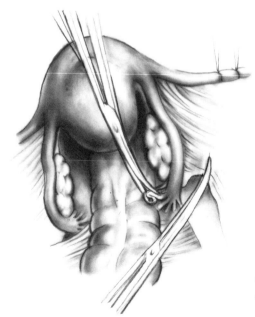

29 The hypogastric artery is sharply dissected and the uterine artery is ligated and divided.

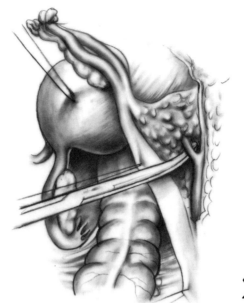

29

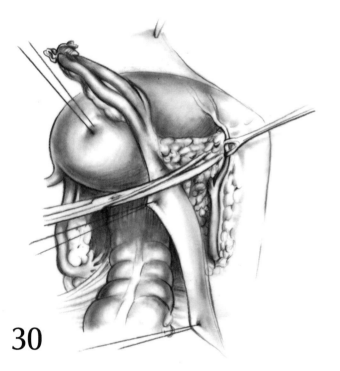

30

30 All of the branches of the hypogastric artery are dissected sharply and preserved.

31 The base of the bladder is dissected from the cervix by scissor or cautery dissection.

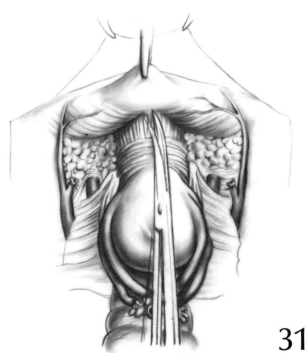

31

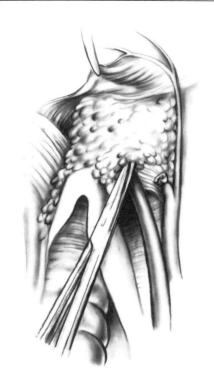

32

32 At this stage the most difficult and potentially dangerous part of the operation involves clearing away all of the tissue overlying the anterior and medial surfaces of both ureters. This is best performed using a right-angle clamp directly on the ureter and serial ligation and division of all vessels until the ureter is seen entering the base of the bladder.

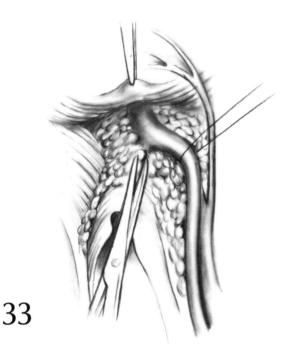

33

33 The entire medial portion of the ureter is now cleared. In order to minimize the risk of ischaemic damage to the ureter the lateral attachments which carry the blood supply should be left intact if at all possible.

34 The posterior and lateral dissection then proceeds as in an abdominoperineal resection. The lateral dissection is performed lateral to the endopelvic fascia.

The vagina and mid-rectum are then separated by sharp dissection, the vagina is divided and is either oversewn or stapled (using absorbable staples). The operation is completed with a formal perineal resection or with a sphincter-saving reconstruction of the distal rectum.

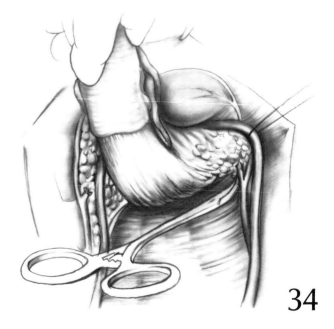

34

Postoperative care

During the immediate postoperative period hypothermia should be corrected and blood, fresh-frozen plasma and platelets given as necessary. If there are signs of continued major pelvic haemorrhage, re-exploration is recommended: if surgical control of bleeding is not possible because of refractory dilutional coagulopathy, the pelvis may be packed beneath pelvic mesh.

Viability of the urostomy and colostomy should be checked daily for the first few days. Ureteric catheters or a large indwelling catheter in the ileal conduit confirm the urinary output. Large amounts of colloid and crystalloid may be required for the first few days.

Complications

The development of a pelvic abscess is the most common major complication, which is not precluded by serous drainage from the pelvic drains. CT scanning with needle aspiration will aid detection of an abscess, and if it is confirmed radiological or surgical drainage is required.

Outcome

Pelvic exenteration

Reports from the Ellis Fischel State Cancer Center suggest that radical approach can be performed in selected patients with acceptable morbidity and mortality rates and 5-year survival in excess of 40%[2,3] (17 primary patients and seven recurrences were reported). In the node-negative patients, 5-year survival was 60%. A group from Hong Kong obtained similar results in 49 patients[4], with 5-year survival of 52% in node-negative cases, and 27% in node-positive. Ledesma and colleagues at Roswell Park reported their experience with 30 primary rectal patients undergoing total pelvic exenteration with a mortality rate of 10%[5]: eight of 17 node-negative patients were alive at 5 years, as were two of eight node-positive patients.

Abdominoperineal resection with in-continuity sacrectomy

This approach has been used on a few patients with primary rectal cancers[6,7], but the numbers are too small to discuss critically. The major experience with the radical extended operations for recurrent rectal cancer has been reported from three centres: Memorial Sloan–Kettering Cancer Center[8,9], University of Virginia[10,11] and the University of Colorado[7,12]. Wanebo and Marcove[8] first reported the integration of the technique of primary sacral resection through the posterior approach with transabdominal visceral exenteration. Of the seven patients who underwent potentially curative resection, recurrence was seen only in two. Wanebo subsequently increased his series to 24 patients, half of whom underwent complete pelvic exenteration. There were three postoperative deaths and five patients were alive over 4 years later[10,11]. Pearlman and associates have resected 21 patients with recurrent rectal cancer; all but three had prior radiation[7,12] and 12 underwent complete abdominosacral exenteration. Of the 16 patients who had potentially curative surgery, eight were free of recurrence with a follow-up of 6–48 months. All authors attest to the excellent pain control associated with these operations, presumably related to the surgically induced hypoaesthesia as well as the tumour control.

References

1. Moriya Y, Hojo K, Sawada T, Koyama Y. Significance of lateral node dissection for advanced rectal carcinoma at or below the peritoneal reflection. *Dis Colon Rectum* 1989; 32: 307–15.

2. Kraybill WG, Lopez MJ, Bricker EM. Total pelvic exenteration as a therapeutic option in advanced malignant disease of the pelvis. *Surg Gynecol Obstet* 1988; 166: 259–63.

3. Salhab N, Jones DJ, Bos JL, Kinsella A, Schofield PF. Detection of ras gene alterations and ras proteins in colorectal cancer. *Dis Colon Rectum* 1989; 32: 659–64.

4. Boey J, Cheung HC, Lai CK et al. A prospective evaluation of serum carcinoembryonic antigen levels in the management of colorectal carcinoma. *World J Surg* 1984; 8: 279–86.

5. Ledesma EJ, Bruno S, Mittelman A. Total pelvic exenteration in colorectal disease. *Ann Surg* 1981; 194: 701–3.

6. Sugarbaker PH. Partial sacrectomy for *en bloc* excision of rectal cancer with posterior fixation. *Dis Colon Rectum* 1982; 25: 708–11.

7. Pearlman NW, Stiegmann GV, Donohue RE. Extended resection of fixed rectal cancer. *Cancer* 1989; 63: 2438–41.

8. Wanebo HJ, Marcove RC. Abdominal sacral resection of locally recurrent rectal cancer. *Ann Surg* 1981; 194: 458–71.

9. Wanebo H. Resection of pelvic recurrence of rectal cancer. *Contemp Surg* 1982; 21: 21–33.

10. Wanebo HJ, Gaker DL, Whitehill R, Morgan RF, Constable WC. Pelvic recurrence of rectal cancer. *Ann Surg* 1987; 205: 482–95.

11. Wanebo HJ, Whitehill R, Gaker D, Wang GJ, Morgan R, Constable W. Composite pelvic resection. *Arch Surg* 1987; 122: 1401–6.

12. Pearlman NW, Donohue RE, Stiegmann GV et al. Pelvic and sacropelvic exenteration for locally advanced or recurrent anorectal cancer. *Arch Surg* 1987; 122: 537–41.

Extended operation with lateral pelvic dissection of lymph nodes in advanced low rectal cancer

Keiichi Hojo MD
Chief of Proctology, National Cancer Center, Tokyo and Professor of Surgery, Tokyo Medical University, Tokyo, Japan

Anthony M. Vernava III MD
Assistant Professor of Surgery, St Louis Medical University, St Louis, Missouri, USA

Principles and justification

The rationale for the extended pelvic lymphadenectomy for rectal cancer is to obtain a better chance for cure by performing a wider resection of perirectal tissues, particularly for advanced, low-lying rectal cancers[1].

There are two main paths of lymphatic drainage of the rectum: first, upward lymphatic drainage of the rectum occurs along the superior rectal vessels up to the origin of the inferior mesenteric artery; and second, lateral lymphatic drainage of the rectum occurs along the middle rectal artery in the lateral ligaments and then along the internal iliac vessels and the common iliac vessels up to the para-aortic lymph nodes[2].

A total of 265 patients with rectal cancer located below the lower edge of the second sacral segment underwent potentially curative surgery between 1979 and 1988 at the National Cancer Center Hospital in Tokyo, Japan. Of these patients 118 (44.5%) were found to have metastasis to regional lymph nodes. Seventy-two patients had metastases only to the pararectal lymph nodes, 16 had metastases to upward lymph nodes and 16 had metastases to lateral lymph nodes, including two with positive para-aortic nodes. In addition, 14 patients had metastases to both lateral and upward lymph nodes.

Metastasis to the lateral lymph nodes therefore occurred in 30 (11.3%) patients. The rate of metastasis to the lateral lymph nodes increases in patients with

tumours located below the peritoneal reflection (14%) and when the carcinoma has penetrated through the bowel wall (20%)[2]. The most common site of positive lateral nodes is near the root of the middle rectal artery. The next most common site of positive lateral nodes is along the internal iliac vessels and then along the obturator vessels. Residual disease in these lateral lymph nodes would result in locally recurrent disease if an extended lymphadenectomy was not performed. The overall 5-year survival rate in these 265 patients was 73.9% (stage I, 86.6%; stage II, 78.3%; and stage III, 51.6%). Survival appears to be improved for patients with either stage II or III disease who undergo extended pelvic lymphadenectomy.

Although the extended abdominoiliopelvic lymphadenectomy has reduced the incidence of locoregional failure and improved survival for patients with advanced stage rectal cancer, the operation is associated with an increased incidence of urinary and sexual dysfunction[3,4]. However, selective sparing of the fourth sacral parasympathetic nerve in patients with stage II and III rectal cancer during the extended pelvic lymphadenectomy preserves both urine voiding function and the survival benefit from the extended operation[3,4]. Unfortunately, sexual function is not preserved unless the entire autonomic pelvic plexus is preserved.

Preoperative

Preoperative examination of the patient is directed at accurately determining the stage of the tumour. Digital rectal examination, barium enema, colonoscopy, computed tomography scan (abdomen and pelvis) and transrectal ultrasonographic examination should be performed in an attempt to stage these patients before operation. Patients with suspected stage II (tumour penetration through the bowel wall) and stage III (tumour metastasis to regional lymph nodes) disease from either preoperative or intraoperative findings are candidates for the extended operation with lateral pelvic lymph node dissection[1, 3, 4].

Operation

1 A long midline incision is made from the pubic symphysis and carried beyond the umbilicus for 6–7 cm. The incision is extended along the right side of the umbilicus to avoid future left lower quadrant colostomy. An abdominal exploration and intraoperative clinical staging of the carcinoma is then performed (the liver is manually and visually examined, the peritoneal surface is examined for any evidence of metastases and the mesentery of the small and large intestine is inspected for any lymphadenopathy). Great care is employed when checking for the existence of lymphadenopathy or lymphatic spread to decide whether or not the patient requires an extended lymphatic dissection.

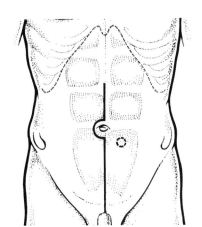

1

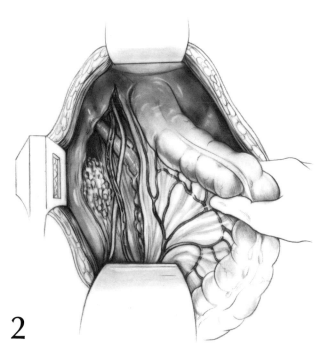

2

2 Mobilization of the sigmoid colon and the mesosigmoid from the retroperitoneum is performed. The colon is lifted out of the abdominal cavity and the left ureter and the testicular (or ovarian) vessels are identified through the thin parietal peritoneum or subperitoneal fascia. The parietal peritoneum is then incised along the medial border of the left ureter, which is dissected cephalad up to the inferior border of the left renal vein: this line constitutes the left border of the para-aortic dissection. The origin of the left psoas major muscle is exposed. The para-aortic fatty connective tissue and lymphatics will be completely resected later.

3 The sigmoid colon is now retracted to the left side, exposing the right side of the retroperitoneum. The right ureter is identified and the retroperitoneum is incised along the medial side of the right ureter, establishing the right border of the para-aortic dissection. The ureter is then retracted laterally and the origin of the right psoas major is exposed. The paracaval tissue is dissected caudad to the common iliac vessels. Finally, the connective and lymphatic tissue surrounding the aorta and the vena cava is dissected caudad from the inferior border of the duodenum. (The dissection completely denudes the vena cava and the right half of the aorta.)

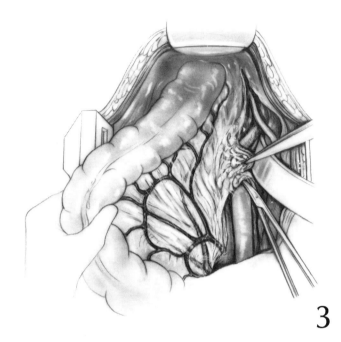

3

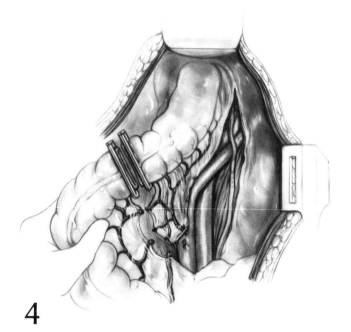

4

4 The sigmoid colon is retracted to the left by the assistant surgeon and the mesosigmoid is placed under slight tension. The sigmoid colon and the mesosigmoid are then divided and the left colic and sigmoid vessels transected. The line of transection is extended proximally to the aorta and the inferior mesenteric vein is divided. In this manner, the dissection is made continuous with the right para-aortic dissection.

The left para-aortic dissection begins at the inferior border of the third portion of the duodenum and is extended caudad to the aortic bifurcation. The inferior mesenteric artery is identified and divided at its junction with the aorta.

5 Dissection of the lymphatic tissues surrounding the aortic bifurcation and the common iliac vessels is performed using small Metzenbaum scissors or with fine cautery.

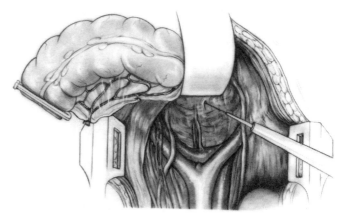

5

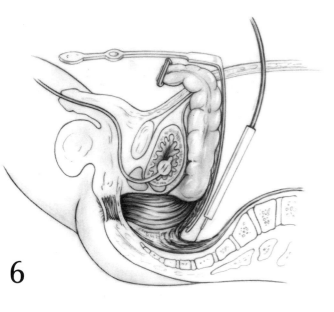

6

6 The rectum is dissected from the presacral fascia from the sacral promontory to below the tip of the coccyx. An electrocautery is employed for the dissection. A retractor is also placed into the retrorectal space to facilitate the dissection by retracting the rectum anteriorly and placing the loose areolar tissue under tension. The proper plane of dissection between the presacral fascia and the mesorectum is bloodless and is usually easily identified. A careful combination of electrocautery dissection and retraction of the rectum anteriorly facilitates complete removal of the mesorectum.

7 After the posterior dissection is completed, the dissection is extended laterally into the pararectal space; scissors are employed for this portion of the dissection to avoid electrical injury to the pelvic autonomic nerves. Great care is taken to identify visually and spare each of the pelvic autonomic nerves.

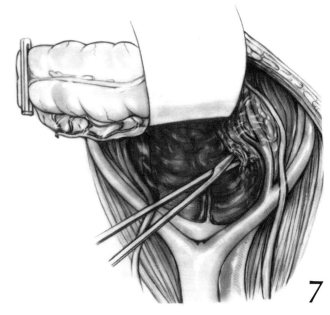

8 After both posterior and pararectal dissections have been completed, an incision is made in the peritoneum anteriorly about 1–2 cm above the peritoneal reflexion. The anterior peritoneal dissection remains outside Denonvilliers' fascia.

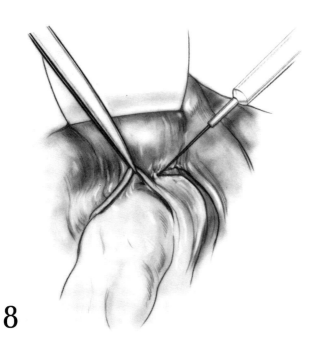

9 The incised peritoneum overlying the rectum is retracted anteriorly and the seminal vesicles are visualized. Dissection is continued in this plane distally as far as possible, usually to just under the posterior surface of the prostate.

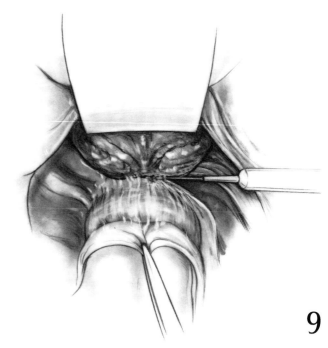

10 The right ureter is retracted anterolaterally with a pair of forceps. The major psoas muscle and external iliac vessels are exposed, and the surrounding fatty connective tissue is resected.

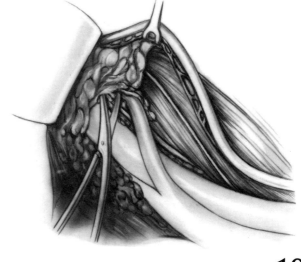

10

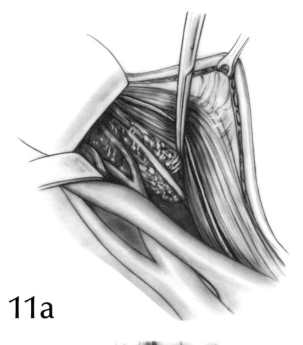

11a

11a, b A small but wide retractor is inserted between the exposed psoas muscle and the external iliac vessels. The iliolumbar space is then opened and dissected free of any lymphatic tissue. During the dissection the obturator nerve and the iliolumbar vessels are identified.

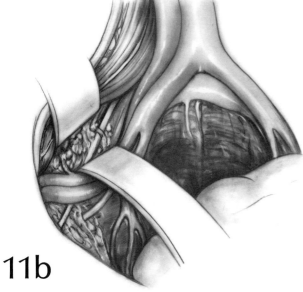

11b

12 The external iliac vessels are then retracted laterally by placing a small retractor in the obturator space between the external and internal iliac vessels. As dissection proceeds laterally the space is further exposed by progressively greater anterolateral retraction. The lymphatics, nodes and fatty connective tissue within the obturator space are then resected with scissors, being careful to avoid injury to the obturator artery and vein.

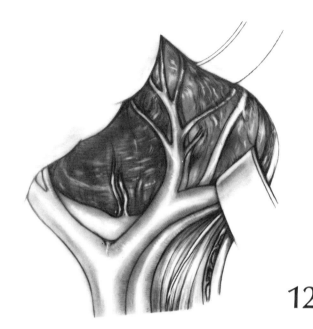

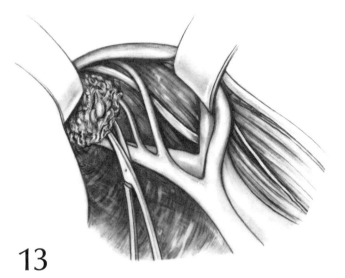

13 After complete dissection of the obturator space, the internal iliac vessels, the superior vesical artery, the obturator vessels and the superior gluteal vessels are exposed, and the connective tissue and lymphatics surrounding these vessels are resected. The superior vesical vein is ligated where it crosses the internal iliac artery.

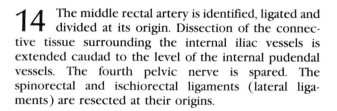

14 The middle rectal artery is identified, ligated and divided at its origin. Dissection of the connective tissue surrounding the internal iliac vessels is extended caudad to the level of the internal pudendal vessels. The fourth pelvic nerve is spared. The spinorectal and ischiorectal ligaments (lateral ligaments) are resected at their origins.

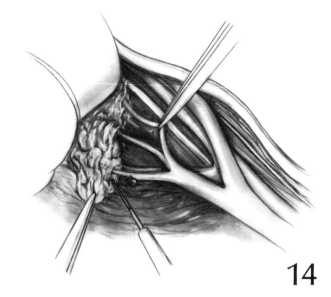

15 The completed right pelvic wall dissection showing the denuded internal iliac vessels, the cut end of the middle rectal artery, the selectively spared fourth pelvic autonomic nerve and the piriformis muscle is visualized.

The remainder of the operation, either low anterior resection (*see* chapter on pp. 456–471) or abdominoperineal excision (*see* chapter on pp. 472–487) is completed. Postoperative care and follow-up are as described in these chapters.

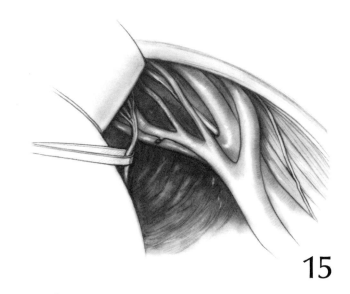

15

References

1. Hojo K, Koyama Y. The effectiveness of wide anatomical resection and radical lymphadenectomy of patients with rectal cancer. *Jpn J Surg* 1982; 12: 111–16.

2. Hojo K, Koyama Y, Moriya Y. Lymphatic spread and its prognostic value in patients with rectal cancer. *Am J Surg* 1982; 144: 350–4.

3. Hojo K, Sawada T, Moriya Y. An analysis of survival and voiding, sexual function after wide iliopelvic lymphadenectomy in patients with carcinoma of the rectum, compared with conventional lymphadenectomy. *Dis Colon Rectum* 1989; 32: 128–33.

4. Hojo K, Vernava AM, Sugihara K, Katumata K. Preservation of urine-voiding and sexual function after rectal cancer surgery. *Dis Colon Rectum* 1991; 34: 532–9.

Illustrations by Denise Smith

Posterior approach to the rectum (parasacral technique)

Takashi Takahashi MD
Chief, Surgical Department, Tokyo Metropolitan Komagome Hospital, Tokyo, Japan

History

Early in the history of surgical treatment for rectal cancer, the main subject of discussion concerned the best approach to the tumour site, particularly for lesions high in the rectum. Two distinct methods were proposed. Kraske originated what is known today as the 'posterior approach' or the 'sacral approach', because the lower part of the sacral bones was excised to gain access to the middle and upper rectum from the posterior aspect. Another approach, known as the 'perineal approach', was developed by Quenu, who incised the anus anteriorly or posteriorly, or on occasion in both directions, to dilate the anus and thus improve access to the lower and middle rectum.

At that time, lymph node dissection as part of 'curative' cancer surgery was not considered necessary. Surgeons were busy developing methods of approaching tumours higher in the rectum. Moreover, surgical pathology, which today plays an important role in deciding on optimum treatment, was still an underdeveloped field.

In 1908, Miles introduced lymph node dissection with his new approach of synchronous total rectal excision, from both the abdominal and perineal aspects. He insisted on the importance of lymph node dissection to help 'cure' these cancer patients and reported better patient survival. The Miles' operation was thought to be the only method of 'radical cure' for rectal cancer, until Dixon in 1939 proposed the possibility of saving the distal rectum and anus in radical surgery for rectal cancer. Thus, today, two distinct and standard methods of radical surgery for rectal cancer are available:

abdominoperineal excision and anterior resection of the rectum which preserves the anal sphincters.

About 20 years ago, the two classical methods of approach to the rectum from a posterior aspect (Kraske's posterior approach and Quenu's perineal approach) were revived in an attempt to reduce the numbers of patients requiring abdominoperineal excision of the rectum, but maintaining the general concepts of a radical procedure for rectal cancer.

Bevan, Mason and Localio revived Kraske's idea and modified it as posterior midline, parasacral transsphincteric and posterior transverse approaches, respectively. Parks restored Quenu's idea and devised the transanal approach, and the method of coloanal anastomosis was developed, which avoided division of the anal sphincter.

These revived methods of approach to the rectum usually have two advantages. They give easier access to small lesions that can be excised locally, and they allow direct vision of an anastomotic site closer to the anal canal during a sphincter-preserving operation. The frequency with which these procedures are now used has diminished; however, the accumulation of pathological knowledge about the spread of cancer (particularly the downward spread of rectal cancer) and the development of new surgical techniques for very low anastomoses using both staples and sutures has greatly increased the use of sphincter-preserving operations. Nevertheless, the posterior approach is indicated occasionally. In this chapter, the technical details of this parasacral approach will be described.

Principles and justification

Indications

Small lesions compatible with local excision

Mucosal lesions, e.g. adenoma, adenocarcinoma and villous tumour, of any size in circumference or on the longitudinal axis are suitable. The upper limit of the tumour, however, must not be more than 12 cm above the dentate line.

Submucosal lesions, e.g. adenocarcinoma, carcinoid, villous tumour and lymphoid polyp, are also suitable provided that there is no chance of lymph node metastasis. This assumption indicates that no more than superficial invasion of cancer cells into the submucosa has taken place, and therefore the lesion must be small and clinically completely mobile.

A lesion that penetrates more deeply into the muscle proper is not suitable for this technique because of the fear of nodal involvement. Local excision of these lesions is indicated only in high-risk patients as a palliative procedure.

Small lesions for excisional biopsy

Local excision is indicated as a means of total biopsy for carcinoma or adenocarcinoma in a broad base polyp with suspicion of submucosal invasion.

Planned anastomosis close to the anal canal

Direct vision for an anastomosis within about 1 cm above the upper limit of the anal canal can be achieved by this method. With increasing experience of very low rectal mobilization from above, however, this indication for a parasacral approach is now seldom needed (described in the chapter on pp. 456–471).

Operations

Position of patient

1 The patient is placed in a prone jack-knife position with the legs apart (described in chapter on pp. 47–50). Two wide tapes are attached to the buttocks on both sides sufficiently lateral not to interfere with the site of the planned skin incision. These tapes are pulled laterally in order to widen and flatten the parasacral area.

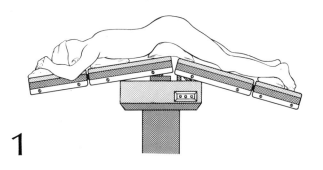

1

Incision

2 Parasacral, transverse and vertical incisions on the posterior perineum over the lower part of the sacrum are the alternatives. The parasacral incision on one side of the sacral bone is often used because of the possibility of modifying its length according to the location and the size of the tumour. When the parasacral approach is extended downwards, the anal sphincter muscles can be divided. This is called the transsphincteric operation and was originated by Mason. It can be extended upwards to incise the lower part of the gluteus major muscle to obtain wider exposure.

The transverse incision, originated by Localio for easier and more direct access to an anastomotic site near the anal canal, can be used for local excision of small lesions located in the lower rectum. The vertical incision, originated by Bevan, is now seldom used in preference to the parasacral approach.

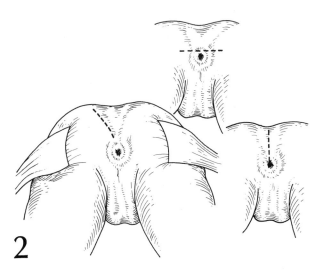

2

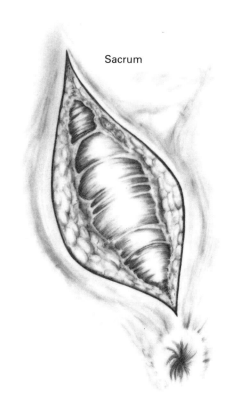

Sacrum

3

Access to the rectum

3 As the subcutaneous fat is divided, the ischiorectal space is entered. The lower border of the gluteal muscle is located in the upper limit of the incision, and the puborectalis muscle bundle and the external sphincter muscle complex are located at the lower limit of the incision.

The incision into the ischiorectal space is placed a little lateral to the anococcygeal raphe in the midline, which extends vertically from the tip of the coccyx to the posterior aspect of the puborectalis muscle. The anococcygeal raphe may need to be divided to expose the posterior circumference of the levator ani muscles.

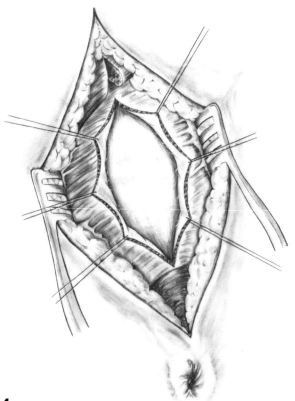

4

4 The levator ani muscles are composed of thin fascicles arranged in an oblique direction; these are too soft and loose to place stay sutures to mark the incision line. Thus, it is recommended that stay sutures are placed into both the levator ani muscles together with the underlying fascia (the parietal endopelvic fascia), which is rather thick and firm. Occasionally, in the lower rectum, a thick adhesion between the two leaves of the fascia (Waldeyer's fascia) may be encountered.

Incision of the muscles is made in the same direction as the skin incision, which will protect nerves and vessels running towards the anal sphincter. The internal pudendal artery, vein and nerve take a descending course in Alcock's canal, which is located laterally to the levator ani muscles (*see Illustration 8*).

5 Under the levator ani muscle and fascia, another firm tissue layer called the visceral endopelvic fascia envelops the complete circumference of the rectum. On this fascia, often called 'proper rectal fascia', a finger can be passed almost around the entire circumference of the rectum, except in the lower part of the rectum near the anal canal where the two leaves of tissue are adherent as Waldeyer's fascia and anteriorly where Denonvilliers' fascia adheres to the prostate or the posterior vaginal wall.

After placing several stay sutures at the cut edge on both sides, the visceral endopelvic fascia is incised. Perirectal fat containing the peripheral part of the superior rectal vessels appears in the wound. Before exposing the appropriate extent of the rectal wall, several vessels must be tied. The fatty tissues must be removed from the posterior rectal wall with coagulation of the small vessels that penetrate the rectal wall.

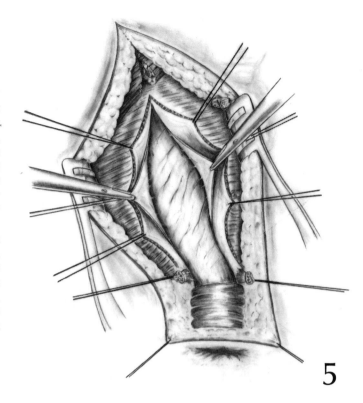

5

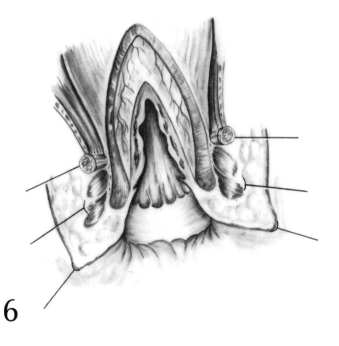

6

6 When the incision in the levator ani muscles is extended downwards, the puborectalis muscle bundles and the main part of the external sphincter muscle complex are easily divided. These muscles are situated in the same plane as the general architecture of the perirectal tissues. Stay sutures must be placed on both cut edges of the muscle bundles. The endopelvic fascia appears thick and firm as it is incised and adheres to the outer layer of the muscle coat of the lower rectum. This layer is often called Waldeyer's fascia or the rectosacral ligament, and it forms a whitish fibrotic coat of tissue. Because it is not possible to separate this layer from the inner sphincter muscle, the fascia and muscle are incised as one layer.

7 Under the muscle the submucosa of the anal canal appears, sometimes with a varix-like appearance of the venous plexus which requires several ligatures before incising the submucosa and mucosa.

The whole thickness of the inner sphincter muscle is penetrated by fine fibrotic bundles, which are thread-like extensions of the outer muscle coat of the rectum. Because they may reach the submucosal layer in this site, it is easy to split the inner muscle and submucosa as one layer instead of separating them.

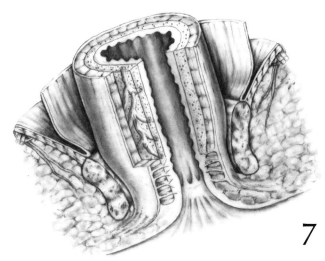

7

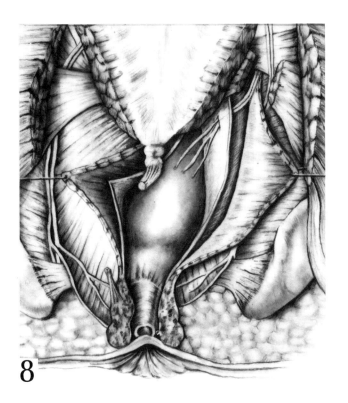

8

8 Alcock's canal, which contains the vessels and nerves, comes closer to the anal canal as it descends and separates the inferior rectal artery and vein and nerve fibres travelling towards the anal sphincter. To prevent damage to these vessels and nerves, the incision line in the anal canal should be kept very near the posterior midline.

9 From the lateral sides of the sacral bones, the gluteal muscles extend laterally and downwards. They limit the upper border of the ischiorectal space. In the prone position, the ischiorectal space lies under the gluteal muscles. Thus, by incising the rather thick bundles of the gluteal muscle along the lateral border of the sacral bones, the real upper limit of the ischiorectal fatty tissue can be opened. The upper limit of the levator ani muscles is also located at the same level. Thus, the incision of the levator ani muscle can be extended a little further upwards where the initial part of Alcock's canal is located close to the sacrotuberous ligament, which is the upper limit of the levator ani muscles (*see Illustration 8*). At this point, the coccyx can be removed to widen the operative field laterally. After peeling off parts of the levator ani muscles from the coccyx, the bone is easily dislocated and removed. A retractor can then open the wound a little more widely.

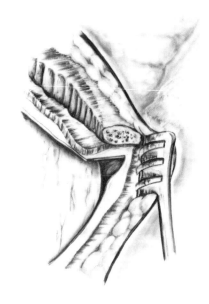

9

10 The lower rectum can easily be isolated by a finger on its posterior aspect, as it is enveloped by the visceral endopelvic fascia (arrow B). Isolation within the fascia can be achieved (arrow A) but with a little difficulty. Laterally, at the level of the mid-rectum, the lateral ligament, the middle rectal artery and vein and pelvic nerves fuse to the fascia and the rectal wall. Further mobilization requires sharp dissection of the ligament from this point.

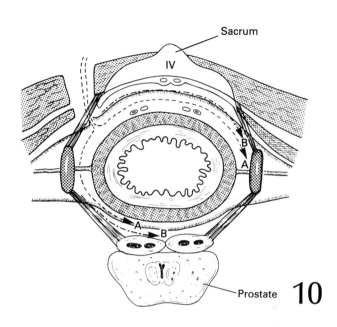

11 By incising the endopelvic fascia sharply with scissors, the middle of the ligament is entered, which leaves the pelvic nerve plexus behind. The dissection then moves to the anterior aspect and reaches the slit-like space under Denonvilliers' fascia.

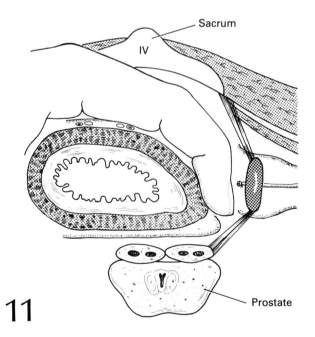

12 When the lateral ligaments on both sides are divided, the isolation of the mid-rectum is completed. A string or a finger can pass around the whole circumference of the rectal tube.

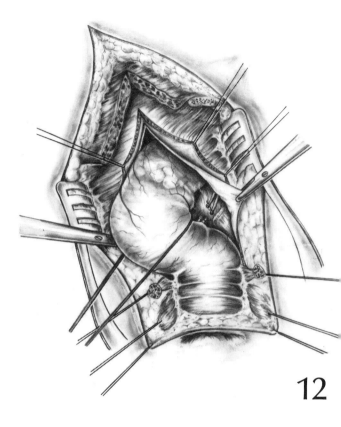

12

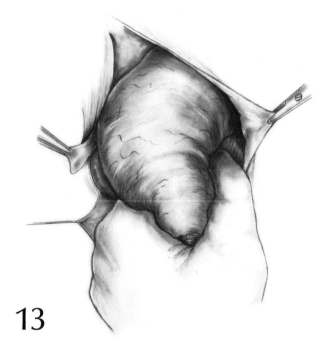

13

13 On the anterior side, in most cases, Denonvilliers' fascia is separated from the rectal wall and is left *in situ*. Sometimes it is necessary to excise this fascia to obtain clear tumour margins (*see* arrow B in *Illustration 10*). In this situation, the nerve supply to the urinary bladder is in danger because of the presence of adhesions between these nerves and Denonvilliers' fascia, and injury to the nerve must be avoided.

LOCAL EXCISION OF A LESION ON THE ANTERIOR WALL

14 The rectum is usually incised in a longitudinal direction. The rectal muscle layers (a thin but firm outer layer and a thick but softer inner layer) are incised as a single layer, guided by traction sutures placed on the incision line in a parallel row.

New stay (fixing) sutures, taking bites of the muscle and submucosa, will prevent the submucosal layer from slipping out of the line of the incision. A properly applied retractor gives wide and direct vision of the inside of the rectum. The mucosal lesion on the anterior side of the rectum can be easily detected and excised with a safe margin around it. Incision of the submucosal layer requires meticulous haemostasis using coagulation or ties; otherwise, bleeding obscures the correct line of the mucosal incision. Stay sutures and ties are placed along the incision line in paired fashion on both cut edges to prevent bleeding and to indicate the correct line for the incision and its later repair.

A full-thickness excision is recommended when submucosal invasion is suspected. Under direct vision, the anterior wall of the rectum is incised in the same way as for the mucosal lesion, but deeply enough to remove the whole thickness of the muscle layer.

To ensure that the muscle layer has been completely incised, the smooth sheet-like extension of Denonvilliers' fascia under the excisional area can be observed. The defect of muscle and mucosal layer is closed by approximating the cut edges horizontally by a Gambee-type one-layer suture.

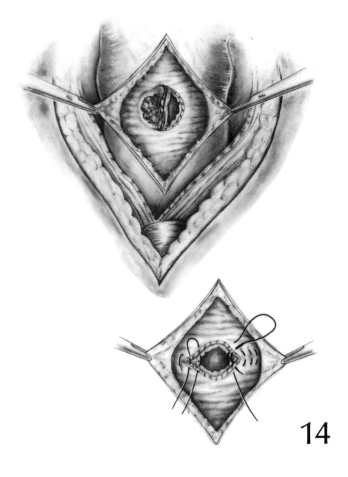

14

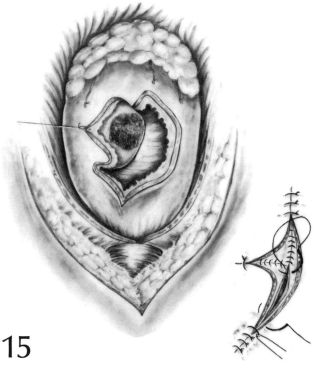

15

LOCAL EXCISION OF A LESION ON THE POSTERIOR WALL

15 For posterior lesions, the initial incision line in the rectal wall can be arranged as part of the line of tumour excision. In this case, perirectal fat tissues adjacent to the site of the tumour should be excised together with the rectal wall. The specimen may contain several lymph nodes. Digital examination through the anus may be necessary to ascertain the correct location of the tumour. Closure of the defect is made part of closure of the rectal wall using a two-layer suture technique.

TUBE RESECTION (SEGMENTAL RESECTION) OF THE LOWER RECTUM

16 For a large mucosal lesion with a circumferential extension and/or possible invasion into the submucosal layer, a segmental resection of the lower rectum can be planned.

As the first step, circumferential isolation of the lower rectum is carried out as already described. Instead of incising the fascia and the rectal wall vertically, however, a horizontal incision is made at a level a little distal to the lower border of the tumour. The location of the tumour should be accurately assessed by digital examination through the intact anus.

Before completing the circular incision, at least four stay sutures should be placed through the whole thickness of the distal cut edge of the rectum, at the anterior, posterior and both lateral sites.

At the estimated proximal incision line, the endopelvic fascia is incised, and fat tissues under it are peeled from the rectal wall. The muscle coat and mucosa are incised in the same way as the distal incision. More than four stay sutures will be required to identify the proximal cut edge of the intestine.

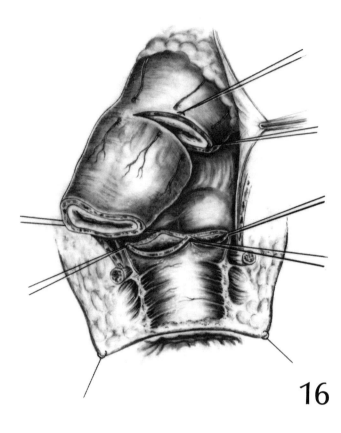

16

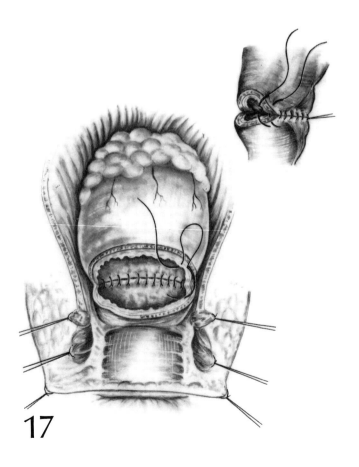

17 The intestinal wall is approximated at both lateral corners. By pulling up the sutures on one side, the anterior aspect of the cut edges of the intestinal wall come into direct vision and are sutured. After the muscle layer has been sutured anteriorly, the inner layers (mucosa and submucosa) are approximated from the inside. This process continues on the posterior aspect until the inner layer of sutures is completed using interrupted absorbable material. Finally, the outer layer of the posterior aspect is sutured.

17

ANASTOMOSIS AS THE FINAL STAGE OF A LOW ANTERIOR RESECTION

As a result of improvements in surgical techniques (mainly the development of stapling instruments), anastomosis very low in the pelvis has become a popular and reasonably secure technique. Even at the lowest level (approximately 2 cm above the anal canal), once the purse-string suture instrument has been applied or a stapling instrument has closed the distal rectal stump, a stapled anastomosis will be possible without the use of a posterior perineal incision. When the distal resection line of the rectum is only about 1 cm or less above the anal canal, however, it may be impossible to fashion an anastomosis at this level (particularly in the narrow pelvis of male patients) without the added assistance of a posterior approach. In almost all cases of very low anterior resections, dissection around the rectum and division of the proximal intestine have already been completed in the abdominal phase of the operation.

In some cases, it may be easier to divide the rectum during the abdominal phase of the operation, and then complete an anastomosis under direct vision with the use of a parasacral approach as described for a segmental rectal resection. Before changing the position of the patient, however, the intra-abdominal portion of the surgery should be completed and the abdominal wound closed.

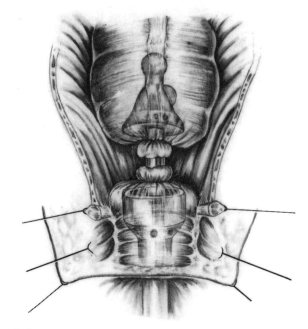

18 It is important to wash out the distal rectum through the anus before the lower rectum is isolated and divided as already described. The distal cut edge of the lower rectum remains without a clamp because this would interfere with fashioning of the anastomosis.

The stapling instrument is inserted through the anus. Both cut ends can be fixed to the shaft and the anvil. Approximation of the intestinal wall and stapling are conducted under direct vision. A hand-sewn anastomosis is sometimes more convenient. A two-layer technique is used as for a segmental resection.

18

Wound closure and drainage

19 After the rectal wall has been sutured or the anastomosis has been completed (being careful not to spill intestinal contents), the whole area is washed with warm normal saline. The wound is closed in layers, making certain that the layers are approximated very accurately, guided by the stay sutures previously placed. A thin, soft drainage tube is inserted through a separate stab wound near the incision line, down into the perirectal space or to the level of the levator ani muscle. The drainage tube will be removed within 4–5 days. In stout and obese patients, a thin Penrose drain is inserted into the ischiorectal space through the incision and removed once serosanguineous drainage ceases at about 48 h.

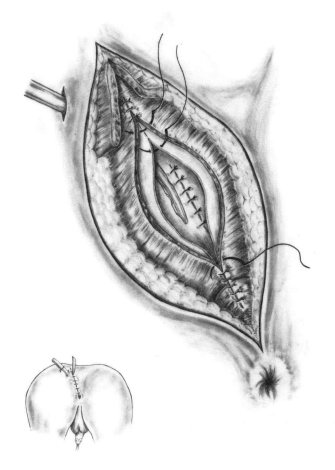

19

Illustrations by Angela Christie

Anorectal injury

Daniel P. Otchy MD, FACS
Assistant Chief, General Surgery Service, Brooke Army Medical Center, and Assistant Professor of Surgery, Uniformed Services University of the Health Sciences, San Antonio, Texas, USA

Daniel Rosenthal MD, FACS
Surgical Consultant, Brooke Army Medical Center, and Clinical Professor of Surgery, Uniformed Services University of the Health Sciences, San Antonio, Texas, USA

Rectal injuries

Principles

Of all patients undergoing laparotomy for abdominal trauma, only 1% will be found to have a rectal injury. Of these injuries, 95% are due to penetrating trauma. The severe consequences of an overlooked injury require that a rectal injury be suspected when the trajectory of a missile crosses the pelvis. Stab and gunshot wounds to the buttocks, perineum and upper thigh may injure the rectum.

Rectal injuries caused by blunt trauma are exceedingly rare: only five cases were seen in a busy US trauma centre over a 10-year period[1]. These injuries are invariably seen in conjunction with deep perineal lacerations and major pelvic fractures. There is often extensive perineal soft tissue damage, urological injury and significant pelvic haemorrhage associated with these rectal tears.

The opinions or assertions contained herein are the private views of the authors and are not to be construed as reflecting the views of the Department of the Army or the Department of Defense.

Preoperative

Preoperative rigid proctoscope examination is mandatory in all patients in whom a rectal injury is suspected because injury to the extraperitoneal portion of the rectum can easily be overlooked during laparotomy for abdominal trauma. Similarly, the pelvic haematoma created by a severe pelvic fracture can obscure the presence of a rectal laceration. Unless the injury is detected proctoscopically, adequate treatment may be delayed, leading to severe pelvic sepsis.

All patients with suspected rectal injury must be assessed and treated for concomitant injuries to other organ systems. These patients should be evaluated and treated according to a resuscitation protocol, an example of which is found in the American College of Surgeons' *Advanced Trauma Life Support Program*[2]. The patient is resuscitated with intravenous crystalloid through large-bore intravenous catheters. A nasogastric tube and a Foley catheter are inserted whenever their use is not contraindicated. As soon after injury as possible, the patient should receive tetanus prophylaxis and an intravenous antibiotic to cover both aerobic and anaerobic enteric bacteria.

Operation

Position of patient

When rectal injury is suspected in a patient with abdominal trauma, the patient should be placed in the Trendelenburg lithotomy position, using leg supports (*see Illustration 3* on page 48). Before opening the abdomen, rigid proctosigmoidoscopy is performed. If blood is seen in the rectal lumen, the site of injury is determined and, if found, its distance from the pectinate line noted. If no definite injury is identified but bleeding from the rectum persists, the site should be treated as if a transmural lesion is present.

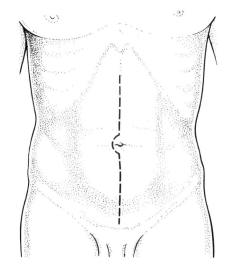

Incision

1 In the majority of cases, a midline laparotomy incision is required to determine the presence or absence of other intra-abdominal injuries. A vertical incision is preferred in trauma cases because of the speed with which it can be made and closed, and the extensive exposure it allows to the rest of the abdomen. In addition, ample areas are available laterally for the construction of stomas.

Rarely, under some circumstances of extraperitoneal rectal injury, the surgeon is confident that no intra-abdominal injury is present. In this case, midline incision can be avoided. The required sigmoid colostomy and distal rectal washing can be accomplished through a properly positioned left lower quadrant incision.

INTRAPERITONEAL RECTAL INJURIES

2, 3 Injuries to the intraperitoneal portion of the rectum are largely managed as colon injuries. Simple lacerations operated upon soon after injury which are not associated with significant pelvic haematoma, major faecal spillage or multiple concomitant organ injuries, can be closed primarily. Neither drain nor diverting colostomy is required in this situation.

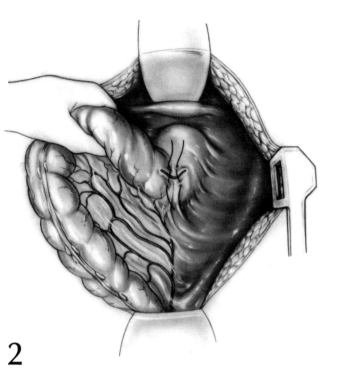

2

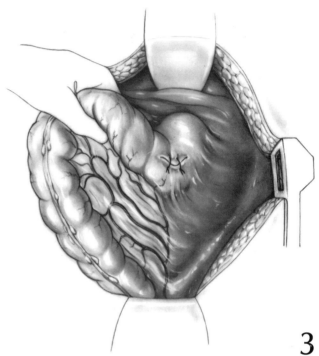

3

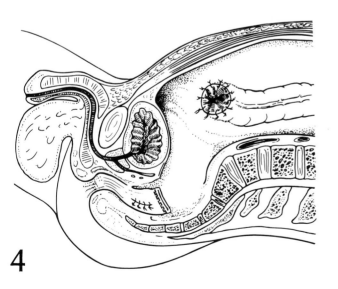

4

4 When the above conditions are not met, the laceration should be repaired and a diverting sigmoid colostomy and distal rectal washing, as described for extraperitoneal rectal injuries, should be performed.

If repair of the laceration is not safe because of its size or the status of the adjacent bowel, resection of the injured segment, stapling of the distal rectum and creation of an end sigmoid colostomy (Hartmann's procedure) should be performed (*see* chapter on pp. 488–496).

EXTRAPERITONEAL RECTAL INJURIES

Exposure and repair

5 Extraperitoneal rectal lacerations are often difficult to locate and expose adequately because of their position deep within the pelvis. Also, the mesorectum is often the site of annoying bleeding which obstructs the view while searching for a tear in that area. Exposure of the extraperitoneal portion of the rectum is obtained by incising the peritoneum lateral to the rectum on each side. The rectosigmoid is lifted forward and the ureters are visualized. The retrorectal space is developed by finger dissection, thereby exposing the posterior circumference of the rectum. In cases of gunshot wounds, single perforations are unusual. Once found, the laceration is closed using interrupted 3/0 Lembert sutures.

More often than not, attempts to expose an injury in the distal rectum are futile and may lead to excessive bleeding. Any attempt to expose rectal injury in the presence of a large pelvic haematoma is contraindicated. In most extraperitoneal injuries treatment relies upon total faecal diversion, cleansing of the distal rectum, drainage and intravenous antibiotics.

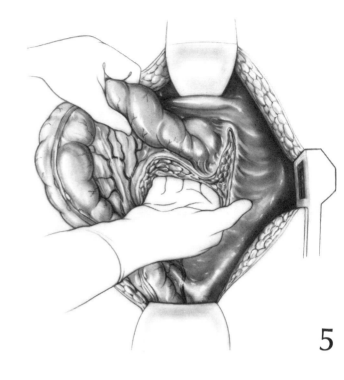

5

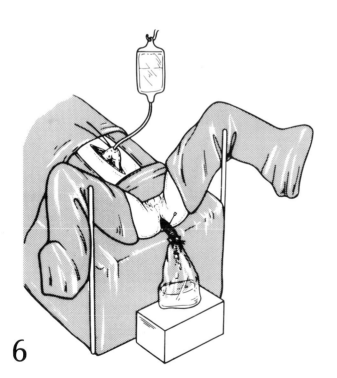

6

Rectal irrigation

6 A large-bore catheter is inserted through a colotomy made in the distal sigmoid colon. A purse-string suture is used to snug the bowel around the catheter. The catheter is connected to a bag of warm sterile saline which is flushed distally. The anus is then dilated and any scybalous faecal material extracted. To allow for the removal of the effluent, a piece of corrugated tube such as that used by anaesthetists on their ventilators is inserted and held inside the anus. A large-bore needle is inserted into the tubing to vent the system and prevent collapse of the bowel. The rectum is then irrigated until the effluent is clear.

Presacral drainage

7, 8 Drainage of the perirectal space is best performed through the perineum through a transverse incision made just posterior to the anal sphincters. The anococcygeal ligament is cut and the presacral space entered. Soft rubber or suction drains can be used.

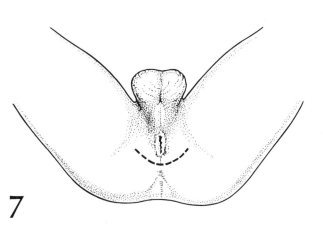

7

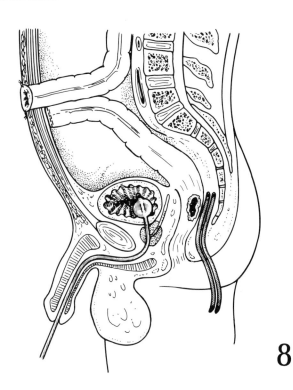

8

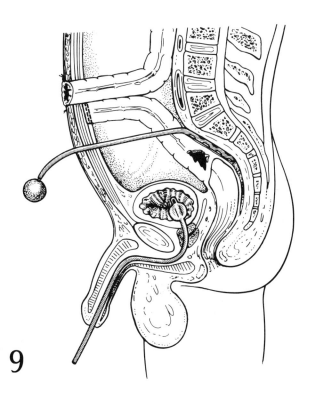

9

9 Retroperitoneal injuries of the rectum, especially those in the upper portion of the organ, can be drained transperitoneally. These are brought out during laparotomy through separate stab incisions in the lower abdomen.

Sigmoid colostomy

10 A completely diverting sigmoid colostomy is mandatory in all patients with an extraperitoneal rectal injury. Since an optimal stoma site is seldom, if ever, marked before operation, selection of a proper spot on the abdomen is a challenge to the surgeon. The stoma site should have 2 inches of intact skin surrounding it and be located over the rectus muscle. In obese patients, placing the stoma too low in the left lower quadrant may result in it being positioned below the patient's abdominal pannus. To avoid this, it is best to err on the side of positioning the stoma somewhat higher, at or above the level of the umbilicus.

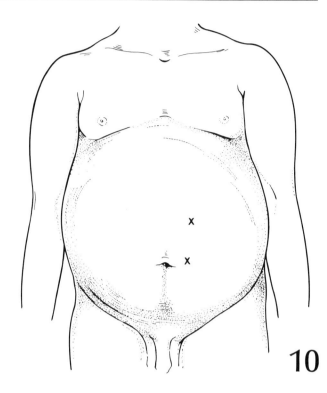

10

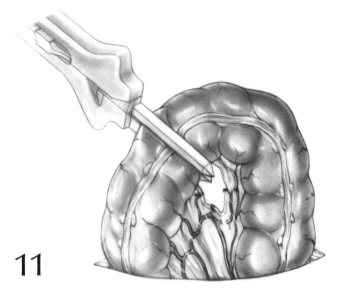

11

11–13 The sigmoid loop is brought without tension through a separate incision, and a short segment of the adjacent mesentery is divided and ligated. The sigmoid loop is transected using a linear stapler. The afferent limb is positioned to extend beyond the efferent limb by a few centimetres. The two limbs of the divided sigmoid are held together by a stitch. After positioning the efferent limb in the subcutaneous tissue, the staple line on the afferent limb is excised and the bowel edges sutured to the skin.

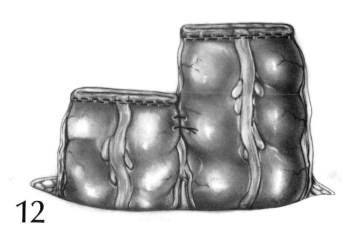

12

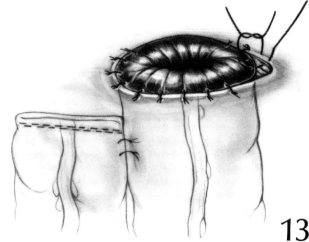

13

Control of rectal and pelvic haemorrhage

14 Occasionally a rectal injury is associated with extensive bleeding. Suture ligation of the damaged vessels is frequently impossible. It is not necessary to resort to heroic solutions such as rectal excision, or ligation of the superior rectal or the internal iliac artery. An expedient way to control such bleeding is to pack the rectum through the anus with gauze. These packs should be removed in the operating room in 48–72 h.

If intrarectal packing does not control bleeding in cases of arterial injuries or major pelvic fractures, a pelvic arteriogram is indicated. Injured arteries identified as the source of bleeding can then be embolized. When an unstable pelvic fracture is present, the application of an external pelvic fixator can help to stop the bleeding. In cases of such extensive blood loss, great care must be paid to replacing essential blood components to prevent or correct coagulopathies.

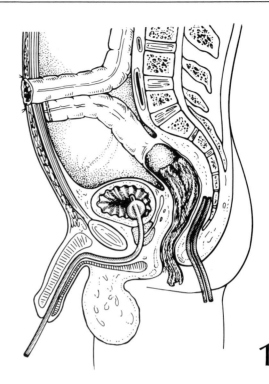

14

Closure of incision

The midline abdominal wound is closed in a single layer using monofilament suture. Because of contamination associated with rectal injuries, the subcutaneous tissue and skin should be left open. A delayed closure can be performed at about 5 days if conditions permit.

Postoperative care

Depending upon the severity of the intra-abdominal and associated injuries the patient is usually initially admitted to the intensive care unit. The prime determinant of survival will be the number and severity of concomitant injuries.

The patient is maintained on nasogastric suction until gastrointestinal function returns as manifested by the passage of flatus and the return of bowel sounds. How long the indwelling urinary catheter should remain in place is determined by the patient's general condition and the presence or absence of associated injuries. In many cases it can be removed by the third postoperative day. However, in the presence of a lower urinary tract injury or a severe pelvic fracture and haematoma, prolonged intubation of the urinary bladder may be warranted.

If soft rubber drains are used, they are withdrawn slightly each day, beginning on the third day. Pelvic sump drains are kept on low suction for 5 days. If the drainage is clear at that time, they are removed.

Control of infection

Development of pelvic sepsis after rectal injury is a dreaded complication. Appropriate management of these injuries, as outlined above, along with intravenous antibiotics, has decreased the incidence of this complication to less than 5%[3].

Patients with rectal injuries associated with deep perineal lacerations or soft tissue injury on or about the buttock may need to be returned to the operating room repeatedly for examination under anaesthesia and further irrigations, debridement and dressing changes. Such aggressive wound care will greatly decrease the incidence of soft tissue infection.

Intravenous antibiotics are administered for 5 days after operation, but are continued longer if complications develop. The antibiotics can be discontinued when the patient is afebrile and the white blood cell count is normal.

If the patient develops fever and leucocytosis after operation, rectal examination is performed to feel for a bulge in the cul-de-sac or other abnormality. An abdominal and pelvic computed tomography (CT) scan should also be obtained. If a localized abscess is identified, it should be drained by CT-guided percutaneous insertion of a catheter. Open drainage should be reserved for multiloculated collections or when percutaneous catheter drainage is unsuccessful.

Colostomy closure

Restoration of intestinal continuity should be deferred for a minimum of 8 weeks.

15 Before colostomy closure, contrast radiography is performed to ensure that the injury has healed. After a standard bowel preparation, the patient is operated on through an elliptical incision encompassing the stoma. Both limbs of the colon are identified and separated from the surrounding tissues. A colotomy is made in each limb, through each of which is passed the jaw of a linear anastomosing stapler (GIA). The instrument is fired, thereby anastomosing the two limbs together longitudinally. The staple line is visualized to be assured of haemostasis. A single permanent suture should be inserted just beyond the distal end of the stapled anastomosis. This will help to decrease any tension on this aspect of the staple line, preventing disruption of the anastomosis.

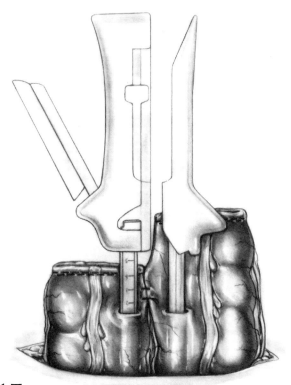

15

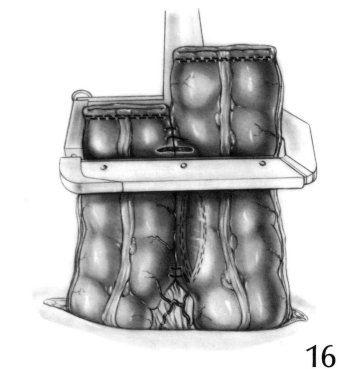

16

16, 17 A linear stapler (TA 60) is placed across both limbs of the bowel just beyond the previously made colotomies. The instrument is fired and the bowel above the staple line is transected and removed. The newly anastomosed sigmoid is placed back in the peritoneal cavity and the fascial defect is closed with a heavy monofilament suture.

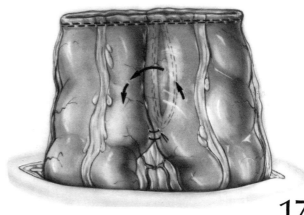

17

Anal injuries

Principles

The extent of anal injury, the mechanism of injury and the presence or absence of associated rectal or perineal laceration will determine the choice of treatment. Assessment of significant injury is best performed in the operating room, with the patient under anaesthesia in the lithotomy position. Rectal, vaginal and rigid endoscopic examination are then performed. If rectal injuries are found, they are treated as outlined above.

18 Anal sphincter injuries associated with motor vehicle accidents are often accompanied by ragged perineal tears, local haematomas and varying degrees of rectal tears. Such extensive injuries are best debrided and left to heal by secondary intention as they do not lend themselves well to primary repair.

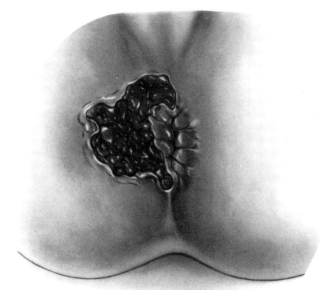

18

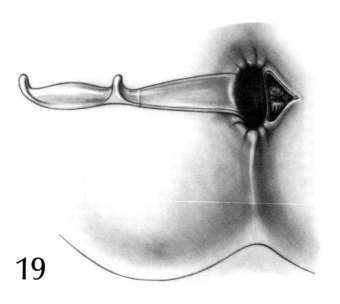

19

Sharp laceration of the sphincter

19 Sharp laceration of the anal sphincter not associated with ragged perineal lacerations can be repaired primarily. If the rectum is not involved, sphincteric lacerations, even extensive ones, do not necessarily require the creation of a proximal diverting colostomy.

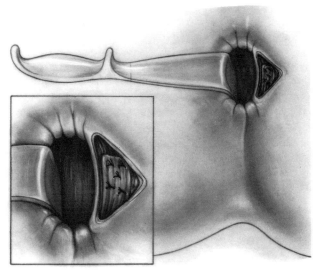

20 The cut ends of the sphincter are identified and reapproximated using monofilament non-absorbable U stitches. The skin overlying the repair is left open.

20

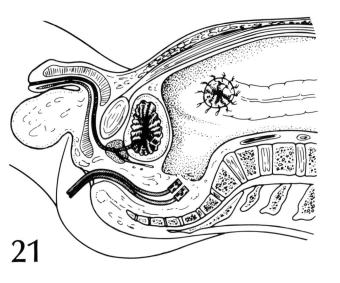

21

Devastating anal sphincter injuries

21 Injuries that are so extensive that abdominal perineal resection is required are rarely seen outside a war zone. Only when the anal sphincter mechanism has been irrevocably destroyed should total proctectomy be performed. A permanent sigmoid colostomy is created. The peritoneal wound is left open and the presacral space is drained with suction catheters.

Injuries caused by sexual assault or erotic misadventures

Forceful anal penetration can produce lesions ranging from mild divulsion of the sphincters to complete disruption of the anal sphincters and rectovaginal tears. When divulsion of the sphincters occurs, the degree of sphincter injury can be difficult to determine because of the local oedema and haematomas that may accompany the injury. The patient is generally found to have either a patulous anus or a distinct delay of anal closure after digital rectal examination. The great majority of these injuries require no specific therapy and most heal with little, if any, dysfunction.

Fist fornication is sometimes associated with more severe forms of anorectal injuries, i.e. rectosigmoid perforations. These obviously required urgent laparotomy and are managed as outlined above.

DELAYED SPHINCTER REPAIR

Preoperative

22 Once the perineal wound has completely healed and the patient has recovered from concomitant injuries, the status of the sphincter can be assessed. If continence is compromised, sphincter repair should be performed. If a diverting colostomy was created for the original injury, it is best to perform the sphincter repair before restoring intestinal continuity.

The degree of sphincter injury is assessed by physical examination. The edges of the torn sphincter will have retracted, and their approximate location can be determined by palpation.

A thorough bowel preparation is necessary in all cases. All patients should receive preoperative intravenous antibiotics directed at the enteric flora.

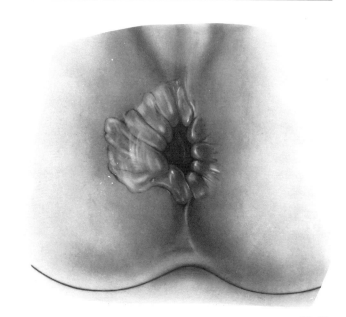

22

Operation

23, 24 The patient is placed in the lithotomy position and the rectum is irrigated with saline solution. A curvilinear incision is made on the perianal skin overlying the sphincter injury. In most cases the incision will need to encompass at least half of the circumference of the anal opening.

With careful fine scissor dissection, the edges of the sphincter are identified in each corner of the wound. The sphincter edge is dissected for a short distance, but no attempt is made to dissect the muscle extensively or to separate the muscle into bundles. Care is taken to preserve the scar on the ends of the sphincter. This scar will be valuable in preventing the sutures from pulling out of the muscle.

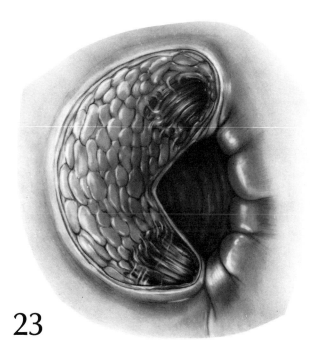

23

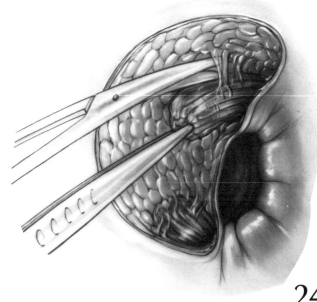

24

25 Atraumatic clamps (Allis' clamps) are placed on each edge of the sphincter. These clamps are then crossed. This manoeuvre should result in tight closure of the anal canal so that only the tip of the surgeon's finger can enter the anus. If the clamps are crossed and the canal remains partially open, then the clamped tissue is not the edge of the sphincters and further dissection is required to identify the muscle accurately.

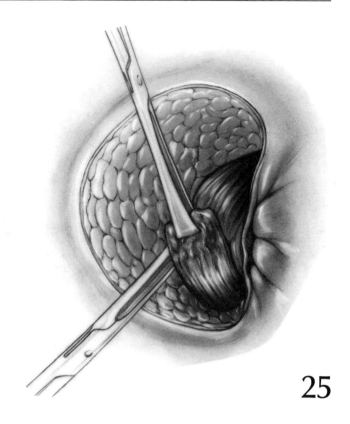

25

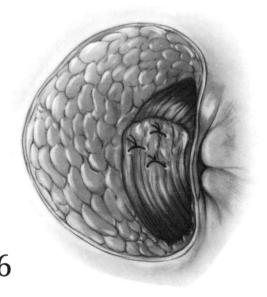

26

26 Once the sphincters are identified, they are sutured together using horizontal mattress stitches of 2/0 polypropylene. Complete haemostasis is of paramount importance, as the development of a wound haematoma can lead to a breakdown or an infection of the repair.

The overlying skin is left open and a perineal dressing is applied.

Postoperative care

If repair is performed without the benefit of a proximal colostomy, the patient is kept on an elemental diet and his bowels are confined for about 5–7 days. With a colostomy in place, the patient can be fed a normal diet.

The perianal wound is irrigated with saline and checked daily. If bowel movement occurs early in the postoperative period, the anus should be washed with water and a mild soap.

FOREIGN OBJECTS IN THE RECTUM

Most foreign objects in the rectum that require surgical attention are inserted by the patient or a partner and have become lodged beyond their reach. These patients present to the emergency department with a host of complaints, ranging from anorectal tenesmus to urinary retention.

Preoperative

The abdomen is examined carefully for evidence of peritoneal irritation. The perianal area is inspected for evidence of trauma and, in the female, a vaginal examination is performed. It may be necessary to insert a catheter into the bladder to relieve urinary retention. Urinalysis is performed to detect the presence of haematuria. Biplanar radiographic films of the abdomen are taken to rule out the presence of pneumoperitoneum if the abdominal findings are equivocal. No attempt should be made to extract the foreign object using sharp or grasping instruments in an uncooperative patient. More damage may be inflicted to the anorectum by attempting to extract a foreign object forcibly than was done during its insertion.

Operation

Although some objects can be retrieved without much difficulty, others will require either local, spinal or general anaesthesia.

The patient is placed in the lithotomy position. For high-lying, impacted or voluminous objects, once anaesthesia has been given the abdomen is palpated and gentle pressure may at times succeed in pushing the foreign body distally. Once the object has descended into the lower rectum it can be grasped and removed.

Besides having to be familiar with the many 'tricks' required to extract a rectal foreign body[4], it behoves the surgeon to remember who among the operating room staff wears a size 6 or smaller glove. Such a diminutive, gentle and well lubricated gloved hand can often retrieve transanally a foreign body that has frustrated all of the surgeon's attempts.

After the foreign object has been retrieved an endoscopic examination of the rectum and distal sigmoid should be conducted to look for injuries. Mucosal lacerations require little or no treatment, while a perforation requires surgery as outlined previously. During endoscopy, air is insufflated into the bowel. Even if the examination is negative, a film of the abdomen is obtained to look for air extravasation.

A rectal foreign body requiring laparotomy is rare. If an operation is needed, antibiotics should be administered before and after operation. The foreign body should be 'milked' into the distal rectum and removed transanally if possible. If this cannot be accomplished, a colotomy is made and the object is extracted. Great care should be taken to avoid peritoneal contamination as the object is being delivered from the bowel. The colotomy is closed in a routine fashion.

References

1. Burch JM, Feliciano DV, Mattox KL. Colostomy and drainage for civilian rectal injuries: is that all? *Ann Surg* 1989; 209: 600–11.

2. American College of Surgeons Committee on Trauma. *Advanced Trauma Life Support Program*. Chicago: American College of Surgeons, 1989.

3. Tuggle D, Huber PJ. Management of rectal trauma. *Am J Surg* 1984; 148: 806–8.

4. Busch DB, Starling JR. Rectal foreign bodies: case reports and a comprehensive review of the world's literature. *Surgery* 1986; 100: 512–19.

Illustrations by Gillian Oliver and the late Robert Lane

Peranal endorectal operative techniques

Ann C. Lowry MD, FACS
Clinical Assistant Professor of Surgery, Division of Colon and Rectal Surgery, University of Minnesota Medical School, Minneapolis, Minnesota, USA

History

The peranal approach offers solutions to several difficult clinical problems, including the local therapy of sessile adenomas and early rectal carcinomas which might otherwise require a permanent stoma. This approach is also utilized for correction of rectocoeles and simultaneous correction of other anorectal pathology.

Parks first described submucosal excision of sessile lesions in the rectum in 1966[1]. The avoidance of a permanent stoma for a benign process appealed to patients and surgeons alike. As reports of low morbidity and acceptable recurrence rates appeared, this approach gained in popularity. Rectal ultrasonography now allows more accurate patient selection, further enhancing the use of this procedure.

Principles and justification

Sessile adenomas are benign lesions involving only the mucosa. Excision is recommended because of their high potential for malignant change. Only the mucosa, however, need be excised. As access is available via the peranal approach, full resection is not necessary. In fact, the potential of a permanent stoma and pelvic nerve injury means resection should be avoided if possible. Other forms of local therapy such as fulguration with electrocautery, laser, or endocavitary radiation are also available, but do not provide an intact specimen for pathological examination. If the patient can tolerate anaesthesia, submucosal excision is the preferred approach.

The introduction of stapling devices and better understanding of distal intramural spread of cancer made low anastomoses possible and appropriate after resection of rectal carcinoma. Cancers in the distal third of the rectum, however, still require abdominoperineal resection when resection is deemed necessary. Well-differentiated superficial carcinomas carry a 6–10% risk of lymph node metastasis, raising doubts about the necessity of resection, particularly if it involves a permanent stoma. Full-thickness excision provides an intact pathological specimen for evaluation of the margins, depth of invasion and histological characteristics. In carefully selected patients, recurrence and survival rates equal to those after abdominoperineal resection have been reported[2, 3].

Preoperative

Sessile adenomas

The entire colon should be assessed for synchronous lesions using the colonoscope; polypectomy is performed for other lesions that appear benign.

Rectal adenomas can be evaluated by digital examination, endoscopy, biopsy and rectal ultrasonography. The purpose is to exclude malignancy and to predict the technical difficulty of transanal excision. Benign neoplasms are soft on palpation. Induration and fixation on digital examination are indicators of malignancy, and biopsy samples should be taken of these areas. Areas of ulceration also require biopsy. Random biopsies are not helpful, however, as the error rate may be as high as 50%[4]. Rectal ultrasonography currently provides the most accurate method of excluding malignancy. Penetration beyond the mucosa indicates a malignant process. Experienced examiners achieve an accuracy of 88% in evaluation of intestinal wall penetration[5]. When rectal ultrasonography is not available, staging depends on digital and endoscopic examination.

The size, extent and location of the lesion determine the technical difficulty, although large and circumferential adenomas can be safely excised using this approach, with lesions up to 10 cm long having been removed. Many lesions in the upper rectum and lower sigmoid colon can be prolapsed into the operative field allowing peranal removal.

A full mechanical bowel preparation, usually a lavage preparation, is used. Intravenous antibiotics are given before operation.

Rectal carcinoma

The entire colon should be examined for polyps and synchronous lesions. Chest radiography and liver function tests should be performed to screen for metastatic disease.

Careful clinical staging of the lesion is imperative. When available, rectal ultrasonography is the most accurate modality[6]. At the University of Minnesota, depth of intestinal wall invasion was correct in 102 of 116 patients (88%). Penetration was overstaged in ten patients (8.6%) and understaged in four (3.4%)[5].

If rectal ultrasonography is not available, various clinical findings help to predict the stage of the lesion. Favourable lesions include exophytic, non-ulcerated lesions less than 3 cm in size. They must be mobile on digital examination and involve no more than one quadrant of the rectum. Poorly differentiated carcinomas carry an increased risk of lymph node metastasis.

A full mechanical and antibiotic bowel preparation is necessary.

Rectocoele

Constipation is the most common complaint associated with a rectocoele. As rectocoeles are a common finding in asymptomatic women, careful evaluation of the patient's complaints is imperative to determine the relationship of the rectocoele to the symptoms. Symptoms of straining to defaecate, incomplete evacuation relieved by anterior perineal support, rectal fullness or pressure are likely to be related to the rectocoele. The necessity of digital vaginal pressure to completely evacuate confirms the relationship of the rectocoele to the patient's symptoms.

Defaecography may present evidence of retention of contrast medium in the rectocoele and exclude internal prolapse as the cause of the patient's complaints. Manometry and electromyography of the anal sphincter will identify hypertonia of the sphincter and anismus. These findings should be appropriately addressed before repair of the rectocoele is considered. If no other pathology is evident, medical management with a high-fibre diet and bulk agents is prescribed. Repair of the rectocoele is indicated if symptoms persist despite adequate conservative management.

Mechanical bowel preparation with enemas is performed. Perioperative antibiotic coverage is recommended by many authors. The perianal area and vagina receive an antiseptic preparation.

Anaesthesia

Low, small sessile adenomas may be excised under local anaesthesia with intravenous sedation, as may small rectal carcinomas. Regional or general anaesthesia, however, is necessary for most lesions.

Local anaesthesia with sedation is adequate for repairing a rectocoele. If used, regional or general anaesthesia is supplemented by a peranal block using a local anaesthetic mixed with adrenaline.

Operations

Adequate exposure is key to the peranal approach. The prone jack-knife position is optimal; a good view is obtained, blood flows away from the operative field, and more room is available for assistants. A Lone Star or other self-retaining retractor allows good visualization and frees the assistant's hands. A headlight provides the best illumination.

SUBMUCOSAL EXCISION OF SESSILE ADENOMAS OF THE RECTUM

Position of patient

The lithotomy position eases the administration of anaesthesia and occasionally provides better exposure of posterior neoplasms (*see Illustration 2* on page 48).

Incision

A Pratt bivalve anoscope is inserted to allow assessment of the lesion. If the lesion is high, Babcock clamps are placed at the edge of the lesion. Traction intussuscepts the intestine, delivering the lesion into the operative field.

1, 2 Occasionally, a rigid sigmoidoscope must be inserted and sigmoidoscopic forceps used to grasp the lesion. The sigmoidoscope and forceps are withdrawn simultaneously, intussuscepting the intestinal wall. If the adenoma cannot be brought into view, a low anterior resection is indicated.

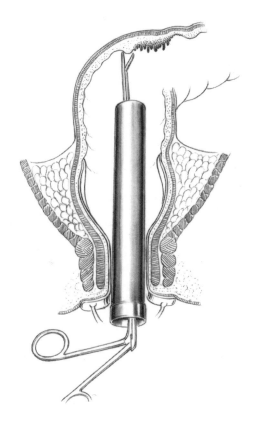

1

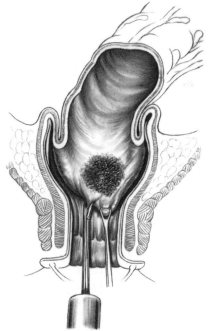

2

3   When the lesion is delivered into the field, stay sutures are placed about 2 cm from the edges. Exposure is maintained with the Lone Star retractor using the accompanying hooks in the anal canal. In addition, the stay sutures are hooked into the Lone Star retractor.

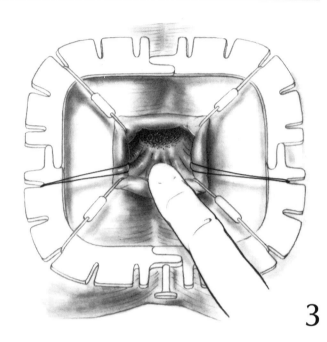

3

4, 5   The submucosal plane under the tumour is infiltrated with saline solution containing 1:200 000 adrenaline. The injection begins several centimetres from the tumour, lifting it from the underlying muscle. It also facilitates identification of the proper plane and aids haemostasis. Small extensions of the adenoma are often more visible after the infiltration.

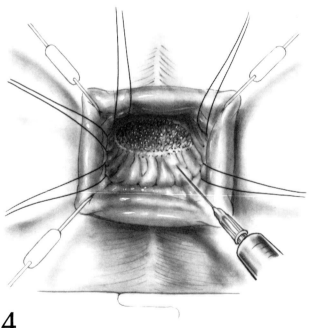

4

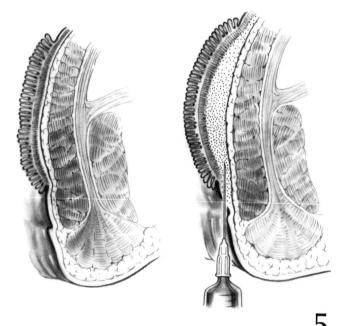

5

6,7 Excision begins in normal mucosa 1 cm from the edge of the tumour using scissors or electrocautery. The submucosal plane is entered and the tumour is lifted off the circular muscle. The lesions are often friable and must be handled with care. The goal is excision in a single piece. It may be necessary to repeat the adrenaline injection as dissection proceeds. Haemostasis must be meticulous to maintain the correct plane of dissection. Traction on the dissected portion of the specimen helps to bring the proximal portion into view.

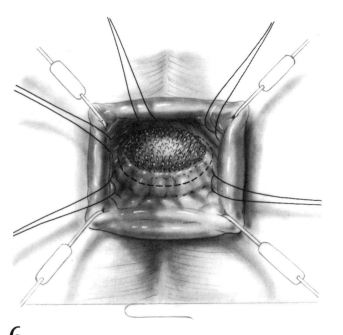

6

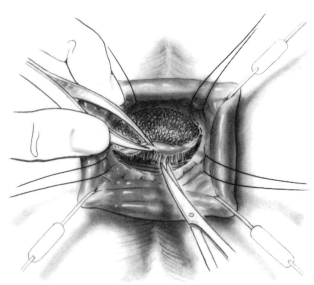

7

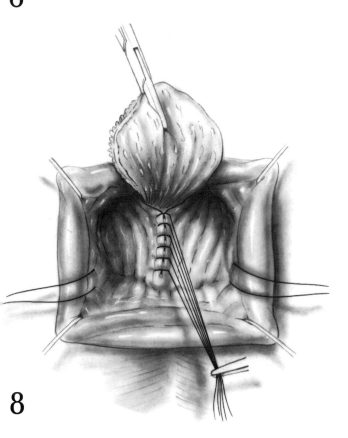

8

8 For large lesions, it is helpful to close the defect as the lesion is excised. Traction on the sutures aids exposure and prevents retraction of the site when the lesion is removed.

9 Small defects may be left open. Healing generally occurs without infection or stenosis.

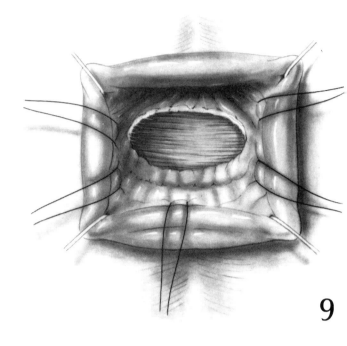

9

10, 11 Circumferential lesions may be excised in a similar fashion. The Lone Star retractor allows exposure to the entire lesion. Beginning distally, the dissection is performed circumferentially and then continued proximally. In this way, a cylinder of mucosa containing the adenoma is excised.

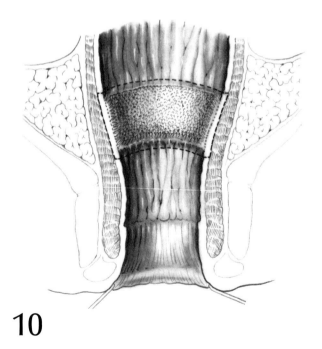

10

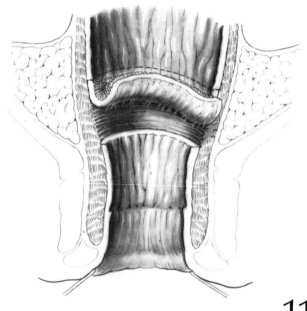

11

12 Stricture formation is likely if the resulting defect is not closed. Circular muscle plication is performed by taking multiple bites in the exposed muscle in each of four quadrants. As the sutures are tied, the rectal wall is plicated bringing the mucosal edges together.

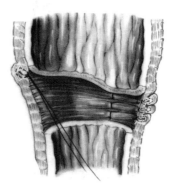

12

13 Absorbable sutures are used to approximate the mucosa.

At completion of the closure, proctoscopy is always performed to ensure patency of the lumen and adequate haemostasis. In dissecting large lesions, it is easy to lose orientation within the rectum. Care must be taken to re-establish exposure to prevent suturing the lumen closed.

The specimen is pinned to a board and labelled to orientate the pathologist. This manoeuvre aids in the detection of malignant foci and inspection of the margins.

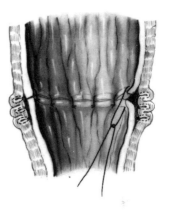

13

MALIGNANCY IN VILLOUS ADENOMAS

Local excision is sufficient for *in situ* carcinoma. If the excised specimen contains invasive carcinoma, more therapy is indicated depending on the depth of invasion. At the minimum, full-thickness excision of the site is necessary. Alternatives include external beam radiation, endocavitary radiation, and abdominoperineal or low anterior resection.

LOCAL EXCISION OF RECTAL CARCINOMA

The essential difference between submucosal excision and local excision of a carcinoma is the depth of the dissection. For malignant lesions, dissection into the perirectal fat is required to ensure complete excision. Positioning and exposure are the same as for submucosal excision. The perianal tissue and extrarectal area are infiltrated with an adrenaline solution to aid haemostasis.

Incision

14 Dissection begins 2 cm from the edge of the tumour. The rectal wall is incised into the perirectal fat. The lesion is progressively excised using the electrocautery for haemostasis. The aim is excision of a disc of intestinal wall including the lesion and 2 cm of surrounding normal rectum.

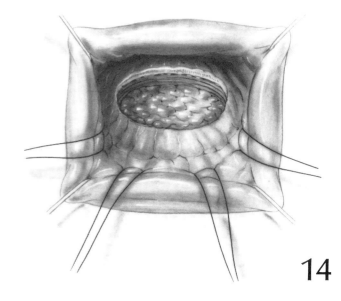

14

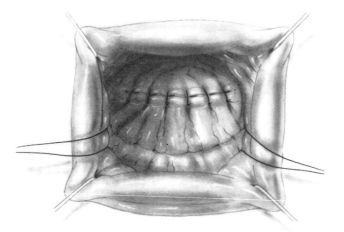

15

Wound closure

15 The wound must be carefully inspected for adequacy of haemostasis. A haematoma increases the risk of septic complications. The wound is closed with a single layer of full-thickness sutures. If tension limits closure, a portion of the defect may safely be left open. Proctoscopy is performed to ensure patency of the lumen. The specimen is pinned to a board to orientate the pathologist.

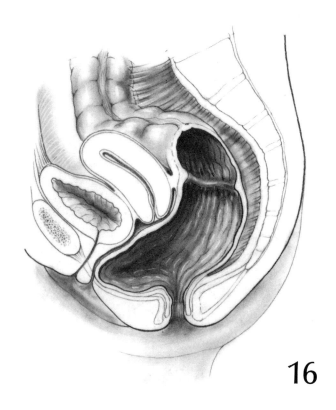

16

RECTOCOELE

16, 17 A rectocoele is a weakness in the rectovaginal septum from attentuation of the submucosa and muscularis of the rectal wall. It is described as low-, mid-, or high-type depending on its location in the rectovaginal septum. Low rectocoeles involve a defect in the anterior sphincter mechanism, mid rectocoeles occur just above the anorectal ring, and high rectocoeles are part of complete genital prolapse. Mid rectocoeles are the most common. Rectocoeles are easily detected by digital rectal examination done while the patient strains or by cinedefaecography.

Repair of rectocoeles can be performed transvaginally or transanally. The endorectal approach is favoured for ease of correction of other anorectal pathology and relief of anorectal symptoms. This approach is appropriate for intermediate rectocoeles. Both low and high rectocoeles require more extensive repair.

The prone jack-knife position provides excellent exposure and allows other anorectal pathology to be easily corrected.

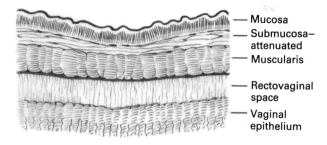

— Mucosa
— Submucosa– attenuated
— Muscularis
— Rectovaginal space
— Vaginal epithelium

17

18 Using a Pratt bivalve anoscope for exposure, a linear incision is made over the excess mucosa. The incision is extended above the palpable weakness. If no redundant mucosa exists, a transverse or vertical incision can be used. The mucosa and submucosa are dissected away from the underlying rectal wall.

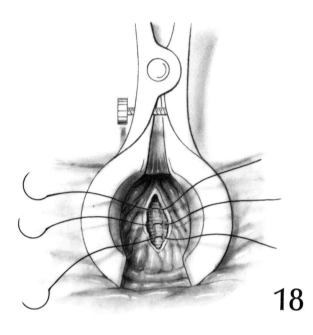

18

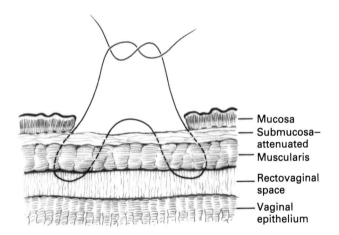

Mucosa
Submucosa–attenuated
Muscularis

Rectovaginal space

Vaginal epithelium

19

19 Imbricating sutures are placed in the rectal wall, levator ani muscles and rectovaginal septum. A guiding finger in the vagina prevents penetration of the vaginal epithelium.

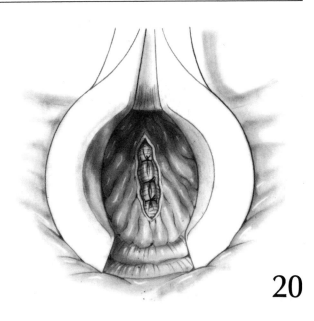

20, 21 These sutures are sequentially tied.

20

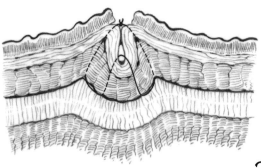

21

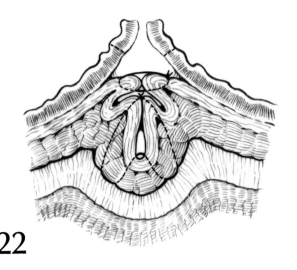

22

22 If laxity persists, a second row of sutures is placed.

23 The excess mucosa is trimmed, and the mucosal defect is closed with a continuous absorbable suture. Other anorectal pathology is appropriately corrected.

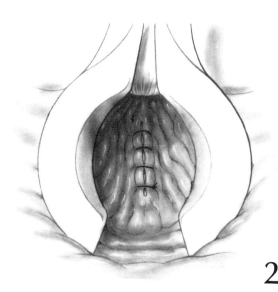

23

Postoperative care

Sessile adenomas

The patient resumes a normal diet. Discomfort is usually relieved by sitz baths and mild analgesics. If a full thickness rectal injury occurs, the patient should have the usual postoperative care following an intestinal anastomosis. Haemorrhage, perforation, peritonitis, urinary tract infection and stricture formation are uncommon complications[7]. Re-exploration is seldom necessary to control haemorrhage. Incontinence has not been a problem.

Recurrences of villous adenomas are relatively common. Previous history of a polyp, size, degree of dysplasia and positive margins increase the risk of recurrence[8]. Most recurrences occur within the first 3 years. Proctoscopy should be performed every 3 months for 1 year and every 6 months for the following 2 years. Yearly examinations suffice after that if there has been no recurrence. Recurrent lesions can be treated with fulguration or repeat excision if no malignancy is found on biopsy. Colonoscopy at regular intervals is required to identify metachronous neoplasms.

Rectal carcinoma

The patient receives perioperative antibiotic coverage. Once intestinal function resumes, the diet is advanced. Significant pain indicates possible perirectal or pelvic sepsis.

Complications include haemorrhage, pelvic infection, peritonitis and urinary tract retention. Pelvic infection usually responds to antibiotic therapy.

If the pathology report indicates a superficial lesion but positive lateral margins, re-excision of the operative site 6 weeks later is recommended. Local recurrence often occurs if observation only is employed. If the report reveals deep invasion, the procedure is viewed as an excisional biopsy. Further treatment options include resection after the perirectal inflammation subsides and external beam or endocavitary radiation. Elderly, high-risk patients may choose observation only.

The excision site is examined every 3 months for the first 2 years. The follow-up evaluation includes digital, endoscopic and, if available, rectal ultrasonographic examination. Early detection of recurrences improves the results of a salvage procedure. Chest radiography, carcinoembryonic antigen, liver function tests and computed tomography screen for development of metastatic lesions. Colonoscopy is performed 1 year later.

Rectocoele

Perioperative antibiotics are prescribed. A regular diet is resumed as tolerated by the patient. Sitz baths are prescribed for comfort. Bulk agents are used to soften the stools.

Urinary retention is the most commonly reported complication. Infection occurs in approximately 5%. Rectovaginal fistula formation has been reported.

Acknowledgements

This chapter was originally written by the late Sir Alan Parks MCh, FRCS FRCP, Consultant Surgeon, The Royal London Hospital and St Mark's Hospital for Diseases of the Rectum and Colon, London, UK

References

1. Parks AG. Benign tumours of the rectum. In Rob C, Smith R, Morgan C, eds. *Abdomen and Rectum and Anus. Operative Surgery Vol. 10.* London: Butterworths, 1966: 541–8.

2. Grigg ML, McDermott FT, Pihl EA, Hughes ES. Curative local excision in the treatment of carcinoma of the rectum. *Dis Colon Rectum* 1984; 27: 81–3.

3. Gall FP, Hermanek P. Cancer of the rectum – local excision. *Surg Clin North Am* 1988; 68: 1353–65.

4. Christiansen J, Kirkegaard P, Ibsen J. Prognosis after treatment of villous adenomas of the colon and rectum. *Ann Surg* 1979; 189: 404–8.

5. Madoff RD, Buenz BA, Jensen IJ, Finne CO, Wong WD. Endorectal ultrasonography: an accurate tool for preoperative staging of rectal neoplasms. Presented at American Gastroenterological Association, San Francisco, USA, 12–13 May 1992.

6. Hildebrandt U, Feifel G. Endorectal sonography. *Surg Annu* 1990; 90: 169–84.

7. Galandiuk S, Fazio VW, Jagelman DG *et al*. Villous and tubulovillous adenomas of the colon and rectum. A retrospective review 1964–1985. *Am J Surg* 1987; 153: 41–7.

8. Sakamoto GD, MacKeigan JM, Senagore AJ. Transanal excision of large, rectal villous adenomas. *Dis Colon Rectum* 1991; 34: 880–5.

Further reading

Arnold MW, Stewart WRC, Aguilar PS. Rectocele repair: four years' experience. *Dis Colon Rectum* 1990; 33: 684–7.

Sarles JC, Arnaud A, Selezneff I, Olivier S. Endorectal repair of rectocele. *Int J Colorectal Dis* 1989; 4: 167–71.

Schapayak S. Transrectal repair of rectocele: an extended armamentarium of colorectal surgeons. A report of 355 cases. *Dis Colon Rectum* 1985; 28: 422–33.

Fulguration of malignant rectal tumours

Eugene P. Salvati MD, FACS
Clinical Professor of Surgery, University of Medicine and Dentistry, Robert Wood Johnson Medical School, New Brunswick, New Jersey, USA

Theodore E. Eisenstat MD, FACS, FASCRS
Clinical Professor of Surgery, University of Medicine and Dentistry, Robert Wood Johnson Medical School, New Brunswick, New Jersey, USA

History

As early as 1889, electrocautery had been reported for the treatment of cancer. During the ensuing 100 years, surgeons have been attempting to evaluate and refine its application in the treatment of rectal carcinoma. For selected patients with rectal cancer, comparable results can be obtained by the application of electrocautery or the classical Miles' operation of abdominoperineal resection.

Principles and justification

Indications

Patient selection for treatment is paramount when considering this form of local treatment for rectal cancer, to decrease the incidence of nodal metastasis to between 10% and 20%.

The authors' patient selection criteria for cure include patients whose tumours are within 7.5 cm of the anal verge, less than 4 cm in diameter, mobile and unattached to local structures. No lymph nodes should be palpable during examination under general anaesthesia. Tumours should be well or moderately differentiated and have no evidence of distant metastasis.

Lesions higher than 7.5 cm from the anal verge are considered suitable for abdominal resectional operations. Patients with demonstrated metastatic disease and patients who are considered inoperable or refuse resectional treatment are considered for palliative treatment.

Preoperative

All patients receive preoperative blood tests, including liver profile, tumour markers, and a computed tomographic (CT) scan of the abdomen and pelvis with oral and intravenous contrast media. Newer modalities such as intrarectal ultrasonography and cell ploidy are being evaluated in the hope of enhancing patient selection.

Operation

Position and anaesthesia

1a–d Patients are admitted to the hospital for initial evaluation under anaesthesia. Should tumour fixation or nodal metastasis be discovered, or the tumour found to be otherwise unsuitable for local treatment, the procedure is abandoned and abdominoperineal excision considered. Under light general anaesthesia, with the patient in the lithotomy position, a local anaesthetic is administered to the anal area. The anaesthetic solution consists of 30 ml of 0.25% bupivacaine with 1:200 000 adrenaline to which has been added 150 turbidity-reducing units of hyaluronidase. The use of a local anaesthetic gives better anal relaxation and permits a lighter general anaesthesia.

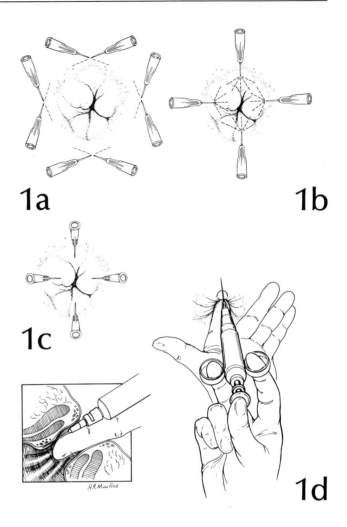

1a

1b

1c

1d

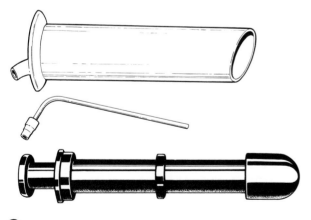

2

2 The use of a special operating proctoscope developed by Salvati has facilitated the procedure. The instrument measures 15 cm in length, has an aperture of 4 cm and an oblique end of 45°. The light source is fibreoptic and there is a built-in suction tube. It is occasionally necessary to perform a lateral internal sphincterotomy to provide adequate space to insert this instrument.

3 A typical tumour seen through the operating
proctoscope is illustrated. The 4-cm aperture
serves as a guide to determine the width of the tumour.

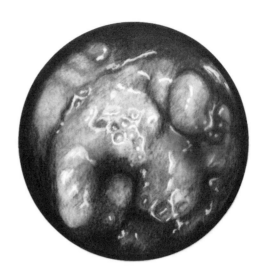

3

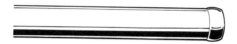

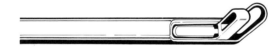

4

4 A Cameron suction-tipped electrode (0.5 cm) is
used to coagulate and evaporate the surface of the
tumour. The charred tumour is then removed by sharp
uterine curettage or biopsy. This procedure is repeated
until the entire tumour and a 1-cm halo of normal tissue
has been coagulated. It is possible to burn deeply into
the perirectal fat laterally and posteriorly, but care must
be taken anteriorly with regard to the vagina and
prostatic capsule.

5 The electrocoagulating tip is applied to the entire
tumour until it turns white.

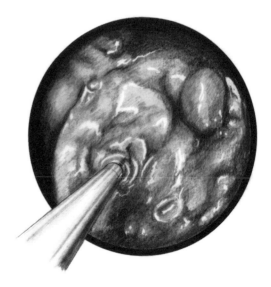

5

6 The angled biopsy forceps is used to excise the charred tumour sharply.

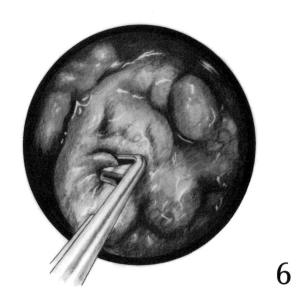

6

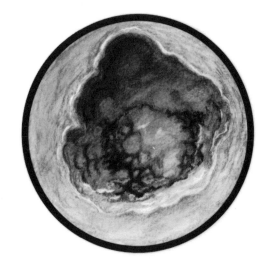

7

7 Electrocoagulation is repeated until the tumour is completely destroyed, as determined by palpation. Posteriorly, this can be carried into the presacral fascia and laterally into the perirectal fat. Much smoke and debris is produced and excellent suction is mandatory, along with frequent saline irrigation via an Asepto syringe. A 1-cm halo of normal bowel is destroyed around the tumour and a final burn is administered.

The operation takes at least 60–120 min under general anaesthesia.

Outcome

The authors' results of electrocoagulation for the treatment of rectal cancer over the past 20 years are shown in *Figure 1*. The results have been consistent and substantiated by other authors.

The majority of patients treated were in their seventh and eighth decades of life.

The overall uncorrected survival rate for all patients treated for cure was 47%. In a group of 50 patients treated for cure with electrocoagulation only, the overall 5-year survival rate was 58%.

The 31 patients who required conversion to abdominoperineal resection had an overall survival rate of 29%. The majority of the patients in this group had Dukes' C lesions on pathological examination of the specimen.

Of 33 patients treated for palliation, only one patient survived for 5 years. However, only one patient required a colostomy before death, while the remainder did not require faecal diversion.

The overall complication rate was 21%. Bleeding occurred in 7% of patients, this being controlled by further electrocoagulation either in the clinic or the operating room. Stricture occurred in 6% and urinary retention in 2.6% of patients. Electrical burns occurred in 2.6% and a perirectal abscess in one patient. A single patient developed perforation requiring urgent faecal diversion. There were three deaths, giving a mortality rate of 3.7%.

Abdominoperineal resection continues to be the 'gold standard' by which treatment of cancer of the rectum is measured. Abdominoperineal resection is associated with significant morbidity and mortality rates as well as the obvious requirement of a permanent colostomy and, commonly, sexual dysfunction. Alternatives for treatment continue to be sought. The development of new instrumentation and procedures has allowed resectional operations on a larger percentage of patients. However, for very low lesions, the Miles' operation continues to be used. The reasons for rejection of electrocoagulation include tradition and personal preference, but are frequently related to scepticism concerning a procedure which violates the classical tenets of extirpation of malignancy for staging purposes.

The authors believe that their results in selected patients are comparable with those achieved by abdominoperineal resection, and continue to advocate the use of electrocoagulation for the curative treatment of rectal cancer in selected patients.

It is hoped that, with the application of appropriate postoperative radiotherapy and chemotherapy, an improvement in survival rate may be obtained for those patients who unknowingly have nodal metastasis.

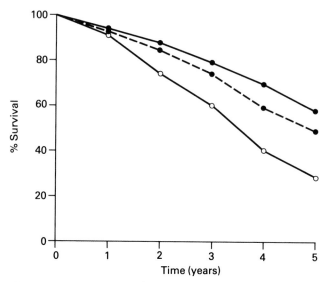

Figure 1.   *Five-year survival rates for patients treated for rectal cancer by electrocoagulation.* ●——●, *Electrocoagulation alone (n = 50);* ○——○, *electrocoagulation with abdominoperineal resection (n = 31);* ●---●, *all patients (n = 81)*

Further reading

Crile G Jr, Turnbull RB Jr. The role of electrocoagulation in the treatment of carcinoma of the rectum. *Surg Gynecol Obstet* 1972; 135: 391–6.

Eisenstat TE, Deak ST, Rubin RJ, Salvati EP, Greco RS. Five year survival in patients with carcinoma of the rectum treated by electrocoagulation. *Am J Surg* 1982; 143: 127–32.

Localio SA, Eng K, Gouge TH, Ranson JH. Abdominosacral resection for carcinoma of the mid-rectum; ten years' experience. *Ann Surg* 1978; 188: 475–80.

Madden JL, Kandalaft S. Electrocoagulation as a primary curative method in the treatment of carcinoma of the rectum. *Surg Gynecol Obstet* 1983; 157: 164–79.

Moertel CG, Fleming TR, Macdonald JS *et al.* Levamisole and fluorouracil for adjuvant therapy of resected colon carcinoma. *N Engl J Med* 1990; 322: 352–8.

Salvati EP, Rubin RJ, Eisenstat TE, Siemons GO, Mangione JS. Electrocoagulation of selected carcinoma of the rectum. *Surg Gynecol Obstet* 1988; 166: 393–6.

Strauss SF, Crawford RA, Strauss HA. Surgical diathermy of carcinoma of the rectum. Its clinical end results. *JAMA* 1935; 104: 1480–4.

Swerdlow DB, Salvati EP. Electrocoagulation of cancer of the rectum. *Dis Colon Rectum* 1972; 15: 228–32.

Pouch procedures: introductory comment

David A. Rothenberger MD
Clinical Professor of Surgery and Chief, Division of Colon and Rectal Surgery, University of Minnesota Medical School, Minneapolis, Minnesota, USA

An ideal operation should eradicate the disease process and restore normal function with minimal rates of morbidity and mortality. Surgeons and their patients have long had to settle for extirpative surgery with permanent stoma construction whenever resection of the rectum and anal canal has been necessary. Although morbidity and mortality rates have steadily decreased during this century, it is only in the past two decades that significant progress has been made in restorative procedures, allowing more normal gastrointestinal function and continence after rectal excision. Today, ileal pouch and colonic pouch reconstructive procedures have assumed a major role in colorectal surgery. The chapters which follow depict techniques of performing these reconstructive procedures and several methods of handling a variety of complications which may arise following such operations.

Evolution of techniques of pouch surgery

The concept of combining a curative total colorectal resection for chronic ulcerative colitis and familial adenomatous polyposis with preservation of anal continence and restoration of bowel continuity by an ileoanal anastomosis is not new. In 1933, Nissen[1] reported a successful anastomosis of the terminal ileum to the anal sphincter after total proctocolectomy for familial adenomatous polyposis in a 10-year-old boy. In 1943, Wangensteen[2] at the University of Minnesota reported an attempt to duplicate this operation in a young man with chronic ulcerative colitis, but this operation failed because of incontinence, requiring re-establishment of a permanent ileostomy. After work in the animal model, Ravitch[3] in 1948 performed a successful total colectomy, mucosal proctectomy and straight ileoanal anastomosis in two patients with ulcerative colitis. Others began to attempt this operation, but postoperative complications were high. This led Goligher[4] in 1951 to suggest the use of a proximal loop ileostomy to protect the healing ileoanal anastomosis. Despite this modification Ravitch[5], in a 1956 review of the world experience with 56 ileoanal anastomosis procedures performed for ulcerative colitis, found that less than one-third were successful. Severe urgency, frequency, perianal excoriation and incontinence typically caused failure of the operation.

The goal of most reconstructive surgery is to mimic normal anatomy in the hope that normal physiology can be duplicated. It seemed clear to some investigators that, although a straight ileoanal anastomosis restored bowel continuity, it did not recreate normal anatomy and function. In 1955, Valiente and Bacon[6] reported laboratory experience with construction of a neorectum using ileum to create a reservoir in an attempt to decrease the frequency of defaecation. Simultaneously, others were experimenting with ileal reservoir substitutes for the urinary bladder[7]. Despite the logic of using an ileal pouch as a neorectum, surgeons did not accept this concept for clinical application until 1969, when Kock[8] reported his initial experience with a continent ileostomy and internal double-folded ileal reservoir in five patients. The Kock procedure created a reservoir and a continence mechanism in the form of an intussusception nipple valve but it required a stoma, albeit flush and theoretically continent, which was intubated 3–6 or more times each day to empty the reservoir. Thus, although it did satisfy some of the requirements of an ideal operation, it did not fully restore bowel integrity. In addition, the operation is technically demanding and significant morbidity results from slippage of the nipple valve. None the less, the Kock pouch experience proved that ileal reservoirs could function in humans and the procedure is still used selectively.

Parks and Nicholls[9] at St Mark's Hospital in London merged all of these concepts into one operation consisting of five basic steps: (1) a total colectomy with proximal proctectomy; (2) distal rectal mucosectomy; (3) construction of an ileal S-shaped reservoir; (4) a pouch–anal anastomosis; and (5) a temporary proximal ileostomy which is taken down at a subsequent operation, thus restoring intestinal continuity. This operation seemingly met the criteria of an ideal operation. It held the promise of allowing a curative resection with reconstruction of a neorectum and preservation of near normal continence, without undue mortality or excess morbidity.

Since the publication of the 1978 landmark article by Parks and Nicholls[9], the restorative proctocolectomy (ileal pouch–anal anastomosis procedure) has become the procedure of choice for chronic ulcerative colitis and familial adenomatous polyposis in many institutions around the world. Not surprisingly, numerous modifications in technique have been advocated to improve the functional outcome or lessen morbidity rates.

Based on the success of the ileal pouch–anal anastomosis procedures, some surgeons began constructing a colonic pouch after extended low anterior resections in the belief that the added reservoir capacity would decrease the frequency and urgency sometimes reported by such patients after a straight, low colorectal or coloanal anastomosis[10].

Current perspectives

Pouch procedures have achieved a high level of acceptance by surgeons and patients, but as their popularity has grown, so too have controversies regarding a variety of aspects of these operations[11]. The following discussion will provide a perspective on new developments and controversies of pouch surgery.

Choice of operation

At present, the various ileal pouch procedures are performed primarily for patients with chronic ulcerative colitis or familial adenomatous polyposis. The basic indications for surgery have not changed, i.e. poor function, toxic megacolon, haemorrhage, perforation, complications of medical therapy, potential cancer risk or development of a cancer. The pros and cons of the various pouch procedures must be compared with the alternative procedures of total proctocolectomy with Brooke ileostomy or total colectomy and ileorectal anastomosis.

Today, most centres restrict the Kock continent ileostomy procedure to those patients requesting conversion of a conventional ileostomy and to patients with functional failure of a pelvic ileal reservoir. Occasionally, a Kock continent ileostomy is performed as a primary procedure in conjunction with a total proctocolectomy.

At present, there are relatively few advocates of a colonic J pouch procedure after rectal excision. Most surgeons are concerned that the added morbidity rates of the J pouch construction and the proximal temporary ileostomy or colostomy will negate the limited advantages theoretically provided to only a relatively small percentage of the many patients undergoing rectal excisions. Some are also concerned that colonic dysfunction with poor emptying of the J colonic reservoir may ultimately develop in such patients. Most surgeons have taken a 'wait and see' attitude before routinely adopting this method for reconstruction after rectal excision.

Staging of operation

Historically, pouch procedures were generally accompanied by construction of a proximal, temporary diverting ostomy. A temporary stoma has its own morbidity, including dehydration and electrolyte imbalance, parastomal skin problems, small bowel obstruction at the stoma, and the morbidity related to the 'take down' procedure. Thus, there is significant advantage in eliminating the temporary stoma but controversy persists as to whether this can be done safely. Selective use of a one-stage procedure is probably safe in an elective setting in a patient whose immunological, nutritional and cardiovascular status is stable, provided that the pouch operation is performed without any technical problems.

Role of mucosectomy

Considerable controversy has arisen regarding rectal mucosectomy; its very necessity is currently being questioned. Traditionally, a complete mucosectomy beginning at the dentate line has been considered an essential step when performing a pelvic pouch procedure. Today, many advocate leaving a 1–2-cm zone of transitional epithelium, which they suggest enhances sensation and improves continence without unduly exposing the patient to an increased risk of colorectal cancer arising in the non-stripped mucosa[12]. As noted in several of the following chapters, a double-stapled non-mucosectomy technique is advocated by several authors.

Reservoir configuration

Most surgeons continue to advocate construction of an ileal reservoir to increase capacity and decrease frequency and urgency after removal of the colon and rectum. The original Parks S reservoir consisted of three 15-cm limbs and a 5-cm efferent spout[9]. The design was criticised as being unduly complicated to construct and difficult for patients to empty spontaneously. The J-shaped two-limbed pouch designed by

Utsunomiya[13] is the most commonly used reservoir because of its ease of construction and its ease of evacuation. A W pouch design as advocated by Nicholls and Lubowski[14], a modified Kock pouch design as advocated by Hulten and colleagues[15] and a new H pouch design suggested by Fonkalsrud and colleagues[16] are other alternatives. Regardless of pouch configuration, it appears best that the ileal reservoir is located within the true pelvis, the outflow tract is short or absent, and there is no tension on the anastomosis.

Morbidity rates and functional results

Although pelvic pouch procedures held the promise of being the ideal operation for patients with chronic ulcerative colitis and familial adenomatous polyposis, the reality is that morbidity rates have been high and functional results are less than perfect[17]. Morbidity has been high, especially early in the learning curve and early in the evolution of these operations when more complex manoeuvres, such as a complete rectal mucosectomy for 6–10 cm, were standard. Modifications of technique, as described in the following chapters, have decreased current morbidity rates to a more tolerable level. Failures continue to occur in 5–10% of patients and some who have not failed must struggle with frequency, urgency, incontinence or pouchitis. The chapter by Dozois discusses management of these issues.

Future directions

To date we have not found the ideal operation for chronic ulcerative colitis and familial adenomatous polyposis[18]. Pelvic ileal pouch procedures give good-to-excellent results for most patients but we must continue to modify techniques to lessen morbidity rates and maximize functional results. Long-term surveillance of this population who have had pelvic reservoirs, generally at a young age, is essential. The long-term risk of cancer developing within ileal pouches is unknown but the Kock pouch experience suggests that the rate will be acceptably low. Whether the recent trend to leave a zone of mucosa in the anal canal will result in a significant risk of developing cancer is also unknown. Similarly, metabolic dysfunction and recurrent pouchitis may become problems in the future. As patients age, progressive incontinence may develop. Whether we can better mimic nature with other pouch designs, or determine the optimal size and motor function characteristics of pouches, remains open to question. Whether colonic pouch procedures are worthwhile awaits long-term follow-up in greater numbers of patients.

Certainly the effort should be made to resolve these questions. Our patients are depending on us.

References

1. Nissen R. Demonstrationen aus der operativen Chirurgie zunachst einige Beobachtungen aus der platischen Chirurgie. *Zentralbl Chir* 1933; 60: 888.

2. Wangensteen OH. Primary resection (closed anastomosis) of the colon and rectosigmoid. *Surgery* 1943; 14: 403–32.

3. Ravitch MM. Anal ileostomy with sphincter preservation in patients requiring total colectomy for benign conditions. *Surgery* 1948; 24: 170–87.

4. Goligher JC. The functional results after sphincter-saving resection of the rectum. *Ann R Coll Surg Engl* 1951; 8 421–39.

5. Ravitch MM. Total colectomy and abdomino-perineal resection (pan-colectomy) in one stage. *Ann Surg* 1956; 144: 758–64.

6. Valiente MA, Bacon HE. Construction of pouch using 'pantaloon' technique for pull-through of ileum following total colectomy: report of experimental work and results. *Am J Surg* 1955; 90: 742–9.

7. Tasker JH. Ileocystoplasty: a new technique: an experimental study with report of a case. *Br J Urol* 1953; 25: 349–57.

8. Kock NG. Intra-abdominal 'reservoir' in patients with permanent ileostomy: preliminary observations on a procedure resulting in fecal 'continence' in five ileostomy patients. *Arch Surg* 1969; 99: 223–31.

9. Parks AG, Nicholls RJ. Proctocolectomy without ileostomy for ulcerative colitis. *BMJ* 1978; ii: 85–8.

10. Parc R, Tiret E, Frileaux P, Moszkowski E, Loygue J. Resection and coloanal anastomosis with colonic reservoir for rectal carcinoma. *Br J Surg* 1986; 73: 139–41.

11. Pena JP, Gemlo BT, Rothenberger DA. Ileal pouch–anal anastomosis: state of the art. *Baillière's Clin Gastroenterol* 6: 113–28.

12. Holdworth PJ, Johnston D. Anal sensation after restorative proctocolectomy for ulcerative colitis. *Br J Surg* 1988; 75: 993–6.

13. Utsunomiya S, Iwama T, Imago M, Matsuo S, Sawai S, Yaegashi K *et al*. Total colectomy, mucosal proctectomy, and ileoanal anastomosis. *Dis Colon Rectum* 1980; 23: 459–66.

14. Nicholls RJ, Lubowski DR. Restorative proctocolectomy: the four loop (W) reservoir. *Br J Surg* 1987; 74: 564–6.

15. Hultén L, Fasth S, Nordgren S, Oresland T. Kock's pouch converted to a pelvic pouch: report of a case. *Dis Colon Rectum* 1988; 31: 467–9.

16. Fonkalsrud EW, Stelzner M, McDonald N. Experience with the endorectal ileal pullthrough with lateral reservoir for ulcerative colitis and polyposis. *Arch Surg* 1988; 123: 1053–8.

17. Wexner SD, Wong WD, Rothenberger DA, Goldberg SM. The ileoanal reservoir. *Am J Surg* 1990; 159: 178–85.

18. Rothenberger DA, Fazio VW, Keighley MRB, Schoetz DJ, Wolff BG. Ileal pouch–anal anastomosis: current controversies. *Perspect Colon Rectal Surg* 1991; 4: 233–64.

Continent ileostomy (reservoir ileostomy)

Jan Kewenter MD, PhD
Department of Surgery, Sahlgrenska Hospital, Göteborg, Sweden

Hans Brevinge MD
Department of Surgery, Sahlgrenska Hospital, Göteborg, Sweden

In this procedure a reservoir for storage of the intestinal discharge is fashioned from the terminal ileum. The outlet from the reservoir is provided with an intussusception valve (nipple valve) and a flush stoma opening is fashioned on the lower anterior abdominal wall. The reservoir has a capacity of around 600 ml and the valve prevents involuntary escape of faeces and gas from the reservoir. The reservoir is easily and quickly emptied by intubation 3–4 times a day. The continent ileostomy provides an alternative to the conventional ileostomy and eliminates the need for an external appliance.

Principles and justification

Indications

The operation may be performed as a primary procedure in conjunction with proctocolectomy for ulcerative colitis, familial polyposis, multiple carcinoma of the colon or after rectal excision in a patient with ileorectal anastomosis for ulcerative colitis. The operation may also be carried out as a second procedure to convert a conventional ileostomy at the patient's request.

If a pelvic pouch is followed by functional failure it can be transformed to a continent ileostomy.

Contraindications

The following patients are regarded as unsuitable for a continent ileostomy.

1. Patients who have had a small bowel resection: 45 cm of the terminal ileum is used in the procedure and serious problems may arise because of biological alteration in the terminal ileum produced by the pouch. Furthermore, should the pouch require excision, the greatly shortened bowel may lead to malabsorption.
2. Patients with Crohn's disease because of the possibility of recurrence in either the remaining small bowel or the reservoir.
3. Patients who are immature or who have low intelligence or psychological instability. Children younger than 10–12 years do not understand the importance of regular emptying and the procedure should be postponed for some years.
4. Patients with fulminating colitis who have undergone panproctocolectomy but who are in poor condition. It is safer to construct a continent ileostomy as a second procedure when the patient has regained full health and requests the operation.

Preoperative

When a continent ileostomy is performed in connection with proctocolectomy no special preparation is needed. Oral fluids are permitted for 2 days before surgery. Mechanical bowel cleansing may be required in patients undergoing colectomy. However, in patients with diarrhoea neither enemas nor other bowel preparations are needed. A patient undergoing conversion from a conventional ileostomy is restricted to fluid only on the day before surgery.

Antibiotics are administered intravenously, starting a few hours before the operation and continuing with daily administration for 3 days.

Operation

Position of patient

The procedure is performed with the patient supine. When proctocolectomy or rectal excision precedes the ileostomy procedure, the lithotomy position is changed and the patient placed supine before the ileostomy procedure is started. This change in position facilitates the operation and may lessen the risk of leg thrombosis. Alternatively, the lithotomy Trendelenburg position may be used throughout.

Incision

1 When the procedure is performed in connection with proctocolectomy, a lower midline incision up to or just above the umbilicus is used. When a conventional ileostomy is converted to a continent ileostomy, a lower midline incision is used and the conventional ileostomy is taken down. The spout eversion is reduced and every centimetre of the distal ileum is saved. The ileostomy opening in the abdominal wall is closed.

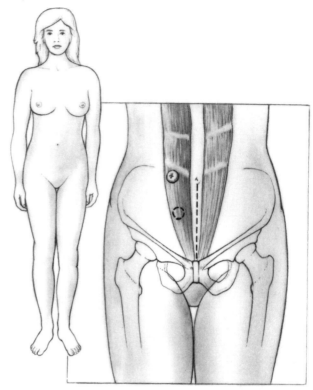

1

Position of gut

In principle the operative procedure is the same whether performed in connection with procto-colectomy or as a conversion of conventional ileostomy to continent ileostomy. In the following text the procedure is described as seen by the operator who is on the left hand side of the patient. It is important to keep this in mind because a number of mistakes can be made if this is not recognized.

2 The terminal ileum is brought out through the wound and placed on the anterior abdominal wall. The gut is formed into a U with the terminal end placed cranially and the bottom of the U to the left hand side of the patient. This positioning of the gut is important, for the later manoeuvres allow the pouch to be positioned in the lower part of the abdominal cavity.

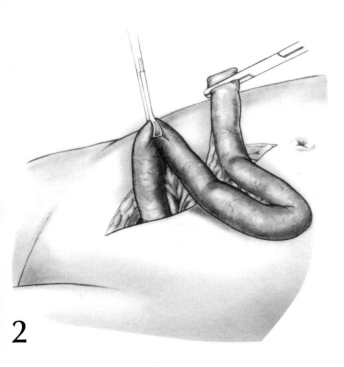

2

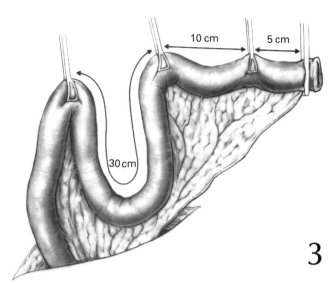

Formation of ileal pouch

3 The terminal 5–10 cm of ileum is used for the outlet. The length of the outlet depends on the thickness of the abdominal wall. Proximal to the outlet, 10–12 cm is preserved for the construction of the nipple valve and the adjacent 30 cm for the reservoir.

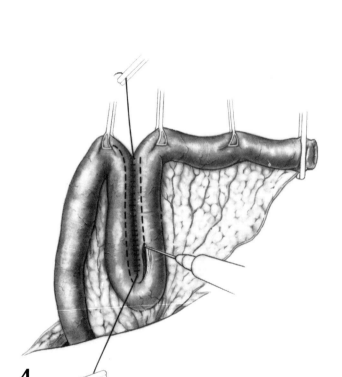

3

4 The antimesenteric border of the U-shaped reservoir segment is sutured with continuous 3/0 absorbable suture. The terminal ileum is positioned cranially.

The U loop is opened along the antimesenteric border on both sides of the suture line with a needle cautery. The incision is extended for 3 cm on the oral limb to separate the outlet from the inlet when the reservoir is formed.

4

5 An absorbable continuous 3/0 suture unites the free edges of the first suture line as a second layer. In the nipple segment the peritoneum and excess fat is removed from a triangular area on both sides of the mesentery, leaving the main vessels intact. This will facilitate the intussusception of the ileum and create adhesions between the mesenteric leaves to preserve the nipple valve.

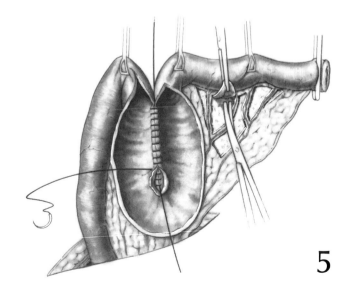

5

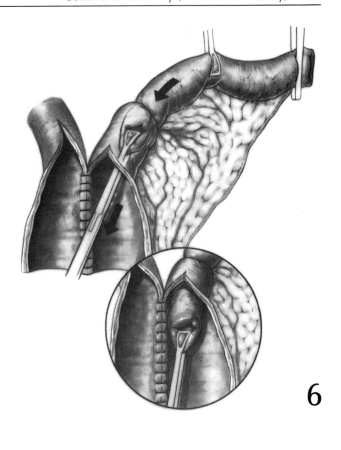

Formation of nipple valve

6,7 By grasping the bowel wall in the middle of the nipple segment through the open lumen, the unsplit nipple segment is intussuscepted into the lumen of the future reservoir. The intussuscepted nipple valve should be approximately 5 cm long. The nipple position is then maintained by the application of four rows of staples, using the 55-mm TA Premium stapler (4.8 mm loading unit). The full length of the arms of the instrument should be used, one on each side of the mesentery and the remainder in the other two quadrants. The most important staples are those at the base of the nipple valve; 8–10 of the 19 staples which are located opposite the opening of the instrument are removed from the loading unit to decrease the risk of insufficient blood supply to the tip of the nipple.

6

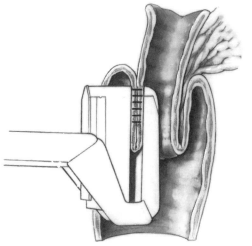

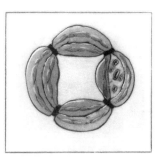

7

Formation of reservoir

8 The open ileal reservoir is folded up and closed by suturing with a continuous, inverted absorbable 3/0 suture. These sutures start at the apex of the future unfolded reservoir and continue towards the corners in both directions. A second seromuscular layer of continuous 3/0 sutures completes the reservoir. One or two layers of interrupted absorbable 3/0 sutures are placed between the reservoir and the outlet around the circumference at the level of the nipple base. These sutures will cover the 'pin-holes' from the staple instrument and fix the nipple base to prevent sliding of the nipple. Special attention is required for the sutures at both sides of the mesentery.

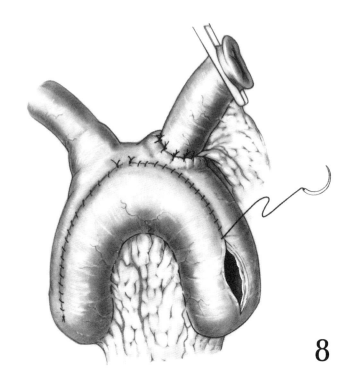

8

Turning and testing the reservoir

9, 10 The corners of the reservoir are pushed downwards between the mesenteric leaves so that the posterior aspect of the reservoir is brought anteriorly. This manoeuvre will allow the reservoir to be positioned in the lower abdominal cavity. After this step the suture lines and the competence of the nipple valve are tested. The afferent ileum is closed with a soft clamp and air is injected into the reservoir by a catheter.

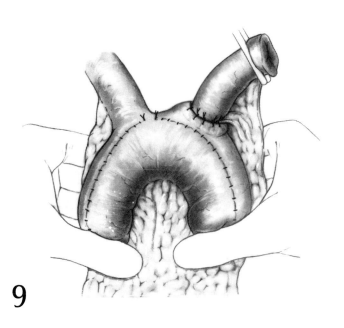

9

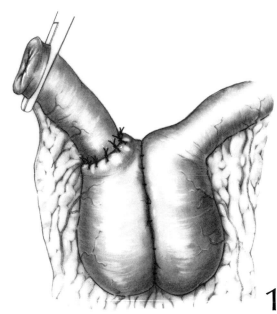

10

Formation of ileostomy channel and securing of reservoir to anterior abdominal wall

11, 12 An opening is made in the skin at the site chosen for the ileostomy. The ileostomy opening is made at a lower and more medial site than is usually chosen for conventional ileostomy. The external fascia is split and a channel is made with the finger through the rectus abdominis muscle and the peritoneum. This channel should pass through the rectus muscle and not at its lateral border as for a conventional ileostomy. The peritoneum around the inner opening of the channel is excised and the rectus muscle is split at the cranial side of the opening to give space for the mesentery supplying the nipple valve and outlet. The inner opening should admit at least two fingers, to prevent compression of the blood vessels supplying the outlet.

The reservoir is positioned with its bottom down in the abdominal cavity and the afferent ileum medially. It is important that kinking of the afferent loop into the reservoir is avoided. Interrupted 3/0 non-absorbable sutures are placed from the lateral aspect of the reservoir to the lateral margin of the split anterior sheet and tied. After the terminal segment of ileum has been pulled through the channel, the medial aspect of the reservoir is sutured to the rectal muscle, also by interrupted sutures. These sutures anchor the reservoir to the inside of the abdominal wall. This step is important because it prevents the creation of a pocket in the outlet in which the emptying catheter can get stuck. It is important to establish that the catheter can easily be introduced into the reservoir after it has been anchored to the abdominal wall.

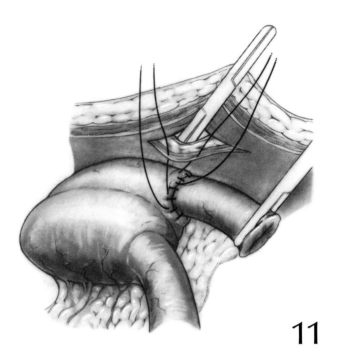

11

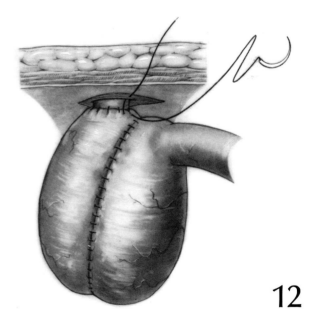

12

Stoma construction

13 Without stretching the outlet, excess terminal ileum is resected by dividing the ileum 1–1.5 cm above the skin level. The intestine is sutured to the skin with mucocutaneous monofilament sutures.

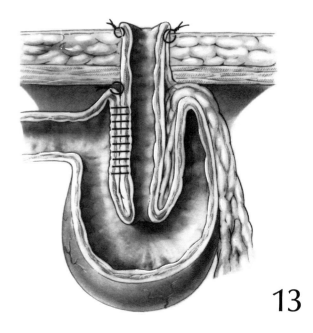

13

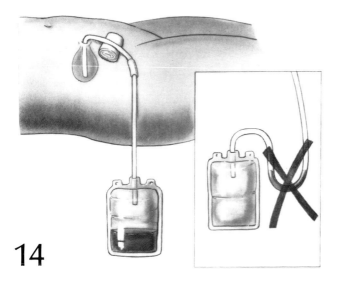

14

Insertion of drainage catheter

14 Before the abdominal wound is closed, a 28-Fr lubricated ileostomy catheter is introduced into the reservoir and anchored with sutures to the abdominal skin so that the tip of the catheter is positioned at the bottom of the reservoir. A protective loop ileostomy is sometimes advisable, especially when this procedure is being performed for the first time. The loop can be closed 4–6 weeks after primary surgery. The abdominal wall is closed and the catheter is connected to a wide-bore tube draining into a bag.

Postoperative care

General principles for management after intestinal operations are followed. Intravenous fluids and electrolytes are administered until the flow of intestinal content through the ileostomy catheter is well established, generally on the third to fifth day, when oral intake is started. Nasogastric suction is not generally used.

Most patients can leave hospital 7–10 days after surgery, after they have been carefully instructed about further postoperative follow-up. The patient is readmitted 27–28 days after operation for 1–2 days, when the catheter is removed and the patient taught how to empty the reservoir.

Management of ileostomy catheter

On postoperative days 1–14 continuous drainage is used. Irrigation with 30 ml saline should be performed every third hour until the flow of intestinal discharge is well established; thereafter three times a day. On days 14–21 the catheter should be clamped for 1-h periods daily, but with continuous drainage at night. From days 22–27 the catheter is clamped for 2-h periods daily but continuous drainage continues at night. On day 28 the catheter is removed. The reservoir is emptied every 3 h during the day and once at night. The time between emptying is gradually prolonged and nightly emptying omitted until ultimately catheterization is performed 3–4 times during the day.

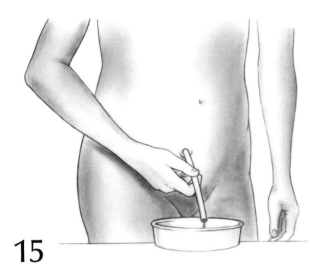

15

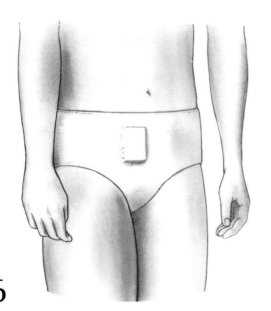

16

15, 16 Before patients leave hospital they are instructed to empty the reservoir at least three times daily and to wash it out at least once daily. Indigestible materials such as fruit skins, mushrooms, peanuts, etc. may block the catheter holes; these are cleared simply by withdrawing, cleaning and reinserting the catheter. Most patients do not require any special diet. The patients are provided with 28-Fr ileostomy catheters, a 60-ml plastic syringe and small pads to cover the ileostomy. The same catheter is used for 1–3 weeks and then discarded.

Complications

Early complications

With careful technique and proper postoperative management leakage from suture lines is unusual. Should a leak occur with peritonitis, laparotomy and repair are required. A diverting proximal loop ileostomy is wise in such cases. If a faecal fistula to the skin surface develops, the reservoir should be continuously drained and the patient fed parenterally. If the fistula persists, surgical repair may be necessary. A proximal loop ileostomy may be advantageous. Necrosis of the exit conduit or nipple valve caused by strangulation of the vascular supply may occur but does not generally need immediate surgical intervention. For proper function of the ileostomy, revisional surgery may be necessary later.

Late complications

These include sliding of the nipple valve, detachment of the pouch from the abdominal wall, fistula through the base of the valve, stomal hernia, prolapse of the nipple valve, stoma stricture and inflammatory changes in the reservoir. These complications occur at varying time intervals after the operation and lead to different degrees of ileostomy malfunction.

1. Sliding of the nipple valve leads to incontinence and difficulties in insertion of the catheter. The complication requires surgical revision by laparotomy.
2. Detachment of the pouch from the abdominal wall can sometimes occur. This results in difficulty in emptying the reservoir, but leakage is unusual.
3. Fistulae can be external, often from the base of the nipple valve to the skin, or internal. This latter fistula is through the base of the nipple and causes incontinence because the contents of the reservoir can bypass the nipple valve. Both types of fistulae necessitate surgical revision.
4. Stomal hernia means that the abdominal opening has widened and the base of the nipple valve, accompanied by the reservoir, is forced into the outlet channel. The configuration of the valve is basically normal.
5. Prolapse of the nipple valve starts with a widening of the inner opening of the outlet channel which leads to eversion of the valve with the tip ultimately delivered through the stoma.
6. Stomal stricture gives rise to difficulties in passing the catheter through the stoma and requires stomal revision.
7. Non-specific inflammatory changes in the reservoir (ileitis) cause diarrhoea with liquid faeces, sometimes containing blood. If the valve is involved in the inflammation the patient may become temporarily incontinent. If the ileitis is severe and long lasting, the patient may become dehydrated and depleted of sodium. Endoscopy reveals an inflamed mucous membrane with contact bleeding and sometimes discrete ulcers. Non-specific ileitis responds to treatment with sulphasalazine or metronidazole. In severe cases, continuous drainage of the reservoir, intravenous fluids and electrolytes may be necessary.

Diagnosis of late complications
For examination of the reservoir and the nipple valve and for diagnosing complications, a small size children's sigmoidoscope or a flexible endoscope should be available. Sliding of the nipple valve, internal fistulae, prolapse of the valve and inflammatory changes in the reservoir may all be diagnosed by endoscopy. Radiological examination after instillation of contrast into the reservoir may also be helpful in some cases.

Revisional surgery

Complications may require surgical revision by laparotomy. The reservoir and its attachment to the abdominal wall are inspected after the abdomen has been opened. The reservoir and the outlet are carefully dissected free from the abdominal wall and mobilized from possible intestinal adhesions. Two sutures are applied on either side of the previous suture line. The pouch is opened and the nipple valve inspected. The cause for the complication is identified.

Correction of nipple prolapse

If eversion of the nipple has occurred, it is usually enough to restaple the existing nipple and anchor the nipple to the inside of the reservoir wall. The channel through the abdominal wall may need to be narrowed.

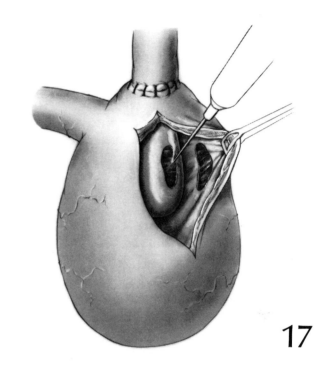

17

Anchoring of nipple tip to reservoir wall

17, 18 The muscular layer at the tip of the nipple valve and a suitable opposing spot of the reservoir wall near the incision are denuded with cautery. The tip of the nipple is then attached by a 55-mm TA stapler to the reservoir wall so that the two areas of denuded muscularis are joined. The reservoir incision is closed and the pouch is sutured to the abdominal wall as described in *Illustrations 11* and *12*.

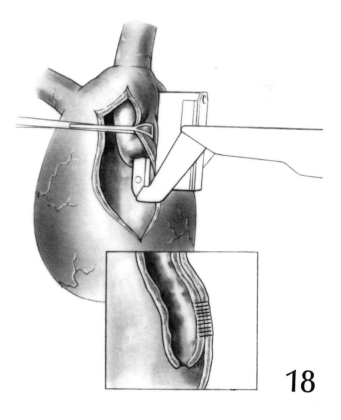

18

Sliding of nipple valve

If sliding has occurred, the existing nipple can usually be used after reduction of the intussusception, provided that the outlet and nipple segment have not been damaged. The nipple valve is reconstructed as shown in *Illustrations 6* and *7* after the mesentery to the nipple segment has been dissected free of its reperitonealization.

Construction of nipple valve of new ileal segment

If the nipple valve and outlet cannot be used at reoperation, or if a pelvic pouch is converted to a continent ileostomy, it is possible to use the reservoir to create a new nipple valve and outlet in two different ways.

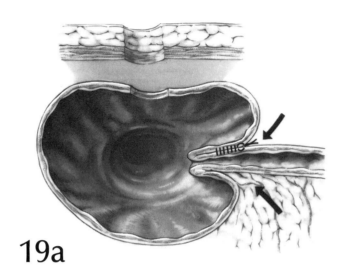

19a

19a–c The existing nipple is removed with its outlet. The intestinal inlet to the reservoir is divided approximately 15 cm from the reservoir at a suitable place, decided by the blood supply. The mesenteric peritoneum of the nipple segment is then removed on both sides, and the nipple segment is intussuscepted into the lumen of the reservoir. The new nipple is constructed in the same way as described in *Illustration 7*. The reservoir is rotated and the oral part of the divided intestine is anastomosed to the place for the former outlet. The reservoir and the new outlet are sutured to the abdominal wall as described in *Illustrations 11* and *12*.

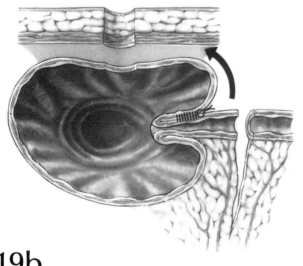

19b

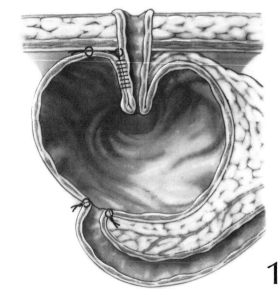

19c

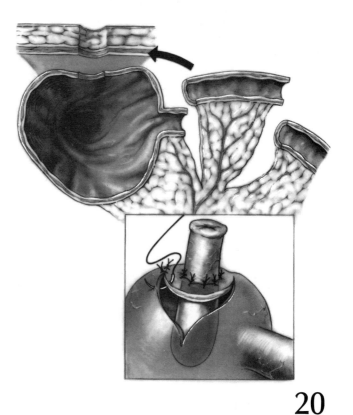

20

20, 21 It can sometimes be difficult or impossible to use the inlet for construction of a new nipple valve. The opening between the afferent ileum and the reservoir can be too narrow or the terminal ileum can be too thick-walled and dilated; this prevents intussusception.

The old outlet and the nipple valve are removed and a suitable segment of ileum is isolated. The peritoneum and excess fat is removed on both sides of the mesentery to the part of the isolated ileum segment that will form the nipple valve. Half of the distal end of the ileal segment is sutured to the pouch with an absorbable suture. A part of the terminal ileal segment is intussuscepted into the reservoir and the nipple valve is constructed as described in *Illustration 7*. The remaining half of the outlet and the pouch is closed with an absorbable suture. The reservoir is sutured to the abdominal wall as described in *Illustrations 11–13*.

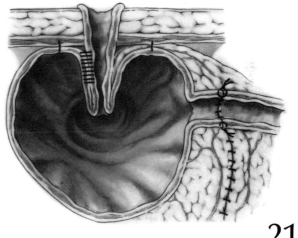

21

Illustrations by Angela Christie

Kock pouch ileoanal anastomosis

Leif Hultén MD, PhD
Professor of Surgery, Surgical Department II, Sahlgrenska Hospital, University of Göteborg, Göteborg, Sweden

Background

Several designs for reservoir construction have been on trial to improve results after proctocolectomy with ileoanal restoration.

Experimental studies suggest that both pouch capacity and pouch motility pattern may be functional determinants, not only for evacuation frequency, but also for continence. Thus, pouch design might have an important impact on ultimate clinical result. There is clinical evidence to show that the S-shaped reservoir attains a larger capacity than the J-shaped pouch, is associated with a significantly lower defaecation frequency, and possibly with better continence. However, the W configuration has been reported to be superior to both the J and S pouches. The favourable expansion properties of the S-shaped pouch have been ascribed to a greater degree of outflow resistance, while the spherical form of the W pouch is considered to be an advantage in providing the greatest volume for any given length of ileum. Whether differences in ultimate pouch volume and function are attributable to the specific properties of the pouch types or to the different lengths of ileum used for their construction is not clear: a longer portion of ileum is required for construction of the functionally favourable W pouch; increasing the length of ileum for construction of a J pouch improves the ultimate result; and the functional results of W pouches are less impressive when compared with J pouches constructed from an equal length of ileum[1].

During experiments with substitutes for the urinary bladder, Kock became impressed by a pouch design proposed by Tasker[2]. The motor activity in the two parts of the ileum split and folded according to this technique was considered to result in large volume capacity and relatively low filling pressures. However, in clinical practice high pressures developed at larger volumes and, although patients generally remained continent during the day, leakage usually occurred during sleep. Therefore, to overcome this problem Kock developed the double-folded reservoir design.

Principles

1a, b

Two limbs of distal ileum are placed in a U shape and united by a continuous suture. The limbs are opened on the antimesenteric border and the bottom of the U is then folded upwards along the transverse axis and the reservoir closed.

Kock proposed that such a pouch configuration should have little or no inherent motility as the peristalsis of the reservoir segments was orientated in four different directions. Moreover, the big initial circumference would create good compliance and volume characteristics because a relatively low pressure within the reservoir should create a wall tension that would favour rapid pouch expansion. This double-folded K pouch design subsequently proved its merits in the continent ileostomy and urostomy. Several recent studies comparing K- and J-configurated pelvic pouches suggest that the K pouch yields superior results[3-6].

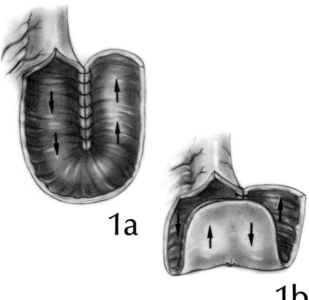

Preoperative

The details of preoperative assessment and preparation are as given in the chapter on pp. 592–604.

Operation

ABDOMINAL PHASE

Position of patient

The patient is placed in a modified lithotomy Trendelenburg position (*see* chapter on pp. 47–50).

Abdominal incision

A midline incision is made from the pubic symphysis to as far above the umbilicus as necessary to give good access and to allow for a careful exploratory laparotomy. A systematic investigation of all viscera should be carried out and the small intestine should be carefully examined and measured.

Bowel mobilization

The technique for colectomy and mobilization of the rectum is standard (*see* chapter on pp. 347–358), but some technical points deserve special mention.

For mobilization of the right colon the parietal peritoneum in the right gutter is incised by diathermy from the caecum to just above the proximal transverse colon. The lesser sac is opened and the greater omentum that is attached to the colon is divided between forceps, saving the gastroepiploic arterial arcade. It appears to be no disadvantage to include the omentum with the colectomy, whereas its preservation will often make the second stage operation time consuming and tedious because of adhesions.

Mobilization of the left colon proceeds as for the right colon, using diathermy for incision of the parietal peritoneum. The colonic vessels are identified (preferably by transillumination) and secured.

The vessels in the ileocaecal area are divided close to the bowel wall and the ileocolic artery is preserved. The ileum is divided close to the ileocaecal valve.

Posterior dissection of rectum

2 The operating table is tilted head-down. A head-lamp is recommended. The superior haemorrhoidal arteries are identified by palpation and/or transillumination. The vessels are ligated and cut at the promontory level, taking great care to identify and sweep back the central root of the presacral nerves.

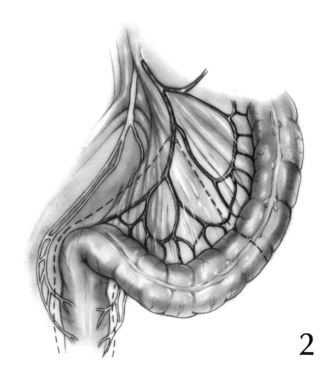

2

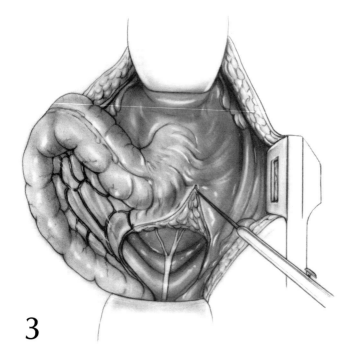

3

3 The presacral space is entered, not by blunt dissection but by cutting the soft connective tissue with diathermy. Using this anatomical plane, the rectum is mobilized posteriorly to the tip of the coccyx, an entirely bloodless manoeuvre allowing the presacral nerves to be clearly identified and safely preserved.

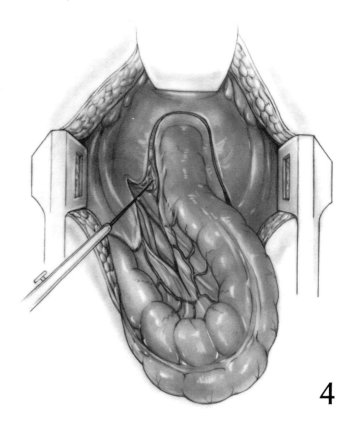

Anterior dissection of rectum

4 With the assistant standing between the patient's legs, a deep pelvic retractor is inserted to lift the bladder forwards. From the point of division of the superior haemorrhoidal artery the peritoneal incision on either side of the mesorectum is prolonged downwards close to the rectum on both sides to meet in the midline anteriorly a few centimetres onto the base of the bladder (or just below the cervix uteri).

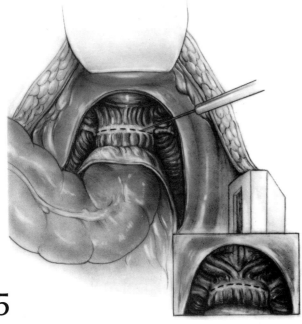

5 The cut is deepened and, by exerting pressure on the retractor, the seminal vesicles are laid bare. The dissection is carried further down to the base of the prostate (or posterior vaginal fornix). Denonvilliers' fascia is incised transversely, exposing the rectal musculature. The use of diathermy makes these procedures virtually bloodless, with perfect exposure of the structures.

The lateral ligaments remain to be severed. There is no need to use clamps because these structures should also be divided by diathermy, keeping close to the rectum and coagulating bleeding vessels as necessary.

Indeed, using diathermy properly requires that only one single vessel is ligated, namely the superior haemorrhoidal artery. In this way the rectum can be fully mobilized down to the levator muscle with perfect exposure and minimal blood loss.

PERINEAL PHASE

6a–c The rectum is carefully washed with chlorhexidine (0.05% solution). A Parks anal retractor is introduced and submucosal injection of adrenaline solution (1:300 000) used to elevate the mucosa and facilitate the dissection (*Illustrations 6a, b*). The mucosa is cored out in four strips, starting at the dentate line (*Illustration 6c*), and is carried to a point a few centimetres above the pelvic floor which has already been reached by the operator, who divides the rectal muscle wall at this level using diathermy. Only a short muscle cuff thus remains. The pelvic cavity is irrigated with chlorhexidine solution and meticulous haemostasis is obtained.

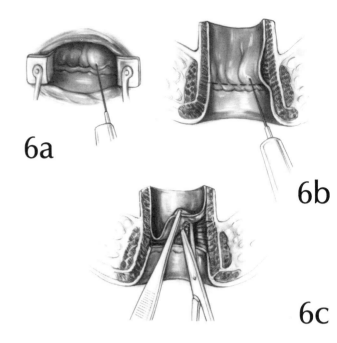

6a

6b

6c

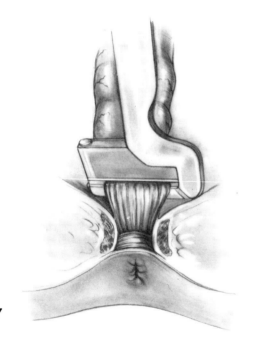

7

7 If mucosectomy is omitted, the rectum is closed with a TA 30 transverse stapler. The level of transection is determined by digital anal examination before firing the stapler and should not exceed 2 cm above the dentate line.

CONSTRUCTION OF RESERVOIR

8 Before constructing the reservoir, the edge of the small bowel mesentery is mobilized up to the duodenum and pancreas to increase the distal reach of the ileum. This is tested by folding the ileum into a J, bringing its apex down to the anal canal by means of a Penrose rubber band passed around the bowel. If the ileum cannot be brought down without tension, multiple transverse incisions in the mesenteric peritoneum and/or division of the ileocolic artery may be required.

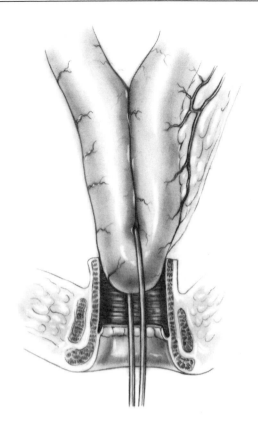

8

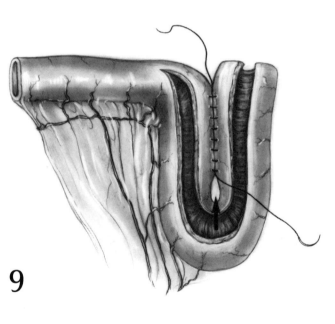

9

9 Two 15-cm ileal segments are sutured side to side along the antimesenteric border with a continuous seromuscular suture of 3/0 polyglactin (Vicryl). The suture is not taken all the way down to the apex of the limb, a finger-wide opening being preserved for the distal pouch anastomosis.

10 The lumen of each loop is opened along the side of the suture line using diathermy, and the intestinal 'plate' is spread out on an operation towel. A second layer of continuous 3/0 polyglactin is inserted through all the layers of intestine from above down to the aperture preserved distally. After being knotted, this last suture is left long and is passed through the inferior opening for future use.

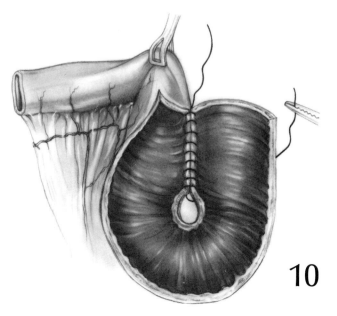

10

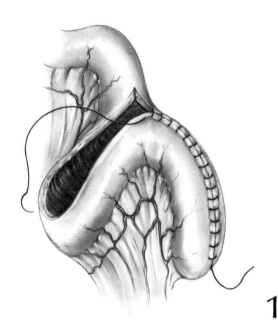

11 The reservoir is formed by folding the intestinal 'plate' upwards along a transverse axis and is closed by suturing the opposing edges with two continuous layers of 3/0 polyglactin.

11

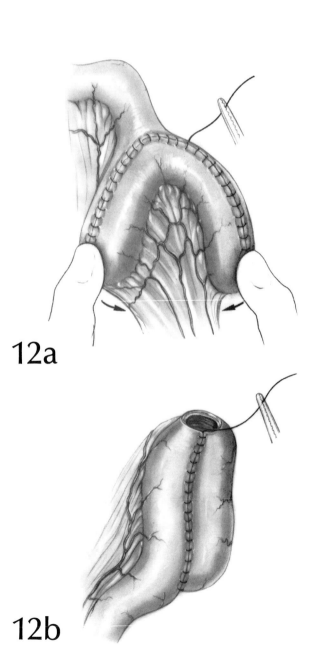

12a

12b

12a, b The corners of the pouch are now pushed inwards between the mesenteric leaves, bringing the posterior aspect of the pouch anteriorly and the opening for the pouch–anal anastomosis distally. The procedure, facilitated by gently pulling the preserved distal suture, is a particularly important step because it increases the distal reach of the pouch, allowing the outlet to be conveniently brought down to the anus for suturing.

POUCH–ANAL ANASTOMOSIS

A Parks anal retractor is inserted through the sphincter, the pelvic cavity is carefully washed from above with chlorhexidine, and complete haemostasis is obtained.

13 The two blades of the retractor are placed anteroposteriorly, allowing exposure of the lateral quadrants of the anal canal. Four interrupted sutures of 3/0 polyglactin are inserted into each lateral quadrant at the pectinate line, a bite of internal sphincter also being taken with each suture. The sutures on the patient's left side are inserted from outside to inside and those on the right side from inside to outside so that the needles can be properly used for the subsequent anastomosis. The sutures are gathered laterally in clamps.

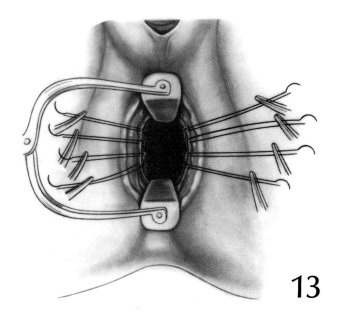

13

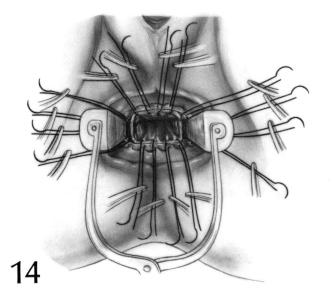

14

14, 15 The anal retractor is then rotated for exposure of the anterior and posterior quadrants. A pair of forceps is passed up through the anal cuff, grasping the suture at the pouch outlet. When it has been properly orientated, the pouch is carefully pulled down in the pelvic cavity and the outlet is taken down through the muscle cuff for suturing.

Four or five interrupted sutures are inserted anteriorly and posteriorly between the full thickness of the pouch aperture and the skin of the anal canal at the pectinate line. To complete the lateral ileoanal suturing, the retractor must be removed. Firm lateral stretching of the perineal skin by the assistant allows these sutures to be safely inserted through the lateral edges of the pouch outlet and knotted without difficulty.

A wide-bore soft Foley no. 24 catheter is inserted into the pouch for postoperative drainage. The catheter is anchored by a silk stitch to the perianal skin, but the balloon is left uninflated.

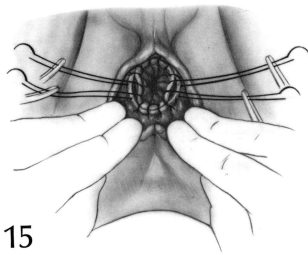

15

16 In patients in whom preservation of the anal canal and its mucosa is considered justified, the pouch–anal anastomosis is accomplished using a Premium CEEA 28 stapler. The cross-stapled top of the anal canal is pierced by the trocar point attached to the instrument shaft (*see* chapter on pp. 74–83).

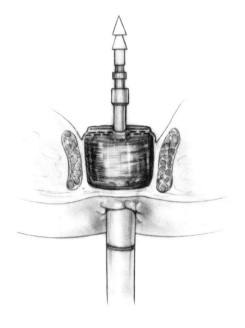

16

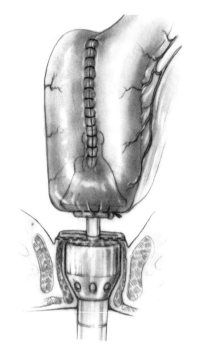

17a

17a, b The anvil is introduced into the pouch (preferably before it has been closed) and the shaft is placed through the pouch aperture. After connecting the instrument and opposing the tissues, the apparatus is fired to establish the anastomosis.

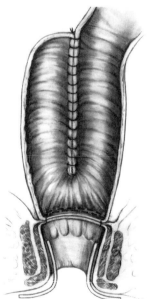

17b

CONSTRUCTION OF LOOP ILEOSTOMY

A 'covering' ileostomy should be used routinely for this operation and its construction deserves special comment. A loop ileostomy constructed under tension will invariably cause problems with retraction as well as other complications. To avoid tension, the loop ileostomy often has to be sited a considerable distance proximal to the pouch so that it can be conveniently

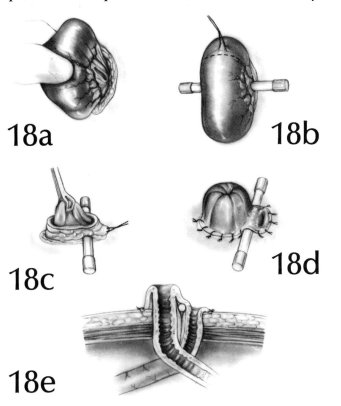

18a

18b

18c

18d

18e

brought out through the abdominal wall. Even if 100 cm or more of ileum is excluded, major problems are rare although ileal fluid losses will increase the need for careful supervision of the stoma. An end ileostomy may sometimes be the alternative. However, the great advantage of a loop ileostomy when compared with an end ileostomy is that the former can usually be closed by a local procedure.

18a–e The loop is turned clockwise so that the future active limb will be located caudad and the distal non-functioning limb superiorly in the wound (*Illustration 18a*). A glass rod should be used to support the bowel (*Illustration 18b*). No anchoring sutures are required. A transverse antimesenteric incision is made superiorly close to the skin level and the wall of the efferent active limb is peeled back and everted, forming a stoma at least 3–4 cm in length (*Illustrations 18c, d*). Mucocutaneous suturing gives good apposition (*Illustration 18e*).

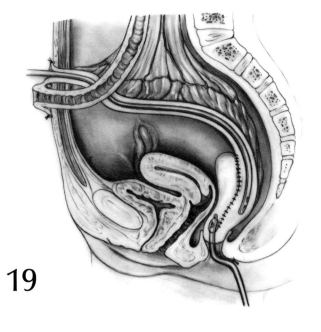

19

19 The ileostomy should be fashioned and completed before abdominal closure (*see* chapter on pp. 243–269). A soft plastic 16-Fr tube is then introduced through the inactive limb and passed down to the pelvic pouch for postoperative irrigation.

Drainage and closure

Before abdominal closure, a Salem sump drain is inserted through a separate incision suprapubically and placed with its tip in the pelvis behind the pouch (15 cmH₂O applied for continuous suction).

A suprapubic bladder catheter is also introduced, preferably by the trocar technique (Cystofix).

A no. 16 Foley gastrostomy catheter is inserted according to the Stamm technique. The balloon is inflated and the catheter carefully anchored to the skin by a stitch.

Postoperative care

General postoperative care is similar to any major pelvic procedure. The reservoir is irrigated with 200–300 ml saline infused daily through the plastic tube. This tube and the Foley catheter draining the pouch are removed on the fifth postoperative day, while the gastrostomy and cystostomy catheters generally remain for 7 days, when the glass rod supporting the ileostomy and the mucocutaneous sutures is also removed.

Before the patient leaves hospital on the ninth or tenth postoperative day, the anastomosis and pouch are examined by endoscopy. This procedure is repeated when the patient is seen 2 weeks later. If there is a tendency towards an anastomotic stricture at this stage, gentle finger dilatation precedes endoscopic examination, after which an 18-mm proctoscope will generally pass. About 8 weeks after operation the patient is taken into hospital for ileostomy closure. A careful manovolumetric study is carried out. Radiological investigation using Gastrografin preferably infused from above through the inactive ileostomy limb is also performed to disclose any leakage or anastomotic defects. Providing that the anastomosis and pouch have healed well, the ileostomy is closed which, in the majority of cases, can be carried out as a local procedure.

References

1. Keighley MRB, Yoshioka K, Kmiot W. Prospective randomized trial to compare the stapled double lumen pouch and the sutured quadruple pouch for restorative proctocolectomy. *Br J Surg* 1988; 75: 1008–11.

2. Tasker JH. Ileocystoplasty: a new technique: an experimental study with report of a case. *Br J Urol* 1953; 25: 349–57.

3. Hultén L, Fasth S, Nordgren S, Öresland T. Kock's pouch converted to a pelvic pouch – a case report. *Dis Colon Rectum* 1988; 31: 467–9.

4. Hallgren T, Fasth S, Nordgren S, Öresland T, Hallsberg L, Hultén L. Manovolumetric characteristics and functional results in three different pelvic pouch designs. *Int J Colorectal Dis* 1989; 4: 156–60.

5. Öresland T, Fasth S, Nordgren S, Hallgren T, Hultén L. A prospective randomized comparison of two different pelvic pouch designs. *Scand J Gastroenterol* 1990; 25: 986–96.

6. Öresland T, Fasth S, Nordgren S, Åkervall S, Hultén L. Pouch size – the important functional determinant after restorative proctocolectomy. *Br J Surg* 1990; 77: 265–9.

Ileoanal anastomosis with ileal reservoir: **S** pouch

W. D. Wong MD
Clinical Assistant Professor of Surgery, Division of Colon and Rectal Surgery, University of Minnesota Medical School, Minneapolis, Minnesota, USA

S. M. Goldberg MD, FACS, FRACS
Clinical Professor of Surgery and Director, Division of Colon and Rectal Surgery, University of Minnesota Medical School, Minneapolis, Minnesota, USA

History

The ileoanal pouch procedure evolved from two concepts: (1) that anal continence could be maintained by preserving the anal sphincters after rectal mucosal stripping; and (2) that anal continence could be enhanced by the addition of an ileal pouch reservoir. Parks and Nicholls in 1978 combined these two concepts and reported the use of a total proctocolectomy with rectal mucosal stripping and a triple-limb ileal pouch with the ileoanal anastomosis, now commonly known as the S ileoanal reservoir procedure[1]. The original S pouch comprised three 15-cm limbs and a 5-cm spout. The main drawback of this initial size of pouch was the need in 50% of patients for the neorectum to be catheterized to evacuate. Several modifications to this reservoir configuration have been made, but the most significant change has been to shorten the spout to 2 cm. This has overcome the need to catheterize, and virtually all patients with a short spout S pouch can evacuate spontaneously. The main advantage of the S pouch over other configurations (e.g. J, W, side-to-side, etc.) has been the additional length afforded to the pouch, making it the easiest pouch to extend down to the anus.

Principles and justification

Indications and contraindications

Chronic ulcerative colitis and familial adenomatous polyposis are the main indications for the ileoanal reservoir procedure, although it has also been applied to patients with severe constipation and associated megarectum. Absolute contraindications are Crohn's disease and significant anal incontinence. Patients with indeterminate colitis may be offered a pouch procedure and generally achieve satisfactory results. Relative contraindications include advanced age (over 65 years) and obesity. Patients with fulminant colitis with sepsis and/or perforation, toxic megacolon, severe malnutrition, shock and immunosuppression may best be managed by a staged approach with subtotal colectomy and ileostomy followed by a restorative ileoanal procedure as a second stage. Patients with a confined colorectal malignancy where long-term curability is likely may still be considered for an ileoanal pouch operation, but most cancers, particularly in the rectum, would preclude a pouch procedure.

Preoperative

A full mechanical and antibiotic bowel preparation is carried out in patients capable of tolerating such preparation; intravenous fluids are administered as indicated. The site for the temporary ileostomy is marked by a stoma care nurse. Once general anaesthesia has been induced, a Foley catheter is inserted and the lower extremities are placed in thigh-high cycled pneumatic compression stockings. The rectum is suctioned clean of faeces through a proctoscope, and the severity of the rectal mucosal involvement is noted. The abdomen and perineum are shaved and prepared in the usual manner.

Operation

Position of patient

The patient is placed in the modified lithotomy position (as described in the chapter on pp. 47–50).

Incision

A midline incision is made and the peritoneal cavity is entered. Abdominal exploration is performed, the wound margins are protected with moist laparotomy sponges, and a Balfour retractor with central bladder blade is inserted. The rectosigmoid is isolated and an umbilical tape passed around it; the intestine is occluded by tying the umbilical tape, preventing intestinal contents from progressing into the rectum, thus minimizing the potential for contamination of the lower dissection.

Mobilization of the left colon

The small intestine is eviscerated and protected with a moist laparotomy sponge. The sigmoid colon is mobilized (as described in the chapters on pp. 347–358 and 359–368). As the splenic flexure is approached, the region of the spleen is inspected and any spleno-omental or splenocolic bands are divided sharply using electrocautery or Metzenbaum scissors to prevent inadvertent traction which might result in a splenic capsular tear. The peritoneal attachments of the splenic flexure are divided by dissection and exposure with the second and third fingers of the surgeon's right hand below the peritoneal attachments, using the thumb to protect the wall of the intestine. The attachments are thinned by finger dissection and divided by electrocautery. When the thicker, fibrofatty attachments of the splenic flexure are reached, these are clamped and ligated. The dissection is carried along the left side of the transverse colon, and the greater omentum is separated and included in the resection.

Mobilization of the right colon

The peritoneal attachments of the right colon are divided with electocautery. The peritoneum over the distal ileomesentery is likewise divided to allow mobilization of the caecum and terminal ileum into the wound. Similar finger dissection is used to isolate the peritoneal attachments of the right colon and this is also divided after being thinned by finger dissection. The duodenum is carefully identified and protected. The hepatic flexure is thus fully mobilized and thicker attachments of the hepatic flexure are clamped and ligated with 2/0 silk ligatures.

Mobilization of the transverse colon

The transverse colon and mesocolon are mobilized down to the root of the mesentery by entering the lesser sac and dividing several congenital adhesions that are present.

Harvesting the colon

1   A small window is made in the ileomesentery and, using a GIA stapler, the ileum is divided flush with the caecum to preserve as much length as possible. The fold of Treves is divided by electrocautery. The ileocolic and right colic vessels are clamped and ligated with 2/0 silk ligatures. The mesentery is thus divided from right to left incorporating the major vessels, including the middle colic and left colic vessels, as the dissection is carried to the left side. Once the sigmoid colon is approached, the dissection is carried down to the level of the superior rectal vessels. The small bowel is packed into the abdominal cavity and the patient is placed in a slight Trendelenburg position.

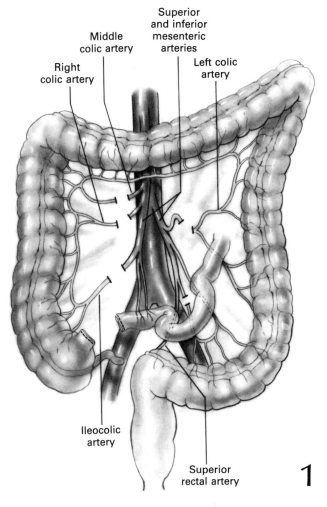

1

Mobilization of the rectum

2   The distal sigmoid colon and rectum are mobilized by a very conservative dissection preserving the main trunk of the superior rectal vessels, thus maintaining the plane of dissection superior to these vessels to avoid injury to the autonomic nerves. The peritoneum on either side of the rectum is scored using electrocautery and the mesorectum is divided anterior to the superior rectal vessels. This requires several applications of Carmault clamps with ligation of the mesorectum using 2/0 polyglycolic acid sutures until all branches of the superior rectal vessels distally have been clamped, divided and ligated.

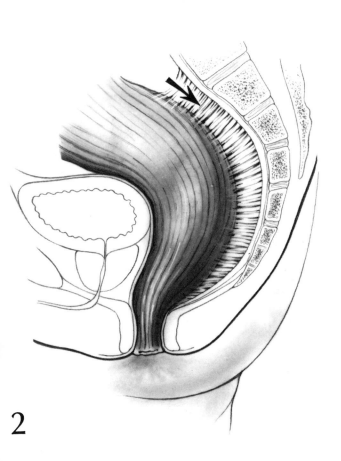

2

3 The dissection is kept as close to the posterior rectal wall as possible and as the mid-rectum is reached the presacral space with its loose areolar tissue is entered. The presacral space is then sharply dissected with electocautery while the rectum is reflected anteriorly and superiorly.

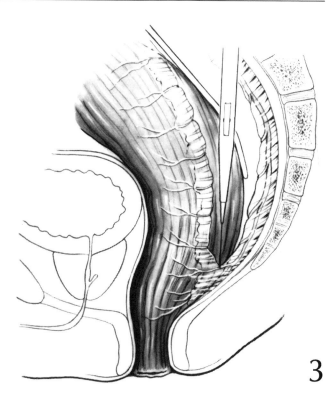

4 The dissection is extended down to the rectosacral fascia which is divided sharply and mobilization to the tip of the coccyx is achieved.

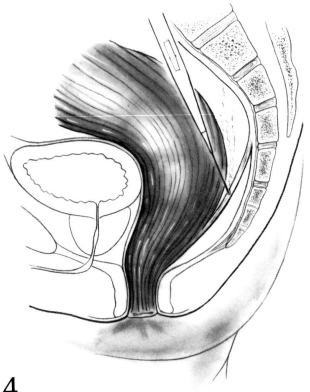

5 The peritoneum over the anterior cul-de-sac is divided and the two laterally scored margins joined. The plane between the rectum, the seminal vesicles and the prostate in men, or the vagina and the rectum in women, is developed by sharp and gentle blunt dissection.

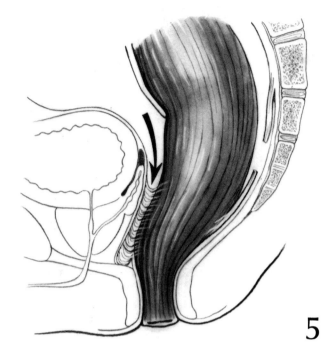

5

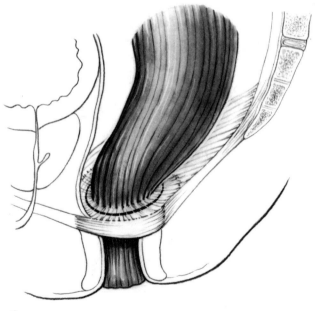

6

6 The lateral stalks are either divided with electrocautery or serially clamped and ligated with polyglycolic acid ligatures. The mobilization and clearance is carried down to the pelvic floor and the levator muscles are exposed.

7 At this point, a decision is made as to whether a rectomucosectomy or a double stapling technique is to be performed. If a rectomucosectomy is chosen the abdominal surgeon can then proceed with construction of the S-shaped reservoir. The length of the ileum is assessed to ensure that it will reach the dentate line without tension once the reservoir is created. This is generally the case if the end of the ileum reaches two fingerbreadths below the pubic symphysis.

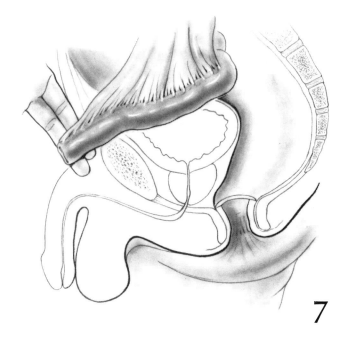

7

8

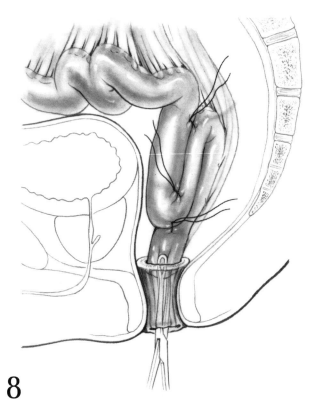

8 If there is any question as to whether the ileum will reach the dentate line, construction of the pouch is deferred until after the rectomucosectomy has been completed. Once this has been accomplished, the S-shaped configuration is held in place with stay sutures and the length of the ileum tested to see if it will reach the dentate line without tension.

Rectomucosectomy

9a–c This dissection is aided by the use of a Lone Star disposable retractor. The submucosal layer is injected with 10–20 ml 1:200 000 adrenaline saline solution, beginning at the dentate line and extending up 4–6 cm. The rectal mucosa is scored at the level of the dentate line circumferentially using electrocautery. The Lone Star retractor is inserted using the hooked elastic retainers to gain exposure. The rectal mucosa is stripped in a cylindrical sleeve fashion beginning at the dentate line posteriorly and progressing circumferentially centimetre by centimetre until the mucosa has been dissected from the underlying circular muscle to a level just above the anorectal ring where the rectum has been previously mobilized from the abdominal approach.

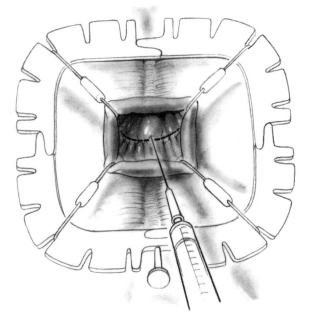

9a

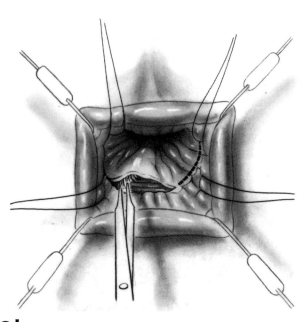

9b

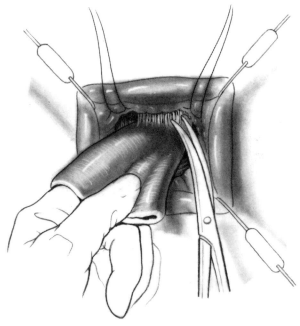

9c

10,11 A purse-string suture of 3/0 chromic catgut is placed in the distal mucosal sleeve which is then pushed into the proximal rectum. This manoeuvre tents the rectal muscular wall which is then divided circumferentially using Metzenbaum scissors or electrocautery. The specimen is then removed by the abdominal surgeon. The pelvis is irrigated and the fluid allowed to wash out through the perineal opening.

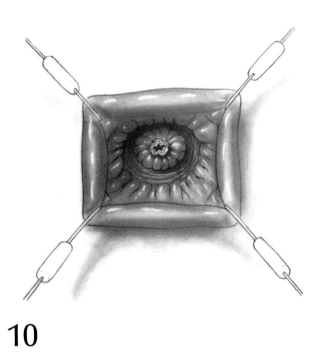

10

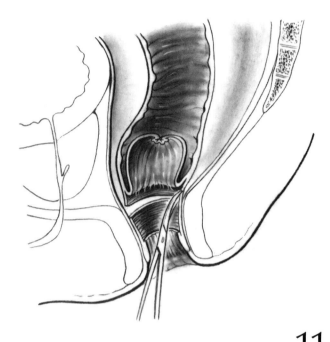

11

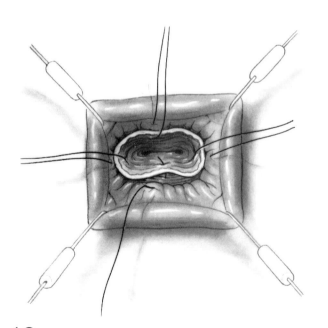

12

12 Four stay sutures of 4/0 polyglycolic acid are placed in the four primary quadrants incorporating anoderm and underlying internal sphincter muscle in the anterior, posterior and left and right lateral locations. These will be used at the time of the anastomosis.

Construction of the S pouch

13 The key to gaining sufficient length for the pouch to reach the dentate line is in adequate mobilization of the mesentery of the ileum. The ileocolic vessels are isolated, clamped and ligated just distal to their origin from the superior mesenteric vessels. The marginal vessel to the terminal ileum is preserved and the mesentery that is supplied by the ileocolic vessel is removed. Small portions of tissue are incorporated in ligating the mesentery to avoid bunching of tissues that shorten the mesentery further. This leaves the terminal ileum supplied solely by the superior mesenteric vascular branch and arcade.

The end of the ileum is drawn inferiorly to ensure that the distal end reaches two fingerbreadths below the pubic symphysis, which will generally ensure that it will reach the dentate line without tension (*see Illustration 7*).

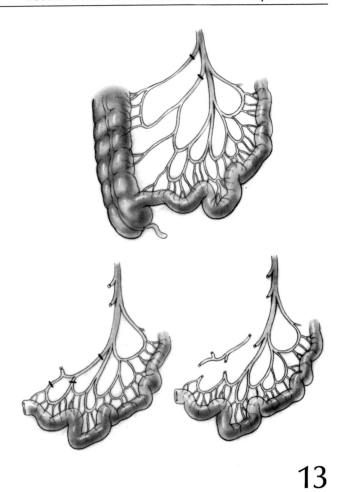

13

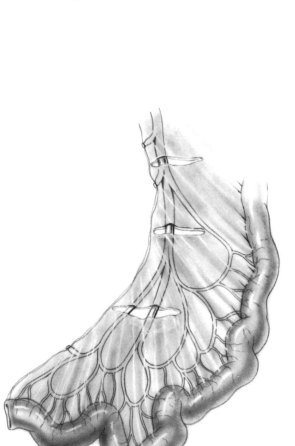

14 If additional length is necessary the peritoneum of the mesentery can be scored transversely at 2–3-cm intervals on both the superior and inferior aspects of the mesentery.

14

15a–c

Once adequate length has been achieved the pouch is constructed. The distal ileum is folded into an S-shaped configuration leaving a 2-cm distal spout and three limbs of 10 cm each folded back and forth in an S-shaped manner. A stay suture of 3/0 polyglycolic acid is placed at either end of the pouch. The wound margins are protected with laparotomy sponges. The proximal ileum is clamped with a linen-shod atraumatic occlusive clamp to prevent contamination of the operative field.

The antimesenteric border of the proximal and middle limb is opened by electrocautery. Residual ileal contents are irrigated to minimize contamination. At the U-shaped corner where the proximal and middle limbs reverse direction, the antimesenteric incision lines are joined. The posterior wall is sutured using a continuous 4/0 polyglycolic acid suture in a running locked manner beginning at the U-shaped end and continuing proximally. Once the proximal end is reached the suture is tied. The distal 10-cm limb is then opened along its antimesenteric border and the U-shaped junction with the middle limb is opened in a similar manner. The inside margin of the antimesenteric border of the distal limb is then sutured to the remaining border of the middle limb with a continuous running locked 4/0 polyglycolic acid suture through its entire length (*Illustration 15b*).

The anterior closure is performed by suturing the two remaining antimesenteric borders of the proximal and distal limb with a running Connell-type suture of 4/0 polyglycolic acid. This completes the pouch construction. The anterior suture line is reinforced with some interrupted 4/0 polyglycolic acid sutures, particularly at the junction of the spout and the pouch (*Illustration 15c*). The exterior portion of the pouch is irrigated with saline before passing it down into the pelvis.

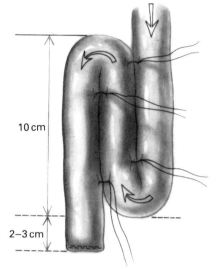

10 cm

2–3 cm

15a

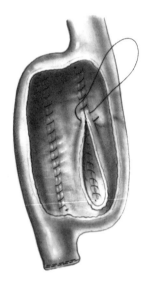

15b

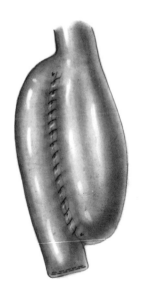

15c

Ileoanal anastomosis

16a, b A ring forceps is passed by the perineal operator into the pelvis and the ileal spout is gently grasped. Downward traction is then applied and the pouch drawn down into the pelvis until the stapled end of the ileal spout reaches the dentate line without tension. This is accomplished with the mesentery positioned either anteriorly or posteriorly. The distal transverse staple line on the ileal spout is excised and the previously placed sutures in the anus are then used to secure the end of the ileal spout in four quadrants. Several interrupted 4/0 polyglycolic acid sutures are placed between the primary quadrant sutures to complete the anastomosis.

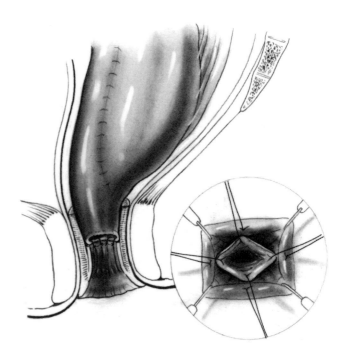

16a

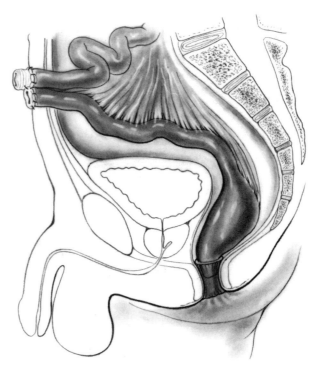

16b

Creation of a defunctioning ileostomy

17 A diverting ileostomy is created approximately 20–30 cm proximal to the pouch by the use of a loop ileostomy or a split ileostomy (as described in the chapter on pp. 243–269).

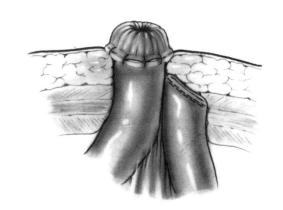

17

Pelvic drainage and abdominal closure

The pelvis is drained transabdominally using a 10-mm Jackson–Pratt drain brought out through a separate stab wound in the left lower quadrant. The abdominal wound is then closed in the usual manner. After abdominal wound closure the ileostomy is completed in a standard fashion.

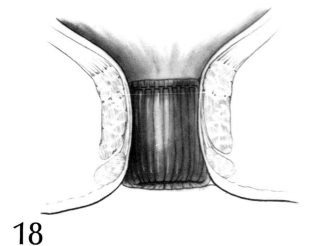

18

Alternative double stapling technique

18 To avoid the rectomucosectomy and any possible stretch injury to the internal sphincter muscle that occurs with it, a double stapling technique may be considered. After complete mobilization of the abdominal colon and rectum, the rectum is transversely stapled just above the levator muscles with a 30-mm or 55-mm linear stapler. After placement of the instrument, the perineal operator inspects the anus and distal rectum to ensure that no more than 1–2 cm of retained transitional mucosa is left. If anything more than this is present a rectomucosectomy is preferred.

19 Construction of the S-shaped ileal reservoir is performed in the manner previously described. Just before completion of the anterior pouch suture line, the anvil and central rod of the circular stapler are inserted into the pouch and the point of the central rod is used to penetrate the end of the ileum just to one side of the transverse staple line. This is then advanced so that the anvil is seated in the ileal spout.

At this point, the perineal surgeon passes the circular stapler, devoid of the anvil, into the anal canal. The central trocar is retracted before placement. The instrument is gradually opened and the trocar thus advanced. It is directed to perforate the distal stump just anterior or posterior to the transverse staple line.

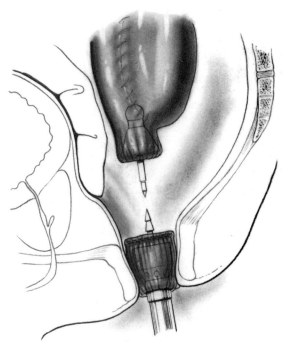

19

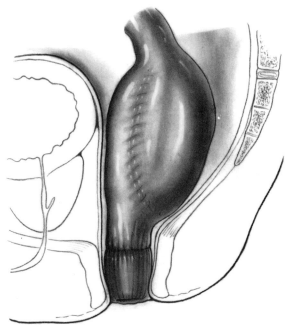

20

20 Once it has been advanced through the apex of the stump, the trocar is removed and the central rod is reattached to the instrument. By closing the instrument, the S pouch is then gradually drawn down into the pelvis and the distal ileal spout is thus anastomosed to the very distal anorectum.

The instrument is opened and gently extracted. The doughnut rings are inspected and the anastomosis checked for haemostasis and integrity. A temporary ileostomy is created as previously described.

Postoperative care

Intravenous steroid coverage and fluid maintenance are administered as required. Postoperative analgesia is obtained either by continuous epidural infusion or by a patient-controlled analgesic pump. Nasogastric suction may be continued in selected instances for 24–48 h. Once ileostomy effluent appears, clear fluids can be initiated, usually 48–72 h after surgery. The Foley catheter is removed on the fourth day after the operation and the Jackson–Pratt drain is removed when the drainage subsides or becomes only serous. The diet is gradually advanced to soft solids 6–7 days after surgery. Once the patient's oral intake is well established, the intravenous steroids and fluids are discontinued and the patient is given oral prednisone, which is then gradually reduced. The patient is generally ready for discharge 7–10 days after surgery.

Outcome

The ileoanal pouch procedure is a satisfactory restorative operation for patients who require total colectomy and who wish to retain gastrointestinal continuity. Mortality has been very rare although morbidity has been moderate. Pelvic sepsis occurs in 5% and can be a devastating complication that may result in ultimate failure. Obstruction of the small intestine remains a very frequent source of morbidity (15–30%) with about one-half of such cases requiring re-exploration and enterolysis. Pouchitis occurs in 20–25% of patients and is seen more frequently in patients with chronic ulcerative colitis than in those in whom the indication for the original operation is familial adenomatous polyposis. Other complications include sexual dysfunction, anal stricture and pouch–anal or vaginal fistulae, as well as the complications that can occur with any major operation. Overall failure is reported in 5–10% of patients. Functional results have been satisfactory.

In a recent review of our own experience at the University of Minnesota, 197 of 250 patients were available for follow-up more than 1 year after operation. The majority of these patients (185) had received an S-shaped reservoir; 88% of patients were able to evacuate spontaneously while 12% required intubation. These latter patients all underwent surgery early in the series and had a long efferent spout. Since shortening of the spout to 2 cm, no patient with an S pouch has required intubation. The mean(s.d.) stool frequency is 7.6(2.5) per 24 h. Major incontinence is rare (2% day, 5% night) but minor incontinence, as defined by faecal or mucous staining not requiring a change of clothes, occurs in 12% of patients during the day and 29% at night; 50% of patients need a pad at night and 38% during the day. Overall patient satisfaction has been greater than 95%.

References

1. Parks AG, Nicholls RJ. Proctocolectomy without ileostomy for ulcerative colitis. *BMJ* 1978; ii: 85–8.

Further reading

Cohen Z, McLeod RS, Stern H, Grant D, Nordgren S. The pelvic pouch and ileoanal anastomosis procedure. Surgical technique and initial results. *Am J Surg* 1985; 150: 601–7.

Nicholls J, Pescatori M, Motson RW, Pezim ME. Restorative proctocolectomy with a three-loop ileal reservoir for ulcerative colitis and familial adenomatous polyposis. *Ann Surg* 1984; 199: 383–8.

Smith L, Friend WG, Medwell SJ. The superior mesenteric artery. The critical factor in the pouch pull-through procedure. *Dis Colon Rectum* 1984; 27: 741–4.

Wexner SD, Wong WD, Rothenberger DA, Goldberg SM. The ileoanal reservoir. *Am J Surg* 1990; 159: 178–85.

Wong WD, Rothenberger DA, Goldberg SM. Ileoanal pouch procedures. *Curr Probl Surg* 1985; 22: 1–78.

Illustrations by Gillian Oliver

Ileoanal anastomosis with ileal reservoir: J pouch

J. Utsunomiya MD
Professor and Chairman, Second Department of Surgery, Hyogo College of Medicine, Mukogawa-cho, Nishinomiya-shi, Japan

History

Terminology and definitions

1a, b The surgical procedure which aims for the total removal of the large bowel mucosa while preserving anal function has been called total colectomy, mucosal proctectomy and ileoanal anastomosis (IAA)[1] or restorative proctocolectomy[2]. These terms should be restricted to an anstomosis of the ileum to the dentate line with mucosa removal, and be distinguished from an operation with an anastomosis near the anorectal line which was previously called ileoanal channelostomy[3] or, more recently, conservative proctocolectomy[4]. The latter procedures do not consistently eradicate all the large bowel mucosa, but because the anastomosis is above the sphincter zone, fewer problems occur with bowel function than with IAA. Therefore, these latter operations can be regarded as variants of very low ileorectal anastomosis (IRA), and the term subtotal proctocolectomy and ileoanal canal anastomosis (IACA) will be used in this text to avoid confusion while discussing the technique of IAA.

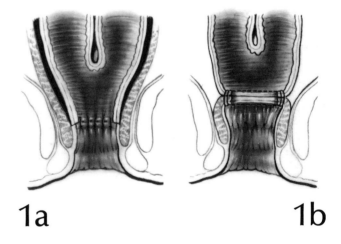

1a **1b**

History of J pouch

2   The initial clinical study on IAA was undertaken by Ravitch and Sabiston in 1947, who reported the first clinical success in patients with ulcerative colitis[5]. Devine and Webb independently performed the procedure using the original technique on patients with familial adenomatous polyposis[6]. In 1952, the overall success rate of IAA without a pouch performed in the USA[7] was 59%. Thus, IAA was not viewed as an acceptable procedure for the treatment of ulcerative colitis or familial adenomatous polyposis because of postoperative bowel dysfunction, technical difficulty and frequent postoperative complications.

IAA supplemented by a pelvic pouch developed from two independent lines of thinking. The first concept involved the collection of intestinal contents in an ileal reservoir, and was initiated experimentally by Valiente and Bacon[8] in 1955, clinically introduced in the form of an abdominal pouch by Kock[9] in 1969, and finally applied as the IAA with S-shaped pelvic pouch by Parks and Nicholls[10] in 1978. The other trend of thought was introduced by Peck[11] who had the idea of replacing the rectal mucosa by a graft of ileum. However, Peck found that the grafted rectum contracted, and therefore created a reservoir by a long side-to-side anastomosis between the grafted neorectum and a segment of ileum at a second laparotomy. Inspired by Peck's idea, the author constructed a similar pouch (later called the H pouch) that was placed within a long rectal cuff. However, this procedure was soon abandoned when it was found that patients experienced problems with evacuation associated with abdominal distension. The same problem occurred in the H pouch developed independently by Fonkalsrud[12] and was solved by shortening the spout. The 'looped pouch' was devised by the author to install a reservoir neorectum located as the natural rectal ampulla with a direct communication to the anal sphincter mechanism, but without creating a spout. This procedure was later called the J pouch, and because patients were found to evacuate easily with less frequency than with other types of pouch, the technique has become the method of choice.

The technical details have evolved in the 177 patients treated so far (49 patients in the Tokyo series and 128 patients treated in the Hyogo series).

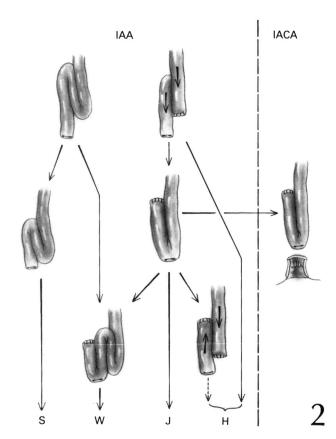

2

Principles and justification

J pouch procedure

3 In the standard J pouch, the superior mesenteric vessels are divided at the terminal trunk to help mesenteric elongation and to preserve the marginal artery to provide bilateral blood flow from both the ileal and the ileocolic arteries. The pouch constructed with bilateral blood supply has a 23% greater blood flow than a short J pouch in which the ileocolic artery is divided.

The portion of the terminal ileum which can reach the dentate line is about 20 cm from the ileocaecal junction. The short form of the J pouch gives a slightly longer reach (by 1–2 cm) than the standard J, but the distal limb of the short J is about 4 cm shorter than in the 20-cm standard pouch[13]. We usually use the standard J pouch because of its superior blood supply and larger capacity. An exception is those patients who have previously undergone total colectomy in which the terminal ileum might have been sacrificed. In Caucasian patients with a fatty mesentery, the short J pouch can be more easily placed in the pelvis.

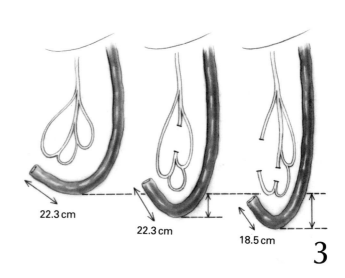

Other types of pouch[14]

The idea of combining the spontaneously evacuable function of the J pouch with the greater capacity of the S pouch led to the development of the W pouch by Nicholls and Pezim[15]. Thus, currently there are four types of pouches in general use: the S, J, W and H types, with the J pouch being reported in 70% of all cases in world literature since 1984. Some studies demonstrated no significant functional differences between the S and J pouches, while other reports conclude that the S pouch has certain slight advantages. The W pouch has been reported to have better bowel function than the J or S types, and this difference was attributed to the larger initial capacity of the pouch (about 300 ml) compared with that of the J pouch (about 200 ml). However, a randomized study revealed that the J pouch was quicker to construct (about 20% less time) and resulted in almost identical bowel function. In our series we have noted that there are functional improvements with the J pouch, even up to 3 years after operation, and conclude that the J pouch is the simplest to construct and functions as well, if not better, than other types of pouch.

Mucosectomy

In IAA mucosectomy is an important component of the operation, but it is the most tedious and difficult part of the procedure. The problem has been to minimize the extent of mucosectomy while preserving anal function.

Lower margin

4 A total mucosectomy starts at the upper border of the dentate line (line *a*) at the top of the columns of Morgagni because function is diminished when the dentate line is removed. An alternative method, starting the mucosal excision above the anal transitional zone (line *b*), remains controversial. In IACA the mucosa and muscle layer are divided at level *c*.

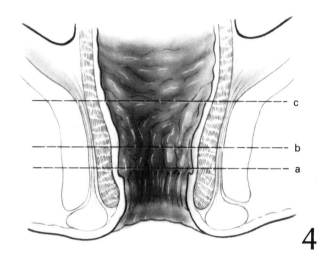

4

Upper margin

5 The rectal cuff is produced after mucosectomy and consists of the muscular rectal stump above the levator muscle and the denuded upper part of the anal canal. The trend has been towards a gradual shortening of this rectal cuff.

Four methods of rectal cuff construction have been developed, according to cuff length.

Long cuff method

The author initially created a muscular cuff of the entire rectum measuring about 15 cm in length in which the resected mucosal layer was to be replaced with the ileal segment or pouch as was originally attempted by Peck[11].

Medium cuff method

This is our method of choice, involving 8–10 cm of the lower rectum, beneath the peritoneal reflection (*see* also 'minimum cuff').

Short cuff method

The long cuff method has been abandoned because of a significant frequency of cuff abscess, long construction time, increased blood loss, technical difficulty and restricted compliance of the pouch in the postoperative period. Thus the short cuff method is currently the most popular and aims to divide the bowel 1–2 cm proximal to the levator ani muscle, leaving the anorectal cuff about 3–5 cm in length with the distal rectal mucosa being removed through the anus.

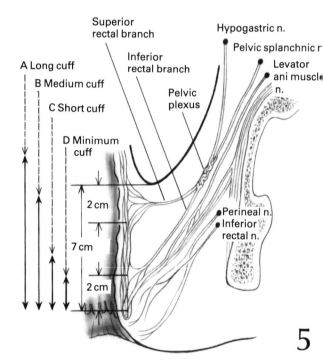

5

Minimum cuff

We have found that, when the rectal stump is totally excised just above the levator ani muscle and the anal canal mucosa is removed, patients were not sufficiently continent and their resting and squeezing anal pressures were reduced when compared with cuffs of a longer length[14]. These differences can be explained on the basis of a more intact innervation in the presence of a longer rectal wall cuff. With a retained but denuded rectal wall, the internal and external sphincters continue to function better by the preservation of the superior rectal branches of the pelvic plexus which enter the rectal muscle wall 2 cm below the peritoneal reflection (medium cuff).

Position of patient

Early in our experience (1978–1982) the operation was started with colectomy, pouch construction and rectal mucosectomy through the abdomen with the patient in the lithotomy position. The procedure was completed by anal mucosectomy and pouch–anal anastomosis through the anus. Since 1982 our procedure has changed and we now start the operation with rectal mucosectomy performed through the anus with the patient in the prone jack-knife position (*see* chapter on pp. 47–50). When this has been performed, the patient is turned and the abdominal phase of the operation continues with the patient supine in the lithotomy position.

It is recognized that damage to the internal sphincter muscles must be minimized to preserve continence, and this goal can only be achieved by meticulous dissection of the anal canal mucosa under the better exposure provided by the jack-knife position. The potential loss of time to allow for the change of operative position can be minimized to about 15 min or less by the involvement of the whole operative team. The blood loss is less with the hips elevated in the jack-knife position and allows, with improved lighting, for a reduction in operative time for this part of the procedure.

Staging the operation

Unlike the recent trend to primary resection for acute obstructive colonic cancer (*see* chapter on pp. 397–415), we do not hesitate to perform IAA by staged surgery to minimize potential dangers that could lead to postoperative morbidity.

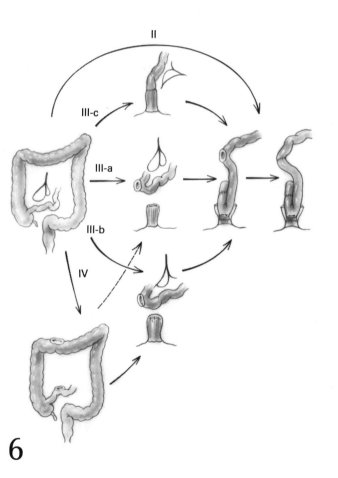

Two staged surgery: IAA with diverting ileostomy

6 In this plan, the anastomosis of the mucosectomized anal canal to the pouch is protected by a diverting loop ileostomy to prevent septic complications which would have long-term deleterious effects on functional results. The omission of the routine use of a diverting loop ileostomy can be considered when the pouch is stapled to the rectal stump above the anal canal (IACA operation). However, we believe that a diverting loop ileostomy is an integral part of the J pouch procedure when associated with mucosectomy.

6

Three or more staged surgery: initial colectomy or ileostomy followed by IAA with diverting loop ileostomy

In patients with ulcerative colitis, IAA has often been performed (80% in our series) in an operation with three or more stages, not only for emergency cases, but also for elective surgery when patients have received long-term steroid treatment or when the patient is nutritionally compromised or when Crohn's disease is suspected. The first stage is total abdominal colectomy, ileostomy and colonic mucous fistula (Schneider's procedure; IIIa). The excluded rectum is always kept open as a suprapubic mucous fistula which is irrigated with steroid-containing solution to reduce mucosal inflammation. The rectal stump is never closed as a Hartmann's operation because the retained inflammation in the rectum is likely to be aggravated by this closed loop situation and may cause pelvic sepsis from stump leakage.

Opening of the mucous fistula is always carried out secondarily to reduce the likelihood of wound infection around the fistula. A loop end ileostomy has been found not to interfere with the later creation of the J pouch when the ileocolic vessels have been preserved in a fashion to be described later in this chapter. If Crohn's disease is confirmed by histology in the resected specimen, the original plan is changed and an ileorectal anastomosis is fashioned.

An initial diverting ileostomy and blow hole(s) in the colon (Turnbull's procedure; IV) to treat severe toxic megacolon is now less frequently used. This is because of greater collaboration with gastroenterologists, who now refer the patient at an earlier stage of disease, and better perioperative care and anaesthesia. An ileorectal anastomosis as the first stage procedure (IIIc) may be indicated for familial adenomatous polyposis and mild cases of ulcerative colitis if the surgeon is not sufficiently experienced in the construction of a pelvic pouch.

Indications

Total mucosal ulcerative colitis

All patients with mucosal ulcerative colitis in whom total colectomy and IRA or colectomy with abdominal ileostomy (AIS) have previously been carried out are candidates for a J pouch (IAA). Major side effects from steroid therapy occurred in 35% of our series, and this association suggests that the timing of surgical intervention in the treatment of this condition should be much earlier than currently practised.

Familial adenomatous polyposis

Patients with familial adenomatous polyposis have a 1% risk of colorectal cancer by the age of 15 years, which rises to a 10% risk at the age of 25 years. By the age of 40 years, the risk is approximately 60%. Prophylactic surgery is therefore justified. Some surgeons recommend an IRA for this purpose because extracolonic tumours (such as desmoid or upper gastrointestinal tract cancers) may cause a lethal outcome more frequently than the risk of death from rectal cancer in the remaining rectal remnant. However, we recommend an IAA because the risk of cancer in the rectal remnant after an IRA has been estimated at 6% during the first 5 postoperative years, whereas the risk of gastric cancer is 2% and for malignant desmoid tumours is also 2%. The J pouch (IAA) provides a functional result similar to that of an IRA, while cancer in a remnant rectum would potentially devastate anal function permanently.

Other indications

Severe constipation associated with megarectum can be treated by a J pouch, but we prefer IACA to IAA because the problem in these patients rests in the muscle layer and not in the mucosa.

A previously performed IRA can be converted to an IAA when the residual rectum becomes dysplastic or is persistently inflamed. Bowel function recovers quickly after the secondary IAA in comparison with that of the primary IAA, presumably because the terminal ileum has already undergone colonization and physiological adaptation to the absence of the colon. Even patients with a Brooke ileostomy or Kock-type abdominal pouch can be successfully converted to an IAA if the anal sphincter has been preserved.

Contraindications

A J pouch (IAA) is contraindicated in patients with Crohn's disease because it involves all muscle layers of the bowel, tends to recur in the intestinal pouch and is often complicated by persisting anal fistulae. For doubtful cases, IAA in three stages is recommended so that the diagnosis may be confirmed on the initially resected colon. Patients with indeterminant colitis might tolerate an IAA, but these patients tend to react similarly to Crohn's disease patients. Internal haemorrhoids and non-Crohn's type anal fistula may not be negating factors if there is little or no sphincter muscle damage from the previous surgery. However, continence disturbance with a reduced maximum pressure ($40 \, mmH_2O$ or less) is a contraindication. Infirm patients (this condition rapidly increases after the age of 70 years) do not adapt well to this procedure and probably should not have the operation carried out.

Subtotal colectomy and ileoanal canal anastomosis (IACA)

Since the circular stapler anastomosis technique has been introduced and, more recently, with the improved Premium CEEA model of stapler becoming available for the double staple technique[16], an anastomosis between the ileal pouch and the upper end of the anal canal without mucosectomy has become popular. This IACA operation provides better continence than the IAA, is simpler and quicker to perform, and also has less risk of anastomotic breakdown. Therefore, the necessity for a covering loop ileostomy has been reduced in these operations. Use of the stapler, however, does not guarantee the total removal of anal canal and lower rectal mucosa, the amount of which varies from 1 to 3 cm above the dentate line. The author does not use IACA for ulcerative colitis or familial adenomatous polyposis because the clinical significance of the retained mucosa with regard to recurrence of the disease and its risk of malignancy is not neglected during the rest of the patient's life. However, the authors do perform IACA for severe chronic constipation with megarectum and hereditary non-polyposis colorectal cancer.

In this chapter, the practical details of our present procedure of IAA with J pouch and medium cuff, which is often performed in three stages on patients with severe ulcerative colitis, is described. However, readers are advised to consult the other chapters in this section which consider additional pouch techniques.

Preoperative

General assessment

Proctological examination is essential to identify anal diseases (haemorrhoid, fistula or fissure) and scars from previous anorectal surgery. Barium enema and sigmoidoscopy associated with biopsy are performed to assess the severity of colitis, the density of polyposis, and the presence of dysplasia or malignant foci. Anal manometry, including maximum resting pressure, maximum squeeze pressure and rectoanal inhibitory reflex, is usually performed. In patients with ulcerative colitis, systemic complications of steroid therapy must be sought, and the extracolonic manifestations and malignancies in patients with familial adenomatous polyposis must be identified.

First stage: colectomy, ileostomy and mucous fistula

Even in an emergency, the proper stoma site must be selected (see chapter on pp. 243–269), but no bowel preparation is carried out to avoid exacerbation of colitis. Broad spectrum antibiotics effective for both aerobes and anaerobes (such as latamoxef sodium) are given intravenously immediately before and during the operation. Increased perioperative steroids are needed.

Second stage: mucosal proctectomy, J pouch–anal anastomosis and diverting ileostomy

This operation is scheduled when the condition of the patient is much improved and a reduction, or preferably a cessation, of steroid treatment has been achieved, which usually requires 2–3 months after the first operation. The rectal remnant is inspected to assess the degree of inflammation, and anal disease and function are assessed. Anaemia, dehydration and nutritional status are investigated and treated as required. All patients with ulcerative colitis who have had previous steroid therapy must be given perioperative steroids.

Patients who are to undergo a primary IAA for familial adenomatous polyposis have orthograde lavage bowel preparation using 400 ml polyethylene glycol solution given orally.

Third stage: ileostomy closure

Three months after pouch construction the IAA is tested by endoscopy and radiographic contrast studies to determine that it is well healed. The maximum resting pressure of the anal canal should have recovered by at least 40% of the preoperative value before the patient is submitted to closure of the loop ileostomy. An enterostomal nurse should help the patient to prepare for perianal sanitation, dietary control, sphincter exercises and the recognition of potential pouch complications.

Operation

First stage: colectomy, ileostomy and mucous fistula

With the patient supine, the abdominal cavity is opened widely with an extended left paramedian incision. The wound is sealed using a plastic sheet (ring drape). The small intestine is *not* placed into an intestinal bag (which is often used in a partial colectomy operation) because the mesentery of the small bowel can be easily rotated, causing intestinal ischaemia with the ileum detached from the colon.

7 After the entire colon has been mobilized from its lateral attachment and gastrocolic ligaments, the ileum is divided close to the ileocaecal junction using a linear cutting stapler, with careful preservation of the ileal branches of the ileocolic vessels.

The entire colon, with the greater omentum attached, is devascularized by dividing the three colic and sigmoid vessels, while preserving the superior rectal vessels. The colon is then exteriorized from the abdominal cavity and removed by dividing the sigmoid colon at a level 2–3 cm above the abdominal surface using a stapling device. (If toxic megacolon is present, the colon is deflated first through a balloon catheter (no. 32) inserted into the transverse colon before starting any manipulation.)

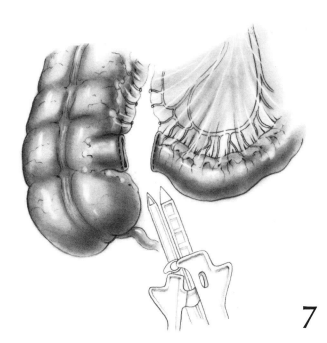

7

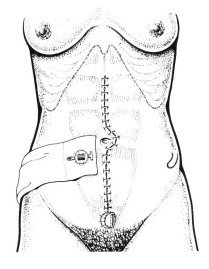

8

8 An end loop ileostomy is then fashioned at the previously marked stoma site using a portion of the ileal loop 10 cm from the distal end (*see* chapter on pp. 243–269). The exteriorized sigmoid colon stump is fixed to the skin with several serocutaneous sutures at the suprapubic end of the incision. The peritoneal cavity is then fully irrigated with a large volume of warmed saline solution. The abdomen is closed using a running suture of 1/0 polyglactin (Vicryl) for the peritoneal layer, a double running suture of 2/0 polypropylene (Prolene) for the fascial layer, and interrupted silk sutures or staples for the skin. No drains are used.

Second stage: mucosal proctectomy, J pouch anal anastomosis and diverting ileostomy

The patient is initially placed in the prone jack-knife position (*see* chapter on pp. 47–50) with the buttocks spread apart using wide adhesive tape.

9 The anal canal is carefully dilated using a paediatric Parks retractor, and the anal orifice is everted by holding the anal edge together with the skin and external sphincter using an Allis' clamp (Glassman model) to expose the mucosal surface of the anal canal. A solution of saline containing adrenaline (1:200 000) is injected submucosally to elevate the mucosal layer, and the mucosa is cut circumferentially using an electrocoagulator at the level of the apex of the pectens which form the dentate line.

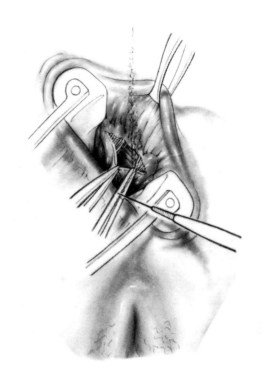

9

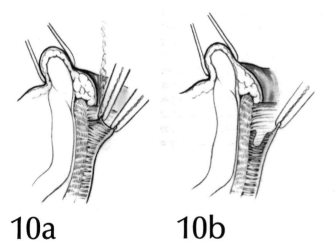

10a **10b**

10a, b While gently holding the cut edge with mucosal forceps (Glassman model), the mucosa is elevated to expose the submucosal connective tissue and bridging vessels. These are severed by picking them up with vascular forceps (Glassman model), and a blended current is introduced from an electrocoagulator. This procedure helps to separate the submucosal layer from the muscular layer selectively and bloodlessly without using scissors or a scalpel (forceps coagulating technique).

11 When the initial circumferential submucosal separation is completed and a mucosal tube of 1–2 cm in length has been created, the intact fibres of the internal sphincter are exposed. Six stay sutures, using 3/0 Vicryl with atraumatic needles, are placed between the perianal skin and the anal margin to include the external sphincter. These sutures will then help to evert the anal orifice and special attention needs to be paid not to damage the internal sphincter. The open end of the mucosal tube is then closed by several fine interrupted sutures. With the mucosal tube gently stretched by tension on the threads, the muscle layer is everted with the aid of muscle retractors to expose the submucosal structures which are gradually separated in a dry field using the forceps coagulating technique. Any small bleeding vessels on the muscle are meticulously coagulated and any holes in the mucosal tube are immediately closed using a fine thread with an atraumatic needle to prevent the holes from enlarging. If the mucosa is completely fused with the muscle, which may happen in the rectum above the anorectal line in patients with longstanding colitis, the superficial fibres of the muscle attached to the mucosal layer are usually removed together with the mucosa.

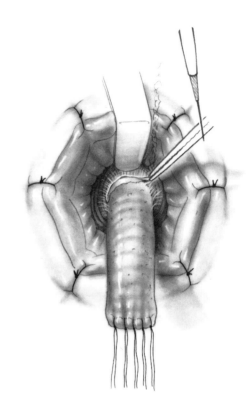

11

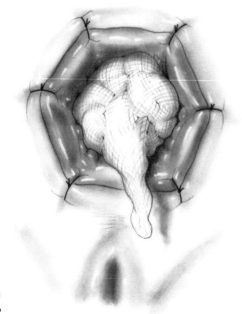

12

12 When the mucosal tube is about 7 cm in length, which is approximately at the level of the seminal vesicles in men and the upper vagina in women, the mucosectomy is stopped and the mucosal tube is ligated to prevent soiling by intestinal contents. The lumen of the denuded anorectal cuff is packed and pushed back with a series of connected gauze sheets to make an additional blunt dissection and to elevate the peritoneal floor.

The patient is then placed in the lithotomy position (*see* chapter on pp. 47–50) to allow simultaneous access to the abdomen and the anus. The position change is performed safely and smoothly by the co-ordinated collaboration between anaesthetists, surgeons and nurses, all of whom are responsible for maintaining lines and tubes and for holding the patient. First, the patient is turned laterally, and then to the supine position onto a stretcher placed to the right of the operating table. The patient is then returned to the operating table in the supine position.

13 The ileostoma and colonic mucous fistula are intitially separated at their junction with the skin and subcutaneous tissue using a cutting electrocoagulator current. The stomas are temporarily closed with several interrupted sutures. The abdomen is then opened through the previous incision, and any peritoneal adhesions, which are usually minimal if the precautions mentioned above have been followed, are carefully dissected. The end loop ileostoma is detached from the abdominal wall by dissecting the peritoneal side, and a clean skin hole is preserved for the diverting ileostomy at the end of the operation.

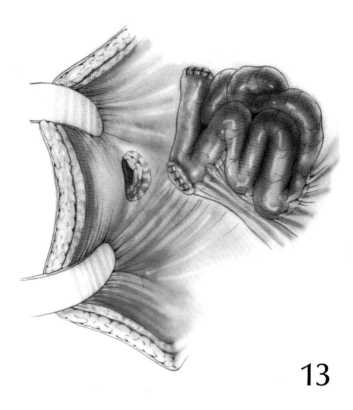

13

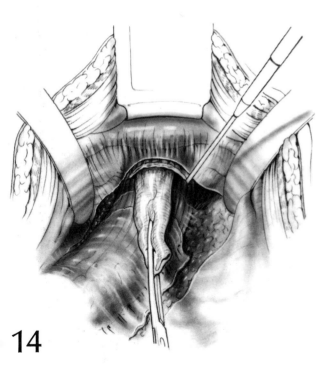

14

14 The distal sigmoid colon and rectum are then separated from surrounding structures, staying as close as possible to the rectal wall to avoid injury to the hypogastric and parasympathetic nerves. The presacral space is bluntly dissected down to the levator muscles and laterally to the lateral ligaments preserving the middle rectal vessels. Anteriorly the peritoneal floor, which has already been elevated by the tamponade effect of the gauze sheets placed in the distal rectum, is opened at its base. The exposed rectal muscle layer is then incised transversely, using the electrocoagulator at the level of the seminal vesicles in men or at the vaginal fornix in women to enter the rectal submucosal space previously created. The gauze packs in the rectum are removed through the abdominal cavity. The rectal mucosal tube is brought out through this anterior opening in the rectum, exposing the posterior inner surface of the rectal muscular wall.

15 The rectal wall is then divided circumferentially to remove the upper rectum attached to the lower rectal mucosal tube. The rectum is thus quickly and bloodlessly removed, leaving a medium sized rectal muscle cuff about 6–8 cm long which is covered by the pararectal pelvic structures. The posterior rectal wall is then cut 2–3 cm longitudinally to enlarge the capacity inside the cuff.

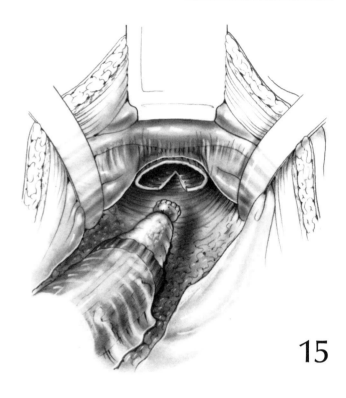

15

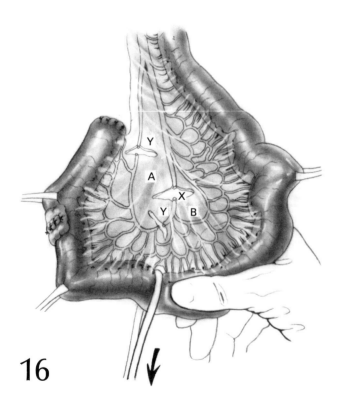

16

16 The ileal mesentery is detached from the retroperitoneum up to the lower border of the duodenum, and the peritoneal sheath covering the superior mesenteric artery is relaxed by several transverse cuts to increase the length of the mesentery. The most inferior portion (the apex) of the ileal loop, which can be brought down to the pubic bone, is carefully selected. At this apex, which is usually found about 20 cm from the ileal end, a Nelaton catheter is inserted through the mesentery for traction. The vessels in the mesentery are examined by palpation and transillumination, and the incision point(s), which can result in a maximal extension of the loop, is determined. This point is usually found on a main trunk of the superior mesenteric vessels (marked X) and forms a vascular connection between the major and minor arcades (marked A and B). The artery and vein are independently divided between double 3/0 Vicryl ligatures, and the avascular area of the mesentery is cut transversely, taking care to preserve the ileocolic vessels. In this fashion, the ileal mesentery can be extended by about 5–8 cm, maintaining a bilateral blood supply both from the ileocolic and ileal arteries to the extended ileal loop (see also *Illustration 4*).

In the event that the ileocolic vessels have been previously divided (as in patients with a past IRA), the ileal vessels should be cut more distally (marked Y) to preserve the terminal mesenteric vascular arcade. Before starting construction of the pouch, the reach of the pouch is tested by a pull-through manoeuvre to ensure that the apex of the loop can indeed reach the anal margin.

17 When the length of the loop is sufficient to provide a tension-free IAA, a side-to-side anastomosis is performed between the limbs of the ileal loop, using two applications of a GIA 90 stapling machine. The stapler is introduced from the opening previously used for the loop stoma on the distal limb and through a small hole created by an electrocoagulator in the opposite ileal limb. The GIA 90 is then fired both distally and proximally to perform the lateral anastomosis.

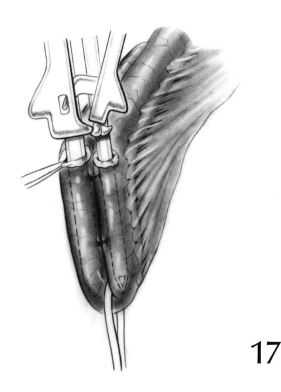

17

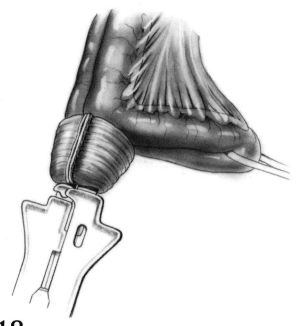

18

18 The stapled suture line within the lumen is exposed by everting the pouch. Any bleeding vessels in the anastomosis are suture-ligated. The holes where the GIA stapler was inserted are debrided and closed transversely by an inverting continuous suture of 3/0 chromic catgut and a continuous seromuscular suture of 4/0 polyglycolic acid. We do not use a TA 50 stapler to fashion an everted closure because, although rare, it can produce an abscess around the suture line which can give rise to sepsis around the pouch. The redundant ileal stump is inverted into the bowel lumen using several seromuscular sutures. This procedure avoids a blind pouch which could give rise to complications.

19 The right side of the peritoneal cavity is emptied by removing all small intestinal loops to expose the mesentery up to the lower margin of the duodenum, thus avoiding bowel rotation. With the patient in the exaggerated lithotomy position, the pouch is brought through the anal canal by pulling down on the Allis' clamps which are attached to the apex of the pouch. The pouch is rotated 180° in a counterclockwise direction to place the antimesenteric side of the pouch against the sacral surface, forming a neorectum similar to the normal rectal configuration. This position also helps to obtain an additional few centimetres of pouch length.

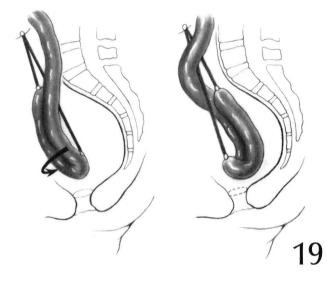

19

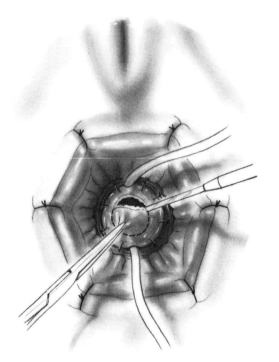

20

20 With the anal orifice already exposed by the six perianal stay sutures, the pouch is anchored to the muscle layer of the anal canal at the level of the anorectal line with approximately eight seromuscular 4/0 polyglycolic acid sutures. The apex of the pouch is then punched out by grasping the bowel wall with a pair of Kelly forceps and cutting a round hole with a diameter of 1.5 cm.

21 The reservoir is directly anastomosed to the anus at the dentate line using 24–32 interrupted atraumatic 4/0 polyglycolic acid sutures. Each suture should incorporate the mucosa of the anal canal, a deep bite of the internal sphincter and the full thickness of the ileal wall. The sutures for the pouch–anal anastomosis are tied after all have been placed so that a uniform distance between each stitch can be achieved. A clean circular anastomotic line will help to promote wound healing by first intention, which is essential to preserve good function. A cardiac surgical suture holder, used for valve replacement, is convenient when performing this anastomosis.

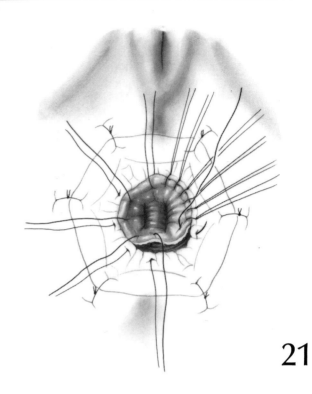

21

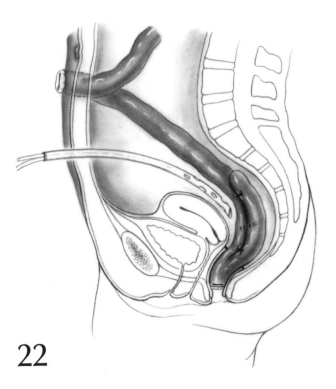

22

22 The most distal loop of ileum which does not cause any tension on the mesentery of the transposed pouch is selected. A Nelaton catheter is then placed through the mesentery for traction and a marking suture is placed to identify the efferent loop. This site is usually 15 cm above the pouch, namely 60 cm from the ileal end. This loop is exteriorized through the abdominal opening used for the previous ileostomy, and a catheter is replaced by a supporting rod. The bowel is then rotated 90° in a counterclockwise direction to place the distal mucous fistula medial to prevent the overflow of mucus into the distal limb of the stoma. The nipple is created (*see* chapter on pp. 243–269). The intestinal loop is never fixed to the peritoneum or fascia; this avoids injury to the intestinal serosa when the stoma is eventually returned to the abdomen.

After the peritoneal cavity has been thoroughly irrigated with saline, a triple sump drain is placed into the presacral area, behind the pouch and then out through the left lower abdominal wall. A stomal appliance attached to a synthetic skin barrier (Varicare system 2) is immediately applied around the stoma. A Malecot catheter (no. 30) is inserted through the anus to decompress the excluded J pouch and to drain the potentially large amounts of serous intestinal fluid that may accumulate immediately after the operation.

Third stage: ileostomy closure

23a–d The patient is given general anaesthesia and the stoma is liberated by incising the peristomal mucocutaneous junction using a scalpel, followed by a cutting electrocoagulator. The nipple is reduced and the opening is temporarily closed by several interrupted sutures. The intestinal loop is completely mobilized from the surrounding subcutaneous fat and fascia by holding the sutured threads. The free peritoneal cavity is entered and the loop is exteriorized for a length of about 5–7 cm. Afterwards, both limbs of bowel are approximated with a suture, and the fork of the linear anastomotic stapler is inserted into each lumen through a stab incision on both limbs of the gut. The stapler is fired to make a side-to-side anastomosis, and the common opening is approximated using a linear stapler. After the fascial layer is sutured, the abdominal wall opening is closed with a subcutaneous purse-string suture using 3/0 Vicryl to minimize the healing area.

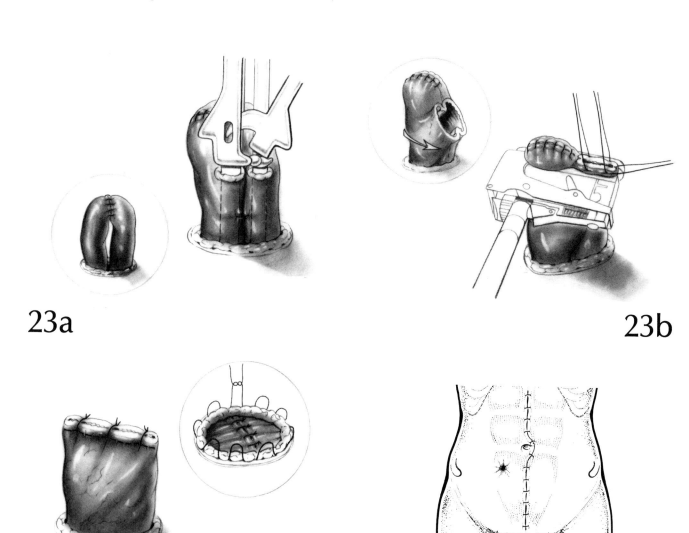

23a

23b

23c

23d

Alternative approach: ileoanal canal anastomosis with J pouch by stapler

24 The first part of the operation is carried out as already described. The distal rectal stump is fashioned by dividing the rectum transversely a few centimetres above the rectoanal line using a rotatable linear stapler (Roticulator 50).

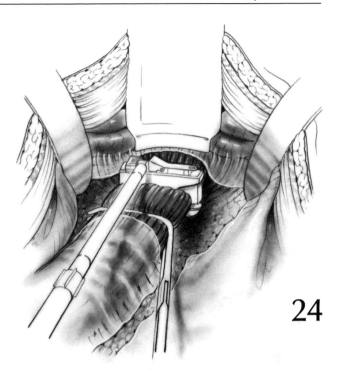

24

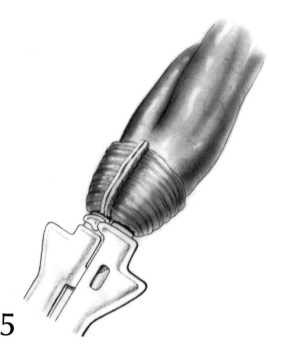

25

25 The pouch is formed by joining the pouch limbs using the GIA 90 inserted through the apex of the bowel.

26 The anvil of the EEA device is then introduced through the opening in the pouch apex and a running edge suture is fixed to the edge using a 2/0 Prolene suture. The body of the stapler is introduced through the anus, which is dilated just sufficiently to allow the stapling device to be inserted. The axis rod is extended to penetrate at the midpoint of the stapled rectal stump on the anterior side. Both lateral edges of the stapled stump are then sutured together onto the rod so that the linear stapler line is totally removed when the EEA stapler is fired. Using this stapling procedure, the J pouch is anastomosed to the rectoanal canal mucosa about 2–3 cm above the dentate line. A diverting ileostomy may not be necessary when the operation is performed by an experienced surgeon.

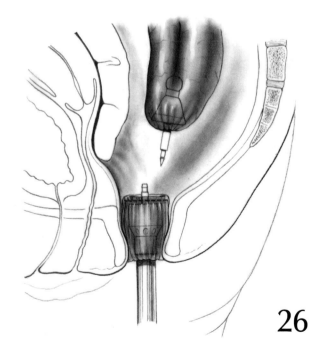

26

Postoperative care

First stage: colectomy, ileostomy and mucous fistula

When the stoma begins to function on the second or third postoperative day, peroral intake is allowed with a gradual increase in the amount and solidity of the food. The closed stump of the sigmoid colon is opened secondarily using an electrocoagulator to create a mucous fistula on postoperative days 5–7, after the abdominal wall has completely adhered to the colonic serosa which seals the wound. The dose of systemically administered steroid is tapered, and the remnant rectum is irrigated daily with 500 ml of saline solution containing 100 mg hydrocortisone and 250 mg metronidazole.

The resected specimen of the colon is carefully examined for the presence of dysplasia, malignancy and Crohn's disease. When the general condition has improved and the steroids have been withdrawn (usually after 3 months), the patient is readmitted to undergo IAA.

Second stage: mucosal proctectomy, J pouch anal anastomosis and diverting ileostomy

No complications

Nasogastric suction is maintained until gradual reduction of gastric drainage confirms that the bowel is beginning to function normally and that the superior mesenteric artery is not obstructing the upper part of the duodenum (superior mesenteric artery syndrome). The transanal catheter in the pouch and the transabdominal pelvic drains are removed on postoperative days 2–5. Ileostomy care is performed as usual. The patient is discharged when recovered and returns to normal social activity.

Early postoperative complications

Cuff abscess An abscess forming inside the rectal cuff between it and the wall of the ileum with the absence of an apparent anastomotic leak usually manifests within 1 month after the operation (the early abscess). The patient becomes febrile, complains of anal pain, notes a pussy discharge from the anus and occasionally has lower abdominal pain and dysuria.

Anoscopy may show a small fistula discharging pus at the anastomotic line. A barium enema might demonstrate a fistula coursing upward from the anastomosis. This complication occurs more frequently (26.0%) when a long rectal cuff is used, but has become rare with a medium cuff (3.9%). Laying open the fistula towards the lumen under local anaesthesia, followed by irrigating the pouch with a solution containing antibiotic agents combined with their systemic administration, may be effective in resolving the problem.

Disrupted ileoanal anastomosis This is a serious complication which might very rarely occur from excessive tension at the suture line (associated with impaired blood circulation to the pouch) or from a fragile ileal wall associated with backwash ileitis. The patient is placed under intensive antibiotic therapy and parenteral nutritional therapy until the lesion becomes stabilized, usually leaving sequelae such as an anastomotic stenosis or a fistula which can then be treated *later* on its merits. In this case, the functional prognosis is pessimistic.

Superior mesenteric artery syndrome This occurs rarely (about 4.3%) and is one of the specific early complications that is caused by excessive tension of the superior mesenteric artery across the fourth part of the duodenum. Patients have excessive belching, prolonged high output drainage from the nasogastric tube, a silent stoma and acute gastroduodenal dilatation on radiography. This complication can usually be successfully treated by returning to effective nasogastric decompression and encouraging patients to turn onto their stomach or side until sufficient elongation of the vessels takes place to allow the duodenum to function.

Transient simple mechanical obstruction is more frequent in patients with familial adenomatous polyposis (43.3%) than in patients with ulcerative colitis (8.3%). An excessive fibroproductive reaction specific to patients with familial adenomatous polyposis may be responsible for this result. All of the general precautions to minimize peritoneal adhesions during operation should be taken.

Intussusception of the proximal ileal segment of the pouch has been reported.

Complications of the diverting ileostomy are discussed in chapter on pp. 292–306.

Urolithiasis A high output of fluid from the stoma may lead to dehydration in about 20% of cases. About 1 litre of intestinal effluent per day is passed, which is six times the normal amount present in faeces and twice as much as from a distal ileostomy. Therefore, urinary volume may be greatly reduced, with a urinary sodium:potassium ratio of 0.8, which is somewhat below the normal limit of 1.0, and there is an increased risk of urolithiasis; this was 1.7% in our series. Loperamide can be administered in an attempt to reduce the faecal output. Bile acid output in the distal effluent with the interruption of the enterohepatic circulation increases eight-fold compared with the four-fold increase found after distal terminal ileostomy. A decrease in serum cholesterol level by 20–30% indicates an abnormal increase in hepatic synthesis of bile acids that may predispose to cholelithiasis; this should be monitored by periodical ultrasonographic examination. Preventive oral administration of ursodeoxycholic acid may be necessary for patients with a longstanding diverting ileostomy. Transient liver dysfunction is often observed during the diverting ileostomy period and this is usually related to this increase in bile acid output.

Third stage: ileostomy closure

An anal catheter is kept in place for a few days to decompress the pouch, which can perforate in patients with ulcerative colitis who have had heavy steroid usage. Watery stools are evident within 48 h of surgery. Patients are advised to evacuate stool as frequently as they wish and to take care of the perianal skin to avoid the development of anal sores. Loperamide is administered orally in doses of 2–3 mg/day.

Bowel dysfunction and management after ileoanal anastomosis

Very frequent liquid stooling and incomplete continence associated with nocturnal soiling and perianal skin irritation seen after IAA is called 'post-IAA bowel dysfunction' and is caused by loss of anal canal mucosa, loss of colonic reservoir and increased amounts of liquid stool. Function gradually recovers during the 12 months after ileostomy closure (the adaptive phase) and then stabilizes (the stabilized phase), as shown in *Figure 1*.

To identify the aetiology of non-recovering bowel dysfunction after IAA, appropriate investigation is essential to analyse the causative components, including maximum resting pressure and maximum squeeze pressure for sphincteric function, pouchography, maximum pouch capacity and distensibility, and amount and viscosity of intestinal contents.

For intractable incontinence, surgical measures are ultimately indicated. Initially, the diverting ileostomy is reopened at the previous stoma site to palliate the problems and to allow time to analyse the patient further. Aggressive diagnostic and therapeutic effort to save the pouch and to maintain function are then attempted.

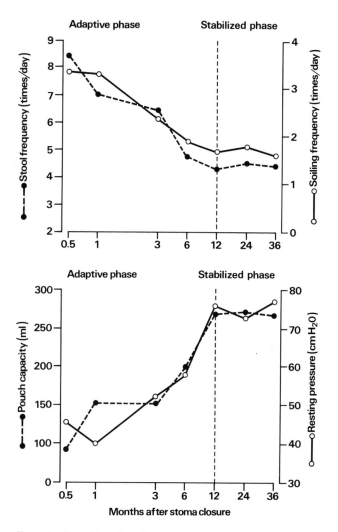

Figure 1   Bowel function after IAA

27 If sphincteric continence is finally abandoned, the metabolically valuable ileum used for the pouch should be salvaged and an attempt made to convert a J pouch to a modified Kock pouch. After the IAA has been carefully detached by meticulous dissection through the anus in the prone jack-knife position, the pouch is dislocated from the pelvic cavity with the patient in the lithotomy position. The nipple valve is constructed using an ileal segment of about 15 cm between the pouch and the diverting stoma. The proximal loop of diverting stoma is then anastomosed to the opening on the pouch apex. The proximal spout of the pouch is fashioned as a flush stoma on the right lower abdomen to create the modified Kock pouch.

Life-long surveillance of patients with familial adenomatous polyposis and ulcerative colitis is strongly advised. Patients with familial adenomatous polyposis should receive yearly endoscopic surveillance of the stomach and duodenum, and examinations for thyroid and desmoid tumours. For patients with ulcerative colitis, systemic manifestation of ulcerative colitis, including pouchitis, should be sought.

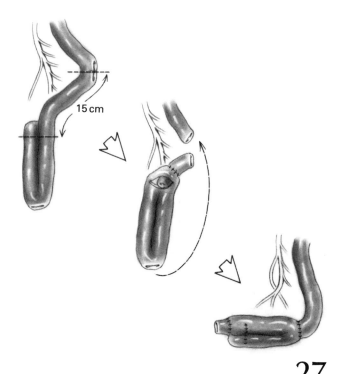

27

Late complications

Pouchitis syndrome

This is a common and important late complication, which is a non-specific inflammation in the pouch and has unknown aetiology. Incidence varies from 10% to 40% in patients with ulcerative colitis and increases with the length of follow-up, whereas this complication has been very rarely found in patients with familial adenomatous polyposis. When the patient complains of malaise, slight fever, increased stool frequency and haematochezia after a period of good bowel function, and when other types of enteritis are excluded, pouchitis is the principal diagnosis. Endoscopy usually shows diffusely fragile oedematous mucosa with multiple erosions or occasionally ulcer. Oral administration of metronidazole usually relieves the syndrome within a few weeks. Steroids may also be effective, but the result is not as definite when they are taken alone. For some cases, hospital management may be required because of diarrhoea, dehydration, malnutrition and anaemia.

Other syndromes

There are several similar syndromes which must be differentiated from true pouchitis. A deep solitary ulcer surrounded by non-inflammatory mucosa in the pouch with similar symptoms can be managed in the same way as pouchitis. If a patient with a stenotic anastomotic ring evacuates mucosal cast, a common aetiology with intractable obstructive enteritis should be taken into consideration. Delayed abscess in the pelvis which can occur around the suture line also manifests as fever, frequent diarrhoea and loss of continence, but may be associated with the peritoneal sign which should then be confirmed by laparotomy. *Salmonella typhimurium* enteritis presents as fever, distended abdomen and diarrhoeal symptoms, and should be differentiated from both pouchitis and intestinal obstruction. Crohn's disease in the ileoanal pouch should also be kept in mind.

Formation of fistulae

Fistulae which can occur from the pouch or the anastomosis to the vagina, urinary tract, vulva or anterior abdominal wall are serious complications that can devastate bowel function. The pouch–vaginal fistula can form after severe pelvic sepsis, and can occur after many months of normal function after ileostomy closure. Repair using the gracilis muscle may be effective (*see* chapter on pp. 758–772).

Sexual functional disturbance

While retrograde ejaculation has not been seen in the series which preserved different lengths of rectal cuff, this has been reported occasionally (9%) in the series with the short cuff (which seems to affect the pudendal nerve).

Late metabolic disorders

Water and electrolytes and bile acid metabolism recover nearer to the preoperative state in patients who have had an IAA procedure than in those who have undergone terminal ileostomy. If iron deficiency anaemia is observed, the Schilling test is performed to identify the blind pouch syndrome associated with bacterial overgrowth in the pouch.

Complications related to steroid withdrawal

After IAA, some patients may start to manifest the steroid withdrawal syndrome with malaise, diarrhoea, fever, anaemia or rheumatoid arthritis.

Outcome

Personal experience by the authors of 177 patients can be divided into two series: the Tokyo series of 49 patients (12 with ulcerative colitis and 37 with familial adenomatous polyposis) that has been followed up since 1978; and the Hyogo series of 128 cases (75 with ulcerative colitis and 53 with familial adenomatous polyposis) that has been followed up since 1983. In the Tokyo series, the operation was successful in 73.5% of patients (58.3% of those with ulcerative colitis and 78.4% of those with familial adenomatous polyposis); in the Hyogo patients, a successful outcome was seen in 92.5% (88.2% of those with ulcerative colitis and 96.9% of those with familial adenomatous polyposis).

References

1. Utsunomiya J, Iwama, T, Imajo M *et al*. Total colectomy, mucosal proctectomy and ileoanal anastomosis. *Dis Colon Rectum* 1980; 23: 459–66.

2. Nicholls RJ, Belliveau P, Neill M, Wilks M, Tabaqchali S. Restorative proctocolectomy with ileal reservoir: a pathophysiological assessment. *Gut* 1981; 22: 462–8.

3. Tosatti E. The ileo-anal-channel-stomy. *Surg Italy* 1973; 3: 201–5.

4. Johnston D, Holdsworth PJ, Nasmyth DG *et al*. Preservation of the entire anal canal in conservative proctocolectomy for ulcerative colitis: a pilot study comparing end-to-end ileo-anal anastomosis without mucosal resection with mucosal proctectomy and endo-anal anastomosis. *Br J Surg* 1987; 74: 940–4.

5. Ravitch MM, Sabiston DC Jr. Anal ileostomy with preservation of the sphincter: a proposed operation in patients requiring total colectomy for benign lesions. *Surg Gynecol Obstet* 1947; 84: 1095–9.

6. Devine J, Webb R. Resection of the rectal mucosa, colectomy, and anal ileostomy with normal continence. *Surg Gynecol Obstet* 1951; 92: 437–42.

7. Best RR. Evaluation of ileoproctostomy to avoid ileostomy in various colon lesions. *JAMA* 1952; 150: 637–42.

8. Valiente MA, Bacon HE. Construction of pouch using 'pantaloon' technique for pull-through of ileum following total colectomy: report of experimental work and results. *Am J Surg* 1955; 90: 742–50.

9. Kock NG. Intra-abdominal 'reservoir' in patients with permanent ileostomy. Preliminary observations on a procedure resulting in fecal 'continence' in five ileostomy patients. *Arch Surg* 1969; 99: 223–331.

10. Parks AG, Nicholls RJ. Proctocolectomy without ileostomy for ulcerative colitis. *BMJ* 1978; ii: 85–8.

11. Peck DA. Rectal mucosal replacement. *Ann Surg* 1980; 191: 294–303.

12. Fonkalsrud EW. Total colectomy and endorectal ileal pull-through with internal ileal reservoir for ulcerative colitis. *Surg Gynecol Obstet* 1980; 150: 1–8.

13. Cherqui D, Valleur P, Perniceni T, Hautefeuille P. Interior reach of ileal reservoir in ileoanal anastomosis. Experimental and angiographic study. *Dis Colon Rectum* 1987; 30: 365–71.

14. Utsunomiya J, Yamamura T. Total colectomy, mucosal proctectomy and ileoanal anastomosis. In: Black GE, Moosa AR, eds. *Operative Colorectal Surgery*. Orlando: Saunders, 1993.

15. Nicholls RJ, Pezim ME. Restorative proctocolectomy with ileal reservoir for ulcerative colitis and familial polyposis: a comparison of three reservoir designs. *Br J Surg* 1985; 72: 470–2.

16. Kmiot WA, Keighley MRB. Totally stapled abdominal restorative proctocolectomy. *Br J Surg* 1989; 76: 961–4.

Ileoanal anastomosis with ileal reservoir: W pouch

R. J. Nicholls MChir, FRCS
Consultant Surgeon, St Mark's Hospital for Diseases of the Rectum and Colon and St Thomas' Hospital, London, UK

History

Restorative proctocolectomy offers total excision of large intestinal mucosa with sphincter preservation. The incorporation of a terminal ileal reservoir is essential to optimize function, and several different designs of reservoir have been described. The outcome of clinical research allows two conclusions: first, capacitance is important (there is an inverse relationship between capacitance and frequency of defaecation); and second, outflow characteristics distal to the reservoir determine whether spontaneous defaecation will occur. Thus, the original S reservoir with a long distal ileal segment which, although of adequate size, often resulted in failure of spontaneous evacuation. This difficulty was largely overcome by reducing the length of the 'spout' or abolishing it altogether as in the J reservoir. However, the J design was often of low capacity. Thus the W reservoir, with its large capacity and better emptying characteristics, was introduced to combine the merits of the S and J reservoirs while avoiding their disadvantages.

The operation can be divided into abdominal and perineal phases. With the exception of the reservoir itself, the technique is common to restorative proctocolectomy in general.

Principles and justification

Indications and contraindications

Patients with ulcerative colitis, familial adenomatous polyposis, and selected cases of functional intestinal disease are suitable. Crohn's disease is a contraindication because the failure rate is high (40% or more). Patients with acute severe colitis should be treated initially with colectomy, ileostomy and preservation of the rectal stump.

The presence of carcinoma is not necessarily a contraindication to the operation. If curative removal of the tumour can be achieved, it is reasonable to undertake operation but disseminated disease is an absolute contraindication. Where the cancer is situated in the rectum, the choice between a restorative or excisional procedure should be based on the same criteria used to decide on either anterior resection or abdominoperineal excision.

Patients undergoing restorative proctocolectomy should receive adequate information on the disadvantages as well as the advantages of the operation. They must know the failure rate, the nature and frequency of complications, and the likely functional outcome. Patients with ulcerative colitis must be informed about pouchitis as a complication.

Preoperative

A complete examination of the large intestine by barium enema or colonoscopy (or both) is essential. The presence of a carcinoma must be known beforehand. In ulcerative colitis, confirmation of the diagnosis by biopsy examination to exclude Crohn's disease should be routine, and the presence of dysplasia will affect the operative technique (*see* below). The patient's general fitness should be assessed and anaemia corrected. A light diet should be taken 2 days before operation, followed by liquids only on the day before the operation. A formal intestinal preparation is not necessary.

A full explanation of the operation should be given and a meeting with a stoma therapist and a patient who has already had the operation should be arranged. The site of a possible stoma is marked.

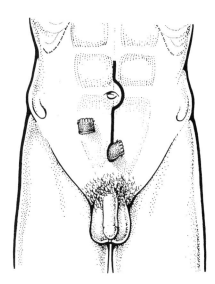

1

Operation

The patient is anaesthetized, and ventilated after tracheal intubation. The bladder is catheterized and electrocardiogram monitoring is established.

The patient is placed on the operating table in the lithotomy position (*see* chapter on pp. 47–50).

The abdomen and perineum are cleaned with an antiseptic skin preparation (aqueous povidone-iodine) and drapes are placed to give access to both.

ABDOMINAL PHASE

Incision

A midline incision is preferable. This gives excellent exposure to the entire abdomen and preserves the skin contour on both sides, permitting the optimal placement of a stoma. The incision should be taken down onto the pubic symphysis to gain full exposure to the pelvis.

1 In patients who have had a previous colectomy with ileostomy and a rectosigmoid mucous fistula, both the ileostomy and mucous fistula are circumcised using sharp dissection and mobilized as much as is possible down to the fascia. Each is then closed by a running suture. The abdomen is re-cleaned with skin preparation and opened through the previous skin incision.

The contents of the abdomen are inspected, paying particular attention to any sign of Crohn's disease in the small intestine.

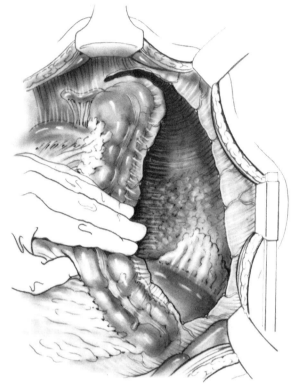

Mobilization of colon (*see* chapters on pp. 347–358 and pp. 359–368).

2 In patients with an intact large intestine, the right colon is mobilized towards the midline, identifying the right ureter and genital vessels. The mesocolon is dissected from the inferior border of the third part of the duodenum.

It is convenient at this point of the operation to divide the intestine. The ileocolic vessels are ligated and branches from the last arcade of vessels in the mesentery are divided to clear the mesenteric border of the terminal ileum just proximal to the ileocaecal junction. The bloodless fold is then removed and the terminal ileum divided between crushing clamps.

The peritoneum lateral to the hepatic flexure is incised and the intestine drawn to the midline by dissecting the mesocolon from the duodenum and head of the pancreas. The right colic vessels are identified and divided.

The surgeon changes to the right side of the patient to mobilize the left colon, safeguarding the left ureter and genital vessels. The peritoneum is incised progressively more proximally towards the splenic flexure to allow separation of the mesocolon from the renal capsule. In ulcerative colitis, the splenic flexure is often drawn down because of shortening which results from the disease and is therefore usually easy to treat. The left extremity of the greater omentum is dissected from the splenic flexure and the flexure is freed after incising the peritoneum laterally and superiorly.

There is no objective information as to whether the greater omentum should be preserved or removed. If preserved, it is dissected from the transverse colon in the avascular plane between the two structures. Adhesions between the omentum and mesocolon are divided.

The vessels supplying the transverse and left colon are then divided. When malignancy or severe dysplasia is present, a radical lymphovascular clearance should be carried out; but when absent, the branches of the middle colic and inferior mesenteric vessels can be divided at points convenient to the surgeon.

2

Rectal dissection

Malignancy absent

In cases with no evidence of malignancy in the rectum, the dissection should be carried out close to the rectal wall in the perimuscular plane. This minimizes both the chance of autonomic nerve damage and the size of the dead space resulting from removal of the rectum.

3 The sigmoid branches of the inferior mesenteric artery are divided close to the mesenteric border of the colon. The first few branches of the superior rectal vessels are then divided at the upper rectal level.

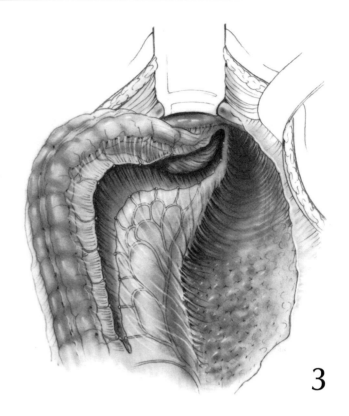

3

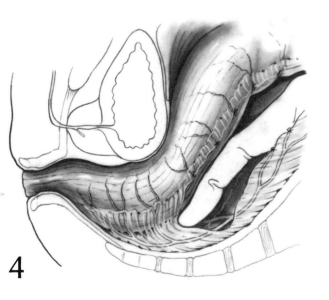

4

4 Beyond this point the superior rectal artery bifurcates, with each branch running down the posterolateral aspect of the rectum. A finger is inserted in the midline immediately posterior to the rectum and, by blunt dissection, an avascular plane between the two branches of the superior rectal artery is developed down the posterior aspect of the rectum.

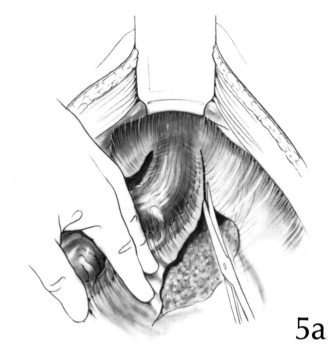

5a

5a, b The peritoneum on each side of the rectum close to its lateral border is then incised longitudinally to the rectovesical or rectouterine pouch. The branches from each division of the superior rectal artery are divided as far as possible distally, either by ligature or diathermy coagulation.

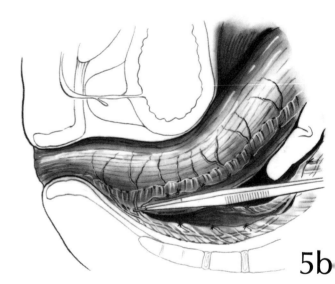

5b

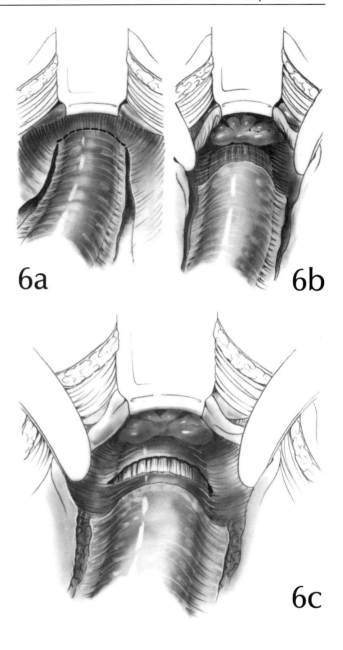

6a

6b

6c

6a–c In men, the peritoneum overlying the base of the bladder is divided transversely in continuity with the most distal points of the two longitudinal peritoneal incisions. A long-lipped retractor (St Mark's pattern) is then placed to elevate the anterior layer of divided peritoneum and, with blunt dissection, the seminal vesicles are identified. These are then mobilized forward from the anterior surface of the extraperitoneal rectum to reveal Denonvilliers' fascia, which is divided transversely at its most proximal point. Further distal dissection anterior to the rectum is then carried out in the plane posterior to Denonvilliers' fascia.

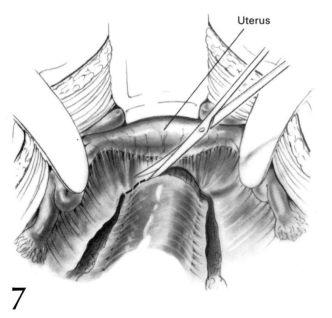

Uterus

7

7 In women, the transverse peritoneal incision is made on the anterior border of the rectum rather than on the vagina. Care is taken to avoid damage to the posterior vaginal venous plexuses. Denonvilliers' fascia can usually be recognized and further dissection is carried out as in men, while maintaining a direct view of the posterior vaginal wall throughout.

8 The branches of the middle rectal vessels become apparent as the mobilization gradually progresses. They are divided close to the rectal wall.

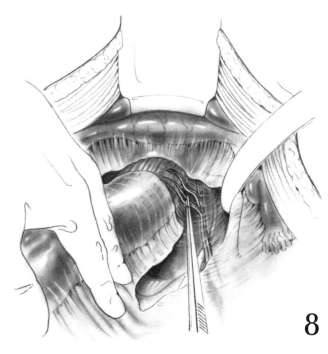

8

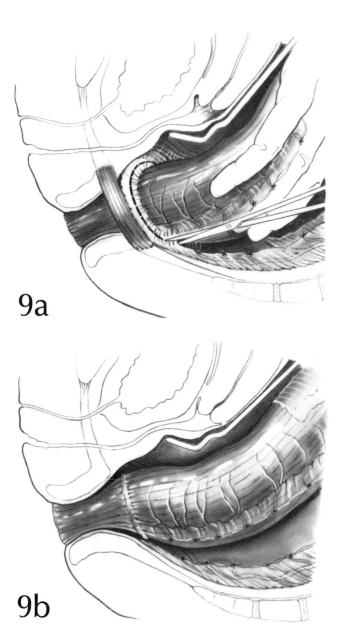

9a

9b

9a, b Below this level the line of reflection of the pelvic fascia covering the levator ani and the side wall of the rectum is often seen. This is a useful landmark because it indicates the most proximal level of the anal canal. The gut is dissected at this point from the levator fascia for a distance of about 1 cm distally. The perimuscular dissection is then complete.

Malignancy present

Dissection of the rectum in the presence of malignancy is identical to that used for anterior resection (*see* chapter on pp. 456–471), and should also be applied in cases of colitis with dysplasia in the rectum, because invasion unrecognized before operation can sometimes be found on histological examination of the operative specimen.

Preparation of rectal stump

It is generally agreed that the gut should be divided at the level of the anorectal junction. A crushing right-angled clamp is placed across the rectum a few centimetres above the proposed level of division.

A perineal operator then cleans the rectal stump below the clamp with gauze swabs soaked in an antiseptic solution (aqueous povidone-iodine) introduced anally.

Sutured ileoanal anastomosis

The level of the anorectal junction can be determined by direct vision or by palpation.

10 In the former case, a perineal operator inserts an anal retractor (e.g. Eisenhammer's pattern) and identifies the dentate line anteriorly. The abdominal operator then pushes the angled point of a diathermy needle through the anterior rectal wall at a point about 2 cm proximal to the dentate line as judged by the perineal operator. The intestine is then divided through the abdomen at this level using cutting diathermy or scissors.

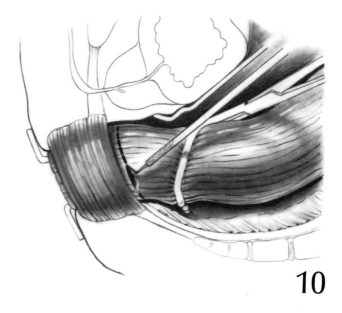

10

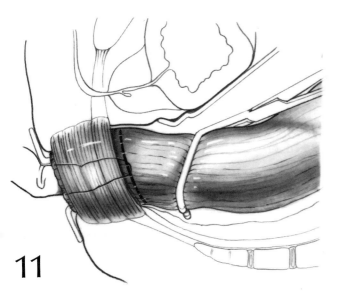

11

11 Alternatively, the tip of an index finger inserted through the anus up to the second interphalangeal joint will be at a similar level.

On dividing the bowel, the surgical specimen is removed. Bleeding from the perimuscular and submucosal vessels in the opened anorectal stump can be brisk and should be secured by diathermy coagulation. A pack is left in the pelvis, firmly applied to the divided stump.

Double-stapled ileoanal anastomosis

12a, b The level of the anorectal junction is determined as described above. A transverse stapling instrument is placed across the intestine at this point. On closing the instrument before firing, care must be taken that all of the intestine is included laterally. In particular, the vagina must be safeguarded by retraction anteriorly.

It is usually possible to use a standard transverse stapler (TA 55), but the pelvis may be too narrow to allow adequate access and then an instrument with rotation in two axes (Roticulator 55 or 30) will be necessary.

After the transverse stapler has been applied, the instrument is fired and the intestine divided immediately proximally. The specimen is then removed.

After previous colectomy

When the rectum or rectosigmoid stump is evident on opening the abdomen, mobilization will proceed as described above. In some cases, however, part of the rectum, along with the colon, will have been excised because some surgeons feel that an intraperitoneal removal of the rectum should be part of the operation of colectomy with ileostomy and preservation of the rectal stump. The surgeon performing a restorative proctectomy may therefore be confronted with the difficulty of finding the rectal stump as a prelude to its removal, although its location is often evident by the presence of scarring just anterior to the sacrum.

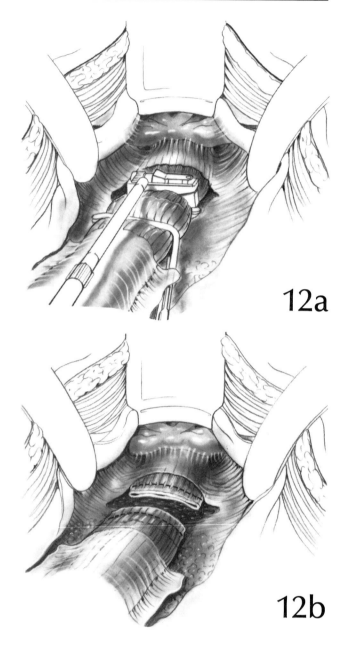

12a

12b

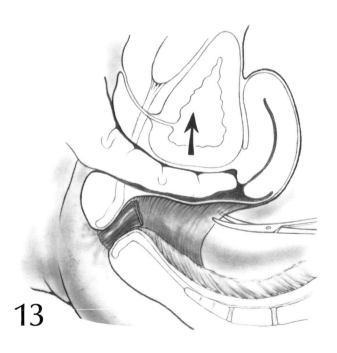

13

13 Dissection should be based on the need to avoid damage to the vagina in women or the urogenital apparatus in men. It is better to open the rectum than to injure the surrounding structures. Before starting, the rectal stump should be cleaned with an antiseptic solution.

The site of the rectum may be made apparent by the simultaneous anal insertion of a finger of the surgeon's left hand. In women, simultaneous vaginal digital examination may be the only way of elevating the posterior vaginal wall anteriorly away from scissor dissection around the rectal stump. With slow dissection, the plane between the rectum and anterior structures will become apparent and further mobilization can be carried out as described.

Mobilization of terminal ileum

Mobility of the terminal ileum to descend to the anal level is a crucial requirement for the success of the operation. The small intestine mesentery is mobilized up to the third part of the duodenum, taking care to identify and safeguard the superior mesenteric vessels. Any intrinsic adhesions within the mesentery should be divided.

14 Where the ileocolic vessels have already been divided, the free edge of the mesentery is incised transversely to within 1 cm of the next branch of the superior mesenteric artery. This will usually produce sufficient mobility.

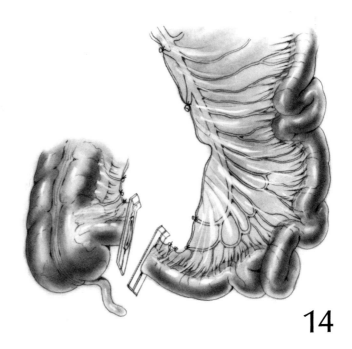

14

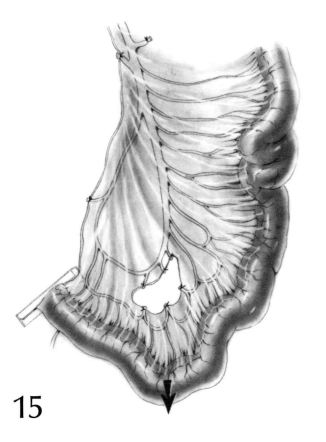

15

15 Some surgeons prefer to preserve the ileocolic vessels, and achieve mobility by division of vessels within the mesenteric arcades nearer to the mesenteric border of the terminal ileum.

Adequate mobility can be confirmed by a trial descent. The pelvic pack is removed and a perineal operator inserts an anal retractor. A stay suture is placed on the antimesenteric border of the terminal ileum chosen to form the ileal component of the ileoanal anastomosis. This will be at the point of greatest mobility determined by drawing the small intestine downwards over the pubic symphysis, and is usually 10–15 cm proximal to the divided intestinal end.

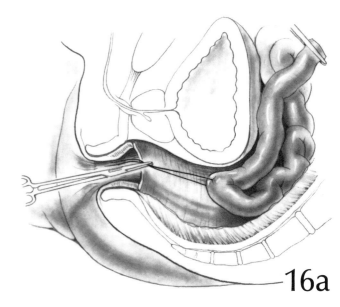

16a

16a–c The perineal operator then advances a pair of long artery forceps through the anus to pick up the stay suture. The forceps are then gently withdrawn, pulling the small intestine downwards through the pelvis into the anal canal. If the apex of the loop of ileum reaches the dentate line, then it will do so subsequently after the reservoir has been constructed. If it does not, further mobilization of the mesentery with division of carefully selected vessels is necessary.

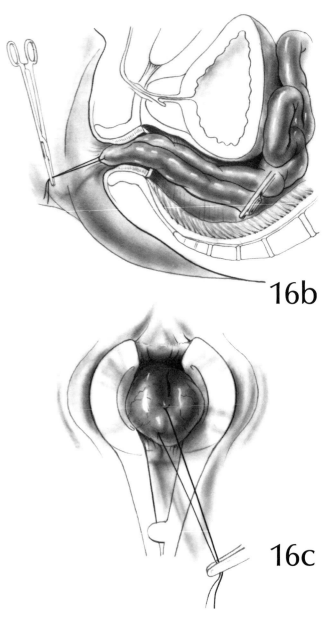

16b

16c

Ileal reservoir construction

The W reservoir is constructed from four loops of terminal ileum, each measuring about 12 cm. The first two and the second two loops are offset by 5 cm.

17 The stay suture at the future site of the ileoanal anastomosis is drawn downwards and the first two loops are approximated with light Babcock forceps.

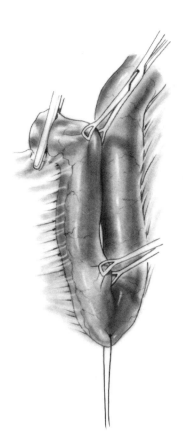

17

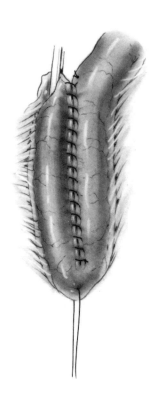

18

18 A continuous seromuscular suture of 2/0 polyglactin (Vicryl) is placed along the antimesenteric border of each loop. This is modified at the line of division of the distal ileum to allow it to be incorporated end-to-side within the reservoir.

19 The third loop is laid along the first two, with its apex about 5 cm more proximal and a second seromuscular suture is inserted.

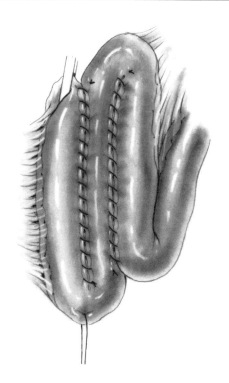

19

20 The fourth loop is then united to the third. All seromuscular sutures are placed close together since the intestine wall between them does not form any useful part of the reservoir.

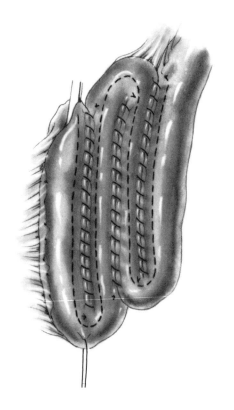

20

21 Packs are placed around the united loops and the intestine is opened between the first two loops using cutting diathermy. A full thickness seromuscular suture is placed along the posterior layer of the opened loops.

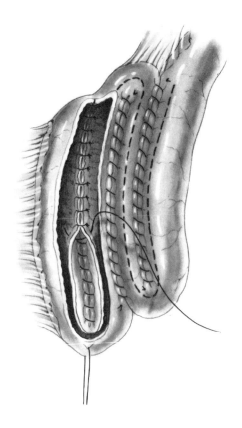

21

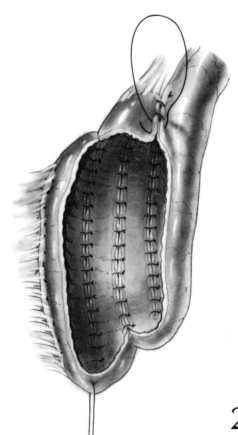

22a–c The third and fourth loops are then opened and sutures in the posterior layer are placed in a similar manner.

The suture between the third and fourth loops is continued onto the anterior surface of the reservoir. Care must be taken not to narrow the lumen of the afferent small intestine.

The anterior layer is sewn to a point which leaves an open end that comfortably takes two fingers. This will serve for the ileoanal anastomosis.

The anterior layer is completed by a seromuscular suture.

22a

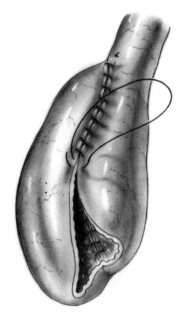

22b

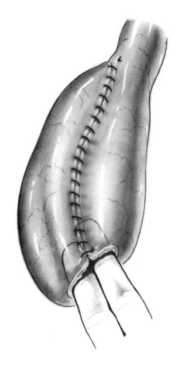

22c

Manual ileoanal anastomosis

23 Two 2/0 polyglactin sutures mounted on a heavy duty 25-mm taper-cut needle are placed at the open end. One suture incorporates each edge of the suture line. The other suture is inserted diametrically opposite. These will subsequently be passed through the pelvis and anal canal to the perineal operator.

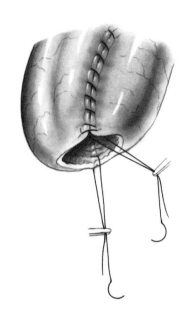

23

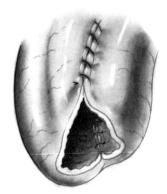

24a

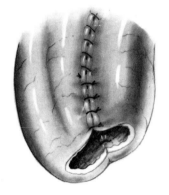

24b

Stapled ileoanal anastomosis

24a, b When a stapled anastomosis is intended, a modification of the anterior layer is necessary. The continuous suture should be terminated about 2 cm shorter than for a manual anastomosis and the remaining part of the reservoir completed with interrupted sutures.

PERINEAL PHASE

Manual ileoanal anastomosis

The perineal operator takes up a seated position facing the perineum. A Mayo table is brought up to the end of the operating table and a skin drape is attached to the leg covers with towel clips. The operating table is adjusted to bring the anus to the level of the surgeon's eyes. A headlight is recommended. Cleaning blood from the operating field is best done by the application of swabs rather than by suction. Long instruments should be used.

An anal retractor is inserted and any obvious bleeding vessels from the divided end of the anorectal stump are coagulated. The abdominal operator simultaneously secures haemostasis in the pelvis. Anal retraction should be gentle and used only when access is needed.

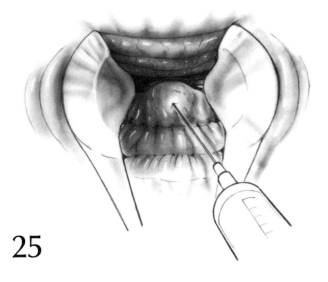

25 An anastomosis just above (5 mm) the dentate line should be planned. A mucosectomy down to this level is necessary. The submucosal plane is infiltrated in the midline posteriorly with a solution of saline containing adrenaline (1:300 000) using a long spinal needle (22-gauge) mounted on a syringe.

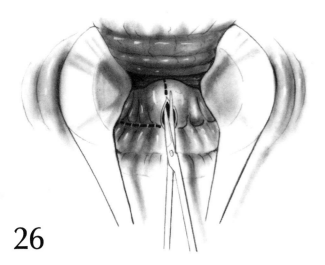

26 A longitudinal incision in the mucosa is made in the posterior midline from the dentate line to its most proximal limit.

27 The retractor is removed and reinserted to expose the right posterior aspect of the anal canal. Further submucosal injection is made and the mucosa is separated from the underlying internal sphincter by sharp scissor dissection.

Miltex scissors (American fistula pattern) are ideal for this manoeuvre. With repeated reinsertion of the retractor and submucosal injection the anal canal is exposed throughout 360° and the mucosa excised to yield a continuous strip of tissue which is sent for histological examination.

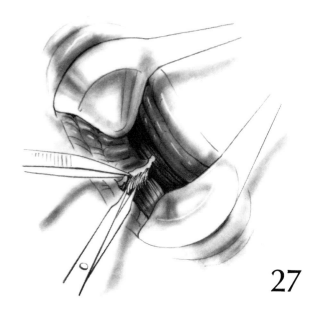

27

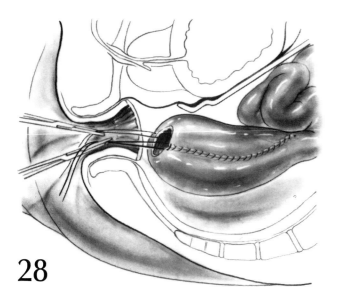

28

28 Two pairs of long artery forceps are then inserted through the anus and their tips advanced into the pelvis. The abdominal operator holds out the sutures previously placed in the end of the reservoir and checks that the mesentery is not twisted. The construction of the reservoir is such that the end suture taking both edges of the anterior layer of the reservoir lies in the left side. The diametrically opposite end suture lies on the right. These sutures are then grasped by the long artery forceps and are drawn down through the anus to the exterior.

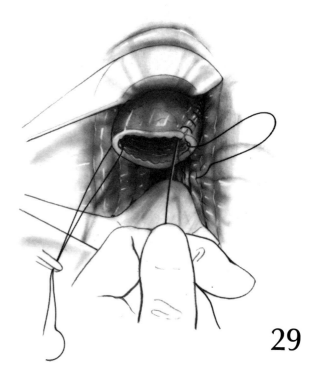

29 The perineal operator then takes the suture corresponding to the left edge of the reservoir in a needle holder. The anal retractor is inserted and the needle is placed through the anal canal epithelium in the left lateral position, taking an ample bite of subepithelial tissue and internal sphincter.

29

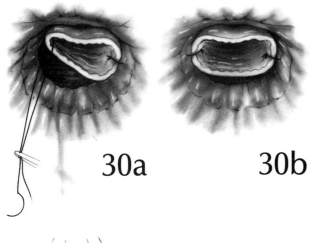

30a   **30b**

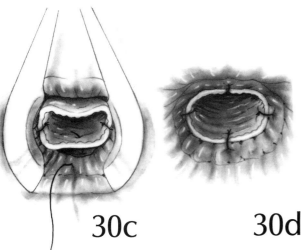

30c   **30d**

30a–d The retractor is withdrawn and the suture is tightened to approximate the left edge of the reservoir with the anal canal epithelium. Apposition judged by palpation is correct when the gap between the two structures can no longer be felt. The suture is tied with four throws and divided.

The suture on the right side of the reservoir is placed through the anal canal in the right lateral position and tied in an identical manner. The anal retractor is reinserted and the field cleared of any blood.

The anterior or posterior (or both) edges of the end of the reservoir will then be seen. The surgeon decides which is more accessible and a suture of 2/0 polyglactin mounted on a 25-mm taper-cut 10 needle is placed between the edge in the midline and the corresponding point of the anal canal.

With sutures now placed at three cardinal points it is easy to insert the retractor directly into the reservoir. This will expose the remaining cardinal point which is sutured.

31 The intervening sectors between the four sutures are then closed in turn. Two to three sutures are usually required for each. The completeness of the anastomosis is tested by palpation and probing using blunt tissue forceps.

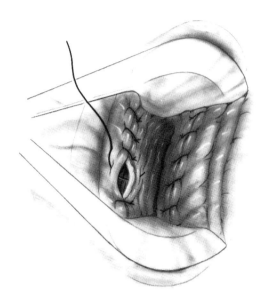

31

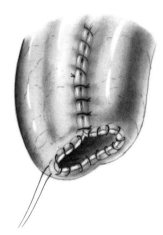

32a

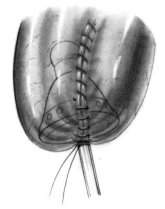

32b

Single-stapled technique for anastomosis

32a, b A purse-string suture using 0 gauge Prolene is placed in the distal anorectal stump in a manner identical to that used in anterior resection. In cases where the stump is inaccessible through the abdomen, the suture can be placed endoanally.

A purse-string suture is placed in the distal end of the reservoir. A circular stapling instrument is inserted through the anus, opened, and the distal purse-string suture tied. The anvil is advanced into the reservoir and the proximal purse-string suture is tied. The instrument is closed, taking care that surrounding structures, especially the vagina, are kept safely away; the apparatus is then fired. The 'doughnuts' are inspected for completeness.

Double-stapled technique for anastomosis

A purse-string suture of 0 gauge Prolene is placed through the end of the reservoir. The anvil, with its trocar having been detached from the circular stapling device, is inserted into the reservoir and the purse-string suture is tied.

33 The head of the instrument is advanced through the anal sphincter, taking care not to rupture the transverse staple line. Counter pressure by the abdominal operator on the closed stump is helpful to avoid damage.

The trocar is advanced through the anal stump just anterior or posterior to the transverse line of staples. The trocar is removed and the anvil is inserted into the head. The procedure is now identical to that used in the single suture technique.

Closure of abdomen

When a defunctioning ileostomy is to be used, the exteriorized ileum should be the most adequately mobile loop nearest to the reservoir.

A drain is placed in the pelvis and is removed 12–18 h later. The abdomen is closed using a mass suture technique.

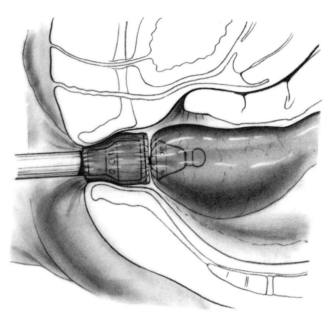

33

Ileoanal anastomosis with ileal reservoir: H pouch

Eric W. Fonkalsrud MD

Professor and Chief of Pediatric Surgery, UCLA School of Medicine, Los Angeles, California, USA

History

During the past 15 years, the endorectal ileal pull-through operation has been used with increasing frequency for patients with ulcerative colitis and polyposis coli. This procedure has the attractive features of curing the disease while avoiding a permanent cutaneous stoma, obviating repeated stomal catheterization as is necessary with the Kock pouch, and provision of a near-normal pattern of defaecation.

During the past decade, almost all surgeons performing the endorectal ileal pull-through have utilized an ileal reservoir to reduce faecal urgency and frequency. The original S-shaped reservoir used clinically by Parks[1] does not provide peristaltic emptying and has a tendency to distend and develop pouchitis. The J-shaped reservoir described by Utsunomiya et al.[2] has the lower end of the pouch at the anus, and thus empties readily. There may be difficulty in achieving sufficient length in the ileal mesentery to allow the side of the ileum to extend to the anus for anastomosis without tension. It is also more difficult to construct a short J reservoir, and to reconstruct the pouch if necessary. Nonetheless, the J reservoir has been used with good success[3].

The lateral isoperistaltic ileal reservoir initially described in 1980 has the two isoperistaltic segments of the reservoir emptying caudally, although it can easily be constructed from a J loop. Furthermore, the end of the spout almost invariably reaches the anus with minimal tension. An end anastomosis of the ileal spout to the anus is easier technically than is the J pouch. The lateral reservoir readily lends itself to construction of a short pouch and provides a tapered, rather than a globular, reservoir in the rectal muscle canal. The lateral reservoir is easier to reconstruct than any of the other reservoirs, if this becomes necessary in subsequent years[4,5].

Principles and justification

Important features of the operation for optimal function have evolved during the past decade. The rectal muscle cuff need not be longer than 4.5 cm; longer cuffs produce narrowing of the reservoir outlet with partial obstruction. The reservoir spout should not exceed 1 cm in length or reservoir outlet obstruction with stasis will often ensue. The length of the reservoir should not exceed 10–12 cm as larger pouches seldom empty effectively. All rectal mucosa should be removed down to the dentate line to minimize the risk of chronic mucosal inflammation, sinus tracts and strictures in the pelvis during the following months. A completely diverting ileostomy is advisable for patients with ulcerative colitis to minimize contamination in the pelvis. A one-stage operation without ileostomy has been performed successfully in several patients with polyposis coli.

Indications

Patients selected for the endorectal ileal pull-through procedure should have biopsy-proven ulcerative colitis and be refractory to medical therapy. A normal small intestinal radiographic series and the absence of perianal sinuses, abscesses, or fistulae help to exclude the presence of Crohn's disease.

Operation

The patient is placed in the semi-lithotomy (Lloyd-Davies) position with the heels and popliteal fossa well padded (*see Illustration 3* on page 48).

1   The site for the ileostomy in the right lower abdomen is selected by the stoma care nurse before the operation to avoid skin creases and the belt line. A nasogastric tube and Foley bladder catheter are inserted under anaesthesia.

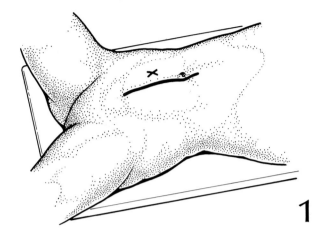

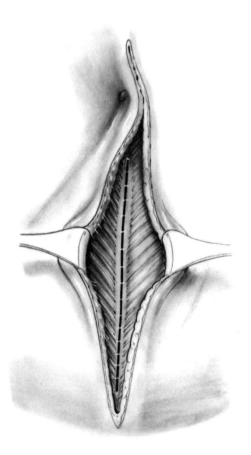

2   The abdomen is opened through a vertical skin incision extending from approximately 3 cm above the umbilicus to the pubic symphysis and slightly to the left of the midline in order to provide more space for the ileostomy. The linea alba is divided in the midline with electrocautery.

3 The intestine is examined from the ligament of Treitz to the ileocaecal valve to exclude the presence of Crohn's disease. The colon, in most cases, will be thickened, somewhat shortened and surrounded by fat with increased vascularity. The ileum is divided approximately 1 cm proximal to the ileocaecal valve to provide sufficient length to reach the anus without tension. It is rare that the distal ileum is involved severely enough to warrant more extensive resection. Active disease in the distal ileum strongly suggests the diagnosis of Crohn's disease.

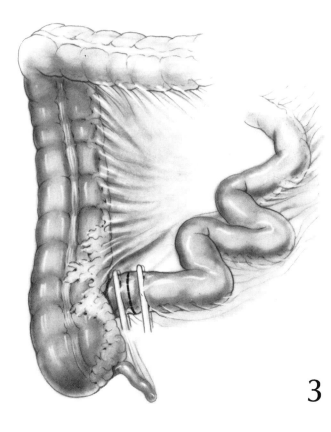

3

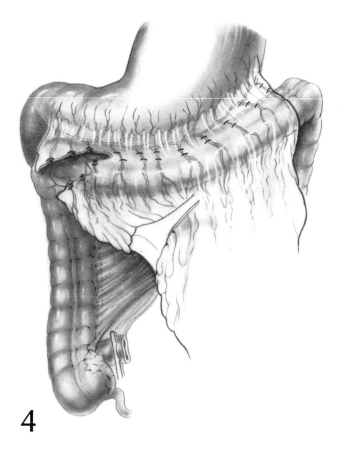

4

4 The colon is resected, taking the omentum with the specimen. Vessels are ligated with polyglactin (Vicryl) rather than silk in order to minimize the risk of stitch granulomas or abscesses.

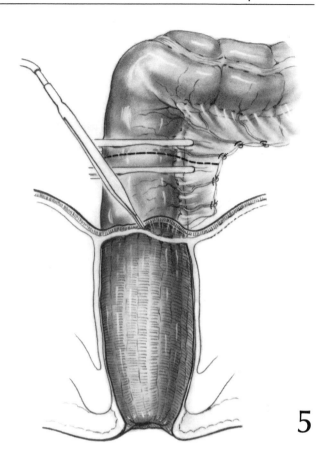

5 The sigmoid colon is transected approximately 10 cm above the peritoneal reflection and the specimen is submitted to the pathologist to examine for carcinoma or Crohn's disease. The sigmoid mesentery is divided and the peritoneal reflection is incised circumferentially around the rectum with electrocautery.

5

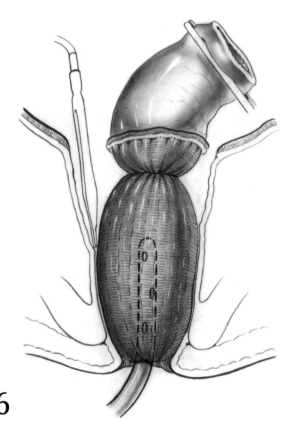

6

6 The rectum is dissected from the adjacent tissues with electrocautery forceps, developing a plane immediately adjacent to the muscularis down to 4.5 cm from the dentate line. The rectum is ligated at the level of the peritoneal reflection and then irrigated copiously with antibiotic solution.

7 The rectal muscle and mucosa are transected with electrocautery approximately 4.5 cm proximal to the dentate line.

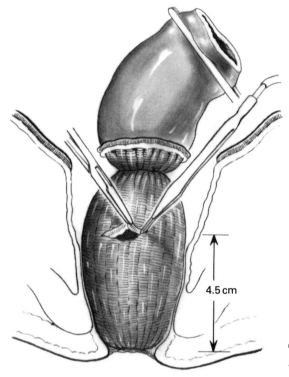

7

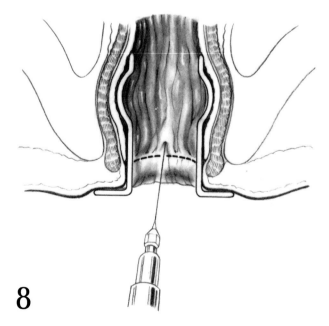

8

8 The rectum is manually dilated and a self-retaining anal retractor is inserted. Dilute adrenaline solution is injected between the mucosa and muscularis to facilitate the dissection. A circumferential incision is made through the mucosa at the dentate line with electrocautery.

9 The mucosa is incised circumferentially at the level of the dentate line and then elevated from the anorectal sphincter muscles using scissor dissection. The mucosa is completely resected up to the line of rectal transection from above. Electrocautery may be necessary to remove fragmented mucosa. Thorough haemostasis is achieved with electrocautery and the pelvis is thoroughly irrigated with antibiotic solution.

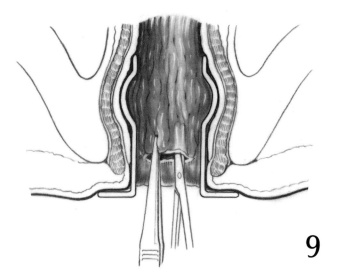

9

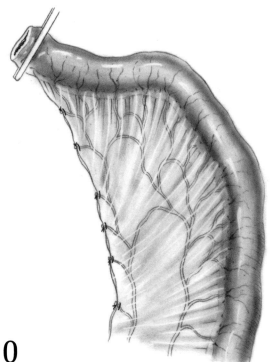

10

10 The ileum is mobilized along the superior mesenteric artery and vein up to a few centimetres above the ileocolic vessels in order to provide sufficient length for the end of the ileum to reach the anus without tension.

11 The ileum is divided approximately 12 cm from the end, carefully preserving the blood supply.

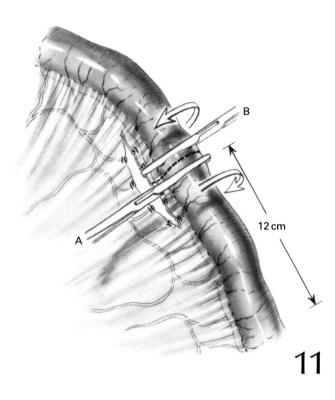

11

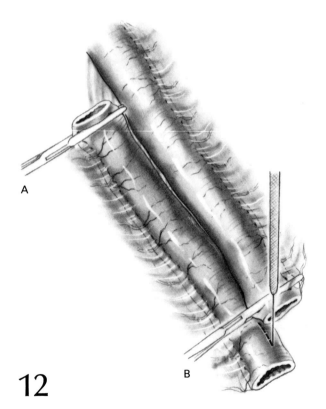

12 The antimesenteric side of the proximal and distal ileum are placed adjacent to each other. A small vertical incision is made on the antimesenteric side of the lower segment 1 cm proximal to the end.

12

13 A long anastomosis is constructed between the proximal and distal ileal segments with a GIA stapler. The upper open end of the reservoir is closed with another firing of the stapler.

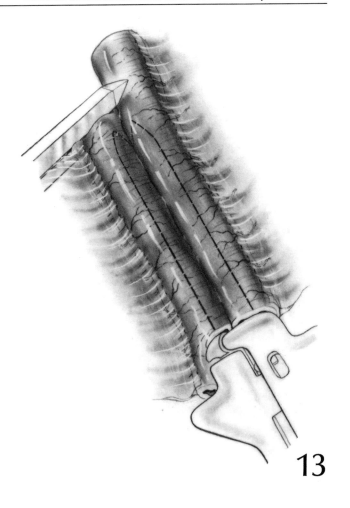

13

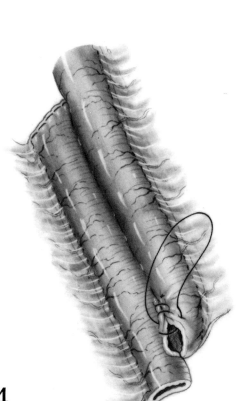

14

14 The distal open end of the reservoir is closed with a continuous inverting 3/0 Maxon suture leaving a spout of less than 1 cm distal to the pouch. The completed reservoir measures 10–11 cm.

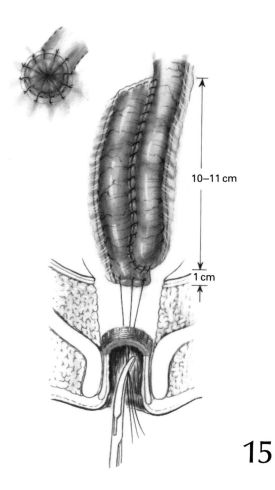

15 The entire staple and suture line is oversewn with a second layer of absorbable suture. The end of the ileal spout is loosely oversewn with silk traction stitches and then drawn through the rectal muscle canal to the anus. Care is taken to avoid twisting the mesentery.

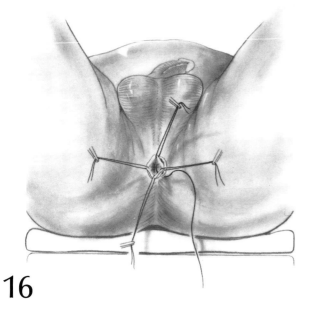

16 The full thickness of the ileal spout is sutured to the anal mucosa and underlying muscularis with interrupted 2/0 polyglactin (Vicryl) (approximately 24 sutures). The ileal mesentery is sutured loosely to the posterior abdomen in the midline to prevent internal herniation.

17 A temporary end ileostomy is constructed approximately 12 cm proximal to the upper end of the reservoir. A disc of skin and underlying muscle is excised from the preselected site in the right lower abdominal wall to construct the ileostomy. The opening is made sufficiently large that two fingers may be easily passed through.

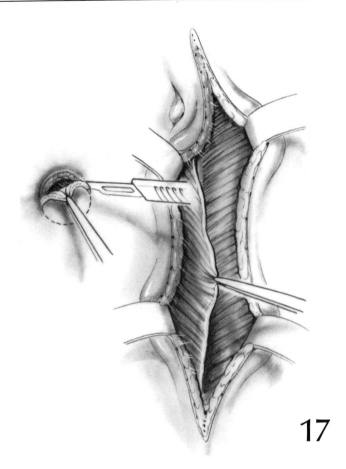

17

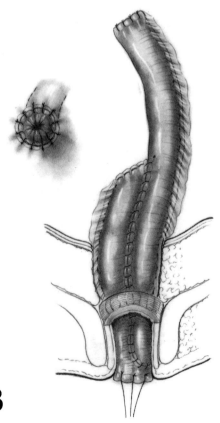

18

18 The ileum is divided approximately 12–15 cm proximal to the upper end of the ileal reservoir with the GIA stapler. The distal end of the divided ileum is loosely oversewn. The proximal end of divided ileum is fashioned into an end ileostomy.

A silicone drain is placed between the ileal reservoir and the rectal muscularis and brought through a separate incision in the left lower abdominal wall. The rectus muscles are closed with heavy interrupted polyglactin (Vicryl) sutures.

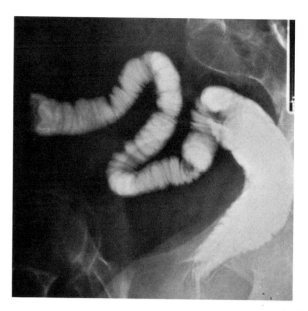

19

19 Approximately 2 months after the operation the reservoir is examined with a water-soluble radiographic contrast enema (Gastrografin) and by sigmoidoscopy to check for leaks or other abnormalities.

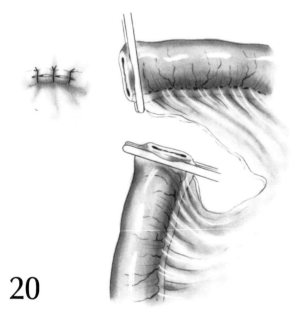

20

20 Approximately 4 months after the operation the ileostomy is closed under general anaesthesia. The rectum is dilated gently with a size 20 Hegar dilator. The abdomen is entered through the previous midline surgical scar. The ileostomy is mobilized from the abdominal wall and the tip resected. The end of the oversewn distal ileal segment is similarly resected.

21 An end-to-end ileal anastomosis is performed in two layers with interrupted absorbable sutures. The mesenteric defect is closed loosely. A size 30 soft rubber catheter is passed up the rectum, placing the tip a few centimetres above the upper end of the reservoir. This catheter is removed 4 days after operation and serves to minimize early liquid drainage onto the perineal skin. The ileostomy wound and the abdominal wound are closed with heavy interrupted absorbable sutures (Vicryl or Maxon).

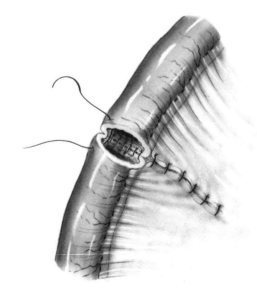

21

Postoperative care

Complications

During the past 14 years, 350 patients have undergone this procedure in the author's hospital. Almost all complications following the endorectal ileal pull-through were surgically correctable when recognized and treated early. The most common complications were associated with stasis and were due to reservoir outlet obstruction and/or construction of a long pouch. Faecal stasis in the pouch causes bacterial overgrowth, faecal urgency, frequency and soiling. Reservoir inflammation (pouchitis) is very uncommon in the absence of stasis. Ninety-two patients have undergone various types of reservoir reconstruction to achieve a short reservoir with short ileal spout, and thus relieve symptoms from stasis.

Routine rectal dilatation with a size 19 Hegar dilator on a daily basis for the first 2 months after operation has virtually eliminated ileoanal strictures which may produce stasis and pouch enlargement.

Of the 350 patients, 11 (3%) underwent subsequent permanent ileostomy construction; three of these patients were shown to have Crohn's disease rather than ulcerative colitis. This low incidence of pouch failure compares favourably with the 6–13% failure rate reported in large series of patients using other reservoir configurations[5, 6]. A temporary diverting ileostomy was constructed in 15 patients following pouch reconstruction, or to permit optimal growth and development in children.

Outcome

Of the 26 patients with carcinoma secondary to either colitis or colonic polyposis, six have died from their disease and two others required removal of the reservoir in the pelvis with wide resection because of recurrent neoplasm.

Of the 339 patients with a functioning endorectal pouch, 319 (94%) are currently progressing well. The majority have between three and five continent movements per 24 h (mean 4.8/24 h). By 6 months after the operation, fewer than 14% experienced nocturnal staining. By 12 months, seepage was rare. Many patients participate in active or vigorous athletic activities. None of the men has suffered impotence. Nineteen women have delivered healthy full-term babies, 11 by the vaginal route.

Follow-up for many years is necessary to recognize some of the more insidious complications of the endorectal ileal pull-through procedure. The operation is technically difficult; however, with close attention to the many details of operative and postoperative care, it is likely to provide gratifying long-term results. The procedure is an excellent alternative to procto-colectomy with permanent ileostomy and should be considered early for the treatment of ulcerative colitis and polyposis coli.

References

1. Parks AG, Nicholls RJ, Belliveau P. Proctocolectomy with ileal reservoir and anal anastomosis. *Br J Surg* 1980; 67: 533–8.

2. Utsunomiya J, Iwama T, Imago N *et al*. Total colectomy, mucosal proctectomy, and ileoanal anastomosis. *Dis Colon Rectum* 1980; 23: 459–66.

3. Dozois RR, Kelly KA, Welling DR *et al*. Ileal pouch–anal anastomosis: comparison of results in familial adenomatous polyposis and chronic ulcerative colitis. *Ann Surg* 1989; 210: 268–73.

4. Fonkalsrud EW, Stelzner M, McDonald N. Experience with the endorectal ileal pullthrough with lateral reservoir for ulcerative colitis and polyposis. *Arch Surg* 1988; 123: 1053–8.

5. Fonkalsrud EW, Phillips JD. Reconstruction of malfunctioning ileoanal pouch procedures as an alternative to permanent ileostomy. *Am J Surg* 1990; 160: 245–51.

6. Wexner SD, Jensen L, Rothenberger DA *et al*. Long-term functional analysis of the ileoanal reservoir. *Dis Colon Rectum* 1989; 32: 275–81.

Management of failed pelvic pouch procedures

Roger R. Dozois MD, MS, FACS
Professor of Surgery, Mayo Clinic, Rochester, Minnesota, USA

History

The ileal pouch–anal anastomosis, by eradicating the underlying colon and rectal disease while restoring anorectal functions reasonably well, provides patients afflicted with either ulcerative colitis or familial adenomatous polyposis with a quality of life superior to that previously expected with conventional panproctocolectomy and ileostomy. Thus, the procedure has become the operation of choice for many of these patients. However, the complexities of the technique to construct the pelvic reservoir, the very nature and severity of the underlying disease, and the therapeutic modalities employed before surgery[1] have all contributed to a significant number of general and pouch-related complications, with significant morbidity

endangering the viability of the ileal reservoir. Despite the extensive experience at the Mayo Medical Center (more than 1300 pelvic pouch operations), nearly 30% of patients will experience some type of postoperative complication. Overall, 10% of pouch-related complications require reoperation because of their persistence and failure to respond to conservative measures and, ultimately, 5% of the pouches will need to be excised. Thus, most pelvic pouch failures can be corrected either by conservative means or by reoperation. In this chapter a classification of postoperative complications is provided, along with their clinical presentation, management, and the anticipated results.

Postoperative complications

Ileoanal pouch procedures are safe and are associated with low operative mortality rates (0.2% at the Mayo Clinic, and less than 1.5%[2] in the literature). In contrast to mortality, morbidity rates after ileal pouch–anal anastomosis remain considerable, having been reported in 13–54% of patients[2,3]. Small bowel obstruction is the most common complication but is not pouch-specific and its incidence is no different than other types of proctocolectomy[4]. Other general complications include wound infection (3%), transient urinary retention (5%), sexual impotence in men (1.5%) and dyspareunia in women (7%) and will not be discussed further. However, sexual dysfunction is less common than is observed after routine proctectomy and complications pertaining to the perineal wound are absent.

Complications specifically related to the pelvic pouch can be broadly categorized as: strictures; perianal sinus/fistula/abscess; abdominal fistula/abscess; unsatisfactory function; and pouchitis.

Strictures

Presentation

Stricturing of the ileoanal anastomosis can be observed before or after closure of the temporary ileostomy. On digital examination at the time of closure of the temporary ileostomy, it is not uncommon to feel a short, soft web of tissue at the anastomosis. This type of 'benign' stricture is asymptomatic, can be treated easily by digital dilatation at the time of ileostomy reversal, and does not recur. True anastomotic stricture is observed late after removal of the ileostomy, and is usually long, dense and non-pliable because of fibrosis. It is more difficult to treat successfully, even by reoperation.

The most common causes of these strictures are tension with ischaemia and perianastomotic sepsis. Undue tension on the anastomosis of the ileal reservoir to the dentate line area may cause the pouch to retract upwards during the postoperative period, leaving portions or all of the underlying internal sphincter and anal canal muscularis denuded and exposed. Usually this will be manifested by the sudden onset of bright red blood through the anus on days 5–7 after surgery, occasionally associated with pain secondary to spasms of the sphincter apparatus, and possibly low-grade fever. Gradual healing of this area results in heavy scarring and the formation of a long, dense stricture. The association of perianastomotic sepsis further compounds these problems, resulting in dense fibrosis and loss of compliance of the surrounding pelvic floor structures.

Prevention

Adequate mobilization of the mesentery, correct construction of the appropriate type of reservoir, and avoidance of sepsis all help to prevent undue tension, ischaemia and disruption of the ileal pouch–anal anastomosis. If necessary, branches of the superior mesenteric vessels and/or the ileocolic vessels may be severed to assure that the apex of the future reservoir will extend well beyond the inferior border of the pubic symphysis, which is a good indication that the reservoir will reach the anus easily. Certain types of reservoirs will reach the anus more readily than others because of anatomical variations of the mesentery and the build of the patient[5]: for instance, a three-loop S-shaped pouch or a quadruple-loop W-shaped pouch may reach the anus better than a J-shaped pouch after transection of the ileocolic vessels. In most situations, however, the easily constructed two-loop J-shaped pouch will reach satisfactorily after proper mobilization, but it may be necessary to use longer ileal limbs (18–20 cm rather than 10–12 cm) and to divide branches of the superior mesenteric or other vessels[5].

Management

At times, simple dilatation of the stricture area may prevent it from progressing, and some of these patients will do well (*Table 1*)[6]. However, such strictures often must be dilated repeatedly or even treated surgically. In such cases the surgeon may choose to excise the strictured segment through a perineal approach and to advance the pouch mucosa distally, sewing it to the dentate line mucosa. It may be necessary to elevate the perianal skin as an advancement flap and move it into the anal canal to meet the pouch mucosa. If this is not feasible, usually because of extreme fixation of the surrounding pelvic musculature, the pelvic reservoir may need to be totally mobilized by an abdominal approach, the strictured segment excised, and the reservoir reanastomosed to the anal canal mucosa. In all of these surgical manoeuvres, great care must be taken to avoid damaging the internal sphincter. Also, depending on the extent and difficulty of the procedure chosen, it may be prudent to establish a temporary diverting ileostomy.

In the author's series of 42 patients reoperated for anastomotic strictures[6], all patients were treated initially by dilatation with graduated Hegar dilators (*Table 1*). Recurrent strictures and other complications were observed in 60% of the patients, all of whom required further operation, including repair of the existing reservoir, especially if the strictures were accompanied by other perianastomotic problems or more complex procedures. Ultimately, of the 42 patients requiring reoperation for stricture, the pouch was excised in six because of recurrent stenosis with poor function (three

Table 1   Operations employed to correct pelvic pouch-related complications at the Mayo Clinic, 1982–1989

	Number of patients			
	Anastomotic stricture (n = 42)	Perianal fistula/abscess (n = 30)	Intra-abdominal fistula/abscess (n = 29)	Unsatisfactory function (n = 13)
Ileostomy at presentation	13 (31)	10 (33)	15 (52)	3 (23)
Frequent procedures performed				
Dilatation of associated stricture	42 (100)	9 (30)		2 (15)
Fistulotomy/excision of fistula tract		17 (57)	4 (14)	
Primary closure of fistula		3 (10)	3 (10)	
Drainage of abscess		5 (17)	18 (62)	
Diverting ileostomy		3 (10)	6 (21)	
Redo ileal pouch–anal anastomosis			5 (17)	4 (31)
Divide pouch septum				4 (31)
Shorten or excise efferent limb				2 (15)
Convert to different type pouch				3 (23)
Postoperative complications	25 (60)	23 (77)	18 (62)	4 (31)
Recurrent stricture	22 (52)	6 (2)		
Perianal fistula	2 (5)	16 (53)		
Perianal abscess	1 (2)	5 (17)		
Intra-abdominal fistula			5 (17)	1 (8)
Intra-abdominal abscess			9 (31)	1 (8)
Other				2 (15)
More than one operation for pouch-related complications	25 (60)	22 (73)	17 (59)	5 (39)

Values in parentheses are percentages.

patients), severe intractable diarrhoea (one patient), and persistent perianal fistula (two patients).

Functional results

In those patients with a functioning ileal pouch–anal anastomosis after reoperation for stricture[6], stool frequency decreased from a mean(s.d.) of 14(11) stools per day before operation to 7(3) stools per day, and from 2(1) to 1(1) stools per night. Continence also improved, and satisfactory functional results were achieved in 69% of patients with functioning ileal pouch–anal anastomoses (*Figure 1*)[6].

Perianal sinus/fistula/abscess

An asymptomatic radiological leak or sinus is occasionally discovered when the patient returns for the temporary ileostomy to be removed and for restoration of intestinal continuity. Such sinuses represent incomplete healing of the anastomosis and are managed by deferring removal of the ileostomy. Persistent sinuses may very occasionally require minor surgical unroofing. True pouch–perianal fistulae have been reported in about 5% of patients and pouch–vaginal fistulae in about 4%[2]. Others have reported a higher incidence. The author has observed perianastomotic fistulae only

in patients with colitis and never in those with polyposis. Pouch–perianal fistulae are most often associated with low-grade fever, perineal, low back or sacral pain, and with intermittent perianal purulent discharge. Preoperative radiographic examination of the fistula and/or the pouch using water-soluble contrast may help to delineate the location and extent of the

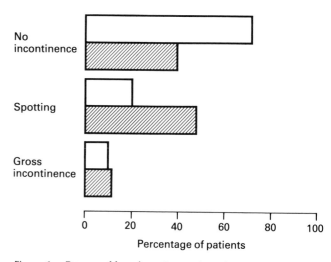

Figure 1.   Degree of faecal continence in patients reoperated for pouch-specific complications after ileal pouch–anal anastomosis. □, Daytime stool frequency; ▨, night-time stool frequency

fistula tract, which most typically originates in the vicinity of the anastomosis and not uncommonly extends behind the pouch. If there is clinical suspicion of a tract, yet clinical examination does not yield conclusive evidence, examination under anaesthesia may be performed to establish the diagnosis. In a significant number of these patients an associated anastomotic stricture may be encountered.

The majority of fistulae occur before or soon after removal of the ileostomy. Occasionally, however, an intersphincteric fistula opening on the perineum near the anus can be seen several years after an otherwise successful pelvic ileal reservoir. These may originate from residual anal glands and should be treated as such.

Treatment

Procedures for perianal complications are listed in *Table 1*. The most common procedure consists of a local perianal operation, including fistulotomy, dilatation of the anastomotic stricture and, in some instances, re-establishment of a diverting ileostomy. Not uncommonly, better local drainage and antibiotics are sufficient. Some low-lying, readily accessible abscesses may be amenable to needle aspiration and drainage guided by computed tomography (CT).

1a–c This tomogram of the pelvis shows a presacral abscess with invasion of ileal reservoir before (*Illustration 1a*) and after CT-guided needle drainage showing expansion of the ileal reservoir (*Illustration 1b*) and decreased size of abscess (*Illustration 1c*).

Complications

Postoperative complications have occurred in over two-thirds of patients, and the reservoir was ultimately removed in 17%[6].

A vaginal fistula may be discovered during routine radiography of the pouch before removal of the ileostomy or once intestinal continuity has been restored. If this is discovered before removal of the ileostomy and is found to originate, as is most often the case, from the dentate line area, the only noticeable symptom may be increased discharge of mucus through the vagina. Deferment of the ileostomy closure for 2–12 months will usually permit spontaneous healing of the fistula tract. Occasionally, especially if it appears after removal of the temporary ileostomy, a vaginal fistula may persist, requiring transvaginal repair using advancement flap or other more complex techniques, usually under the coverage of an ileostomy. In these instances, there is a significant increase in the need for excision of the reservoir.

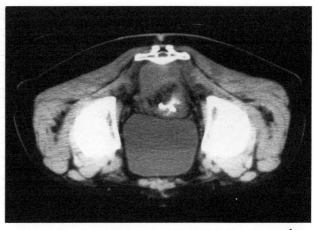

1a

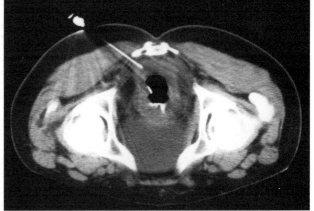

1b

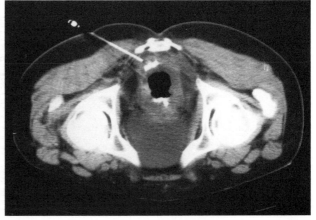

1c

Functional results

Postoperative stool frequency decreases and continence improves compared with preoperative values. Satisfactory functional results were achieved in 70% of patients with a functioning ileal pouch–anal anastomosis in the author's series.

Pelvic phlegmon and abscess/fistula

This complication may be expected to result from contamination of the presacral space during or after the operation or if there is partial disruption of the pouch suture line, but it has not been observed after construction of an ileal pouch–anal anastomosis in polyposis patients, suggesting that other disease-related (rather than surgeon-related) factors may cause such problems in patients with inflammatory bowel disease. These factors include the preoperative status of the patient, the severity of underlying disease, and the type and duration of the preoperative treatment of the colitis with cytotoxic agents.

Pelvic sepsis presents with fever, local or generalized peritonitis, abdominal pain, and diarrhoea. The pain may be located in the abdomen, lower pelvis or lower back, sometimes radiating into one or both legs. A leucocytosis is usually found. A fistula may be demonstrated during radiographic examination of the pouch, and computed tomography may help to define the nature of the infectious process: a frank abscess is usually associated with distortion of the ileal reservoir rather than an ill-defined early phlegmon.

Prevention

Measures used to minimize the potential for postoperative pelvic/perianastomotic infections include:

1. Adequate preparation of the patient, with bowel cleansing, oral neomycin and metronidazole, and perioperative parenteral antibiotics.
2. Condition of the patient/timing of surgery. Critically ill patients, such as those with fulminant coliitis or toxic megacolon, may be better served by a three-stage procedure. After total colectomy and ileostomy, the entire rectum is left behind, reserving pouch construction and ileoanal anastomosis for a later second stage. Earlier referral for this type of complex surgical therapy may help to reduce septic complications, as suggested by the absence of postoperative sepsis in polyposis patients.
3. Irrigation of the rectum with 5% povidone-iodine (Betadine) before a laparotomy and perioperative antibiotics may help combat intraoperative contamination and reduce the infection rate.
4. Meticulous technique, avoiding tension on the reservoir, intraoperative contamination, and using absorbable sutures in the pelvis cannot be overemphasized.
5. A short muscular cuff helps to reduce the infection rate.
6. A soft Silastic drain should be routinely placed behind the reservoir to aspirate serum, blood and debris from the presacral space.
7. A diverting ileostomy helps to prevent pelvic sepsis, at least in patients with colitis. The author has been less concerned with sepsis in healthy young patients with polyposis and has not observed this complication with this diagnosis even if an ileostomy is not used.

Treatment

Treatment consists of draining the abscess via the abdominal route. In doing so, care must be taken not to disrupt the integrity of the pouch itself. Even if a fistula is identified, it is unlikely that the surgeon will be able to repair the defect primarily because of the friability of the surrounding tissues. A previously removed ileostomy should be re-established. If a loop ileostomy is in place but diversion of the faecal stream has been incomplete, the loop ileostomy should be converted into a Brooke-type end ileostomy at the time the pelvic abscess is drained. Rarely, the ileal pouch–anal anastomosis may need to be removed, a new reservoir constructed, and a new anastomosis performed[6]. This should be reserved for a later operation when sepsis is under control.

Complications

Complications are frequent and may include recurrent intra-abdominal abscess(es), intra-abdominal fistula and stricture. In the author's experience, 59% of these patients will require further operations, and eventually about 34% of the pouches will need to be excised (*Figure 2*)[6].

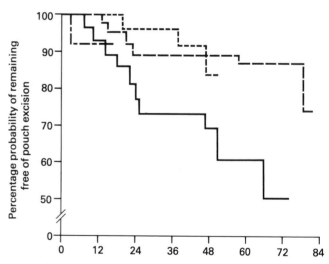

Time after operation for pouch-related complications (months)

Figure 2.   Probability of pouch excision among patients with pelvic pouch-specific complications requiring reoperation after ileoanal anastomosis. ––– Stricture; ---- perianal abscess/fistula; —— intra-abdominal abscess/fistula; ·—·— functional problems

Functional results

Galandiuk *et al.*[6] reported that postoperative stool frequency at follow-up had decreased from a mean(s.d.) of 15(12) to 5(2) stools during the day and from 2(0) to 1(1) stools at night, and that continence improved. Eventually, pouch function was satisfactory in 83% of patients with functioning ileal pouch–anal anastomoses.

Unsatisfactory function

Adequacy of functional results is subjective and such results may depend on a variety of factors that are independent of technique. In general, patients who have the better results are young, male or female with few or no children, those with fewer stools before surgery, and those with polyposis. Functional failure may result from poor patient selection and a variety of physiological factors. Age is no contraindication to the construction of an ileal reservoir, but patients over 55 years and multiparous women should be assessed carefully before surgery. Anal manometry may be used to eliminate patients with inadequate or borderline sphincter function.

Patients suspected of having Crohn's colitis should be discouraged from having an ileoanal anastomosis and their expectations clearly discussed before operation.

Patients with unsatisfactory neorectal functions would include those with poor neorectal emptying due to a long efferent limb after construction of an S-shaped or an H-shaped (lateral–lateral) pouch; incontinence related to a reservoir which is too small or too large; obstruction secondary to a J-pouch septum; outlet obstruction caused by mucosal prolapse; and recurrent pouchitis associated with poor neorectal emptying[6].

Treatment

Patients with an S-shaped or H-shaped reservoir or a long efferent limb may require shortening or total amputation of the efferent limb. If this is technically not feasible, the reservoir should be excised and a new one constructed. A transperineal approach can be (and has been) used in some patients, but the author and others[7] prefer a transabdominal approach for such difficult reconstructive operations. Some authors have described transanal division of the septum between the long efferent limb and the S pouch using a GIA stapler (described in the chapter on pp. 615–628)[8], but the author has no experience with this approach. In patients with a J-shaped pouch and a retained septum which is obstructing defaecation, transanal transection of the septum can be easily accomplished using a GIA stapler (described in the chapter on pp. 629–649). Partial or total reconstruction of the reservoir may be necessary for those patients with reservoirs that are too small or too large, or reservoirs that need revision for other reasons.

Functional results

In the author's experience of revisional operations of 13 malfunctioning reservoirs, stool frequency decreased from a mean(s.d.) of 14(7) to 8(6) stools per day and from 3(2) to 2(2) stools per night. Postoperative continence also improved. Function was satisfactory in 60% of patients with functioning ileal pouch–anal anastomoses. One reservoir had to be excised and could not be repaired or replaced.

Among all patients with pouch-related complications requiring reoperation after ileal pouch–anal anastomosis, the overall probability of pouch excision is high (>20%), and is even higher when the indication for surgery is an intra-abdominal abscess/fistula (*Figure 2*)[6].

Pouchitis

The symptoms and signs of pouchitis, characterized by the sudden onset of watery (sometimes bloody) diarrhoea, cramps in the lower abdomen, urgency, malaise and fever, are reminiscent of the colitis that the patient experiences before surgery and can be considered a temporary dysfunctional 'failure' of the operation. Patients with colitis, especially those with extracolonic manifestations, are at greatest risk; those with colitis alone are at lesser risk. Pouchitis is rare in polyposis patients. Most patients are treated successfully with antibiotics, especially metronidazole, even if the pouchitis recurs. Pouchitis alone has rarely been a cause of pouch failure; moreover, in these rare instances the possibility of Crohn's disease cannot be ruled out.

Conclusions

In the author's experience with more than 1300 operations, the ileal pouch–anal anastomosis has been successful in most patients (94%), but in 6% the operation has ultimately failed and excision of the pouch and/or establishment of a permanent ileostomy has been required[3]. The most frequent causes of failure have been pelvic sepsis, poor functional results (gross incontinence at night and/or multiple stools), later appearance of granulomatous disease and, very rarely, recurrent, recalcitrant pouchitis (2% of all failures)[8]. Salvage operations for pouch-specific complications are safe[8] in that none of the reoperated patients has died. The risk of further complications and reoperation, including pouch excision, is high, and reoperation should not be undertaken unless the surgeon has already gained considerable experience in primary construction of the ileal pouch–anal anastomosis. In experienced hands, reoperation can restore pouch function in two-thirds of the patients, and 70% of these can be expected to have a stool frequency and degree of continence that does not differ greatly from patients who have had no major complications after construction of the original pelvic reservoir.

Acknowledgements

Table 1, Figures 1 and *2* are reproduced from Galandiuk et al.[6] with permission of the publishers. *Illustration 1a–c* is reproduced from Dozois[1] with permission of the publishers.

References

1. Dozois RR. Pelvic and perianastomotic complications after ileoanal anastomosis. *Perspect Colon Rectal Surg* 1988; 1: 113–21.

2. Wong WD, Rothenberger DA, Goldberg SM. Ileoanal pouch procedures. *Curr Probl Surg* 1985; 22: 1–78.

3. Pemberton JH, Kelly KA, Beart RW Jr, Dozois RR, Wolff BG, Ilstrup DM. Ileal pouch–anal anastomosis for chronic ulcerative colitis: long-term results. *Ann Surg* 1987; 206: 504–13.

4. Francois Y, Dozois RR, Kelly KA *et al.* Small intestinal obstruction complicating ileal pouch–anal anastomosis. *Ann Surg* 1989; 209: 46–50.

5. Dozois RR. Technique of ileal pouch–anal anastomosis. *Perspect Colon Rectal Surg* 1989; 2: 85–94.

6. Galandiuk S, Scott NA, Dozois RR *et al.* Ileal pouch–anal anastomosis: reoperation for pouch-related complications. *Ann Surg* 1990; 212: 446–54.

7. Nicholls RJ, Gilbert JM. Surgical correction of the efferent ileal limb for disordered defaecation following restorative proctocolectomy with the S ileal reservoir. *Br J Surg* 1990; 77: 152–4.

8. Schoetz DJ Jr, Coller JA, Veidenheimer MC. Can the pouch be saved? *Dis Colon Rectum* 1988; 31: 671–5.

Illustrations by Antoine Barnaud and the late Robert Lane

Excision of the rectum with colonic J pouch–anal anastomosis

R. F. Parc MD
Chairman, Department of Surgery, Hôpital Saint-Antoine, Paris, France

J.-L. Faucheron MD
Chief Resident, Department of Surgery, Hôpital Saint-Antoine, Paris, France

M. T. El Riwini MB, BCh
Faculty of Medicine, University of Alexandria, Egypt

Principles and justification

The use of sphincter-saving operations is now widely accepted for the treatment of tumours in the middle third of the rectum[1,2]. Long-term survival and local recurrence rates after anterior resection[3] are similar to those obtained by total excision when the length of rectum removed below the tumour is at least 2 cm. After rectal excision with very low colorectal or straight coloanal anastomoses, there is frequently a degree of urgency and increased bowel movements resulting from the loss of the rectal reservoir[4–7]. In order to improve the functional results, we have proposed a modification of the original technique of coloanal anastomosis described by Parks and Percy[4], in which a J-shaped colonic reservoir is constructed and the anastomosis is performed between the end of the reservoir and the anal canal.

Indications

This technique is indicated especially for malignant tumours situated at a distance of 2–4 cm from the dentate line, and in some cases of benign lesions of the rectum such as circumferential villous tumours where the lower edge extends 0–2 cm above the dentate line.

Preoperative

A low residue diet is commenced 2 days before surgery. Bowel preparation is carried out using 3–5 litres polyethylene glycol the day before surgery. Enemas are given if necessary to complete bowel cleaning. The abdomen is shaved from the nipple to the pubic symphysis, as is the perineum, and the patient showers with povidone-iodine the day before the operation. General anaesthesia with muscle relaxants is routinely used. Systemic antibiotics are given at the induction of anaesthesia. A nasogastric tube is introduced into the stomach.

Operation

Position of patient

The patient is positioned in the modified lithotomy Trendelenburg position (*see* chapter on pp. 47–50), with the hips flexed at 30° for the abdominal phase and 100° for the perineal phase. Great care should be taken in positioning the legs to avoid deep vein thrombosis, compartment syndrome or external tibial nerve paralysis. The legs are protected with a spongy cover and mobilized every hour during the procedure. A Foley catheter is placed into the bladder and strapped to the right thigh. The anus is gently dilated and the rectum washed with a mixture of normal saline and povidone-iodine.

The skin of the abdomen and perineum is prepared with povidone-iodine and drapes are adjusted, excluding the penis and scrotum (in males) and the vulva (in females) from the operative field. When the skin is dry, sterile drapes are placed over the abdomen.

The surgeon stands on the left of the patient, the first assistant on the right, the second assistant between the patient's legs and the instrument nurse on the right of the surgeon.

The operation includes an abdominal phase and a perineal phase.

Incision and abdominal exploration

1 A long midline incision is made, extending from the pubic symphysis to the mid-epigastrium. The lower part of the incision should reach the pubic symphysis to give good exposure into the pelvis. The upper part of the incision may reach higher than the mid-epigastrium if required for better exposure for mobilization of the splenic flexure.

A self-retaining retractor is used to retract the edges of the abdominal wall. The peritoneal cavity is explored to assess the location, size and fixity of the lesion, and to seek a synchronous colonic lesion, invasion of mesenteric or para-aortic lymph nodes, peritoneal spread or hepatic metastases. Ascitic fluid, if present, is collected for cytological examination.

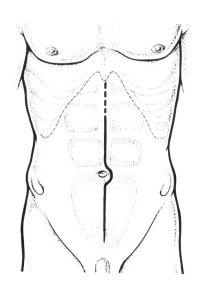

1

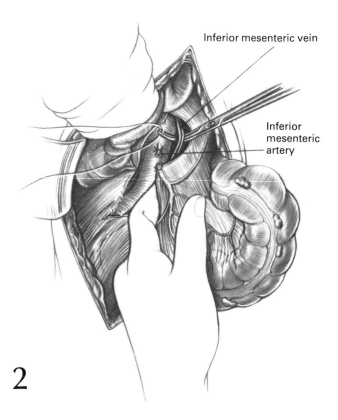

Inferior mesenteric vein

Inferior mesenteric artery

2

Exposure, ligature and division of the inferior mesenteric vessels

2 The small intestine is packed in moist pads and kept to the right of the abdominal cavity by the first assistant. The sigmoid colon is lifted up by the surgeon.

The lower part of the abdominal aorta is then exposed and the peritoneum incised on its right border. The inferior mesenteric artery is ligated and divided close to its origin. The peritoneal incision is then extended upwards to the base of the transverse mesocolon until the inferior mesenteric vein is exposed at the lower border of the pancreas. The inferior mesenteric vein, which lies some 2–3 cm lateral to the aorta, is ligated and divided at this level.

An essential part of the technique is sectioning of the inferior mesenteric artery at its origin and the inferior mesenteric vein at the border of the pancreas which permits good mobilization and further descent of the left colon to the pelvis without traction. However, in elderly patients the artery can be ligated distal to the left ascending colic artery to assure a good arterial supply to the descending colon.

Mobilization of the left colon

3 Once the inferior mesenteric vessels are divided, the sigmoid colon is mobilized by division of the developmental adhesions on the left side of the sigmoid colon. The first assistant holds the sigmoid colon in a forwards direction, while the surgeon incises the peritoneum on its left lateral side at the 'white line'. At this stage in the procedure, the left ureter must be visible but needs only to be visualized, not mobilized.

Mobilization of the descending colon continues by division of the peritoneal reflection in the left paracolic gutter towards the spleen. There is a good avascular plane for this dissection which passes between the perinephric fat and the mesocolon. The first assistant pulls the colon to the right and the surgeon, using blunt and sharp dissection, separates the mesocolon from the perinephric fat. Care should be taken not to injure the mesocolon and to keep the vascular arcades intact.

The surgeon changes position to the right of the patient for mobilization of the splenic flexure, which is an essential step that permits the colonic reservoir to reach the pelvis without tension. The splenic flexure is easier to mobilize after dissection of the left third of the transverse colon from the great omentum, which opens the lesser sac. Care should be taken not to damage the middle colic artery and its arcades. Once the left part of the transverse colon is free, the surgeon holds the two limbs of the splenic flexure in the left hand, exerting slight traction on the suspensory ligament, and begins the dissection from the posterolateral abdominal wall. Adhesions between the spleen and the flexure should be divided gently before proceeding to fully mobilize the flexure. The mesentery of the left part of the transverse colon must be mobilized at the lower border of the tail

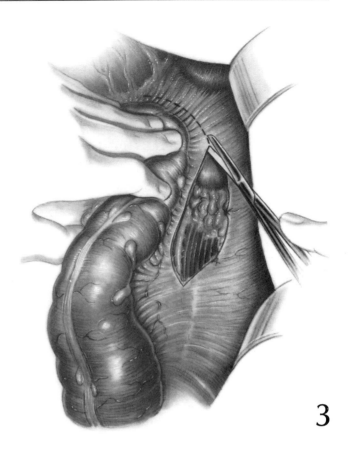

3

of the pancreas. Two technical points that help to mobilize the splenic flexure are retraction of the left costal margin and tilting the table into the reverse Trendelenburg position.

The left colon thus mobilized is attached to the posterior abdominal wall by a thin peritoneal fold of mesocolon crossing in front of the abdominal aorta. This peritoneal attachment is incised 2 mm from the aorta from the level of the transverse mesocolon downwards to the level of the aortic bifurcation. Bleeding from the fine vessels crossing this peritoneal fold may be electrocoagulated.

Mobilization of the rectum and growth

4 The table is tilted into the Trendelenburg position and the self-retaining retractor is moved towards the upper part of the incision. Two further retractors are fixed to the self-retaining retractor and used to keep the small intestine packed with moist pads in the upper part of the abdominal cavity. The surgeon should be on the left side of the patient, the first assistant on the right. The second assistant stands between the patient's legs holding a retractor to keep the bladder (and uterus in females) forward. These arrangements give good exposure into the pelvis. At the bifurcation of the aorta, the lower end of the peritoneal incision is extended downwards to the right side of the rectum, crossing the common iliac vessels and taking care not to injure the right ureter. An important point is not to skeletonize the bifurcation of the aorta to preserve the genitourinary plexus. The left rectal gutter is thus opened and the presacral space entered. The surgeon, using blunt and sharp dissection, separates the rectum from the sacrum in a plane anterior to the sacral fascia, avoiding injury to the presacral veins.

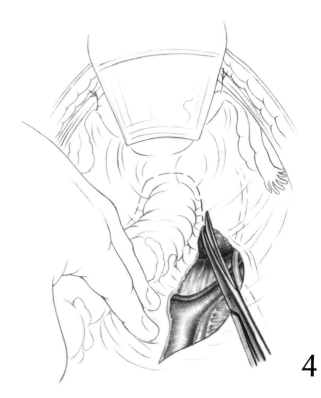

4

It is very important to carry out the dissection laterally as close as possible to the pelvic wall, with the hypogastric vessels as the lateral landmark, to ensure wide removal of lymphatic tissues from the pelvis. Postoperative recurrence depends to a great extent on widespread lateral pelvic dissection.

The peritoneum of the pouch of Douglas is incised, and the dissection is carried downwards in the plane between the rectum and the urinary bladder and prostate after opening Denonvilliers' fascia in men or between the rectum and the posterior wall of the vagina in women. In the latter, great care should be taken not to injure the vagina, particularly when using electro-coagulation. The dissection is continued as low as possible below the level of the seminal vesicles in men and far along the posterior vaginal wall in women. The lateral ligaments of the rectum are then identified on each side, clamped, divided and ligated. Dissection proceeds downwards to the level of the levator ani, which must be cleaned completely of all perirectal fat, again to avoid recurrence of tumour. It is important to avoid grasping the rectum at the tumour site, because this squeezes the lesion and separates tumour cells

which may result in intraluminal seeding, especially at the anastomosis.

Several technical points aid the dissection in the lower pelvis:

1. Bimanual examination: the surgeon introduces the left index finger into the rectum, holding the rectum with the right hand, thus assessing the remaining distance between the level of rectal dissection that has been reached and the upper limit of the anal sphincter. The surgeon then changes gloves aseptically and continues to mobilize the rectum if necessary.
2. Pressure should be exerted on the perineum (by the fist of the second assistant) to push the whole pelvic floor upwards.
3. The application of a malleable retractor behind the rectum will pull it anteriorly and to the right or the left.
4. A right-angle crushing clamp applied below the lower margin of the lesion may be used for traction on the lower rectum.

Choosing colorectal or coloanal–pouch anastomosis

5 The whole rectum is thus mobilized with the crushing clamp applied just below the lower border of the lesion. Using a ruler, a safety margin of 2 cm is measured from the crushing clamp distally where a right-angle (Satinsky) clamp is applied across the rectum. The distance between the Satinsky clamp and the upper border of the anal sphincter is measured. A coloanal–pouch anastomosis is used if the distance between the level of resection and the upper border of the anal sphincter is less than 2 cm; otherwise a standard low anterior resection with colorectal anastomosis using a CEEA stapling device is performed. We believe that coloanal–pouch anastomoses give better functional results than direct coloanal anastomoses constructed just above the sphincter.

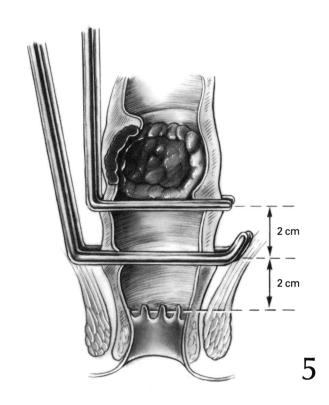

5

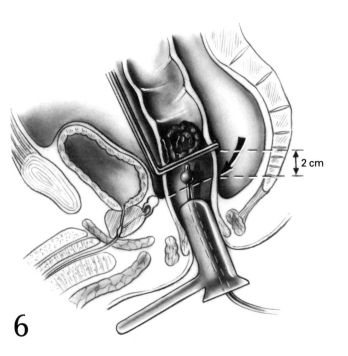

6

Rectal irrigation and rectal wall incision

6 If the coloanal–pouch anastomosis is chosen, the Satinsky clamp is removed and the rectal stump washed out with povidone-iodine solution through a Foley catheter until returns are clear.

The muscular wall of the rectum is transected circumferentially at the level of the sphincter ring and levator muscles. Bleeding is prevented by cautious diathermy coagulation. The mucosa is visible but should not be incised.

From this stage the procedure can be conducted by two teams: the abdominal team prepares and divides the colon and manufactures the J-shaped colonic pouch while the perineal team accomplishes the mucosectomy of the anal stump. If only one team is used the mucosectomy must be performed first to permit the removal of the specimen.

Mucosectomy of the rectal stump

7 Once the rectal stump has been irrigated two Gelpi retractors (Aesculap) are applied perpendicular to each other with prongs at 3, 6, 9 and 12 o'clock on the anal verge, resting on the external sphincter. Severe retraction must be avoided as this may cause damage to the anal sphincter and subsequent poor functional results.

An injection of saline containing lignocaine and adrenaline (1:10 000) is made into the submucosa to 'float' the mucosa away from the underlying muscle. The mucosa is removed from 5 mm above the dentate line in a circumferential manner using sharp-pointed scissor dissection and simultaneous coagulation of all bleeding points. The mucosectomy continues upwards until the section of the muscle is reached. This allows the specimen to be removed from the abdomen. Haemostasis of the anal muscular stump is reviewed as well as haemostasis in the lower pelvis, after irrigation with warm saline from the abdomen.

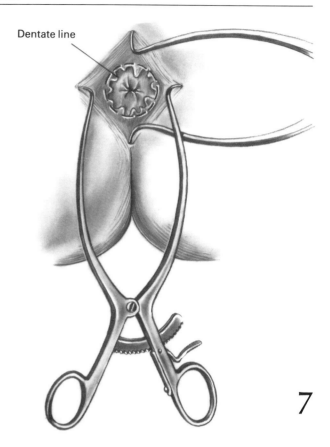

Dentate line

7

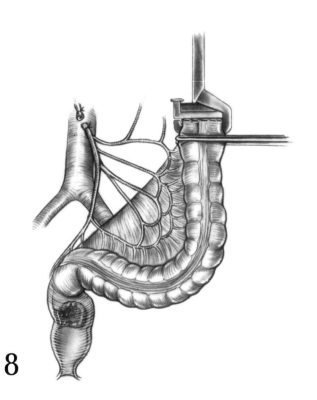

8

Preparation and division of the colon

8 A suitable site for division of the colon is chosen to ensure a good blood supply and which allows manufacture of a pouch that will descend easily into the pelvis without tension; the pouch apex should come very easily to the level of the lower border of the pubic symphysis without traction. Usually the site for division is in the descending colon just proximal to the sigmoid. The mesocolon is spread out to display the vessels, then divided obliquely from the site of ligation of the main vessels to the chosen site of colonic division. While doing this, great care should be taken not to jeopardize the vascularity of the colon: before division, any arterial branch coming from the left ascending colic artery should be temporarily clamped and the pulsation in the arcade checked to be sure that vascularity is preserved. The colon is then divided at the selected site after application of a TA55 stapling device on the proximal part and a crushing clamp distally. The resected specimen is removed from the operative field and opened so that the distance between the lower border of the tumour and the level of muscular division can be measured to make sure that a margin of 2 cm has been achieved. Frozen-section examination should be requested at this time if dealing with a very low lesion. The stapled end of the colon is underrun by a continuous 4/0 suture of polyglycolic acid. Its vasculature is assessed by arterial pulsation.

Manufacture of the J-shaped colonic pouch

9a, b The distal 15 cm of the colon are brought together in a J-shaped manner to construct the pouch. Each pouch limb measures 7–8 cm. The descending limb must be on the left, the ascending one on the right and the mesentery behind the pouch. A pair of Allis' forceps is applied on the antimesenteric border of the colon at the apex of the future pouch. Two other Allis' forceps are placed equidistant from the first (7–8 cm) at the base of the pouch: one on the stapled end of the colon and the other on the descending limb of the pouch. Two adjacent holes are made by stab puncture on the antimesenteric border of each limb of the pouch, at equal distance from the top, close to the Allis' forceps. The two forks of a GIA 90 stapler are introduced into the lumen of the colon, each through one hole, towards the apex of the pouch. The two proximal pairs of Allis' forceps are applied to the border of the holes posterior to the stapler to maintain slight traction upwards while the instrument is fired in a caudad direction. Care must be taken while firing not to include the mesentery between the two limbs: this must be checked by looking behind the stapler. The mesentery must be kept away from the stapler, usually by the index finger. The bowel is then everted to expose the remaining bridge, which is sectioned with a GIA 50 stapler. Haemostasis is secured at the site of anastomosis and the pouch inverted. The pairs of Allis' forceps are removed and the hole is closed by a continuous 4/0 polyglycolic acid suture. The upper stapled end of the short limb is fixed to the adjacent descending limb by an interrupted suture of 4/0 polyglycolic acid. The pouch is again tested to ensure that its apex can reach the lower border of the pubic symphysis. If traction is present, more length can be gained by dividing the mesocolon between the vessels, this manoeuvre giving both length and laxity. The Allis' forceps at the top are then removed.

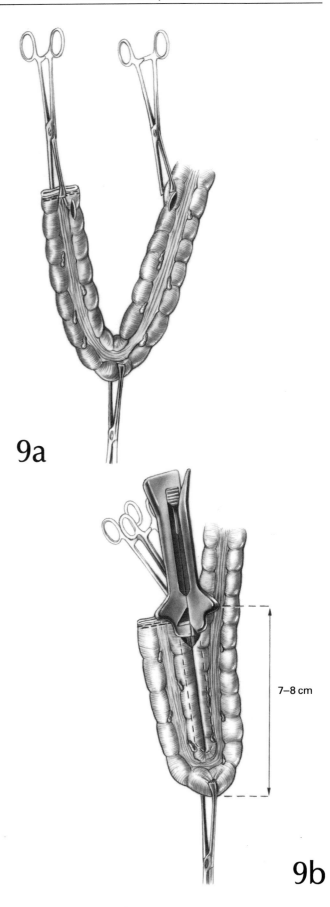

9a

7–8 cm

9b

Coloanal anastomosis

10 The pouch is directed towards the lower pelvis, with great care not to twist the mesentery. At the perineum a pair of Babcock forceps is introduced through the anus to catch the apex of the pouch, and is guided through the anal stump aided by gentle squeezing from above. The pouch is then fixed to the anal sphincter by four interrupted sutures of 4/0 polyglycolic acid, each at one cardinal point just above the mucosal section. The apex of the pouch is opened, and the anastomosis is performed between the mucosa of the anal canal and the full thickness of the colonic pouch, using interrupted sutures of 4/0 polyglycolic acid. Four stitches are initially placed at 3, 6, 9 and 12 o'clock and then four further stitches are added to each of the quadrants thus formed.

The Gelpi retractors are removed, and a Penrose drain is inserted into the reservoir through the anastomosis. Care should be taken to ensure that the mobilized colon does not compress the duodenojejunal junction; if this occurs the latter should be mobilized by division of the ligament of Treitz to avoid postoperative obstruction. The free border of the mesentery is sutured to the posterior peritoneal wall using 4/0 polyglycolic acid to avoid postoperative small bowel obstruction.

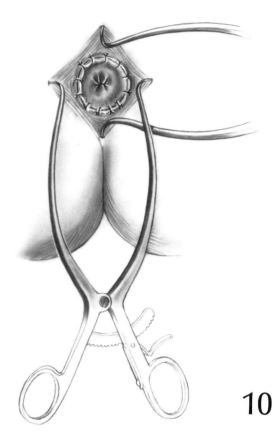

10

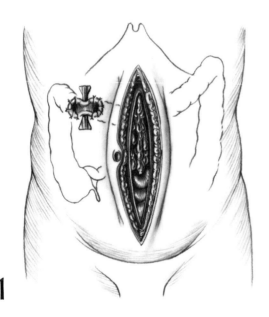

11

Drainage, temporary transverse loop colostomy and closure

11 Two fine-bore suction drains are positioned in the pelvis anterior and posterior to the pouch and brought out through lateral abdominal stab wounds. The right third of the transverse colon is prepared for the construction of a temporary transverse loop colostomy, which is brought out through the anterior abdominal wall by a transverse incision in the upper right quadrant of the abdomen. The abdominal wall is then closed in two layers of continuous sutures: 0 polyglycolic acid on the peritoneal layer and 1 on the aponeurosis.

Variations

The reservoir can be constructed using the sigmoid colon in case of very low malignancy or benign rectal tumour.
    The reservoir can be constructed after extended colectomy (for vascular reasons or the presence of a synchronous colonic lesion) using the right transverse colon to form the reservoir, after which a loop ileostomy is performed.

Postoperative care

Postoperative care is similar to that following any abdominopelvic restorative procedure. Antibiotics (cefoxitin, netilmicin, metronidazole) are given during, and for 2 days after, surgery. An intravenous infusion and a nasogastric tube are maintained in place until the return of normal peristalsis. The Penrose drain is kept for 1 day to reveal any bleeding in the pouch, and the two abdominal drains are removed on days 3–6 after surgery. The Foley catheter is usually left in place for 7–10 days postoperatively to avoid urine retention. However, we advocate placement of a suprapubic urinary catheter at the end of the procedure, which seems to decrease postoperative urinary complications such as urethral strictures, urinary retention or infection. Spontaneous bladder function returns more readily during the postoperative course. The patient learns to manage the colostomy bag before discharge from hospital (usually between days 10 and 12 after surgery). The closure of the transverse loop colostomy is carried out about 8 weeks after the operation.

Outcome

Between January 1984 and September 1990, 162 consecutive patients were treated. The overall mortality was 0.6%; one patient died from myocardial infarction on the seventh postoperative day. Surgical complications occurred in 15 cases (9.2%). Of these, five developed pelvic sepsis (none required surgery) and three had small bowel obstruction (one required laparotomy), one rectovaginal fistula, one haemorrhage of the stoma, one stoma prolapse, one ureteric stenosis requiring operation, one urethral stenosis and two wound infections. At 1-year follow-up, 52% were fully continent and 44% had minor problems. Among the five patients (4%) with frequent faecal incontinence, three had a local recurrence. The mean number of bowel movements was 2.1 per 24 h (range 0.3–8), urgency being absent. Nearly 25% of patients (40) had to simulate reservoir evacuation with a suppository or an enema. The improved function compared with straight coloanal anastomosis is probably related to the presence of a reservoir function.

References

1. Williams NS, Johnston D. Survival and recurrence after sphincter saving resection and abdominoperineal resection for carcinoma of the middle third of the rectum. *Br J Surg* 1984; 71: 278–82.

2. Goligher JC. Current trends in the use of sphincter-saving excision in the treatment of carcinoma of the rectum. *Cancer* 1982; 50: 2627–30.

3. Pollett WG, Nicholls RJ. The relationship between the extent of distal clearance and survival and local recurrence rates after curative anterior resection for carcinoma of the rectum. *Ann Surg* 1983; 198: 159–63.

4. Parks AG, Percy JP. Resection and sutured colo-anal anastomosis for rectal carcinoma. *Br J Surg* 1982; 69: 301–4.

5. Cugnenc PH, Grassin P, Parc R, Loygue J. Place et résultats de l'opération de Babcock dans le traitement du cancer du rectum. *J Chir* 1981; 118: 121–6.

6. Drake DB, Pemberton JH, Beart RW, Dozois RR, Wolff BG. Coloanal anastomosis in the management of benign and malignant rectal disease. *Ann Surg* 1987; 206: 600–5.

7. Nicholls RJ, Lubowski DZ, Donaldson DR. Comparison of colonic reservoir and straight coloanal reconstruction after rectal excision. *Br J Surg* 1988: 75: 318–20.

Further reading

Berger A, Tiret E, Parc R *et al*. Excision of the rectum with colonic J pouch–anal anastomosis for adenocarcinoma of the low and mid rectum. *World J Surg* 1992; 16: 470–7.

Parc R, Tiret E, Frileux P, Moszkowski E, Loygue J. Resection and coloanal anastomosis with colonic reservoir for rectal carcinoma. *Br J Surg* 1986; 73: 139–41.

Procedures for rectal prolapse: introductory comment

D. C. C. Bartolo MS, FRCS
Consultant Surgeon, The Royal Infirmary of Edinburgh, Edinburgh, UK

There are several surgical options in the management of complete rectal prolapse which are described in this section. Their number indicates that we do not, as yet, have the ideal procedure which suits this heterogeneous patient population. Abdominal rectopexy corrects the prolapse in most patients, but incontinence may persist. In this respect, the transabdominal approach is superior to the perineal approach[1,2].

Abdominal procedures

Review of results

Overall, approximately 75% of patients can expect improved continence after abdominal rectopexy, but many patients are far from satisfied with their functional outcome. The most obvious causes for patient dissatisfaction are recurrence of the prolapse, faecal incontinence, and constipation.

Mann and Hoffman reported that 47% of patients were constipated after Ivalon sponge rectopexy and they considered that this complication might explain the recovery of continence[3]. Duthie and Bartolo did not find that bowel frequency was significantly altered after four different types of rectopexy[4]. Specifically, postoperative constipation, incomplete evacuation, and straining at stool did not differ from preoperative status. None of their patients required regular laxatives, but some remained on a high-fibre diet to maintain a regular bowel habit. Similarly, McCue and Thomson[5] reported that bowel function was generally unchanged after rectopexy although 15% developed significant postoperative constipation. Their results suggest that constipation is more common after Ivalon rectopexy than after other forms of prolapse surgery. In Thomson's hands, the low incidence of constipation was attributed to preserving part of the lateral ligaments of the rectum. Thomson's figures contrast with the much higher incidence of constipation reported by Mann and Hoffman, where the whole of the lateral rectal ligaments were divided.

Madoff *et al.*[6] reviewed the functional results of colonic resection and suture rectopexy for complete rectal prolapse in 47 patients followed up for more than 3 years. Sigmoidectomy was performed in 33 patients; the prolapse recurrence rate was 6.3% and rectal mucosal prolapse occurred in 8.5%. In the 20 patients who presented with constipation, only ten improved after surgery. By contrast, in seven of the eight patients who underwent subtotal colectomy, constipation was improved. For those patients who presented with incontinence, only 38% had significant improvement, while in six patients continence worsened, and in an additional four patients significant diarrhoea developed. These authors expressed some anxiety regarding the outcome of colonic resection and suture rectopexy and stress that continence may actually deteriorate. However, these poor results have not been seen in other reports of resection and suture rectopexy in which the majority of patients found that continence was significantly improved after surgery.

The above results show a very mixed picture with different explanations for the various outcomes. In an attempt to address some of the issues, the results of rectopexy were reported in 68 patients using four different techniques[4]: (a) simple suture rectopexy; (b) Ivalon sponge; (c) anterior/posterior Marlex mesh; and (d) resection rectopexy. (The resection rectopexy differed from the Frykman–Goldberg procedure in that the splenic flexure was routinely mobilized and thus the resection was more extensive.) This was not a randomized trial but an observation review of four different operations carried out in a single surgical unit.

Preoperative anal resting pressures were found to correlate inversely with the overall improvement in continence but did not predict which patients would improve. Those with the lowest pressures appeared to have the most to gain. Anal resting pressures rose except after implant surgery, with the most significant increases being identified after resection rectopexy.

Anal sensation did not change dramatically in the study overall, but after resection rectopexy the volume required to stimulate rectal sensation diminished significantly. This change allowed patients to perceive an urge to defaecate at a lower volume of rectal distension, leading to appropriate action by the patient to avoid incontinence. Thus in this series the best results were achieved when implants were avoided. Improvement in continence occurred most frequently after suture rectopexy (89%) and resection rectopexy (79%), but less so after Marlex rectopexy (67%) and Ivalon sponge procedures (40%).

Farouk et al.[7] reported an additional series of 22 patients who had undergone resection rectopexy. Continence to solid and liquid stool improved significantly in all but one patient. Resting anal canal pressures rose and this was associated with a significant increase in the frequency of electrical activity in the internal anal sphincter seen on the electromyogram. However, despite these improvements, anal pressures remained within the range seen in unselected patients with faecal incontinence. Thus, sphincter pressure recovery does not fully explain the reasons for improved continence in these patients.

Postoperative continence

The improvement in postoperative continence may be explained by three mechanisms:

1. Effects on resting anal pressures. There appears to be general agreement that resting anal pressures rise in patients in whom continence is restored and this improvement results from an increase in the activity of the internal anal sphincter. A plausible explanation for the benefits of this operation is that the presence of the prolapsed bowel within the lower rectum and anal canal induces reflex relaxation of the internal sphincter. Removal of the prolapse from this area allows internal sphincter tone to recover.
2. Rectal motility. Before surgery patients have abnormal rectal motility with high pressure waves in the rectal wall probably caused by the presence of the prolapsed gut within the rectum. After surgery these high pressure waves disappear.
3. Relationship between resting anal pressure and rectal motility. The interrelationship between resting anal pressure and rectal motility may provide the most plausible explanation for the recovery of continence after successful rectopexy. Duthie and Bartolo[4] found that preoperative anal canal pressures were exceeded by rectal pressures, but after surgery the lowered rectal pressure no longer exceeds that generated in the anal canal. Although the resting anal canal pressure remains relatively low when compared with normal values, it is able to cope with the lowered pressures generated in the rectum once successful rectopexy has been achieved.

Postoperative constipation

Disordered bowel habit is considered to be one of the predisposing factors in the aetiology of rectal prolapse in some patients, and this long-term disorder may contribute to postoperative constipation. Furthermore, because constipation frequently complicates both Ivalon and Marlex rectopexy, there is a case for adopting an operation which specifically aims to minimize the risks of this postoperative complication. However, the precise mechanisms of constipation following rectopexy are uncertain.

Preoperative slow colonic transit

Most studies reviewing the outcome of rectal prolapse surgery do not report the results of preoperative colonic transit studies. It may be that those reports with their high incidence of constipation may have contained subjects with slow colonic transit. The efficacy of subtotal colectomy in those patients with slow colonic transit in association with rectal prolapse is consistent with this hypothesis.

Mechanical effects of surgery

High fixation of the rectum allows the redundant sigmoid colon to lie in the pouch of Douglas and this configuration may create a mechanical obstruction at the site of rectopexy. Indeed, Ripstein now favours posterior rectal fixation to try to avoid this complication, the original Ripstein procedure being complicated by a 16.5% incidence of faecal impaction. Despite this modification, if the sigmoid loop is redundant it may also become kinked at its junction with the rectopexy. The placement of Ivalon sponge behind the rectum causes fixation by fibrosis. This fibrosis decreases rectal compliance which may explain the high rate of postoperative constipation following Ivalon sponge rectopexy.

Bowel denervation

An alternative or additional hypothesis for postoperative constipation is that rectal mobilization divides the autonomic neural inflow to the left colon thereby altering bowel function. Resection rectopexy, as advocated by Frykman and Goldberg[2], aims to prevent constipation by removing this partially denervated sigmoid and furthermore avoids rectosigmoid distortion which is a mechanical problem common to the other fixation procedures.

Perineal procedures

There has been a recent resurgence of interest in the Délorme procedure which is remarkably well tolerated by frail patients who suffer almost no postoperative discomfort. However, from the functional point of view there is a long recovery period because of the loss of rectal capacity which gives rise to urgency and incontinence. Furthermore, prolapse recurrence rates tend to be higher than with transabdominal rectopexy, but this rate can be minimized by adhering to the specific technical details described in Kennedy's chapter. The Gant–Miwa technique described by Muto has many similarities to the Délorme procedure and its principal advantage is that it is so well tolerated by elderly, frail patients.

Conclusion

Transabdominal rectopexy appears to be the 'best buy' for the fit patient in whom the objective of surgery is to achieve a low prolapse recurrence rate and a restoration of bowel continence. In these patients the most important preoperative investigation is colonic transit time. In those patients with significant clinical constipation or a slow colonic transit time, a resection is indicated and subtotal colectomy should be considered for the most severe cases. However, the anastomosis should take place at the sacral promontory because low anterior resection is associated with an increased anastomotic leak rate and loss of the compliant rectal reservoir which is an important component of the continence mechanism. (Removal of the rectum and its replacement by non-compliant and often diverticular sigmoid colon may explain the lower continence rates following perineal rectal excision in the treatment of prolapse.)

In those patients with normal colonic transit time, suture fixation or the Orr–Loygue operation are options. The use of Ivalon sponge or Marlex mesh is not advocated because they appear to increase rectal fibrosis and thus reduce rectal compliance associated with postoperative constipation and faecal incontinence.

In the frailer, elderly patient, where the objective is simply to remove the sticky, smelly perineal mass, one of the perineal procedures described in this section is to be commended.

In the future rectal prolapse operations will, in a selected proportion of patients, be carried out laparoscopically and resection rectopexy is relatively straightforward using this minimally invasive technique. Long follow-up is mandatory after all operations for rectal prolapse so that the long-term effects of these different operations can be defined.

References

1. Solla JA, Rothenberger DA, Goldberg SM. Colonic resection in the treatment of complete rectal prolapse. *Neth J Surg* 1989; 41: 132–5.

2. Watts JD, Rothenberger DA, Buls JG, Goldberg SM, Nivatvongs S. The management of procidentia: 30 years experience. *Dis Colon Rectum* 1985; 28: 96–102.

3. Mann CV, Hoffman C. Complete rectal prolapse: the anatomical and functional results of treatment by extended abdominal rectopexy. *Br J Surg* 1988; 75: 34–7.

4. Duthie GS, Bartolo DCC. Abdominal rectopexy for rectal prolapse: a comparison of techniques. *Br J Surg* 1992; 79: 107–13.

5. McCue JL, Thomson JPS. Clinical and functional results of abdominal rectopexy for complete rectal prolapse. *Br J Surg* 1991; 78: 921–3.

6. Madoff RD, Williams JG, Wong WD, Rothenberger DA, Goldberg SM. Long-term functional results of colon resection and rectopexy for overt rectal prolapse. *Am J Gastroenterol* 1992; 87: 101–4.

7. Farouk R, Duthie GS, Bartolo DCC, MacGregor AB. Restoration of continence following rectopexy for rectal prolapse and recovery of the internal anal sphincter electromyogram. *Br J Surg* 1992; 79: 439–40.

Illustrations by Gillian Oliver

Rectal prolapse: intra-abdominal repair with or without resection

Robert D. Madoff MD
Clinical Assistant Professor of Surgery, Division of Colon and Rectal Surgery, University of Minnesota Medical School, Minneapolis, Minnesota, USA

J. Graham Williams MCh, FRCS
Lecturer in Surgery, University of Birmingham, Queen Elizabeth Hospital, Birmingham, UK

Stanley M. Goldberg MD, FACS, FRACS
Clinical Professor of Surgery and Director, Division of Colon and Rectal Surgery, University of Minnesota Medical School, Minneapolis, Minnesota, USA

History

Abdominal prolapse repairs were first described at the turn of this century[1]. Jeannel described colopexy in 1896[2], and Pemberton and Stalker advocated anterior sigmoid fixation following posterior rectal mobilization in 1939[3]. Direct suture fixation of the mobilized rectum to the sacrum was first described by Cutait in 1959[4]. Numerous rectal fixation procedures have since been described, with and without foreign material, all emphasizing the importance of adequate rectal mobilization[1]. In 1969, Frykman and Goldberg combined rectal mobilization with both suture rectopexy and sigmoid resection for the treatment of rectal prolapse[5].

Principles and justification

Abdominal fixation procedures for rectal prolapse are widely popular. These techniques involve securing the mobilized rectum to the presacral fascia with or without foreign material. Variations of this approach include the anterior rectal sling (Ripstein), the posterior rectal sling (Wells) and simple suture fixation (Cutait). Suture fixation can be combined with sigmoid resection, and this operation has been the procedure of choice at the University of Minnesota Division of Colon and Rectal Surgery for patients fit to undergo transabdominal prolapse repair. The avoidance of foreign material for fixation lessens the risks and consequences of postoperative infection, particularly when an intestinal resection is included as part of the procedure.

The original rationale for resection in addition to fixation was to prevent early recurrence by suspending the left colon from the splenocolic ligament. Concomitant sigmoidectomy also eliminates the risk of postoperative volvulus of the characteristically redundant sigmoid colon that becomes even longer following rectosigmoid mobilization. Furthermore, recent evidence has suggested that the addition of sigmoidectomy to rectopexy may prevent or alleviate postoperative evacuation disturbances, particularly constipation[6, 7]. Finally, the combination of subtotal colectomy with rectopexy has been successful in the treatment of patients suffering from severe and intractable slow transit constipation in addition to rectal prolapse[8]. Care must be taken that associated anal incontinence is not present.

701

Preoperative

The diagnosis of full-thickness rectal prolapse should be obvious from the history and physical examination. The prolapse is demonstrated by asking the patient to strain seated on a commode or in the squatting position. It is difficult to demonstrate rectal prolapse with the patient in the prone jack-knife position. Full-thickness rectal prolapse can be differentiated from rectal mucosal prolapse by the presence of characteristic concentric (as opposed to radial) rectal folds, and by the presence of a palpable anal sulcus in full-thickness prolapse. A patulous anus is characteristic of rectal prolapse.

Preoperative assessment of the colon by barium enema or colonoscopy is required to exclude an associated lesion. Colonoscopy may be performed immediately before surgery. Anorectal physiology testing and defaecography are seldom helpful in establishing the extent of full-thickness rectal prolapse. Anorectal physiology, however, is a useful research tool for assessing objectively the effect of the operation on the pelvic floor and anal sphincters. Colonic transit studies should be performed on patients with severe constipation.

Full mechanical and antibiotic bowel preparation is required. Appropriate regimens include liquid diet with enemas, laxatives such as magnesium citrate or sodium picrosulphite, and polyethylene glycol-based oral lavage solutions. Care should be taken to avoid dehydration in elderly and poor-risk patients. Prophylactic intravenous antibiotic cover is administered for 24 h, commencing at induction of anaesthesia. A second-generation cephalosporin provides broad-spectrum cover against colonic organisms and is a rational choice. The bladder is emptied with a Foley catheter. A standard operative preparation of the abdomen is performed.

Anaesthesia

Transabdominal prolapse repair requires general anaesthesia. Patients medically unfit for general anaesthesia are best served by perineal rectosigmoidectomy (as described in the chapter on pp. 730–735).

Operation

Position of patient

1 The patient is placed in the modified lithotomy position described on page 48. The authors' strong preference is for Allen stirrups, which are easily adjustable and whose short foot rests apply no pressure to the peroneal nerve. Pneumatic compression stockings are routinely used for deep venous thrombosis prophylaxis; these stockings also help to prevent compression of the peroneal nerve as it courses over the lateral head of the fibula. The foot of the table is then dropped.

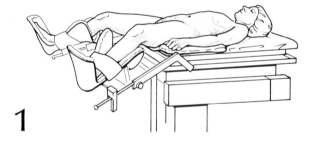

Incision

2 While a lower midline incision is acceptable, the authors prefer an infraumbilical transverse incision, which is more comfortable for the patient, less liable to cause respiratory disturbance, provides excellent exposure, and leads to a superior cosmetic result.

A self-retaining retractor is placed and routine abdominal exploration is performed. The small and proximal large intestine are packed away in the upper abdomen.

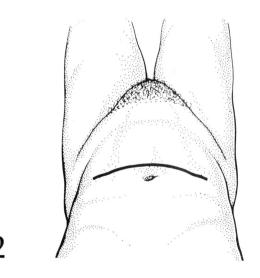

Rectosigmoid mobilization

3 The sigmoid colon is mobilized along the line of Toldt using an electrocautery blade mounted on a tip extender. The rectosigmoid junction is retracted to the right, and the left peritoneal reflection is scored approximately 1 cm from the intestinal wall. The rectosigmoid junction is then retracted to the left for scoring of the right peritoneal reflection. Care is taken throughout dissection and rectopexy to avoid injury to the ureters and gonadal vessels on either side of the pelvis.

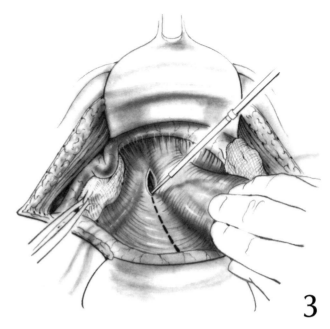

3

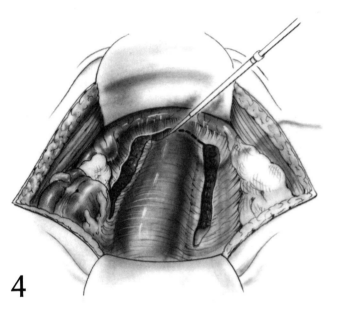

4

4 The uterus is retracted anteriorly and the peritoneal scoring is completed at the base of the cul-de-sac.

5 The presacral space is entered at the level of the sacral promontory, and posterior mobilization in the avascular plane is completed under direct vision with blade electrocautery. This dissection is facilitated by anterior retraction of the rectum with a long curved retractor, such as a Harrington retractor. Mobilization is complete when Waldeyer's fascia has been divided and the levator ani muscles have been reached. Anterior dissection is carried out to the upper third of the vagina in women and to the seminal vesicles in men. The lateral stalks are preserved. A typical mobilization gains 10–15 cm of intestinal length.

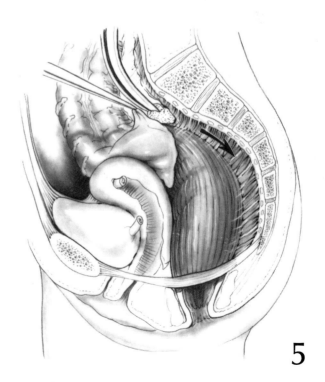

5

Rectal fixation

6 The rectum is fixed to the presacral fascia with 2/0 silk horizontal mattress sutures. Each bite is taken in three parts through the lateral stalk (anterior to posterior), across the presacral fascia of the sacral hollow (off the midline to avoid the middle sacral artery), and back through the lateral stalk (posterior to anterior).

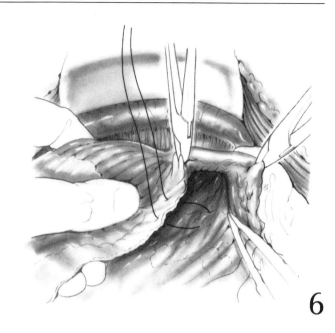

6

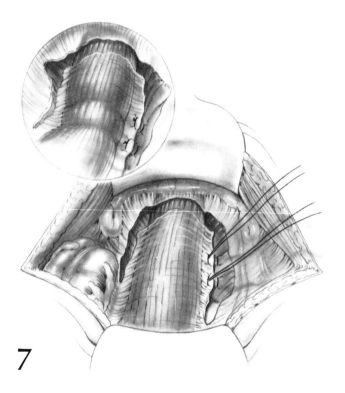

7

7 Two sutures are placed on one or both sides of the rectum and are positioned to draw the distal rectum cephalad and posterior. Placement of the fixation sutures immediately adjacent to the rectal wall minimizes the risk of bleeding from branches of the middle rectal artery. Each suture is individually tagged, and they are tied only after all have been placed. Occasionally, a constricting band will become evident when the sutures are drawn tight; under these circumstances, the offending sutures must be removed and repositioned.

Sigmoid resection

A resection is performed to remove the redundant sigmoid colon with the anastomosis at a comfortable level utilizing peritoneal intestine. If subtotal colectomy has been carried out for associated severe constipation, ileosigmoid anastomosis is performed at the 20–25-cm level. The authors' preference is for a hand-sewn, single-layer anastomosis using a semiclosed technique with interrupted 4/0 silk sutures. Stapled anastomosis can also be carried out.

Postoperative care

Nasogastric or orogastric tubes are used during the operation for gastric decompression, but they are removed in the recovery room. Patients are given nothing by mouth until intestinal function returns. The authors now routinely use intravenous opiates with patient-controlled analgesia during the postoperative period.

Outcome

The recurrence rate after suture rectopexy with or without resection ranges from 0%[9] to 9%[10]. The authors' recurrence rate, with a mean follow-up of 65 months, is 6%[8]. While concomitant sigmoid resection does not seem to improve the recurrence rate of abdominal rectopexy, there is preliminary evidence that resection may alleviate prolapse-associated constipation[6,7]. Subtotal colectomy with suture rectopexy should be performed in patients with documented severe slow transit constipation, rectal prolapse and adequate rectal evacuation. In the authors' series[8], 70% of severely constipated patients with prolapse improved following rectopexy and subtotal colectomy (either in one or two stages).

Restoration of continence is reported in 70–90% of incontinent patients undergoing suture rectopexy, and in 40–90% of patients undergoing resection/rectopexy[11]. It is possible that intestinal resection compromises the ability of abdominal rectopexy to restore normal continence, but the answer to this question awaits completion of ongoing randomized trials.

References

1. Goligher JC. *Surgery of the Rectum and Colon.* 5th edn. London: Baillière Tindall, 1984.

2. Jeannel D. Du prolapsus du rectum. *Clin Fac Med Toulouse II* 1896; 101: 121–37.

3. Pemberton J, Stalker LK de J. Surgical treatment of complete rectal prolapse. *Ann Surg* 1939; 109: 799–808.

4. Cutait D. Sacro-promontory fixation of the rectum for complete rectal prolapse. *Proc R Soc Med* 1951; 52(Suppl): 105.

5. Frykman HM, Goldberg SM. The surgical treatment of rectal procidentia. *Surg Gynecol Obstet* 1969; 129: 1225–30.

6. Sayfan J, Pinho M, Alexander-Williams J, Keighley MRB. Sutured posterior abdominal rectopexy with sigmoidectomy compared with Marlex® rectopexy for rectal prolapse. *Br J Surg* 1990; 77: 143–5.

7. McKee RF, Lauder JC, Poon FW, Aitchison MA, Finlay IG. A prospective randomized study of abdominal rectopexy with and without sigmoidectomy in rectal prolapse. *Surg Gynecol Obstet* 1992; 174: 145–8.

8. Madoff RD, Williams JG, Wong WD, Rothenberger DA, Goldberg SM. Long term functional results of colon resection and rectopexy for overt rectal prolapse. *Am J Gastroenterol* 1992; 87: 101–4.

9. Graham W, Clegg JF, Taylor V. Complete rectal prolapse: repair by a simple technique. *Ann R Coll Surg Engl* 1984; 66: 87–9.

10. Husa A, Sainio P, Von Smitten K. Abdominal rectopexy and sigmoid resection (Frykman–Goldberg operation) for rectal prolapse. *Acta Chir Scand* 1988; 154: 221–4.

11. Madoff RD, Watts JD, Rothenberger DA, Goldberg SM. Rectal prolapse: treatment. In: Henry M, Swash M, eds. *Coloproctology and the Pelvic Floor.* 2nd edn. London: Butterworths, 1992: 321–50.

Rectal prolapse: rectopexy with synthetic circular net (Ripstein's operation)

B. F. Holmstrom MD
Department of Surgery, Karolinska Institute, Danderyd Hospital, Danderyd, Sweden

S. A. Dolk MD
Department of Surgery, Karolinska Institute, Danderyd Hospital, Danderyd, Sweden

Principles and justification[1-3]

Rectal prolapse starts as an intussusception, which begins approximately 7 cm up the anterior wall of the rectum at the sacral promontory. The operation fixes this part of the intestine into the posterior concavity of the sacral curve and thus prevents the intussusception from occurring. In the postoperative period, fibrosis will develop which maintains the rectum in the desired position. The Marlex mesh will heal so completely that it will be difficult to find by inspection but can be palpated if further surgery is required.

Preoperative

The patient showers on the night before and the morning of surgery. Two bisacodyl suppositories are given early in the morning on the day of surgery. No laxatives or enemas are recommended so that the first bowel movement is not delayed.

Operation

Incision

1 The abdomen is opened through a left paramedian incision which is covered by moist gauze packs and a plastic cover sheet to avoid contact between the patient's skin and the synthetic mesh.

The abdominal contents are examined to exclude unexpected pathology. The small intestine and caecum are packed away from the pelvis. The urinary bladder, which was filled with 200 ml saline before the operation began, is punctured with a Cystofix set to create a cystostomy and the saline is evacuated. The urethral catheter is removed after the operation.

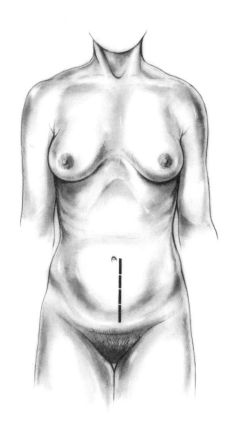

1

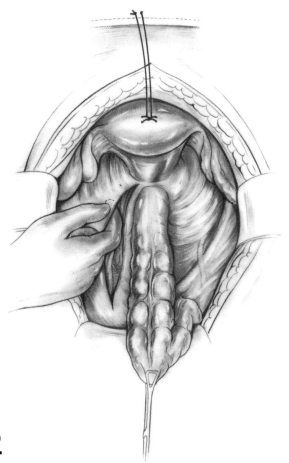

2

2 A polyglactin (Vicryl) suture is placed through the uterus at two points, knotted, and then stitched to the dressings below the incision to keep the uterus and the vagina stretched anteriorly and thus removed from the operative field. The pouch of Douglas is usually deeper than normal in patients with rectal prolapse. The rectosigmoid junction is pulled up into the incision, and the peritoneum is incised on the left side a few centimetres above the sacral promontory. The incision is extended along the rectum, 1–2 cm lateral to it, down to the peritoneal reflexion. The lateral part of the peritoneum is mobilized on both sides and is left as a flap, which will later cover the synthetic mesh. The left ureter is identified.

3 The same procedure is repeated on the patient's right side.

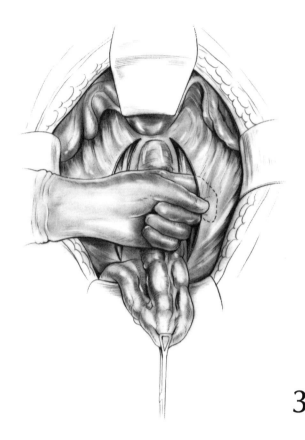

3

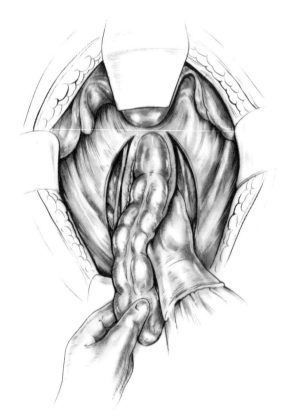

4

4 The rectum is mobilized dorsally from the sacrum by incision of the fascia of Waldeyer; the incision is carried down to the apex of the coccyx in a bloodless plane. There will now be a passage between the rectosigmoid mesentery and the sacrum. The mobilization is continued laterally on both sides of the rectum, but the lateral ligaments are not divided.

The rectum can now be pulled up and straightened; the peritoneum at the bottom of the pouch of Douglas is divided and the rectovaginal septum is dissected about 3–4 cm downwards.

5 While a pack is left in the pelvic operative field, the sterile Marlex mesh is cut with scissors to the shape shown. This shape prevents the sigmoid colon from angulating over the upper border of the Marlex mesh down into the pelvis.

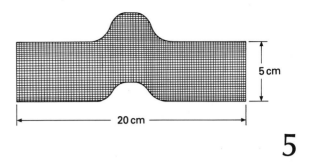

5

6a, b The mesh is sutured as far down on the rectovaginal septum as possible with the first suture of 2/0 Ti-Cron, while the rectum is held stretched upwards. The two wings of the mesh are then swung around the rectum to form a ring.

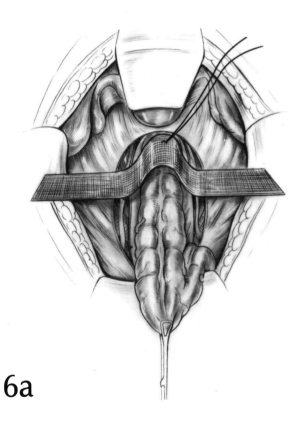

6a

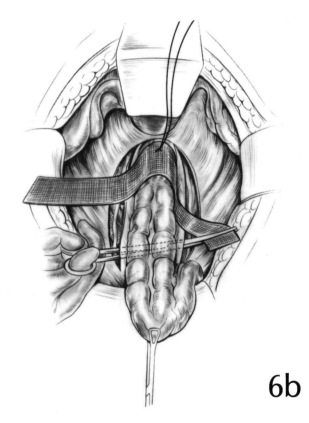

6b

7 The ring is held together with two artery forceps and should have a diameter of 8–10 cm corresponding to at least four fingers in diameter. This ring cannot be too wide, but it can certainly be too narrow! The redundant parts of the wing are cut away. The first suture between the ring and the sacrum is placed in the presacral fascia, which must be exposed by the removal of fat and connective tissue, about 3 cm below the sacral promontory. The suture must be well placed into the fascia, and this can be ascertained by pulling upwards on it and feeling that it is securely anchored. The suture is then placed through the two wings of the Marlex mesh between the two artery forceps. It must be ensured that both wings are caught by the suture, which can then be tied.

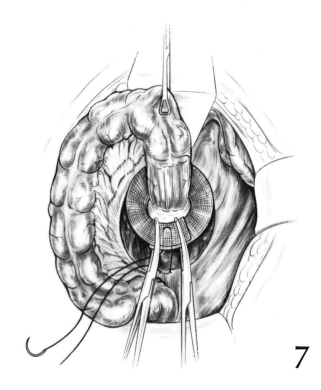

7

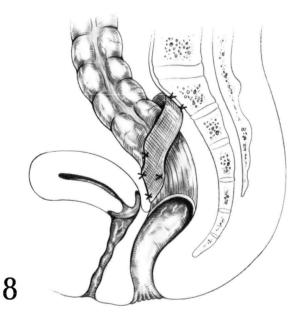

8

8 The third suture is placed 1–3 cm above the second. The posterior intestinal wall should be movable within the mesh ring with no tissue caught in the sutures.

The fourth suture is placed 1–3 cm above the first in the rectovaginal septum. The fifth and sixth sutures are placed on the right side between the mesh and the rectal wall, and the seventh and eighth sutures similarly placed on the left side. When the stretch on the rectum is relieved, the bowel should not fall back into the pelvis.

Wound closure

9 A suction drain is placed retroperitoneally and brought out in the right iliac fossa. The two peritoneal flaps are united in front by a continuous 2/0 polyglactin suture, beginning at the posterior vaginal wall and moving towards the rectum. Having reached the rectum, the suture is then continued on both sides ending at the point where the incision in the rectosigmoid peritoneum began.

The suture in the uterine fundus is cut above the knot, thus avoiding bleeding. The abdominal incision is closed by a continuous 2/0 polyglactin suture in the peritoneum. The anterior rectus fascia is closed by a 0 polyglactin suture and the skin with a continuous non-absorbable suture.

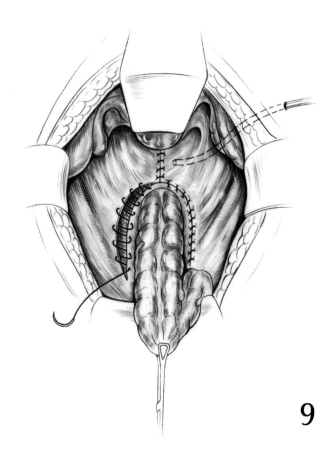

9

Postoperative care

Prophylactic antibiotics are not given on a routine basis. The patient is allowed to drink *ad libitum* on the first day after operation and to eat on the second day. The first bowel movement may be delayed in some patients and simple laxatives are given. The patient can usually leave the hospital between the fifth and eighth day after operation.

Complications

In the authors' series of approximately 150 operations[4], the overall complication rate is low (approximately 5%). The following complications have been observed: intrapelvic haematoma; wound infection; incisional hernia; recurrence of rectal prolapse (approximately 5%); constipation (the reason for which is not clear, but slow intestinal transit seems to be an important factor);

and incontinence, which is usually present before surgery and is often but not invariably improved by the procedure.

References

1. Ripstein CB. Treatment of massive rectal prolapse. *Am J Surg* 1952; 83: 68–71.

2. Ripstein CB. Surgical care of massive rectal prolapse. *Dis Colon Rectum* 1965; 8: 34–8.

3. Jurgeleit HC, Corman ML, Coller JA, Veidenheimer MC. Procidentia of the rectum: Teflon-sling repair of rectal prolapse, Lahey Clinic experience. *Dis Colon Rectum* 1975; 18: 464–7.

4. Holmstrom B, Broden G, Dolk A. Results of the Ripstein operation in the treatment of rectal prolapse and internal rectal procidentia. *Dis Colon Rectum* 1986; 29: 845–8.

Rectal prolapse: abdominal rectopexy with posterior fixation

Michael R. B. Keighley MS, FRCS

Barling Professor of Surgery, Department of Surgery, Queen Elizabeth Hospital, Birmingham, UK

History

Classically, posterior abdominal rectopexy, as described by Wells, utilized Ivalon sponge sutured to the presacral fascia and to the mobilized rectum to fix the rectum within the sacral hollow[1]. Alternative methods of fixation have been used with great success with materials such as polytetrafluoroethylene (Teflon) and polypropylene mesh[2]. There is now substantial evidence that a foreign body is not necessary and might be associated with some of the complications of the procedure, particularly constipation and chronic sepsis. Sutured rectopexy is therefore gaining popularity[3].

Abdominal rectopexy may be combined with sigmoid colectomy[4], which is indicated in the patient with rectal prolapse and associated constipation or where there is a long redundant sigmoid loop after rectal mobilization. Concomitant pelvic floor repair has been advocated for patients with rectal prolapse with severe faecal incontinence, particularly when certain predictive parameters are identified before operation; these are low resting anal pressures, short anal canal and gross perineal descent[5]. In such patients, rectopexy may be combined with a pelvic floor repair, either from above or from the perineum, the latter giving a more secure reconstruction[6].

Principles and justification

Indications

Abdominal rectopexy is regarded as the operation of choice for most fit patients with a full-thickness rectal prolapse. Posterior abdominal rectopexy is preferred to the anterior methods of rectal fixation, because anterior rectopexy is often complicated by constipation and stenosis at the rectopexy site[7].

Secondary indications for abdominal rectopexy include solitary rectal ulcer and incomplete rectal intussusception. Rectopexy is only advised in the treatment of a solitary rectal ulcer if the patient has incapacitating symptoms, particularly bleeding and coexisting rectal prolapse. Symptomatically, the results of rectopexy for solitary rectal ulcers are disappointing. Rectopexy has also been advocated to correct an incomplete rectal intussusception demonstrated by video proctography. Although the operation successfully corrects the anatomical abnormality, symptoms tend to persist and the author does not advise abdominal rectopexy for incomplete intussusception alone.

Contraindications

The approach may be contraindicated for individuals who represent a high anaesthetic risk or who are particularly frail. Under these circumstances, a perineal procedure might be preferable.

Preoperative

Preoperative anaesthetic assessment is advised in elderly patients. Complex anorectal function tests may help to identify patients requiring a coexisting colectomy or pelvic floor repair[5]. Preoperative bowel preparation is performed.

Anaesthesia

General or spinal anaesthesia may be used[2].

Operation

Position of patient

The patient is catheterized and placed in the Lloyd-Davies position, as described in the chapter on pp. 47–50.

Incision

1 A midline incision is used. The small intestine is retracted out of the pelvis and secured with wet abdominal mops.

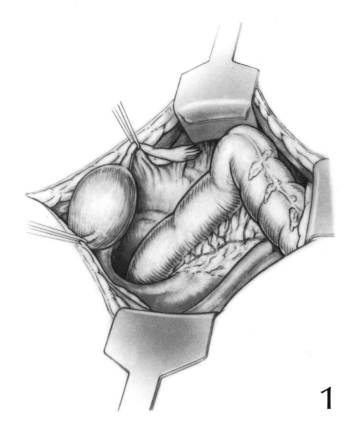

1

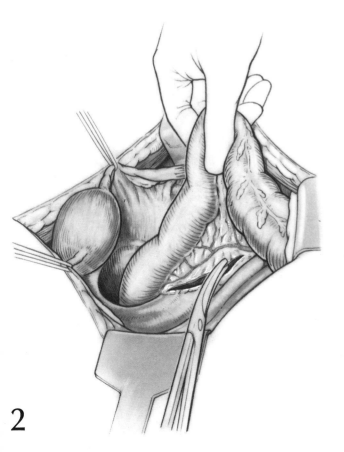

2

2 The surgeon grasps the sigmoid colon in the right hand; the peritoneum over the left side of the sigmoid colon, crossing the pelvic brim, is divided. The sigmoid colon is then returned to its normal anatomical position, and the right side of the pelvic peritoneum is divided. A pelvic retractor is placed in the midline to retract the uterus anteriorly. The superior haemorrhoidal vessels are identified and the loose areolar tissue behind the vessels is divided so that a window is created from one side of the pelvis to the other.

3 Dissection now proceeds downwards in the midline posteriorly behind the superior haemorrhoidal vessels, and behind the mesorectum to the tip of the coccyx. The rectum is then retracted to the left, in order to divide the right lateral ligaments. In rectal prolapse the lateral ligaments are attenuated, and seldom contain blood vessels that require ligature. The same manoeuvre is performed on the opposite side.

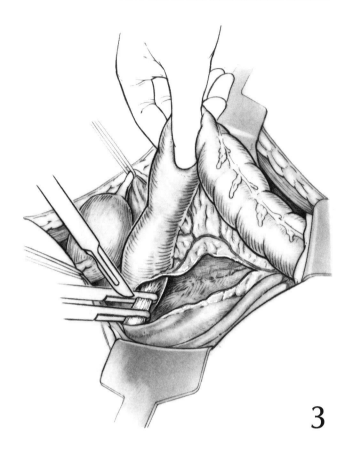

3

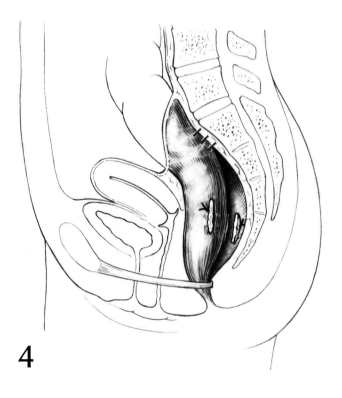

4

4 The anterior pelvic peritoneum is not divided, because the deep rectovaginal pouch in rectal prolapse makes this manoeuvre unnecessary and it increases the risk of bleeding from vaginal veins. Once the rectum has been fully mobilized it is forcibly pulled upwards to fix it to the presacral fascia.

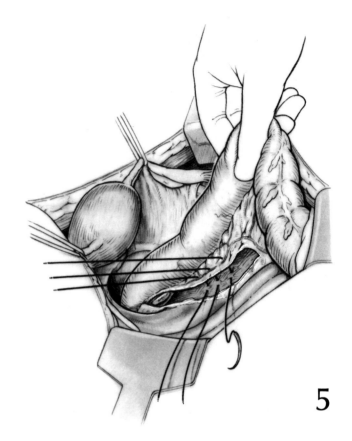

5 Three polypropylene (Prolene) sutures are placed in the midline just below the sacral promontory, through the presacral fascia and through the mesorectum in the midline. It is important to avoid the presacral veins which lie on either side of the midline and can be associated with catastrophic haemorrhage if they are damaged.

5

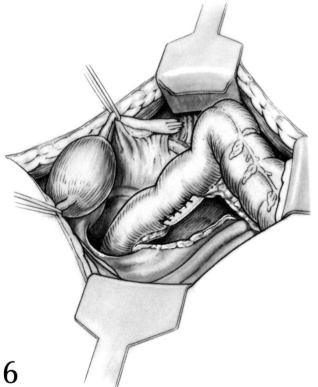

6 A polypropylene mesh may be used as an alternative method of fixation. A small rectangle of mesh is cut, three sutures are placed through the centre of the mesh and the presacral fascia in the midline. The two free lateral leaves of the mesh are then used for attachment to the lateral aspect of the mesorectum.

6

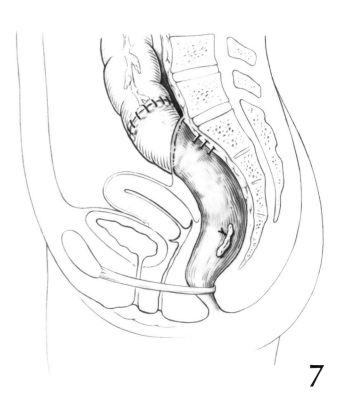

7 If the sigmoid colon is grossly redundant after full rectal mobilization and rectopexy, or if the patient complains of constipation, a sigmoid colectomy may be included. The sigmoid mesocolon is divided, ligating the vessels, and an end-to-end colorectal anastomosis is performed just above the rectopexy site. Haemostasis is achieved in the pelvis. Two closed suction drains are inserted, and the abdomen is closed in the usual way.

7

Postoperative care

Intravenous infusion is continued until the ileus has resolved, and early ambulation is encouraged.

Complications

Immediate complications include bleeding and pelvic sepsis. Catastrophic haemorrhage may occur from damaged presacral veins. Alternatively, a slow ooze may be associated with a pelvic haematoma, which may become infected. Pelvic infection may occur, particularly if there is contamination around a foreign body, or if there is a leak from the colorectal anastomosis. Late complications are persistent incontinence and constipation. Approximately 30% of patients who initially present with incontinence and a rectal prolapse have persistent incontinence, despite an abdominal rectopexy[8]. This may be managed by a subsequent pelvic floor repair. Approximately 60% of patients who have a rectopexy alone develop postoperative constipation[8]. This complication has now been significantly reduced by combining sigmoid colectomy with abdominal rectopexy[9].

Outcome

Abdominal rectopexy is an extremely successful method of controlling a rectal prolapse. The incidence of recurrent prolapse depends on the duration of follow-up, but in most large series does not exceed 5%[1-4,8,9].

References

1. Penfold JCB, Hawley PR. Experiences of Ivalon-sponge implant for complete rectal prolapse at St. Mark's Hospital, 1960–1970. *Br J Surg* 1972; 59: 846–8.

2. Keighley MRB, Fielding JWL, Alexander-Williams J. Results of Marlex mesh abdominal rectopexy for rectal prolapse in 1000 consecutive patients. *Br J Surg* 1983; 70: 229–32.

3. Loygue J, Huguier M, Malafosse M, Biotois H. Complete prolapse of the rectum. A report on 140 cases treated by rectopexy. *Br J Surg* 1971; 58: 847–8.

4. Frykman HM, Goldberg SM. The surgical treatment of rectal procidentia. *Surg Gynecol Obstet* 1969; 129: 1225–30.

5. Yoshioka K, Hyland G, Keighley MRB. Anorectal function after abdominal rectopexy, parameters of predictive value in identifying return of continence. *Br J Surg* 1989; 76: 64–8.

6. Altemeier WA, Giuseffi J, Hoxworth P. Treatment of extensive prolapse of the rectum in aged or debilitated patients. *Arch Surg* 1952; 65: 72–80.

7. Gordon PH, Hoexter B. Complications of the Ripstein procedure. *Dis Colon Rectum* 1978; 21: 277–80.

8. Yoshioka K, Heyen F, Keighley MRB. Functional results after posterior abdominal rectopexy for rectal prolapse. *Dis Colon Rectum* 1989; 32: 835–8.

9. Sayfan, J, Pinho M, Alexander-Williams J, Keighley MRB. Sutured posterior abdominal rectopexy with sigmoidectomy compared with Marlex rectopexy for rectal prolapse. *Br J Surg* 1990; 77: 143–5.

Rectal prolapse: Loygue operation

Bernard Nordlinger MD
Professor of Surgery, Centre de Chirurgie Digestive, Hôpital Saint-Antoine, Paris, France

Philippe Wind MD
Assistant Professor, Centre de Chirurgie Digestive, Hôpital Saint-Antoine, Paris, France

History

In 1947, Thomas Orr[1] from Kansas City described a new technique for treatment of complete prolapse of the rectum, in which the rectum was suspended from the sacral promontory using strips of fascia lata without dissecting the rectum. This technique appeared to be associated with a high risk of recurrence. In 1957 Loygue and Cerbonnet[2] added two major changes to Orr's technique: first, the rectum was dissected as far down into the pelvis as possible; and second, the peritoneum of the pouch of Douglas was resected. A few years later the method was improved by the use of nylon strips instead of fascia lata for rectal suspension[3].

Principles and justification

Rectopexy to the sacral promontory is a simple procedure for the treatment of complete rectal prolapse. The operation combines mobilization of the rectum down to the levator ani muscles without devascularization or denervation, with suspension to the prevertebral fascia in front of the sacral promontory with strips of non-resorbable material. The peritoneum of the pouch of Douglas is resected and obliterated.

Preoperative

Clinical examination should confirm the exteriorization of a total rectal prolapse and exclude a purely mucosal or haemorrhoidal prolapse. The tone of the anal sphincter is assessed by rectal examination. In most cases, electromyography of the anal sphincter or rectal manometry is not necessary. A colonoscopy is advisable to exclude other colorectal pathology. Although the bowel is not opened during rectopexy, a mechanical preparation of the bowel is carried out with 3 litres of polyethylene glycol solution (PEG) the day before surgery. Prophylactic antibiotics (metronidazole and gentamicin) are given on the day of surgery.

Anaesthesia

Rectopexy to the promontory is generally performed under general anaesthesia, but an epidural anaesthetic can also be used in elderly or debilitated patients.

Operation

Position of patient

The patient is placed supine on the operating table, with the surgeon on the left side and the first assistant on the right.

Incision

A midline incision extending from the pubic symphysis to the epigastric region is performed. The patient is tilted in a moderate head-down position. A self-retaining retractor is placed and the small gut is packed into the upper abdomen. Exploration of the abdomen usually confirms the abnormal mobility of the rectum, which is not fixed to the sacrum, and the unusual depth of the pouch of Douglas.

Full mobilization of the rectum

1, 2 The first step is the mobilization of the sigmoid colon and mesocolon from the posterior parietal peritoneum. The rectum is then mobilized as far down as possible anteriorly and posteriorly by dissection in its sheath. The rectal peritoneum is first incised along its line of reflection from the pelvic wall to the rectum. The incision has the shape of an inverted U. The peritoneal incision begins on the right side of the base of the mesosigmoid immediately lateral to the inferior mesenteric artery and continues, close to the right side of the rectum, to the pouch of Douglas and then comes back up on the left side. The presacral connective tissue is opened just in front of the presacral fascia on the right side at the beginning of the peritoneal incision immediately behind the inferior mesenteric vessels which are carefully preserved. The presacral nerve remains posteriorly. The rectum is then mobilized posteriorly down to the levator ani muscle, taking care not to tear the presacral veins. Anteriorly, dissection exposes the posterior vaginal wall or the fascia of Denonvilliers. Laterally, the lateral ligaments can usually be preserved. If any vascular ligatures are necessary to ease the mobilization of the rectum, they should be carried out close to the bowel wall so as not to injure the parasympathetic nerves. Dissection can be more difficult in patients with a previous hysterectomy.

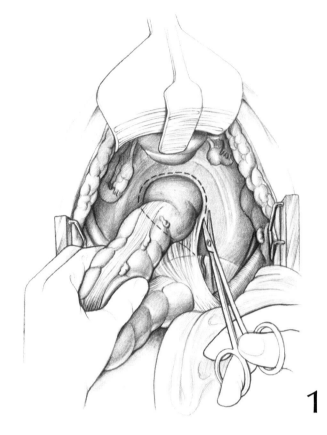

1

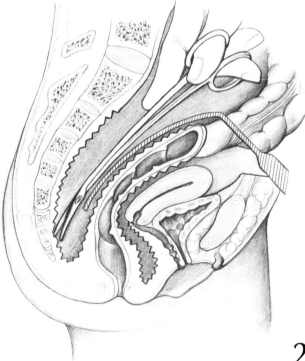

2

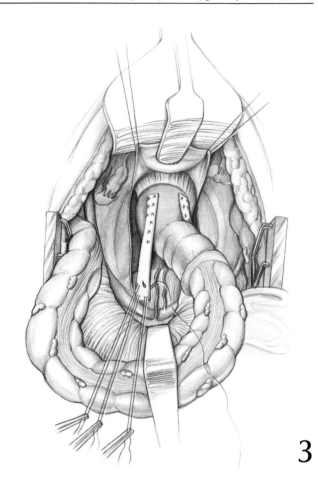

3

Rectopexy

3,4 A 1-cm wide nylon strip is then sutured as far down as possible on each side of the rectum using a double row of four or five non-resorbable stitches over a length of 5 cm. Sutures are placed directly into the muscularis of the rectum and not into the perirectal fat. Gentle traction on the rectum must be able to pull up the anterior reflection line of the peritoneum to the level of the sacral promontory. The two nylon strips are then sutured under moderate tension, and as far from the midline as possible, to the prevertebral fascia, but not to the intervertebral disc itself. Four non-resorbable stitches are used. Care must be taken not to tear the iliac vein during this step of the procedure.

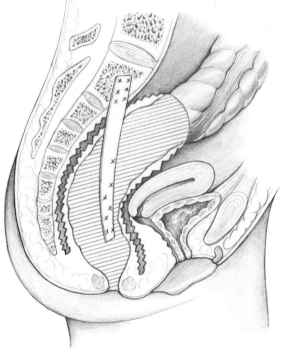

4

Resection of pouch of Douglas

5   The posterior peritoneum of the uterus in women and of the bladder in men is resected and the pouch of Douglas is obliterated by suturing the peritoneal edges together. One or two closed suction drains are left in place in the retroperitoneal space for 2–3 days. The posterior peritoneum is closed, covering the nylon strips, and then the abdominal wall is closed.

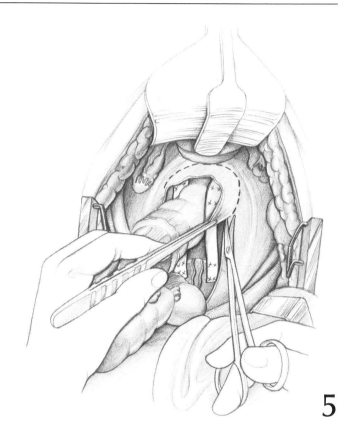

5

Postoperative care

Patients are given intravenous fluid until they pass flatus. Stool softeners may be required to ease the first bowel movements and reduce the tendency for constipation during the first few days after surgery. The patient can usually be discharged by the seventh or eighth postoperative day.

Complications

Damage to the presacral nerve or its branches can be avoided by maintaining dissection in the plane close to the rectum, which should also prevent tearing of any presacral veins. The iliac veins can be injured when suturing the nylon strips to the prevertebral ligament, particularly with the lateral stitches. Intervertebral disc infection is avoided by suturing the nylon strips to the anterior vertebral ligament and not to the intervertebral disc itself. Pelvic sepsis may be caused by a tear of the rectum or haematoma and, in very rare cases, this requires a temporary diverting colostomy.

Outcome

Recurrence

Because of the risk of late recurrences, the results of any surgical procedure used for the treatment of rectal prolapse should be judged after long-term follow-up. In a series of 257 patients undergoing rectopexy by this technique, the incidence of recurrent prolapse was 4.3%, with a minimum follow-up of 5 years[4].

Faecal incontinence

Faecal incontinence is often associated with rectal prolapse and is caused by the distension of the anal sphincter by the prolapse. In 84% of patients with faecal incontinence, the cure of the prolapse was sufficient to restore normal continence[4]. Surgery of the sphincter should be considered only if incontinence persists after rectopexy.

References

1. Orr TG. A suspension operation for prolapse of the rectum. *Ann Surg* 1947; 126: 833–40.

2. Loygue J, Cerbonnet G. Traitement chirurgical du prolapsus total du rectum par la rectopexie suivant le procédé de Orr. *Mem Acad Chir* 1957; 83: 325–9.

3. Loygue J, Huguier M, Malafosse M, Biotois H. Complete prolapse of the rectum. *Br J Surg* 1971; 58: 847–8.

4. Loygue J, Nordlinger B, Cunci O, Malafosse M, Huguet C, Parc R. Rectopexy to the promontory for the treatment of rectal prolapse. Report of 257 cases. *Dis Colon Rectum* 1984; 27: 356–9.

Rectal prolapse: perineal approach (Délorme operation)

Harold L. Kennedy MD, FACS
Assistant Clinical Professor of Surgery, University of California, Sacramento, California, USA

History

Since the original work of Moschcowitz, surgeons have attempted to define better the pathophysiology of rectal prolapse and have continued to search for the most appropriate surgical procedure to treat this condition. The consensus is that the prolapse is a rectorectal intussusception, and the surgical procedures currently available are designed to correct or prevent this intussusception. Bowel dysfunction and incontinence are frequently associated with rectal prolapse, and their pathophysiologies are poorly understood. Transabdominal procedures of treatment have been associated with the lowest rates of recurrence but are accomplished with the associated morbidity of a major abdominal procedure so frequent in poor-risk elderly patients. Thus, surgeons have sought a reliable perineal procedure with a lower rate of morbidity.

Several perineal operations have been advocated, the most familiar of which is the Thiersch procedure. Initially, this was performed with a wire suture but recently a sling of Dacron-impregnated Silastic has been used. Unfortunately, complications (infection, extrusion and faecal impaction) have limited the usefulness of this procedure. Perineal rectosigmoidectomy has been popularized and is certainly a viable alternative, but a significant rate of recurrence has been experienced. In 1900 Délorme introduced a procedure whereby the rectal mucosa is stripped from the muscular wall and the redundant muscular wall plicated.

Principles and justification

Indications and contraindications

Repair of rectal prolapse is advised in any patient in whom full-thickness external prolapse occurs, because incontinence may develop or worsen. If the patient is reluctant to proceed with surgical treatment and is fully continent (which usually is not the case), an alternative is to follow the patient with the understanding that when incontinence occurs, a repair should be carried out. This author does not routinely operate on 'internal prolapse' unless it is associated with incontinence, and does not use the Délorme procedure for this condition. However, in the elderly patient with external prolapse, the Délorme procedure is the procedure of choice. In the middle-aged patient, who otherwise could tolerate an intra-abdominal procedure, the author offers the Délorme procedure as long as the patient understands that in exchange for a simpler procedure with less morbidity, a higher recurrence rate must be accepted. Patients tend to have frequent stools in the early postoperative period, presumably secondary to the diminished rectal reservoir, and this author is therefore reluctant to utilize this procedure in patients who have the 'diarrhoeal' form of irritable bowel syndrome. An abdominal procedure is advised in patients who do not wish to accept a higher recurrence rate, have significant irritable bowel syndrome, or have a distal rectum that is relatively 'fixed', i.e. the superior sulcus of the prolapse is several centimetres from the dentate line.

Preoperative

All patients undergo routine flexible sigmoidoscopy and barium enema, but routine manometric examination of the sphincter is not performed. Mechanical and antibiotic bowel preparation is carried out with a standard peroral lavage solution and oral neomycin and metronidazole. Patients are admitted on the day of surgery and receive perioperative systemic antibiotics.

Anaesthesia

The procedure can equally easily be carried out under general or regional anaesthesia. In very poor-risk patients local anaesthesia can be used but this is not preferred by the author because, when delivering a long segment of mucosa, traction on the mesentery produces discomfort.

Operation

Position of patient

A Foley catheter is inserted and the patient is placed in the prone jack-knife position (*see* page 49).

Mucosal dissection

1 Using a Pratt bivalve speculum, the submucosa of the rectum is infiltrated circumferentially with 0.5% lignocaine containing a 1:100 000 solution of adrenaline. Beginning approximately 1 cm above the dentate line, the mucosa is stripped circumferentially with Debakey tissue forceps and Metzenbaum scissors. This is facilitated by the assistant sequentially rotating the speculum and simultaneously applying outward traction on the anal verge. Haemostasis is obtained with electrocautery. The mucosal/submucosal plane is somewhat scarred in the distal rectum, but the proper plane can generally be identified. Once the dissection is under way, the mucosa is grasped with Pennington forceps. Dissection is continued by the application of traction on the Pennington forceps by the surgeon and countertraction on the muscular tube utilizing forceps by the assistant.

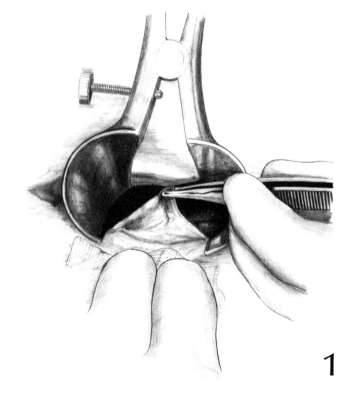

1

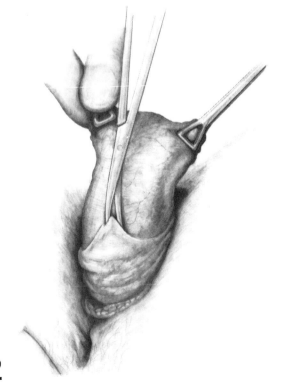

2

2 As the dissection proceeds, it may be possible to deliver the intussusceptum out of the rectum, which will further ease the mucosal stripping. Placing the index finger behind the mucosal tube aids in the dissection. Metzenbaum scissors or electrocautery may be used to dissect the mucosa from the muscular tube. As the dissection proceeds proximally, some tension is commonly encountered: by continuing the mucosal dissection the tension temporarily disappears, allowing the surgeon to remove additional amounts of mucosa.

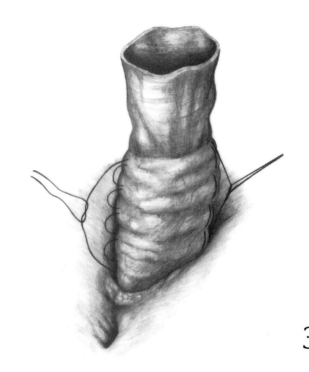

Technical mistake

3 Many articles describe placing the plication sutures while the muscular tube is prolapsed. In the author's opinion this represents a 'technical mistake'. In this position, the proximal extent of the mucosal dissection will generally be below the level of the dentate line and when the muscular sleeve is returned to the pelvis, this will predispose to recurrent prolapse. By returning the muscular sleeve to its normal position in the pelvis and then continuing the mucosal dissection, the surgeon is able to eliminate all of the redundancy and thus reduce the potential for recurrence.

3

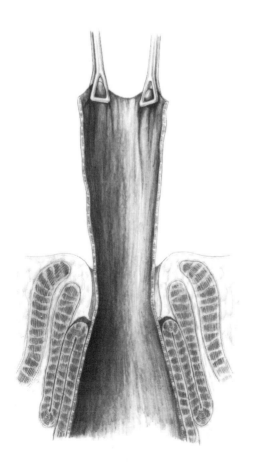

Replacing the muscular tube

4 When the upper limit of the dissection is reached, it is imperative that the section of the rectum which has been prolapsed during this initial part of the procedure be replaced inside the pelvis. The surgeon is then usually able to continue the dissection and to remove additional amounts of mucosa. The dissection continues until the tension on the muscular sleeve continues despite additional mucosal dissection (generally 12–25 cm of mucosa can be removed). Haemostasis is now achieved in the muscular sleeve.

4

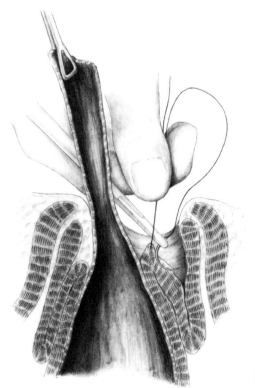

Muscle plication

5a, b Beginning at the junction of the mucosa and the muscular sleeve, 0 polyglactin sutures are placed in a superior fashion along the inner layer of the muscular tube. Traction on each suture as it is placed will deliver the muscular tube towards the anus to allow placement of the next. Once the apex is reached, the process is continued inferiorly along the outer layer of the muscular tube, placing one suture in each of the four quadrants. At this stage all the sutures should be tagged but not tied. Four additional sutures are then placed, one between each of the original sutures. Before tying the sutures, the muscular sleeve is irrigated with an antibiotic solution containing kanamycin, 1 g, and bacitracin, 50 000 units, in 200 ml saline.

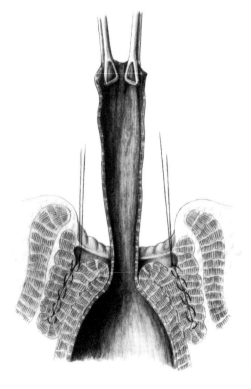

5b

Coloanal anastomosis

6 Longitudinal incisions are then made in each of the four quadrants of the stripped mucosa up to the muscle. A 4/0 polyglactin suture is placed at the apex of these incisions, incorporating mucosa, rectal muscle and anal mucosa. The mucosal strips are then excised, and the remainder of the anastomosis carried out using interrupted 4/0 sutures using the quadrant sutures for traction.

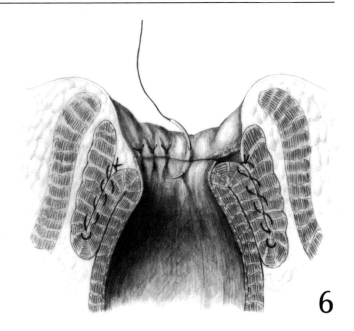

6

Postoperative care

Full oral liquids are started 12 h after surgery and a regular diet is commenced on the second postoperative day. Most patients are ready for discharge by the third day on a bulk agent and sitz baths. It is most unusual for the patient to encounter any significant pain and this suggests the development of a complication. Frequent stools are common, as is occasional incontinence, which is presumably the result of pre-existing incontinence coupled with loss of rectal reservoir function. In most patients the stool frequency gradually decreases and in time their bowel function becomes relatively normal. Any perianal irritation usually responds to topical administration of hydrocortisone and ketoconazole cream.

Complications

Complications are few. Postoperative bleeding requiring return to the operating room has occurred in only one patient encountered by the author. Haematoma may occur in the muscular sleeve and become infected, but this is uncommon. Because the dissection takes place in the intraperitoneal portion of the rectum a full-thickness perforation is possible, especially if the surgeon is not operating in the proper plane: this has not, however, been seen by the author, and it may be that the muscle plication affords some protection from the development of peritonitis from any small unrecognized area of full-thickness dissection.

Outcome

In 26 patients treated by the author there have been two (4%) cases of recurrent prolapse. Because many patients are elderly, this may not be an accurate estimate of the long-term potential for recurrence but it compares well with the reported recurrence rate of 6–17%[1–5]. Continence reportedly improves in 50% of cases, a figure which compares well with the results obtained with intra-abdominal procedures[1,3,4].

References

1. Christiansen J, Kirkegaard P. Délorme's operation for complete rectal prolapse. *Br J Surg* 1981; 68: 537–8.

2. Gundersen AL, Cogbill TH, Landercasper J. Reappraisal of Délorme's procedure for rectal prolapse. *Dis Colon Rectum* 1985; 28: 721–4.

3. Houry S, Lechaux JP, Huguier M, Molkhou JM. Treatment of rectal prolapse by Délorme's operation. *Int J Colorectal Dis* 1987; 2: 149–52.

4. Monson JRT, Jones NAG, Vowden P, Brennan TG. Délorme's operation: the first choice in complete rectal prolapse? *Ann R Coll Surg Engl* 1986; 68: 143–6.

5. Uhlig BE, Sullivan ES. The modified Délorme operation: its place in the surgical treatment for massive rectal prolapse. *Dis Colon Rectum* 1979; 22: 513–21.

Rectal prolapse: Gant–Miwa operation

Tetsuichiro Muto MD, DMSc
Professor of Surgery, University of Tokyo, Tokyo, Japan

Preoperative

Patient assessment

The general condition of the patient is assessed and routine investigations (blood count, serum electrolyte determination, chest radiography, electrocardiography and urinalysis) are determined by the presence of concomitant morbid conditions and the type of anaesthesia to be used.

Bowel preparation

A full mechanical bowel preparation is advised, using the method of choice of the surgeon. Perioperative systemic antibiotics are also given.

Anaesthesia

The operation can be performed under local anaesthesia in poor-risk or elderly patients. Otherwise, general or lumbar anaesthesia is used.

Operation

Position of patient

The patient is placed in the lithotomy or jack-knife position as described in the chapter on pp. 47–50.

Procedure

1 The rectal mucosa is pulled by Péan's clamp to make a complete assessment of the rectal prolapse.

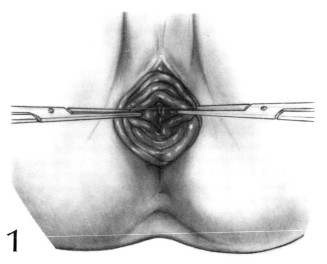

1

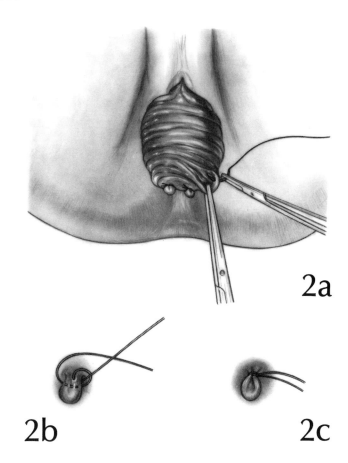

2a–c The most distal part of the prolapsed mucosa is seized with a Péan's clamp; and a needle with an absorbable thread (3/0 coated polyglycolic acid (Dexon) or 3/0 polyglactin (Vicryl)) is inserted deeply enough to incorporate a large amount of submucosal tissue at the tip of the clamp. The thread is ligated around the clamp to form a 'mucosal tag' 5–7 mm in diameter. The needle is inserted deeply into the submucosa to make as large a mucosal tag as possible. This procedure is started distally making several tags in a line and is continued towards the anal margin.

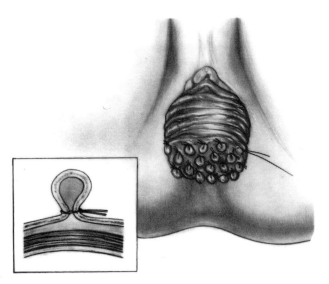

3 The procedure is carried out stepwise in a circular fashion. In order to reduce the redundant mucosa, the mucosal tags are made as numerous as possible (> 100); wherever the redundant mucosa is present it is ligated to form a mucosal tag. The prolapsed rectum is gradually shortened towards the anus until the dentate line is reached). The end of the prolapsed rectum is pushed back into the anus by gentle manual pressure.

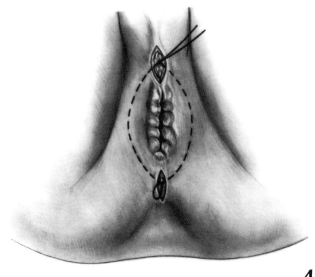

4 A purse-string suture of 1 Surgilon is added around the anus like a Thiersch wire. Small incisions are made at anterior and posterior sites in the perianal skin. A large needle with Surgilon is inserted at the subcutaneous level in a semi-circular fashion from anterior to posterior and then posterior to anterior.

4

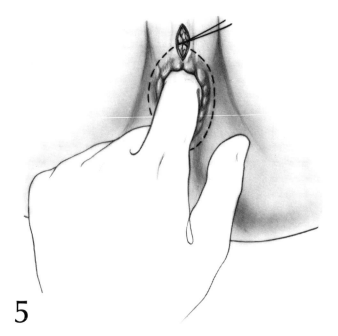

5

5 The thread is ligated sufficiently tightly that the assistant can feel the strength of the thread around the index finger. Fascia lata can be used for the purse-string suture.

Wound closure

6 The skin incision is closed to complete the procedure.

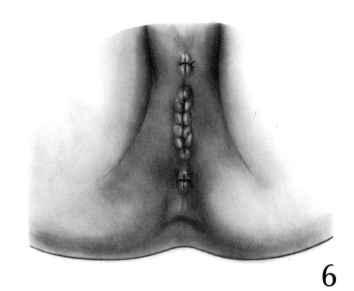

6

Postoperative care

The patient is treated as for haemorrhoidectomy (as described in the chapter on pp. 784–788). After a few days of liquid diet, a normal meal can be served. Mild laxatives and stool bulking agents are administered to prevent straining and constipation.

Further reading

Arakawa K. Procidentia of the rectum in Japan. *J Jap Soc Colo-Proctol* 1979; 224–9 (in Japanese, summary in English).

Gant SG. *Disease of the Rectum, Anus and Colon*. Vol. 2. Philadelphia: WB Saunders, 1923: 22–57.

Miwa T. *Treatment of Anal Disease*. Tokyo: Nanzando, 1962: 102–7 (in Japanese).

Muto T, Konishi F, Kamiya J, Sawada T, Sugihara K, Morioka Y. Gant–Miwa technique (mucosal plication of prolapsed rectum) with Thiersch operation in the treatment of rectal prolapse. *Coloproctology* 1984; 6: 310–14.

Rectal prolapse: perineal rectosigmoidectomy with levatoroplasty

J. Graham Williams MCh, FRCS
Lecturer in Surgery, University of Birmingham, Queen Elizabeth Hospital, Birmingham, UK

Robert D. Madoff MD
Clinical Assistant Professor, Division of Colon and Rectal Surgery, University of Minnesota, Minneapolis, Minnesota, USA

History

The first description of perineal rectosigmoidectomy was provided by Mikulicz. The first operation he reported was for an incarcerated, gangrenous prolapse, but he also treated five other patients with uncomplicated rectal prolapse by perineal 'amputation'[1]. The operation was popular during the first part of this century, but recurrence rates of over 50% reported from St Mark's Hospital for Diseases of the Rectum and Colon, London, lessened surgeons' enthusiasm for this procedure[2, 3]. Altemeier from Cincinatti published a large series of patients with rectal prolapse treated by perineal rectosigmoidectomy with few recurrences, reviving interest in this procedure[4]. A number of other groups have reported series of patients treated by rectosigmoidectomy with recurrence rates between 0% and 10%[5-7]. Furthermore, marked improvement in associated faecal incontinence has been reported when levatoroplasty is performed at the same time.

Principles and justification

The principle of the operation is to excise the prolapsing segment of the rectum from below, thus avoiding abdominal exploration. The operation entails more than merely amputating the prolapse flush with the anus. Mobilization of the rectum and pelvic colon is essential to adequately resect the redundant prolapsing intestine. Circumferential, full-thickness rectal prolapse is required for the operation to be technically feasible. The operation is associated with very low morbidity and mortality rates and traditionally has been indicated for elderly or high-risk patients. Recent reports of low recurrence rates, however, make the operation an attractive alternative to transabdominal repair for all patients with rectal prolapse.

Unlike most abdominal approaches, perineal rectosigmoidectomy avoids dissection at the pelvic brim, and hence avoids the potential for pelvic nerve damage and presacral haemorrhage. The operation is particularly appropriate for treating incarcerated or gangrenous rectal prolapse. Pelvic floor repair is easily performed during rectal excision, which is not the case with the Délorme operation (mucosectomy and rectal wall plication). The potential disadvantage of perineal rectosigmoidectomy is that the rectum is excised with loss of reservoir capacity. Care should be exercised in patients who have undergone previous sigmoid or rectal excision as the blood supply to the rectum may be compromised by ligation of the inferior mesenteric vessels, and an ischaemic segment of rectum may result if perineal rectosigmoidectomy is then performed.

Preoperative

Preoperative assessment and preparation are dealt with in the chapter on pp. 701–705.

Anaesthesia

Perineal rectosigmoidectomy can be performed under general or regional anaesthesia. Regional neural block by spinal or epidural anaesthesia is appropriate for frail, poor-risk patients who form the majority of candidates for this operation.

Operation

Position of patient

The operation can be performed in the lithotomy position or the prone jack-knife position (*see Illustrations 2* and *4* on pp. 48–49). The prone jack-knife position necessitates endotracheal intubation if general anaesthesia is used, but has several major advantages over the lithotomy position. First, it is easier to position assistants around the operating table, and all the surgical team have an excellent view of the operative field. Secondly, bleeding is less because the perineum is the uppermost part and venous congestion is less. Thirdly, exposure and illumination within the pelvis are easier to achieve.

The patient is turned prone with the hips flexed over a large, firm hip roll. The knees are padded and slightly flexed with the feet supported by two pillows. The chest is supported by a small round pad on either side. The arms are brought forward and placed on padded arm boards. The head is turned to one side and rests on a padded ring. The buttocks are taped apart with 7.5-cm adhesive tape. The operating table is tipped with the patient's head down.

Incision

1 The rectal prolapse is delivered by gentle traction on the rectal wall using Babcock forceps passed through the anus. As the prolapse appears, the Babcock forceps are removed to grasp more proximal rectal wall. Once delivered, the rectal wall is infiltrated with 1 : 200 000 adrenaline solution circumferentially, about 1 cm from the dentate line. An incision is made at this level using a scalpel or the electrocautery blade through all layers of the rectal wall. This is thicker than might be anticipated, and the incision is deepened until extrarectal fat is reached. This incision is then continued circumferentially keeping 1 cm above the dentate line. Initial scoring of the mucosa with electrocautery is helpful in keeping the incision at the right level around the whole circumference of the rectum.

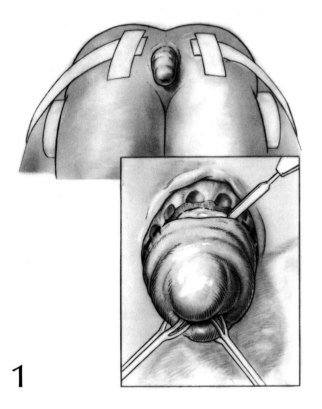

1

Mobilization of the rectum

2   Rectal mobilization is performed by dividing the tissues of the mesorectum, working around the full circumference of the prolapsed bowel. A small right-angle clamp, such as a Lahey clamp, is useful. Strands of mesorectal tissue are elevated and electrocoagulated or divided and ligated with 3/0 absorbable sutures. When the muscular coat of the inner tube of prolapsed rectum is reached, the dissection continues cephalad, dividing the mesorectal tissues close to the intestinal wall. This dissection should proceed circumferentially.

A surprising length of bowel may be mobilized as the dissection proceeds. The mobilization is complete when more than gentle traction is required to pull more colon down. During this phase, an anterior sliding hernia is often opened. It is possible to palpate the pelvic contents through this hernia, and formal repair of the pelvic peritoneum is unnecessary. If the pelvis has been entered, it is possible to palpate the straightened colon in the pelvis.

A Lone Star self-retaining ring retractor is useful during this dissection. The ring is placed over the prolapse against the buttocks, and eight hooks, attached to the self-retaining ring by elastic tubing, are placed circumferentially around the cut edge of the rectal wall to splay it out and expose the operative site.

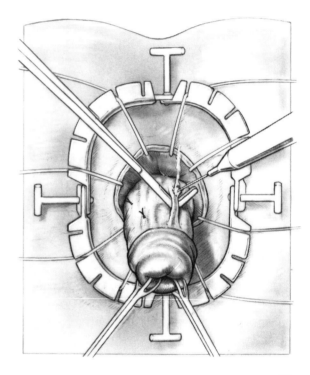

2

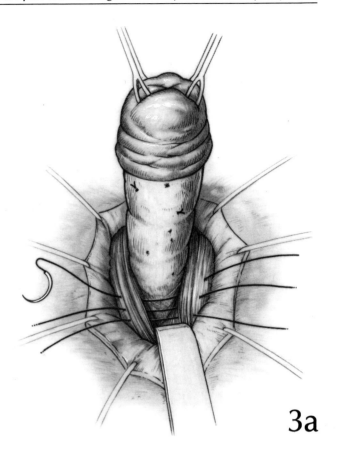

3a

Levatoroplasty

3a, b Levatoroplasty is easily performed during perineal rectosigmoidectomy. The repair can be anterior or posterior to the rectum, or both. Levatoroplasty appears to have a beneficial effect on postoperative continence. The levator ani muscles are identified by using a narrow retractor, such as a Dever retractor, to pull the outer tube of rectum and the perineal body anteriorly. At the same time, the fully mobilized rectum is drawn posteriorly. The levator ani muscles are visible on either side of the pelvis. Drawing the mobilized rectum anteriorly allows the levators to be identified posterior to the rectum.

Levatoroplasty is performed by placing a series of interrupted 2/0 polypropylene sutures through the levator ani muscle on each side and tying the sutures loosely when all have been placed. The levatoroplasty should be tight enough to allow a finger to be passed into the pelvis alongside the rectum.

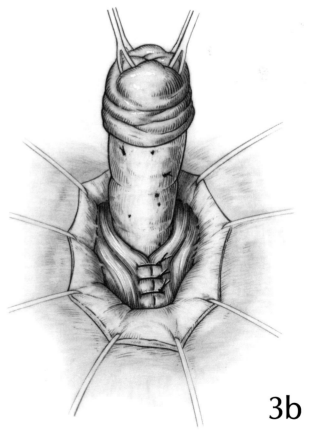

3b

Anastomosis

4a–c The final phase of the operation is to resect the mobilized, prolapsing rectum and perform the anastomosis. The level of proximal resection should be at the limit of mobilization to maintain a good blood supply to the proximal intestine.

A small incision is made into the proximal intestine at the site of resection, and a stay suture of 3/0 polyglactin (Vicryl) is placed through the full thickness of the cut edge of the rectum and the proximal intestinal wall. This is tied, and the incision in the proximal intestine is extended to one side for one-quarter of the circumference. A further stay suture is placed at the end of this incision through both edges of intestine and tied. A further series of full-thickness polyglactin sutures are placed between the two stay sutures to complete the anastomosis in the first quadrant. The diameter of the distal rectum is usually considerably greater than that of the proximal intestine and the anastomosis requires tailoring appropriately.

The next quadrant of proximal intestine is incised, and a further stay suture is inserted. The anastomosis in this quadrant is completed as previously. The procedure is repeated for the remaining circumference of the intestine. It is important to perform the anastomosis in segments, because the proximal intestine may retract into the pelvis if the intestine is simply excised before stay sutures are placed. When complete, the anastomosis retracts into the pelvis where it is examined with a bivalve speculum to check for gaps or bleeding.

The anastomosis can be performed with a circular stapler[8]. The anvil is passed into the proximal intestine, a purse-string suture is placed and tied round the shaft, and a second purse-string is placed round the distal rectal edge and tied. The gun is closed within the pelvis and fired. It is difficult to perform a stapled anastomosis if levatoroplasty has been performed.

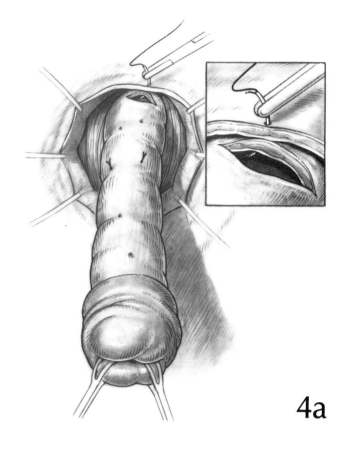

4a

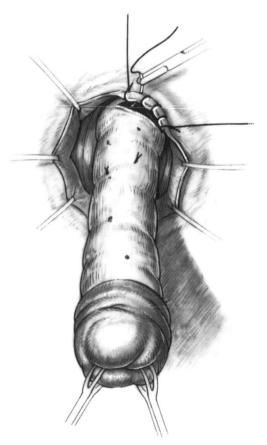

4b

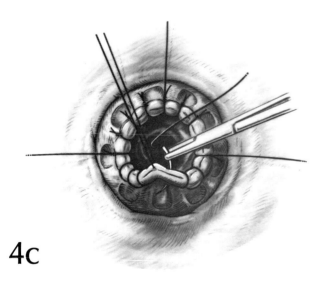

4c

Postoperative care

The postoperative course after perineal rectosigmoidectomy is usually very smooth. Patients have minimal pain, easily controlled by mild opiates. Oral intake can be commenced after 24–48 h, and the bowels function within a few days of surgery. Most patients are ready for discharge by day 4. Potential complications include anastomotic bleeding and pelvic sepsis. Anastomotic bleeding that requires intervention is easily controlled by transanal suture ligation of the bleeding point.

Outcome

The recurrence rate after perineal rectosigmoidectomy depends, in part, on how long the patient is followed. Reported recurrence rates vary; however, recent series document recurrence rates of between 5% and 10%[6,7]. Recurrence probably reflects inadequate resection, and care should be taken to mobilize all the redundant rectum and to perform the anastomosis within the pelvis rather than at the surface. Improvement in faecal incontinence is less likely following perineal rectosigmoidectomy than following abdominal repair of rectal prolapse. Concomitant levatoroplasty, however, is associated with marked improvement in continence, with many patients regaining full continence[5,7].

References

1. Mikulicz J. Zur operativen behandlung des prolapsus recti et coli vaginati. *Arch Klin Chir* 1889; 38: 74–97.

2. Porter N. Collective results of operations for rectal prolapse. *Proc R Soc Med* 1962; 55: 1087–91.

3. Hughes ESR. Discussion on rectal prolapse. *Proc R Soc Med* 1949; 42: 1007–11.

4. Altemeier WA, Cuthbertson WR, Schowengerdt C, Hunt J. Nineteen years' experience with the one stage perineal repair of rectal prolapse. *Ann Surg* 1971; 173: 993–1001.

5. Prasad ML, Pearl RK, Abcarian H, Orsay CP, Nelson RL. Perineal proctectomy, posterior rectopexy and postanal levator repair for the treatment of rectal prolapse. *Dis Colon Rectum* 1986; 29: 547–52.

6. Ramanujam PS, Venkatesh KS. Perineal excision of rectal prolapse with posterior levator ani repair in elderly high-risk patients. *Dis Colon Rectum* 1988; 31: 704–6.

7. Williams JG, Rothenberger DA, Madoff RD, Goldberg SM. Treatment of rectal prolapse in the elderly by perineal rectosigmoidectomy. *Dis Colon Rectum* 1992; 35: 830–4.

8. Vermeulen FD, Nivatvongs S, Fang DT, Balcos EG, Goldberg SM. A technique for perineal rectosigmoidectomy using autosuture devices. *Surg Gynecol Obstet* 1983; 156: 84–6.

Surgery for anal incontinence: introductory comment

M. M. Henry MB, FRCS
Consultant Surgeon, Central Middlesex Hospital, Honorary Consultant Surgeon, St Mark's Hospital for Diseases of the Rectum and Colon and Senior Lecturer, Academic Surgical Unit, St Mary's Hospital, London, UK

The surgical management of the patient with severe anal incontinence has never been entirely satisfactory. Although anal function can be restored in many patients initially, it is frequently not sustained over a prolonged period. Interpretation of published results for the various procedures described is hampered by the lack of objective detail about the indications for surgery and also the poor assessment of function after surgery. In spite of intensive research into the physiology of anorectal function over the last decade, we do not have a 'gold standard' by which function may be assessed and compared globally. It is always worth recalling, however, that if reconstructive pelvic surgery is deemed to have failed, a colostomy may not necessarily be a disaster for the patient. Many patients prefer the management of an incontinent stoma sited on the anterior abdominal wall to one situated in the perineum. It is the author's view that all patients should undergo a detailed assessment of anorectal function before the decision to proceed with surgery is made. Having said this, there is no evidence that the functional outcome of surgery correlates with any of the preoperative physiological tests which have been devised. The only exception is in the treatment of anal sphincter repair, where it has been clearly shown that the demonstration of denervation in the external anal sphincter before surgery strongly points to a poor functional outcome following such surgery[1].

Currently used methods

Postanal pelvic floor repair

This procedure, originally described by the late Sir Alan Parks, sets out to restore the anorectal angle and is principally indicated for patients with denervation of the pelvic floor and external anal sphincter muscles. As Bartolo has indicated in his chapter, there is little experimental evidence that the 'angle' was effectively altered by this procedure, but there is some evidence that the length of the anal canal was increased and that the mechanical advantage to these muscle fibres was improved. The technique is attractive because of its simplicity once the operator has become adept at the dissection of the intersphincteric space (the avascular plane between the internal and external anal sphincters). The incidence of complications is low in all series, with only minor sepsis being a relatively common problem. There has been one recorded death, from unrelated causes. As Bartolo has stated, good results are achieved in only approximately 60% of patients and these results are not sustained. However, it is important to recall that, in most series, the procedure has been performed for patients with severe incontinence in the presence of extensive pelvic floor denervation. There is a suggestion that good results have been claimed for other procedures because patients with lesser functional disabilities have been presented for surgery.

Anal sphincter repair

In the absence of denervation, simple repair of the external anal sphincter can be expected to generate good results. It has become accepted practice to perform an overlapping rather than end-to-end repair since Parks originally demonstrated that there was a lower risk of disruption with the former procedure. It is essential to perform the repair with suture material which is slowly absorbable or non-absorbable. Gynaecologists frequently achieve poor results with this operation because they use catgut. Dr Thorson comments that a colostomy is not necessary. This statement is undoubtedly true in the majority of cases where repair is contemplated at a late stage. In the presence of acute trauma or where complications such as sepsis or local stenosis develop, it may be necessary to defunction the repair temporarily.

Repair procedures in patients with pelvic floor descent

Patients with pelvic floor failure may present with descent of the pelvic floor and gynaecological and urological disorders, as well as with loss of anal continence. In such patients it is often necessary to embark on vaginal repair procedures, which can be performed synchronously with the anal surgery. Such techniques are described elegantly in the chapter by Professor Hudson.

Recent developments

Artificial anal sphincter

One of the two new and exciting approaches to the management of anal incontinence, namely the use of a prosthetic device, is described in the chapter by Wong. The concept is based on the use of prosthetic devices similar to those used for treating urinary incontinence. The problem is that the device is not cheap and wherever prostheses are employed the risk of sepsis is high. It is too early to comment on how valuable a contribution this will make because the numbers reported here are too small to draw conclusions, but there is some cause for optimism.

Electrically stimulated gracilis neosphincter

Professor Williams' operation is the second advance in the surgery of anal incontinence to have been developed within the last decade. The technique employs the principle that striated muscle can alter its physiological behaviour if subjected to long-term low-frequency electrical stimulation. The gracilis sling procedure, originally described by Pickrell, suffered from poor results because the transposed muscle possessed no resting electrical tone. Using an implanted electrode and stimulator the gracilis muscle is continuously electrically active and its muscle fibres become more adapted to function in a similar way to the pelvic floor. The technique is technically complex, has to be performed in three stages and employs technology which, at this developmental stage, remains expensive. Nevertheless, this procedure for the moment represents the operation of choice for those patients who have developmental atrophy of the pelvic floor musculature and for those in whom previous conventional techniques have failed.

Reference

1. Laurberg S, Swash M, Henry MM. Delayed external sphincter repair for obstetric tear. *Br J Surg* 1988; 75: 786–8.

Postanal pelvic floor repair for anal incontinence

David C. C. Bartolo MS, FRCS, FRCSEd
Consultant Surgeon, Department of Surgery, University of Edinburgh, Royal Infirmary, Edinburgh, UK

Principles and justification

Anorectal incontinence is a distressing condition that primarily affects women; in the majority of cases it is related to trauma during parturition. Although there are indications for postanal repair, its use has diminished in recent years since the results of the procedure have been more fully analysed.

1 The original objective of this operation was to re-create the double right angle that normally exists between the anal canal and the lowermost rectum and mid-rectum. The force of abdominal pressure was considered to act on the anterior rectal wall, thrusting it onto the closed anal canal and effectively occluding it. Recent studies, however, have failed to confirm the flap valve theory of continence[1], suggesting that improvement after postanal repair is less related to the angle and more to improved muscular contractility[2, 3].

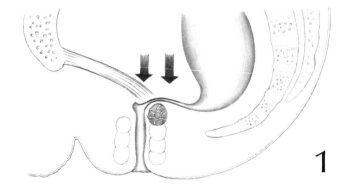

1

The principle of postanal repair is to enter the relatively avascular space between the internal sphincters and the rectal smooth muscle centrally, and the external sphincters and levator ani muscles peripherally. The pelvic floor sphincters, including the puborectalis, are circular and when they weaken, the diameter of the circle they describe enlarges. Therefore, the circumference of the circle formed by the sphincters should be reduced by half, leading to the area described by the sphincters being reduced to about one-quarter. It is necessary to approach the sphincter from its inner surface (i.e. within the circle) because: (1) these stitches are best placed across the sphincter from one side of the circular muscle to the other to imbricate the muscle and reduce the diameter; (2) no important nerves or blood vessels reach the muscle from this aspect, except from S3 and S4 direct branches to the levator ani and puborectalis muscle. The pudendal nerves enter from the perineal surface and therefore should not be at risk with this approach.

This anatomical approach is relatively straightforward once the basic anatomy of the region is understood. Thus, the structures that pass through the pelvic floor muscles (i.e. the termination of the intestinal and genitourinary tracts) must be displaced anteriorly before the sphincter is plicated.

Preoperative

Patient assessment

In the assessment of patients with faecal incontinence, it is necessary to determine whether rectal prolapse, either complete or incomplete, is present. If prolapse is found, it should be corrected by surgery first and postanal repair reserved for those patients in whom incontinence persists. If there is doubt about the presence of an incomplete rectal prolapse, then defaecography should be used to visualize the intussusception and document its severity.

Attention should then be turned to the integrity of the sphincter complex. Overt obstetric tears may be obvious on clinical examination because of scarring and extreme deficiency of the anterior perineum. Formerly, the only way to diagnose less severe sphincter defects was by electromyographic mapping, in which multiple needle punctures with a concentric needle electrode were used to map areas of myoelectric activity and inactivity. This is a particularly unpleasant investigation, which is often poorly tolerated by patients. In contrast, endoluminal ultrasonography is relatively non-invasive and provides a 360° image of the anal sphincter complex. Detailed analysis of the internal anal sphincter and external sphincter integrity is possible. When defects are found, the procedure of choice is direct sphincter repair.

Patients with so-called 'idiopathic faecal incontinence' (with no rectal prolapse and intact sphincters) have been shown to have neuropathic degeneration of the external sphincter and puborectalis muscle. The most potent cause of such nerve damage is prolongation of the second stage of labour. Operative intervention with forceps, particularly involving mid-cavity rotation of the fetal head, will obviously exacerbate these neurological injuries. In addition, various abnormal presentations of the fetus, e.g. breech or occiput posterior, may have damaging effects because of possible direct trauma and/or traction injury to the nerves produced by the excessively prolonged perineal descent associated with delay in the second stage of labour.

Therefore, patients selected for postanal repair are those in whom muscle weakness has arisen because of nerve damage. The objective of the operation is to tighten the sphincter and pelvic floor musculature, although such coapting of denervated muscle has its limitations in terms of functional results.

Patient preparation

The patient is given laxatives the day before the operation, but it is very important that the rectum is completely clear, otherwise liquid faeces will contaminate the operative field.

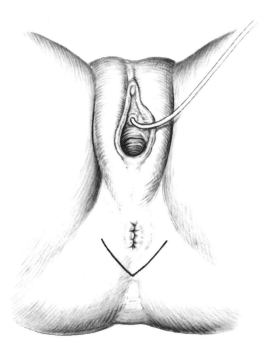

2

Operation

Position of patient and incision

2   The author prefers to place the patient in the prone jack-knife position, but the lithotomy position is equally acceptable (*see* chapter on pp. 47–50).

A V-shaped or hemispherical postanal incision is made about 6 cm behind the anal canal. The reason for placing the wound so far behind the anus is that in the course of the repair the skin of the anal region is drawn into the anal canal and if the wound were put too close to the orifice, it would be pulled up into the anal canal, thereby increasing the chances of sepsis.

The skin anterior to the incision is raised, and care is taken to keep the flap thick to avoid postoperative necrosis of the skin.

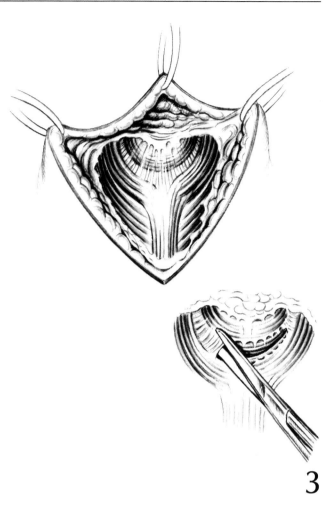

3

3 The posterior fibres of the external sphincter and the lower border of the internal sphincter are exposed. The plane between the two is relatively bloodless and can be identified anatomically. The longitudinal fibres guide the operator to the correct site. The external sphincter is usually red and easily identified, whereas the internal sphincter is white. If the external sphincter has degenerated, the distinction between the two muscles becomes blurred. Stimulation of the tissue with diathermy current, however, will usually cause contraction in the external sphincter. By gentle scissor dissection the internal sphincter is displaced from the lower part of the external sphincter for about half its circumference.

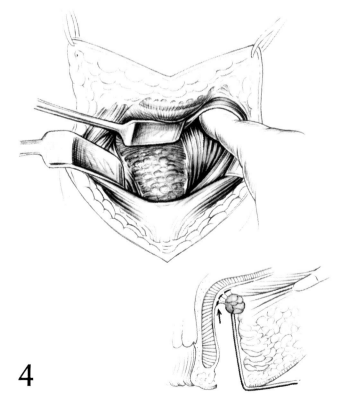

4

4 As the dissection progresses, the viscus is lifted off the upper part of the external sphincter, progressively onward and upward until the puborectalis is reached. It is necessary to avoid straying from this plane because it is not difficult to enter the rectum and somewhat easier to dissect through the external sphincters into the ischiorectal fat. Throughout the dissection, the separation between the two layers is carried as far forward on each side of the anal canal as possible. Waldeyer's fascia is encountered above the puborectalis muscle and is divided, exposing the mesorectal fat.

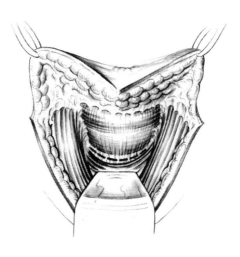

5 A deep retractor is placed into the pelvis to hold the rectum forwards, so that the origin of the levator ani muscles on both sides can be seen.

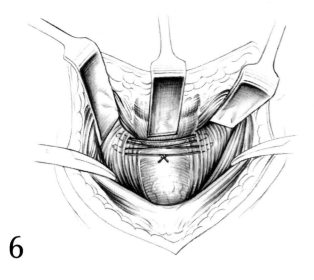

6

6, 7 Sutures of 2/0 polypropylene (Prolene) are placed across the muscle. The highest and most lateral point of the levator group is identified by blunt dissection, close to the spine of the ischium, which is readily palpable. A small curved needle is passed under a fairly large bundle of the levator on one side. The retractor is then moved to expose the exactly corresponding site of the muscle on the other side. About three sutures are placed at this topmost level and are tied only lightly, without tension, to form a lattice across the pelvis.

The next layer of sutures is placed on the upper part of the pubococcygeus muscle and again each is tied only lightly with the formation of a lattice. The lower part of the pubococcygeus, however, is a stronger bar of muscle and its origin is much nearer the midline on the pubic arch. Sutures are placed as close to its origin on each side as possible, and again about three are used.

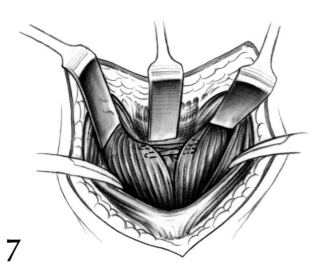

7

8 The puborectalis suture is the most important layer. This muscle is the strongest and thickest of all those encountered and can be seen with ease. Once more the sutures are placed as near to the origin on the pubic symphysis as possible. Each is tied so that the muscle is approximated, but a small gap is left to take into account any swelling that may occur in the tissues following surgery.

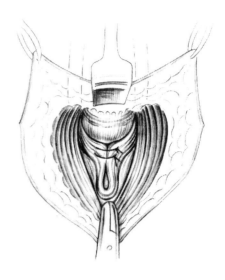

8

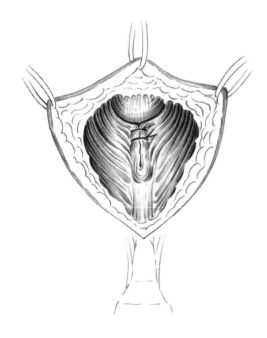

9

9 Another layer of sutures is placed in the external sphincter below the puborectalis and finally, at the anal margin, a layer of absorbable sutures is used to avoid putting non-absorbable polypropylene too near the skin.

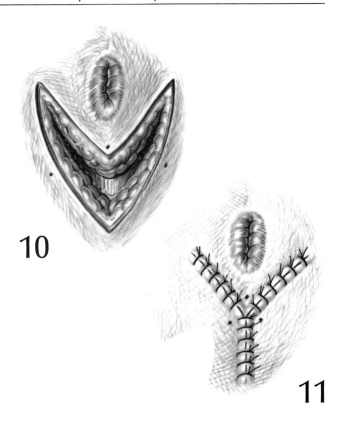

10

11

10, 11 As a result of the repair, the anterior skin flap is drawn forwards and cannot be resutured to the posterior skin edge without undue tension. The wound is therefore reconstituted in the shape of a Y. It is not uncommon for local necrosis to occur at the apex of the anterior flap but this always heals uneventfully.

Postoperative care

A catheter is normally placed in the bladder because most patients are given caudal anaesthetics for postoperative pain control, and if sensation is reduced, retention may occur. It is very important to avoid straining because constipation can disrupt the whole repair. The two ways to avoid complication are either to fashion a temporary colostomy or to produce liquid stools. Neither alternative is pleasant, but the liquid stool regimen is prescribed in sufficient doses to maintain about three semiliquid stools per day. Once a normal bowel habit has been achieved, laxatives can gradually be withdrawn. Some patients find they have difficulty with evacuating the rectum following postanal repair and require the use of regular suppositories. This regimen may be needed indefinitely, and it is often necessary to remind patients of this during follow-up visits.

Outcome

Recent studies have shown variable success rates for this procedure; approximately 60% show significant improvement in the short term[4]. Unfortunately, follow-up shows that these results are not sustained. This has been one of the most disappointing aspects of the management of patients with anorectal incontinence. Furthermore, studies in which the anorectal angle has been measured before and after surgery have reported no change in anorectal angulation, despite improvement in continence. It appears that restoration of faecal continence is more related to improvement in sphincter pressures than to changes in the angle.

It must be emphasized that in a situation where the muscles have partly degenerated, it is unlikely that any operative procedure can restore total normality. The majority of patients have some difficulty in controlling flatus and may have soiling if they have an attack of diarrhoea. To keep matters in perspective, however, even a normal person can have problems under such circumstances, and many of these patients can be helped. When surgery has not been successful, constipating drugs can prove extremely useful, particularly if used in association with suppositories to aid rectal emptying.

References

1. Bartolo DCC, Roe AM, Locke-Edmunds JC, Virjee J, Mortensen NJM. Flap valve theory of anorectal continence. *Br J Surg* 1986; 73: 1012–14.

2. Orrom WJ, Miller R, Cornes H, Duthie G, Bartolo DCC, Mortensen NJ. A comparison of anterior sphincteroplasty and postanal repair in the treatment of idiopathic fecal incontinence. *Dis Colon Rectum* 1991; 34: 305–10.

3. Miller R, Orrom WJ, Cornes H, Duthie G, Bartolo DCC. Anterior sphincter plication and levatorplasty in the treatment of faecal incontinence. *Br J Surg* 1989; 76: 1058–60.

4. Womack NR, Morrison JFB, Williams NS. Prospective study of the effects of postanal repair in neurogenic faecal incontinence. *Br J Surg* 1988; 75: 48–52.

Surgical repair of anal sphincters following injury

Alan G. Thorson MD, FACS
Associate Professor of Surgery and Program Director, Section of Colon and Rectal Surgery, Creighton University School of Medicine and Clinical Assistant Professor of Surgery, University of Nebraska College of Medicine, Omaha, Nebraska, USA

History

Direct surgical repair of anal sphincters following injury may be approached by one of three basic methods: (1) the injured muscle ends may be brought together by direct apposition; (2) the muscle may be plicated, thereby transposing functional muscle over non-functional fibrous scar tissue; or (3) the muscle may be overlapped during a sphincteroplasty type of repair.

The advantages of an 'overlapping' sphincter repair include utilization of fibrous scar on both ends of the muscle, which provides substantial tissue to hold sutures, and increased surface areas of muscle tissue in contact with each other, thereby decreasing the chance of suture disruption. These advantages, plus the improved functional results, make the overlapping sphincteroplasty the preferred method.

Principles and justification

The most common cause of sphincter disruption is obstetric injury[1,2]. Other injuries that may result in sphincter dysfunction include previous anorectal surgery, trauma, or congenital abnormality. Classically, direct sphincter repair has been utilized for incontinence when a clear-cut anatomical defect can be demonstrated. More recently, however, sphincteroplasty has also been proposed in the management of idiopathic faecal incontinence[3,4]. Although results are not as good as for anatomical disruption, it appears that sphincteroplasty provides as good a result for idiopathic incontinence as any other operation.

Preoperative

The best results from an 'overlapping' sphincteroplasty are obtained in those patients who have an anatomical injury. In most instances, these injuries can be readily evaluated on physical examination. More subtle injuries may require more specialized testing, including anorectal manometry, vector symmetry analysis, electromyography, or transanal ultrasonography. Most patients with sphincter injuries should wait at least 3 months before repair to allow local oedema and inflammation to resolve. In addition, this period will allow more mature scar tissue to form, which can provide a sound foundation for the sutures. Evaluation of the colon by radiographic contrast studies or endoscopy should also be performed to rule out the possibility of complicating or contributing factors, such as inflammatory bowel disease.

Patients undergoing sphincteroplasty are given a complete mechanical bowel preparation on the day before surgery. Oral antibiotics are not necessary. Intravenous prophylaxis with a broad-spectrum antibiotic, such as a second generation cephalosporin, should be used. A colostomy is not necessary.

Anaesthesia

Complete relaxation of the perineum is critical, therefore general or regional anaesthesia is necessary. This may be supplemented with local anaesthetic for immediate postoperative pain relief.

Operation

Position of patient

1 The patient is placed in the prone jack-knife position with the buttocks taped apart to provide maximum visualization (*see Illustration 4* on page 49). A Foley catheter is inserted.

The critical anatomy includes the location of the innervation of the external sphincter. This innervation approaches the sphincter bilaterally from the postero-lateral position via branches of the pudendal nerve as they reach the anal canal.

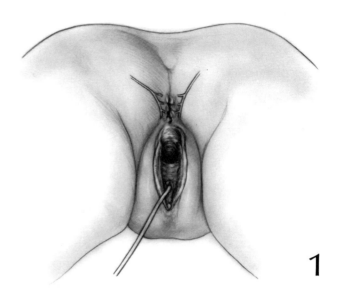

1

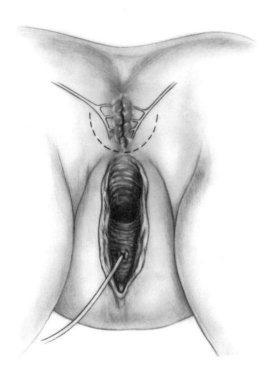

2

Incision

A local anaesthetic solution of 0.5% lignocaine hydrochloride with 1:200 000 adrenaline is sometimes helpful in developing the planes of dissection over that portion of the anal canal that has been scarred by the injury.

2 An incision is made around the anus anteriorly for an arc of 200–240°. Further extension posteriorly is not advised because of the risk of injury to branches of the pudendal nerve. Laterally, the incision is placed 1.0–1.5 cm beyond the anal verge. Anteriorly, it must go through the middle of the perineal body which may be nearly non-existent. It should then follow along the lateral border of the subcutaneous external sphincter. Care should be taken to preserve all muscle fibres so that they can be incorporated into the repair.

Developing flaps

3 As the incision is deepened into the ischiorectal fat, it is important to preserve as many small neurovascular bundles as possible. The dissection is carried lateral to all identifiable fibres of the subcutaneous sphincter. In the area of the previous injury, the vaginal mucosa is dissected carefully off the residual scar. In some cases, the only perineal body remaining may be the vaginal and anal mucosa with little intervening scar. Alternately placing a finger in the vagina and anus will provide helpful tactile sensation during this difficult dissection. In severe cases, a true cloaca may exist.

Once the lateral borders of the external sphincter are clearly identified, the anoderm is also elevated as a mucosal flap. It is easiest to start this dissection laterally and work medially, because this allows planes of dissection to be developed in tissues that have not been previously injured. Early in the course of this dissection, the fibrous scar connecting the two functional limbs of the sphincter mechanism should be identifiable. The use of a Pratt bivalve anal speculum or a Fansler operative anoscope may be helpful when initiating the dissection. It is better, however, to avoid stretching the sphincter any more than is necessary. Once the flaps are defined, appropriately placed single or double skin hooks will provide adequate exposure.

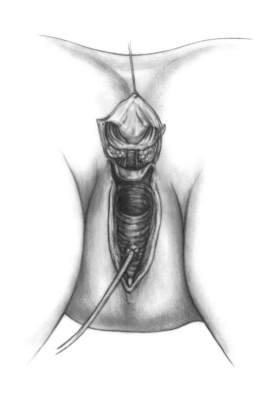

3

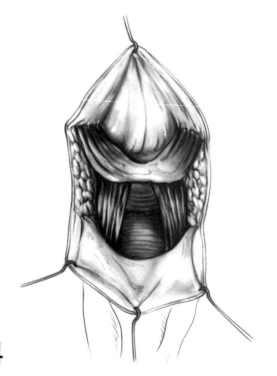

4

Identifying the levator ani

4 As the vaginal and anal mucosal flaps are further developed, the dissection will ultimately lead to normal planes of dissection cephalad to the injury. This should allow separation of the rectal–vaginal septum with much greater ease. As the point is reached where all that remains between the rectum and the vagina is the septum without intervening sphincter, the levator ani will be identified laterally to either side of the rectum.

Levatoroplasty

5 The dissection is carried to completion reaching the most cephalad point of the dissection. At this time the fibrotic portion of the sphincter can be sharply divided. An attempt should be made to leave equal parts of fibrous tissue on each of the ends of the sphincter.

A levatoroplasty can now be performed by placing several interrupted sutures of 0 polydioxanone or 0 polypropylene. The sutures will plicate the levators to the midline, which can be helpful in providing some additional length to the anal canal.

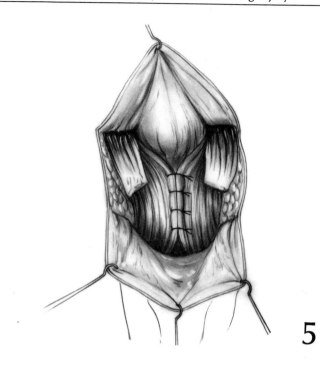

5

Overlapping sphincteroplasty

6, 7 The sphincteroplasty may now be performed. Six mattress sutures of 2/0 polyglycolic acid are placed to bring each fibrous end as far as possible to the opposite side. Three sutures are placed in each end of the sphincter. The sutures should be placed so that the sphincter can be tightened to allow the entrance of just the tip of the index finger into the anal canal. The sutures are then tied, completing the wrap. At this time, any tears that have occurred in either the vaginal or the rectal mucosa should be meticulously repaired with fine chromic catgut sutures.

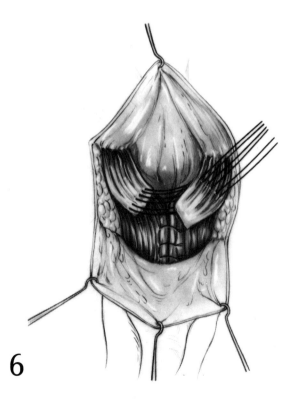

6

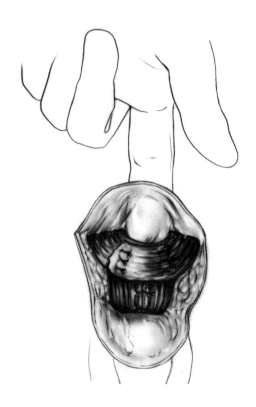

7

Wound closure

8 The wound is closed with interrupted simple sutures of 3/0 chromic catgut. The circumferential wound is converted into a V–Y plasty to allow closure over the broadened perineal body without undue tension. The wound is not closed tightly in the midline, and 0.25-inch Penrose drains are placed on both sides of the repair extending cephalad to the extent of the dissection. The drains are secured to the skin with 3/0 chromic catgut. The wounds are dressed lightly with a gauze sponge.

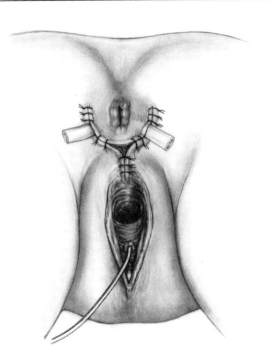

8

Postoperative care

After operation, clear liquids and intravenous antibiotics are given for 3 days. Bowel confinement can be aided by loperamide hydrochloride or diphenoxylate hydrochloride. Sitz baths are initiated on the first day after surgery. After 3 days of bowel rest, the patient is placed on a high-fibre diet and bulk laxatives. The Foley catheter is removed on days 3–4 after operation. The Penrose drains, which were secured with chromic catgut sutures, usually dislodge spontaneously on days 3–5 after operation. Once the patient begins passing flatus, tap water enemas are initiated and are used during any 24-h period in which no spontaneous bowel movements occur.

It is not uncommon for the loosely approximated wound to dehisce. This should not cause undue concern to the patient or to the physician provided that the muscular sutures stay in place. Even massively open wounds will granulate and close secondarily, given appropriate wound care and hygiene.

Outcome

Satisfactory functional results using sphincteroplasty for traumatic injury are obtained in 80–90% of patients[1,5]. When used for idiopathic incontinence, sphincteroplasty will provide a satisfactory result in about 60% of patients[3,4].

References

1. Fang DT, Nivatvongs S, Vermeulen FD, Herman FN, Goldberg SM, Rothenberger DA. Overlapping sphincteroplasty for acquired anal incontinence. *Dis Colon Rectum* 1984; 27: 720–2.

2. Abcarian H, Orsay CP, Pearl RK, Nelson RL, Briley SC. Traumatic cloaca. *Dis Colon Rectum* 1989; 32: 783–7.

3. Miller R, Orrom WJ, Cornes H, Duthie G, Bartolo DCC. Anterior sphincter plication and levatorplasty in the treatment of faecal incontinence. *Br J Surg* 1989; 76: 1058–60.

4. Orrom WJ, Miller R, Cornes H, Duthie G, Mortensen NJ, Bartolo DCC. Comparison of anterior sphincteroplasty and post anal repair in the treatment of idiopathic fecal incontinence. *Dis Colon Rectum* 1991; 34: 305–10.

5. Wexner SD, Marchetti F, Jagelman DG. The role of sphincteroplasty for fecal incontinence reevaluated: a prospective physiologic and functional review. *Dis Colon Rectum* 1991; 34: 22–30.

Illustrations by Patrick Elliott after Cathy Mayes

Pelvic floor descent

C. N. Hudson MChir, FRCS, FRCOG, FRACOG
Director, Clinical Academic Department of Obstetrics and Gynaecology, Medical College of St Bartholomew's Hospital, London, UK

Principles and justification

Posterior colpoperineorrhaphy is a standard gynaecological operation, commonly performed for laxity and overstretching of the vaginal introitus following childbirth. This laxity is often, though not invariably, accompanied by an anterior bulge of the middle third of the posterior vaginal wall, termed rectocoele. The latter is often made larger, as well as more prominent, by deficiency of the fibromuscular perineal body. This term is used to describe the entire wedge-shaped tissue between the vagina and anal canal. It contains the anterior segments of the external anal sphincter muscle and the medial 'attachments' of the superficial transverse perineal muscles.

This condition, to a minor degree, is very common in parous women and often requires no treatment. Symptoms attributable to it are a feeling of perineal insecurity, a palpable bulge, ineffective coital performance, and occasional difficulty in faecal evacuation, overcome by digital pressure on the posterior vaginal wall during defaecation. Women with uterine as well as vaginal prolapse quite commonly require digital pressure to complete defaecation. Backache and perineal pain should not be regarded as features of rectocoele; the former alone may occasionally be ascribed to second-degree uterine prolapse with obvious stretching of the posterior limb of the cardinal ligaments (uterosacral ligaments). Dyschesia is not a feature and tenesmus seldom so, except when a prolapsing retroverted uterus presses on the anterior rectal wall producing a sensation reminiscent of that induced by a descending fetal head during labour. These symptoms are elaborated as they must be distinguished by rectal surgeons dealing with problems of excessive pelvic floor descent, and indeed of rectal prolapse.

Gynaecological displacements and their corrective surgery may actually aggravate problems of defaecation. Overacute angulation at the anorectal junction may prevent adequate descent of the faecal bolus. Overstretching and impairment of the 'levator sling' may render incompetent the pelvic floor elevation necessary to complete evacuation. Furthermore, alteration of the anatomy of the uterosacral ligaments and pouch of Douglas may facilitate invagination of the anterior rectal wall into the anal canal with the formation of a solitary rectal ulcer, and indeed actual intussusception, which may develop into rectal prolapse.

Many patients with rectal prolapse give a history of straining during defaecation with consequent inhibition of the pelvic floor muscles, leading to traction neuropathy and eventually incontinence. This sequence may sometimes also be found in women with uterovaginal prolapse, together with an excessively deep pouch of Douglas, which often becomes a regular feature of both rectal and uterine procidentia.

The need for a modified form of gynaecological pelvic floor repair is sometimes apparent in women whose symptoms may be primarily rectal. If the associated or underlying cause of straining is uterine prolapse, the pelvic floor repair operation may conveniently be accompanied by vaginal hysterectomy. If, however, uterine removal is inappropriate but there is significant uterine descent, posterior sacral hysteropexy may be preferable. Manchester repair, on the other hand, may aggravate the rectal situation, because plication of the cardinal ligaments in front of the cervix inevitably opens the posterior gap between the uterosacral ligaments and thus predisposes to vaginal enterocoele or rectal prolapse in a susceptible patient if appropriate additional steps are not taken.

749

Objectives of the operation

These are:

1. Excision of a redundant pouch of Douglas (enterocoele).
2. Reduction by 'keel' repair of redundant rectal wall that has previously constituted either a high rectocoele or anterior rectal wall prolapse (with or without solitary ulcer).
3. Reduction of the overstretched urogenital hiatus by artificially approximating the puborectalis and pubococcygeus muscles to form a new apex to the perineal body together with such supralevator fascia as may be obtained.
4. Optional endoanal sphincteroplasty to reduce a patulous anus and displace it posteriorly, thus accentuating the anorectal angle.

Indications

These objectives, which may be achieved by the vaginal route, roughly correspond to those of the abdominal Roscoe–Graham operation and are subject to the same limitations.

The operation should be considered as a second stage if a standard operation for rectal prolapse (e.g. polyvinyl alcohol (Ivalon) sponge repair) has not been completely successful. Its main place, however, is in the treatment of early rectal prolapse and pelvic floor descent, associated with a degree of vaginal rectocoele and enterocoele. It can be combined with transperineal anterior plication of the anal sphincter muscle, if there is either a defect or the anus is patulous.

In cases of solitary rectal ulcer, the operation is unlikely to be successful if persistent mucous discharge remains.

Special contraindications

These include:

1. Anal incontinence associated with marked loss of the anorectal angle and with gross pelvic floor neuropathy. Some such cases may respond better to a postanal repair.
2. Intrinsic rectal disease responsible for local ulceration including lymphopathia venereum.
3. Habitual anal coitus.

Preoperative

The general evaluation and care of any patient undergoing vaginal surgery is necessary. Special packs and douches are not usually necessary, but prophylactic imidazole therapy (e.g. tinidazole) is recommended.

Special attention must be paid to the elimination of intrinsic intestinal disorders by sigmoidoscopy and, if appropriate, contrast radiographic studies, including defaecating proctography. The degree of genital prolapse, coital status (actual or prospective), and future reproductive requirements must also be evaluated, as must associated general pathology, such as chronic bronchitis and obesity. Examination, including cervical cytology and often pelvic ultrasonography, must exclude any associated gynaecological pathology. In particular a history of hysterectomy might mandate an abdominal approach.

Local vaginal pathology and infections may require topical treatment, including oestrogen creams. Some surgeons advocate a short course of systemic oestrogen, but the possible increased risk of thromboembolism has to be balanced against the therapeutic advantage.

The presence of stress incontinence may be a factor requiring additional individual evaluation and Thiersch wires should be removed and the bowel emptied.

Operations

POSTERIOR COLPOPERINEORRHAPHY

The standard lithotomy position is used. Caudal or lumbar epidural anaesthesia as an adjuvant is often helpful.

1 Bimanual examination should be performed, and traction applied to the cervix with a volsella to assess descent. The degree of descent provides the information on which a decision is made whether to proceed first to a vaginal hysterectomy. In any event, diagnostic curettage should be carried out. The labia should be distracted.

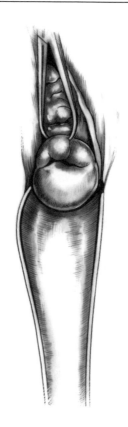

1

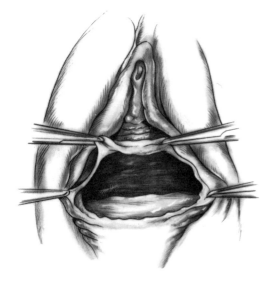

2

Incision

2,3 An individual decision should be made as to the approach to the perineal body. If the introitus is lax, a measured standard transverse incision should be used. Otherwise, if retention of coital ability is desirable, a midline episiotomy is preferred.

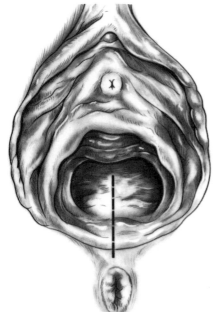

3

4 The cut edges of the midline incision must be elevated with small clips and dissected free from the perineal body and above the apex from the underlying rectum. It is helpful to keep an index finger in the vagina against the flap, so that the correct thickness of flap may be judged.

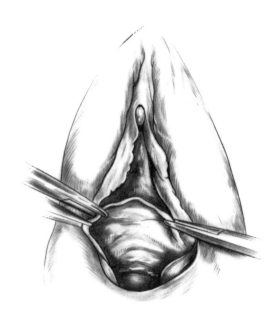

4

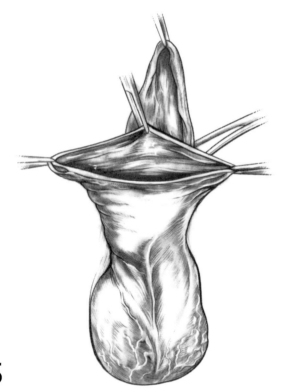

5

5 Once the attachment of the prerectal fascia to the apex of the perineal body is passed, a plane of cleavage may be established as far as the peritoneal attachment of the pouch of Douglas to the anterior rectal wall. The vagina should be incised up to the back of the cervix or the equivalent, and the pouch of Douglas opened.

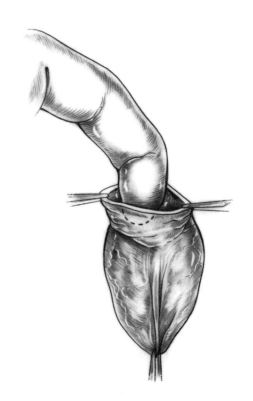

6 At this stage a finger should be inserted into the pouch of Douglas to palpate for ovarian or other pathology and then to evaluate the size of the redundant sac as in any other hernia repair. When freed right to the rectal attachment, the sac should be transfixed, closed and excised. The point of attachment is recognized by the appearance of the longitudinal muscle of the rectal wall.

6

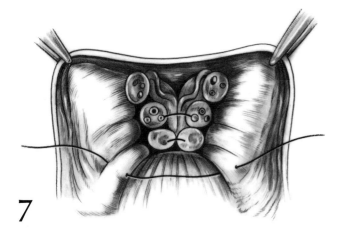

7

7 If the uterus has been removed, it is desirable to approximate the uterosacral ligaments with one or two interrupted catgut sutures. Caution should be exercised, because the ureter may have been drawn down by peritoneal mobilization.

8 The redundant intraperitoneal rectal wall should now be infolded in a manner comparable to the 'keel' repair of abdominal wall hernia. Full-thickness wedge excision of the rectal wall has been advocated, but this is not usually regarded as necessary. A continuous suture of polyglycolic acid is suitable.

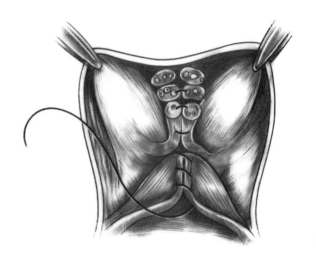

8

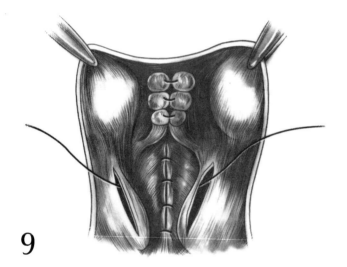

9

9 At this stage, further mobilization of the rectal wall from the levator muscles and pelvic sidewalls may be necessary. When these are clear, a stab incision with scissors is made under the fascia on the superior surface of the pubococcygeus muscle. This layer may be united with its fellow in front of the rectum without producing too much vaginal constriction and joining with the posterior uterosacral stitch.

10 Thereafter, two or three interrupted sutures can be placed in the puborectalis/pubococcygeus muscles to approximate them at the apex of the new perineal body, a position which they do not normally occupy. It is most important to insert two fingers into the vagina to test whether an undue 'hourglass' constriction has been induced. For the repair, 0 or 1 polyglycolic acid sutures are suitable, though some surgeons have used non-absorbable wire or nylon sutures; there are, however, inherent risks of sinus formation and polyglycolic acid seems preferable.

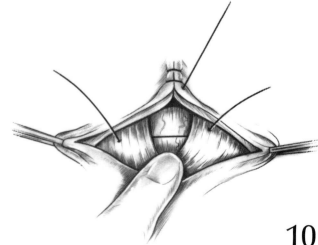

10

11 Once these sutures have been checked they can be tied. It then remains to build up a new perineal body in such a way that the vaginal lumen reforms in a tubular rather than an 'hourglass' fashion. Buried sutures are best inserted from within outwards into the halves of the recently or previously divided perineal body.

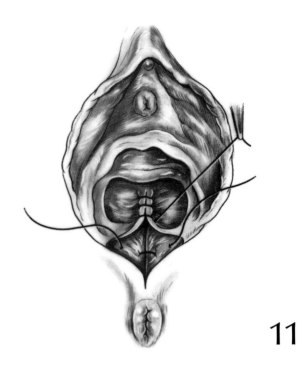

11

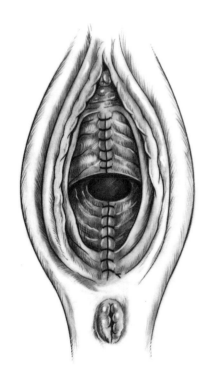

12

12 It should be noted that unless there is significant redundant vaginal skin over a rectocoele, there need be no trimming of the vaginal wall incision. Merely opening and closing such an incision reduces the available lumen slightly, and coital function can as easily be impaired by excision of too much vaginal skin as by overzealous suture of the pubococcygeus muscle. The original episiotomy should be repaired with interrupted polyglycolic acid sutures.

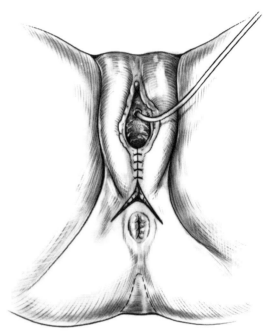

13

ENDOANAL SPHINCTEROPLASTY

13 This is an optional 'extra' if there is a patulous anus. The median 'episiotomy' is extended posteriorly as an inverted Y to expose the subcutaneous and superficial external anal sphincter muscles.

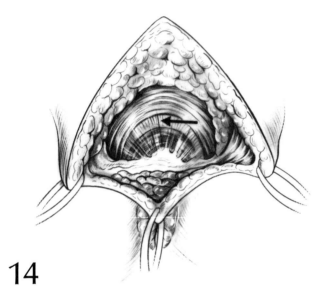

14

14 The intersphincteric plane is developed to allow the smooth muscle and anal canal wall to be displaced centrally.

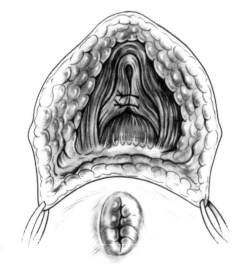

15

15 The redundant loop of external sphincter is reduced by 'racquet handle' closure with interrupted polyglycolic acid sutures, displacing the anal aperture posteriorly.

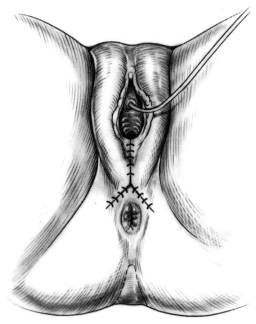

16 Cruciform closure of the inverted Y is carried out with fine polyglycolic acid sutures.

16

Postoperative care

In view of the fairly extensive infraperitoneal dissection, haematoma formation from branches of the internal pudendal vessels is common. A vaginal pack for 24–48 h is prudent, and suction drainage through a perineal stab wound has much to commend it.

Even without anterior repair, many patients will have retention of urine, and a suprapubic catheter is required for a few days, with prophylactic nitrofurantoin. If there is extreme bruising, antibiotic treatment is preferable.

This is a painful operation, and the insertion of diclofenac sodium suppositories is strongly recommended. Gentle digital examination of the vagina before discharge from hospital is desirable to break down any soft adhesions.

Care of the bowels is important. Constipation and straining are most harmful, but liquid paraffin as a laxative is unsatisfactory. If a sphincteroplasty has been performed, purgation to produce diarrhoea (and incontinence) for 2 weeks is suggested. Early resort to bran or its substitutes is recommended. Coitus should be avoided until after a postoperative visit at 6 weeks.

Further reading

Hudson CN. Female genital prolapse and pelvic floor deficiency. *Int J Colorectal Dis* 1988; 3: 181–5.

Illustrations by Gillian Lee Illustrations

Construction of an electrically stimulated gracilis neoanal sphincter

Norman S. Williams MS, FRCS
Professor of Surgery and Director, Surgical Unit, The Royal London Hospital, London, UK

History

Efforts to create a neoanal sphincter have relied principally on the transposition of skeletal muscle, usually the gracilis, around the anal canal. Pickrell et al.[1] were the first to use this technique in man, and although satisfactory results were reported, other investigators have found the technique unreliable[2]. To improve the procedure, Cavina et al.[3] stimulated the gracilis muscle intermittently for several weeks after operation to prevent atrophy.

The original technique and subsequent modifications may fail because the gracilis, a fast-twitch muscle, is incapable of prolonged contraction without fatigue. Salmons and Henriksson[4] showed that in animals, long-term low-frequency electrical stimulation could convert a fast-twitch, fatiguable muscle to a slow-twitch, fatigue-resistant organ. Using this principle, the author's initial studies in animals[5] and in man[6-8] showed that, although the technique was practicable, the results were inconsistent. The technique was then modified to make it more reliable.

Principles and justification

Indications

The neosphincter can be used for several types of patients:

1. Incontinent patients who have a deficient anal sphincter mechanism as a result of trauma or neurogenic damage and have an intact rectum and anal canal. Construction of a neosphincter is indicated if a conventional operation, such as postanal repair, has failed or is contraindicated.
2. Some patients with anorectal agenesis who have had an unsuccessful pull-through procedure and in whom electromyographic mapping indicates the absence of any functioning anal sphincter (thus ruling out a re-routing procedure) are suitable.
3. Some patients who have undergone an abdomino-perineal excision of the rectum for cancer are suitable provided they have no evidence of local recurrence or distant metastases. The colon must be brought down to the perineum and sutured to the perineal skin several weeks before neosphincter construction[8]. Similarly, patients who have low rectal cancer and are about to undergo abdomino-perineal excision of the rectum may be considered for the procedure. In such individuals, the colon will be sutured to the perineal skin at the time of the resection.

Contraindications

1. Damaged gracilis muscle: in practice this includes patients with spina bifida and those with generalized neurological diseases such as multiple sclerosis. Similarly, patients with myopathic disease affecting the limb muscles are unsuitable for the procedure. If there is any doubt about gracilis muscle function, it should be tested by electromyography.
2. Disseminated malignant disease or local pelvic recurrence.
3. Lack of sufficient manual dexterity to use the magnetic controls of the electrical stimulator.
4. Persistent perineal sepsis or Crohn's disease.
5. A cardiac pacemaker *in situ*.

Preoperative

Counselling

This is a most important part of the preparation in which the procedure must be fully explained. It must be stressed that there are usually three stages to the procedure, and that a leg wound will result. The latter is an important consideration, particularly for women. The pros and cons of the procedure compared with a permanent colostomy must be discussed, and it must be made clear that success cannot be guaranteed. The prospective patient should meet a patient of similar age and same sex who has had the procedure for a similar indication. The patient should be shown the stimulator and magnet and provided with appropriate literature. He/she must be given sufficient time to make a decision and encouraged to return for further discussion.

Marking the site of the stimulator and covering stoma

Having made the decision to undergo the operation, a site is chosen where the stimulator is to be implanted. This is usually in a subcutaneous pocket overlying the lower ribs anteriorly. This will be on the left side if the covering stoma is to be on the right. In women, the site must be chosen so as to avoid rubbing by the brassiere. Once chosen, the site must be marked with indelible ink. Similarly, the stoma care nurse must site the position for the covering stoma. In those patients in whom a colonic pull-through procedure is not to be performed, either a loop ileostomy in the right iliac fossa or a transverse colostomy can be used. In those who are to have a colonic pull-through, a loop ileostomy is essential.

Bowel preparation and prophylactic antibiotics

A full bowel preparation is required for all operative stages apart from stage 1, unless this stage is to include a colonic pull-through. It is usually sufficient to give a liquid diet for 48 h and 2 sachets of sodium picosulphate/magnesium citrate (Picolax) during the 24 h before the procedure. Antibiotic prophylaxis is provided by metronidazole and cefuroxime sodium. For stages 1 and 3, one dose is given with the premedication and two more are given at 6 h and 12 h after the procedure. For stage 2, the same antibiotics are continued for 5 days after the operation.

DVT prophylaxis

Patients should be given subcutaneous heparin, 5000 units twice or three times a day, depending on their body weight.

Anaesthesia

It is imperative that the anaesthetist uses no muscle relaxants during stage 2 of the operation. If muscle relaxants are used, they will make it impossible to observe muscle contraction during nerve stimulation.

Operations

INCONTINENT PATIENTS WITH AN INTACT ANORECTUM BUT DEFICIENT ANAL SPHINCTER

Stage 1: mobilization of gracilis muscle

This stage is performed to ensure an adequate blood supply to the distal half of the gracilis muscle when it is subsequently transposed to the perineum. The patient is placed in the modified Lloyd-Davies position (as described in the chapter on pp. 47–50). The skin of the perineum, groin and inner aspect of the thigh on the side chosen for mobilization of the gracilis is prepared with povidone-iodine. If the covering stoma is to be eventually sited on the right side of the patient's abdomen, the left gracilis muscle is chosen for mobilization.

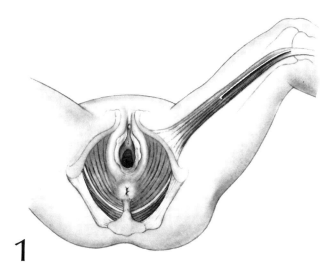

1 A longitudinal incision approximately 10 cm in length is made on the innermost aspect of the thigh along a line from the medial femoral condyle towards the inferior pubic ramus, commencing approximately 2 cm proximal to the femoral condyle.

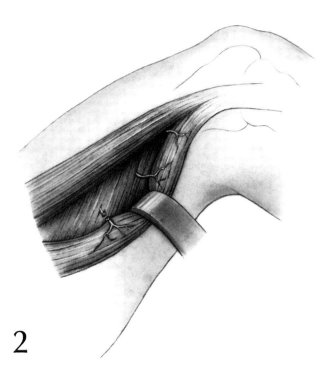

2 The skin incision is deepened through the superficial and deep fascia, and the gracilis muscle is identified. The gracilis is the most superficial muscle on the medial side of the thigh. Its tendon is easily identified in the lower part of the incision by the fact that its upper edge is overlapped by the tendon of the sartorius muscle as the latter arches over it to be inserted into the upper part of the medial surface of the shaft of the tibia below the tibial condyle. The tendon of the gracilis muscle is inserted into the tibia just behind the insertion of the sartorius tendon.

The gracilis muscle is mobilized in its distal half by division and ligation of the two or three distal vessels that supply it on its lateral surface. The intervening and overlying areolar tissue is also cleared from the muscle, but at this stage the tendon is not divided.

The wound is closed using a continuous 2/0 chromic catgut suture for the subcutaneous tissue and a subcuticular continuous 3/0 polypropylene suture for the skin.

Stage 2: transposition of gracilis muscle, implantation of electrode and neurostimulator and construction of covering stoma

Stage 2 is carried out 4–6 weeks after stage 1.

3 The previous thigh incision is extended proximally to the point where the tendinous origin of the adductor longus muscle can be palpated. At this point, the direction of the incision moves more laterally to curve over the tendinous origin of the adductor longus muscle.

The tendon of the gracilis muscle is traced down to its insertion in the tibia, after dividing any fibrous tissue or adhesions that have developed since the 'delay' procedure. The tendon is divided with strong scissors as close to its insertion as possible. It is also necessary to separate the gracilis tendon from the sartorius tendon by dividing the tissue that binds the two tendons together.

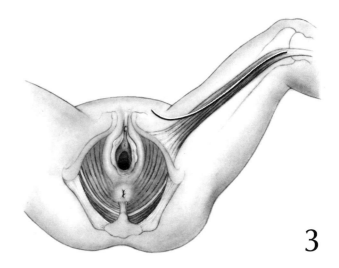

3

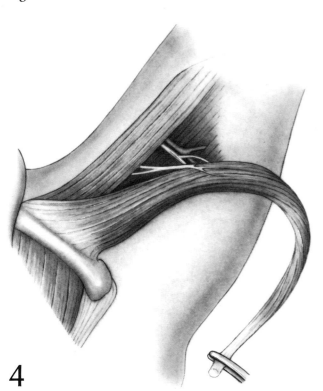

4

4 Once the tendon has been divided, it is clamped in a pair of small artery forceps, which is then used as a retractor. By exerting traction in a proximal direction, the muscle can be mobilized upwards towards the main vascular pedicle. Any peripheral vessels not previously divided during the delay procedure are now divided and ligated. All areolar tissue overlying the muscle and binding it to the deeper muscles is divided.

The main vascular pedicle is identified entering the lateral border of the gracilis, usually at the junction of the proximal and distal two-thirds of the muscle.

The pedicle consists of an artery and two venae commitantes. The artery is a branch of the obturator artery and emerges from beneath the medial border of the adductor longus to supply the gracilis muscle. Once identified, the vascular pedicle is carefully cleared of areolar tissue and freed to its point of exit beneath the adductor longus. The peripheral branches of the nerve to the gracilis lying above the main vascular pedicle can be identified using a nerve stimulator, to ensure their preservation.

Mobilization of the muscle continues proximally by dividing the areolar tissue overlying its medial surface on the upper third to its origin from the lower half of the body of the pubic symphysis and the inferior pubic ramus.

5 The main nerve to the gracilis is sought by entering the plane between the adductor longus and adductor brevis muscles approximately 3 cm proximal to the main vascular bundle.

The main nerve is a continuation of the anterior branch of the obturator nerve. It traverses the superior surface of the adductor brevis muscle in a lateral to medial direction. In its upper part, it gives off a branch to the adductor brevis and then emerges from beneath the medial border of the overlying adductor longus to split into several branches, which enter the upper part of the lateral border of the gracilis muscle. By exerting downward traction on the upper part of the gracilis muscle, the main nerve is stretched. Identification of the nerve is confirmed by stimulation with a disposable nerve stimulator (set at 0.5 V), observing an *en masse* contraction of the gracilis muscle.

The areolar tissue on either side of the nerve binding it to the adductor brevis muscle is cleared. The tissue overlying the nerve is left undisturbed, and the site for electrode implantation is selected distal to the branch to the adductor brevis, but proximal to the main nerve division into its peripheral branches.

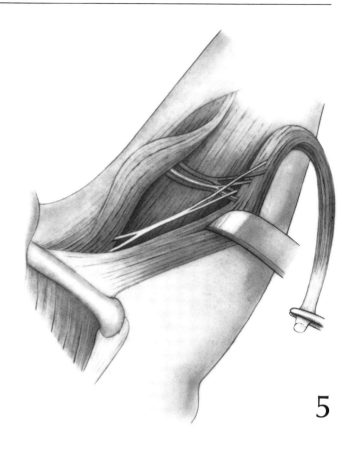

5

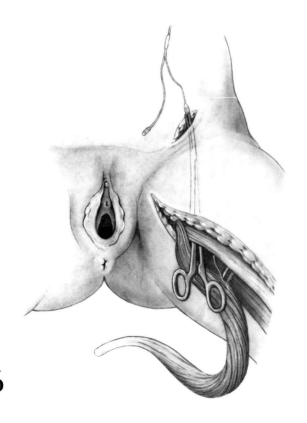

6

6 A 2-cm incision is made approximately 5 cm above the mid-inguinal point on the side on which the muscle has been mobilized. A pair of long artery forceps (Lloyd-Davies type) is passed under the adductor longus muscle in the plane between it and the adductor brevis muscle, and is tunnelled subcutaneously until its tip emerges through the skin incision above the inguinal ligament. The track that has been created is enlarged by opening and closing the artery forceps several times. The tip of the electrode (NICE) on the shorter lead is grasped in the jaws of the artery forceps and gently brought through the subcutaneous tunnel, so that it emerges parallel to the main nerve. The bifid nature of the electrode lead is designed so that two muscles can, if necessary, be transposed and stimulated simultaneously. For most patients, however, only one muscle is required. Thus, if only one muscle is to be used, the second electrode on the longer lead is also brought through the same subcutaneous tunnel and anchored to the superior surface of the adductor longus, so that it can be located easily at a later date if required.

7 A transverse incision approximately 5 cm in length is made over the anterior lower ribs in the mid-clavicular line at the position that has previously been identified. This incision is deepened to create a subcutaneous pocket large enough to take the purpose-designed implant (NICE device).

The tunneller with the trocar *in situ* is then introduced through the lower incision above the groin and advanced in the subcutaneous plane to emerge through the upper incision.

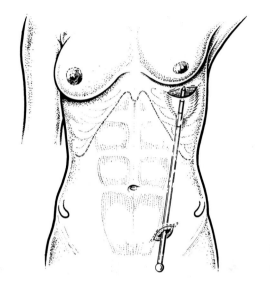

7

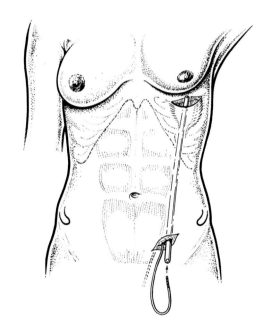

8

8 The trocar is removed from the plastic tube, and the proximal end of the lead with its connector destined for connection to the implant is threaded through the plastic tube to emerge in the upper incision. The plastic tube is withdrawn through the upper incision, leaving the lead ready for connecting to the implant.

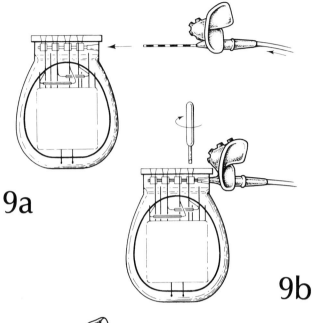

9a

9b

9a–e The connector part of the lead is passed through the silicone boot, which is then turned inside out. The connector is inserted into the port on the superior surface of the implant after first releasing the four screws at each connector point. It is essential to ensure that the connector part of the lead is fully pushed into the port of the implant. Only then is it fixed in place by screwing the four screws down so they abut firmly against the connector part of the lead. The silicone boot is then levered over the superior part of the implant and pressed home using the roller. The implant is programmed at 1 V and 10 Hz (pulse width 210 μs) using the radiotelemetry programming unit.

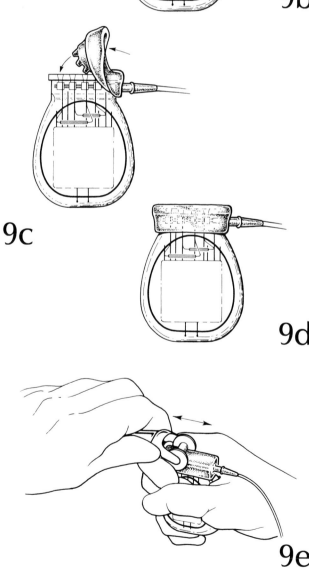

9c

9d

9e

10 The electrode plate is sutured over the main nerve in its long axis. The plate has precut holes for non-absorbable sutures. The sutures should all be placed before they are tied. Six interrupted 3/0 non-absorbable silk sutures on a round-bodied needle are used. Each suture passes through the hole on the periphery of the electrode plate, through the underlying adductor brevis muscle, taking care not to damage the nerve, and back through the plate, so that when tied the knot lies on the superior surface of the plate. From time to time the implant is turned on by using the programmer so as to ensure that the electrode lies on the main nerve and that an *en masse* contraction of the gracilis muscle is achieved. Once the position of the electrode is correct, all the sutures are tied.

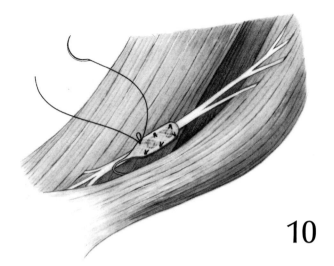

10

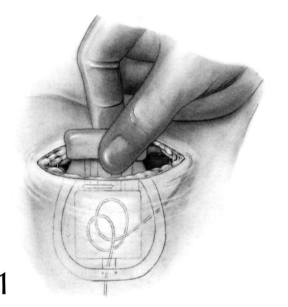

11

11 The implant is turned off with the programmer and is placed in the subcutaneous pocket, ensuring that any redundant lead is placed behind the implant. The transverse skin wound is closed with subcuticular polypropylene.

The small wound above the groin is closed after first ensuring that a loop of excess lead no less than 1.5 cm in length is left in a small subcutaneous pocket at this point. This will relieve strain on the system and provide for patient growth and mobility.

12 Transposition of the gracilis muscle around the anal canal is started by two curvilinear incisions approximately 2 cm from the right and left margins of the anal verge. A circumferential subcutaneous tunnel around the anal canal, external to any remaining external anal sphincter, is created. This is deepened to ensure that it can easily accommodate the gracilis muscle when it is transposed. The skin bridges anteriorly and posteriorly are preserved. Care must be exercised in creating the space anteriorly between the anterior wall of the anorectum and the posterior vaginal wall in women. In many of these patients there is considerable scarring in this region, and the vaginal and rectal walls are closely applied to each other. This dissection is aided by infiltration of the plane with a weak solution of adrenaline in saline (1:300 000).

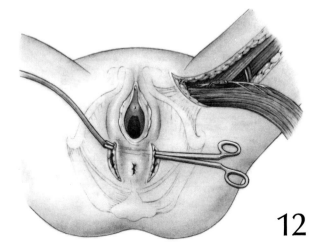

12

13 By gentle dissection with scissors, the plane is opened sufficiently to allow the insertion of a Jacques catheter, which can then be used to retract the anorectum downwards and allow the plane to be further dissected under direct vision. A headlight is particularly useful for this part of the procedure.

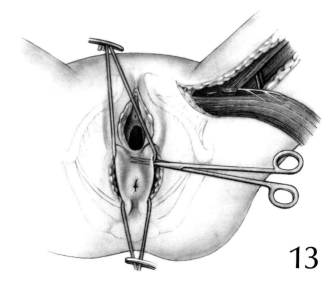

13

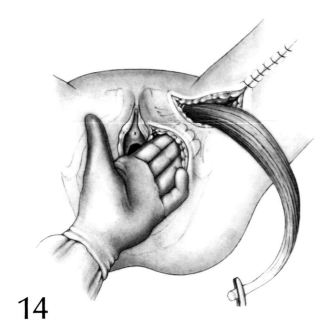

14

14 An incision is made in the skin crease between the thigh and the buttock on the side of the muscle to be transposed. Through this incision, a tunnel is created into the thigh to emerge close to the upper part of the mobilized gracilis muscle. It is necessary in creating this tunnel to divide Scarpa's fascia with scissors. The tunnel must be at least three finger-breadths wide. A similar tunnel is created from this incision to that on the lateral side of the anal verge.

15 Using a pair of long artery forceps attached to the free tendon of the gracilis, the muscle is brought into the perineum through the tunnel that has been created, ensuring that the muscle is not twisted.

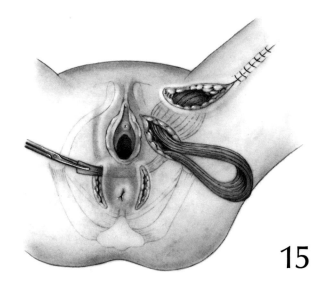

15

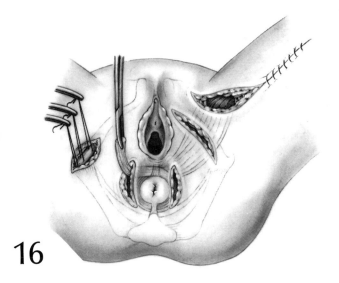

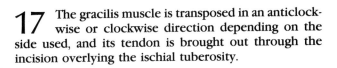

16

16 The muscle is brought round the anal canal in a gamma configuration. A small incision is made over the contralateral ischial tuberosity. The incision is deepened down to bone, and three interrupted 0 Ethibond sutures are attached to the underlying periosteum. The sutures are left long and clipped with the needles attached.

17 The gracilis muscle is transposed in an anticlockwise or clockwise direction depending on the side used, and its tendon is brought out through the incision overlying the ischial tuberosity.

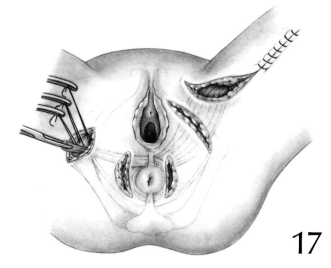

17

18 The ipsilateral leg is then adducted to the midline, and the muscle is pulled through its tunnels so that it fits snugly around the anal canal, which should allow insertion of the tip of the index finger. The tendon of the gracilis muscle is then sutured to the ischial tuberosity using the previously placed interrupted Ethibond sutures.

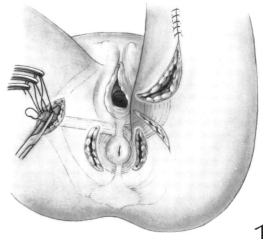

18

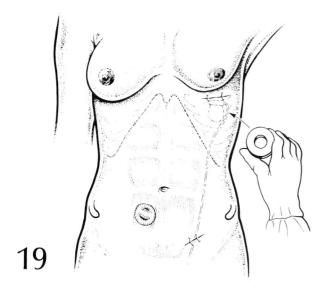

19

19 Once positioned, the stimulator is turned on with the programmer to ensure that contraction of the gracilis muscle occurs and occlusion of the anal orifice is achieved. The magnet is then used to check that it is able to turn the stimulator off.

All wounds are closed after first spraying them with an antibiotic spray (Tribiotic). Subcuticular polypropylene (Prolene) is used for the leg wound and interrupted 2/0 polyglactin (Vicryl) for the perineal skin wounds.

A covering loop stoma is then constructed. The author usually uses a loop ileostomy sited in the right iliac fossa and performs the operation laparoscopically (as described in the chapter on pp. 243–269 and the section on pp. 122–239).

TOTAL RECONSTRUCTION OF THE PERINEUM AFTER RECTAL EXCISION

This part of the operation differs from that previously described, in that the 'delay' procedure for the gracilis muscle is also accompanied by a colonic pull-through operation with a coloperineal anastomosis.

20 Rectal excision is performed by an abdomino-perineal approach (as described in the chapter on pp. 472–486). Before the perineal dissection is commenced, however, the position of the anal verge is marked with indelible ink, so that the neoanal canal can be positioned correctly. The perineal incision is elliptical in shape and commences anteriorly midway between the anus and the bulb of the urethra in the male or the posterior vaginal fourchette in the female, extending backwards to a point midway between the coccyx and posterior anal verge. Laterally, the incision lies approximately 1–2 cm from the anal verge.

The incision is deepened through the para-anal tissue and ischiorectal fossa up to the plane of the pelvic floor muscles. The extent of radial dissection is not usually as wide as previously advocated, provided that this is compatible with lateral clearance of the tumour and the coccyx is not routinely removed. The dissection continues cranially, and the muscles of the pelvic floor and the lateral ligaments of the rectum are divided closer to the rectum than described previously, although it is essential to remove all the mesorectum.

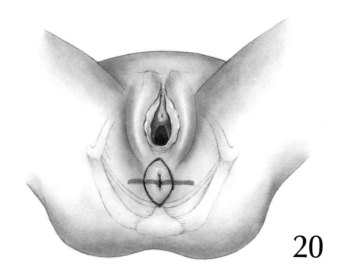

20

After the rectum and sigmoid colon have been fully mobilized, the descending colon is transected using the GIA stapler at a convenient point, ensuring that the proximal side has an adequate blood supply. The rectum and sigmoid colon are removed. The descending colon is mobilized proximally around the splenic flexure to the mid-transverse colon. Care is taken to preserve the left branch of the middle colic artery which supplies the distal colon.

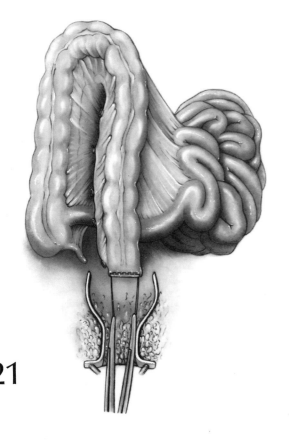

21

21 Stay sutures of different colours are attached to each end of the stapled line of the transected distal colon. The perineal operator then passes two pairs of long artery forceps via the perineal wound into the pelvis. The abdominal operator attaches the ends of the stay sutures into the jaws of the artery forceps in such a way that when the colon is brought down to the perineum it is not twisted. The perineal operator then gently pulls the colon down through the perineal wound; the abdominal operator assists in this process by gently guiding its passage.

The abdominal operator tacks the colon to the sacrum with three or four non-absorbable sutures, which pass from the promontory of the sacrum through the serosa. Care must be taken not to damage the blood supply to the colon during this manoeuvre.

22, 23 The perineal operator repairs any muscle that remains in the perineum and tacks the cut levator ani muscles to the serosa of the colon. The stapled end of the colon is cut off. Redundant colon is excised to prevent prolapse and the mucosa is sutured circumferentially to the perineal skin at the previous site of the anal verge. Interrupted polyglactin sutures on a taper cut needle are used for this anastomosis in the same manner as for a colostomy construction. The remainder of the perineal wound is then closed with interrupted polyglactin sutures.

A loop ileostomy is constructed in the right iliac fossa (as described in the chapter on pp. 243–269). The abdomen is closed in the usual manner, leaving two suction drains positioned in the pelvis emerging through the abdominal wall.

About 2 months after all wounds have healed, the electrically stimulated gracilis neosphincter is constructed around the neoanal canal as previously described.

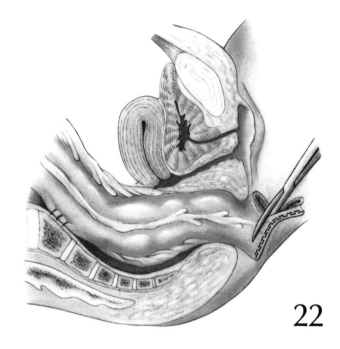

22

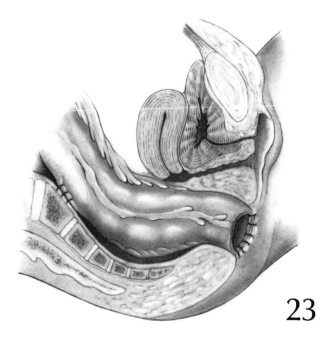

23

Postoperative care

The patient is nursed with the legs together for the first 3 days and is then encouraged to become mobile. Oral fluids are started after flatus has been passed. Long-term electrical stimulation commences on the tenth day, provided all wounds are healing satisfactorily. The stimulator is programmed using the programming unit. The 'training' protocol at present is as shown in *Table 1*.

Table 1 Training protocol for electrical stimulation of gracilis neoanal sphincter

	Weeks 1 and 2	Weeks 3 and 4	Weeks 5 and 6	Weeks 7 and 8	After week 8
Pulse width (μs)	210	210	210	210	210
Frequency (Hz)	12	12	12	12	12
Time on (s)	2	2	2	2	4
Time off (s)	6	4	2	1	1

After 8 weeks, some conversion of 'fast-twitch' to 'slow-twitch' muscle should have occurred, which can be demonstrated by anorectal manometry using a microtransducer (*Figure 1*). With the probe positioned

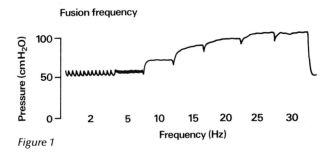

Fusion frequency

Figure 1

in the anal canal at the site of the neosphincter, the frequency of stimulation can gradually be increased until a smooth (fused) contraction takes place. The minimum frequency that produces such a tetanic contraction is known as the tetanic fusion frequency (TFF). Immediately after the operation, TFF is usually 25 pulses/s; after 8 weeks, it invariably decreases to about 10–15 pulses/s. When this reduction has occurred, the 'off' time can be reduced to zero, so the stimulator is working in continuous mode and the neosphincter is also contracting continuously, thus occluding the anal canal.

At this point, the patient is admitted for stage 3, i.e. closure of the covering stoma (as described in the chapter on pp. 243–269.)

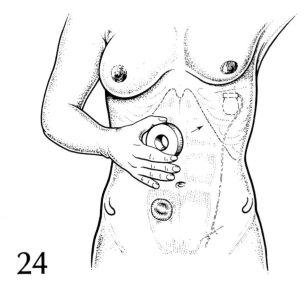

24 After closure of the stoma, the patient should be instructed on how to turn the stimulator off or on by passing the magnet over it.

Initially, there may be problems in rectal evacuation. This often occurs in patients who previously 'strained' before they developed incontinence. No doubt the straining was to some extent responsible for the incontinence, but when continence is improved, the old habits return. It is essential in such cases to institute a suppository regimen as soon as possible. If patients lack the sensation of impending evacuation, they should be encouraged to try to evacuate every 6–8 h intitially, gradually increasing the interval, depending on the results of such a regimen.

References

1. Pickrell KL, Broadbent TR, Masters FW, Metzger JL. Construction of a rectal sphincter and restoration of anal continence by transplanting the gracilis muscle: a report of four cases in children. *Ann Surg* 1952; 139: 853–62.

2. Yoshioka K, Keighley MRB. Clinical and manometric assessment of gracilis muscle transplant for faecal incontinence. *Dis Colon Rectum* 1988; 31: 767–9.

3. Cavina E. Seccia M, Evangelista G *et al.* Construction of a continent perineal colostomy by using electrostimulated gracilis muscles after abdominoperineal resection: personal technique and experience with 32 cases. *Ital J Surg Sci* 1987; 17: 305–14.

4. Salmons S, Henriksson J. The adaptive response of skeletal muscle to increased use. *Muscle Nerve* 1981; 4: 94–105.

5. Hallan RI, Williams NS, Hutton MRE, Scott M, Pilot MA, Swash M. Electrically stimulated sartorius neosphincter: canine model of activation and skeletal muscle transformation. *Br J Surg* 1990; 77: 208–13.

6. Williams NS, Hallan RI, Koeze TH, Watkins ES. Construction of the neorectum and neoanal sphincter following previous procto-colectomy. *Br J Surg* 1989; 76: 1191–4.

7. Williams NS, Hallan RI, Koeze TH, Pilot MA, Watkins ES. Construction of a neoanal sphincter by transposition of the gracilis muscle and prolonged neuromuscular stimulation for the treatment of faecal incontinence. *Ann R Coll Surg Engl* 1990; 72: 108–13.

8. Williams NS, Hallan RI, Koeze TH, Watkins ES. Restoration of gastrointestinal continuity and continence after abdominoperineal excision of the rectum using an electrically stimulated neoanal sphincter. *Dis Colon Rectum* 1990; 33: 561–5.

Illustrations by Angela Christie

Artificial anal sphincter

W. D. Wong MD
Clinical Assistant Professor of Surgery, Division of Colon and Rectal Surgery, University of Minnesota Medical School, Minneapolis, Minnesota, USA

D. A. Rothenberger MD
Clinical Professor of Surgery and Chief, Division of Colon and Rectal Surgery, University of Minnesota Medical School, Minneapolis, Minnesota, USA

History

Anal incontinence can be devastating for patients and conservative measures often fail to control the problem. However, selected patients may benefit from surgical repair. Traditional surgical procedures include sphincteroplasty for traumatic sphincter disruption, postanal repair for neurogenic incontinence, prolapse repair for procidentia-associated incontinence, and the Silastic Thiersch operations. In general, patients who fail these traditional methods are often faced with the incapacitating symptoms of faecal incontinence or must live with a diverting colostomy. A new technique using an artificial anal sphincter has provided very encouraging results in a limited clinical trial. This procedure remains experimental and has not yet been approved for general use. Its initial application has been reserved for patients who have failed conventional management of severe anal incontinence and whose only reasonable alternative is a permanent stoma.

Components

The artificial anal sphincter is made by American Medical Systems and is a modification of the AMS-800 urinary sphincter device. It consists of three Silastic components: an inflatable cuff, a pressure-regulating balloon, and a control pump. The cuff is available in 2.0–2.5-cm widths and in lengths varying from 9 to 14 cm. The pressure-regulating balloon is available in several pressure ranges varying from 60 to 90 mmH$_2$O. The control pump is a sophisticated device which can be activated and deactivated.

Mechanics and function

The inflatable cuff is placed circumferentially around the anus and is connected to the pressure-regulating balloon and the control pump. In its activated state, the cuff is filled with fluid and the pressure is maintained by the pressure-regulating balloon. This occludes the anus and maintains continence. When the patient wishes to defaecate, the control pump is compressed several times, which displaces the fluid out of the cuff and into the pressure-regulating balloon. This empties the cuff and allows defaecation to proceed. Over the ensuing 7–10 min, the control pump allows refilling of the cuff from the pressure-regulating balloon back into the cuff, thus reactivating the device and restoring continence.

Preoperative

All patients undergo a complete mechanical and antibiotic bowel preparation. The patient is placed in the modified lithotomy position with legs in Allen stirrups with the lower portion of the operating table retracted (*see* chapter on pp. 47–50). Many candidates for this surgery have pre-existing colostomies. If so, the stoma is carefully isolated from the lower operative field. If a colostomy has not been previously established, the procedure begins with a midline, lower abdominal incision and establishment of a sigmoid end-loop colostomy (*see* chapter on pp. 274–283) with the distal end stapled to form a Hartmann's pouch. Once this is accomplished, the abdominal incision is closed, and a stoma bag is applied to the colostomy. The lower abdomen and perineum are re-prepared and draped, keeping the newly established colostomy isolated from the lower operative field. The patient is then ready for a synchronous approach to the implantation of the artificial anal sphincter.

Operation

Perineal procedure

Incision

1 Bilateral 3 cm pararectal incisions lateral to the external sphincter are made. The incisions are deepened within the ischiorectal fat superiorly to the limits of the inferior aspects of the levator ani muscle.

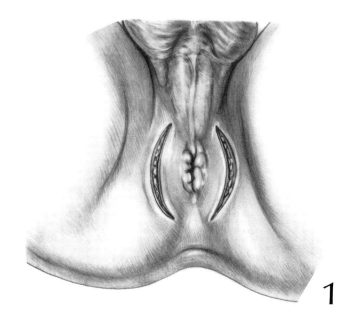

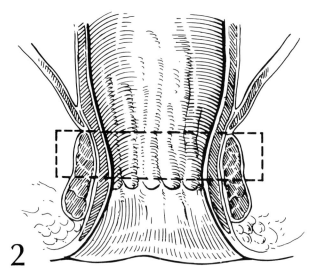

2 A circumferential tunnel is then created by incising the anal coccygeal raphe posteriorly, leaving the distal portion of the raphe intact to prevent distal migration of the cuff. Anteriorly, the tunnel is created as proximal as possible to allow for a relatively high placement of the cuff. The level of the circumferential tunnel corresponds to a location just distal to the anorectal ring.

Sizing the cuff

3 Once a circumferential tunnel has been created, an elastic sizer with centimetre markings is wrapped around the anus and distal rectum at the site of the proposed cuff placement. The sizer is wrapped snugly around the enclosed tissue and the circumference is noted; 1 cm is added to the measured value, and this sum determines the length of the cuff selected.

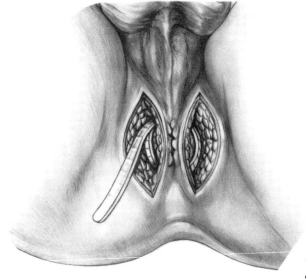

Cuff placement

4 Once the proper cuff length has been selected, the space is inspected to determine whether a 2.0-cm or 2.5-cm wide cuff will fit best. The appropriate cuff is then wrapped around the anus at the tunnel site. A silastic holed tab locks over a securing knob on the outer surface of the cuff to hold this in a secure circumferential position. The cuff is placed so that the connecting tubing is directed superiorly to either the right or left side depending on the planned placement of the control pump.

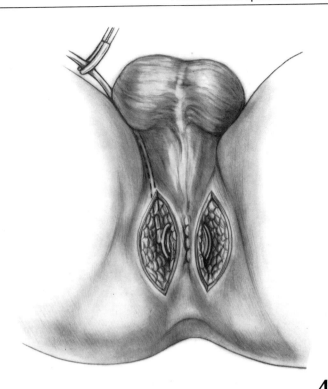

4

Abdominal procedure

5 While the perineal surgeon is placing the cuff, the abdominal operator simultaneously prepares for placement of the pressure-regulating balloon and the control pump. A short Pfannenstiel incision is made two fingerbreadths above the pubic symphysis, and the anterior rectus fascia is divided transversely. The rectus muscles are separated in the midline and retracted laterally. The space of Retzius is identified and the bladder is pushed inferiorly, creating a space large enough to accommodate the balloon. A pressure-regulating balloon of suitable capacity is selected and instilled with 40 ml of isotonic radio-opaque solution. The connecting tubing is atraumatically occluded with a Silastic-shod mosquito clamp.

The perineal and abdominal operators work together to tunnel the connecting tubing between the cuff and pressure-regulating balloon by passing a tunnelling trocar connected to the cuff tubing superiorly from the pararectal incision along the perineum, progressing above the superior pubic ramus just lateral to the pubic tubercle. The trocar is drawn into the abdominal wound subcutaneous tissue just above the anterior rectus fascia. Approximately 5–7 ml of isotonic radio-opaque solution is then injected through the cuff tubing into the cuff to fill it to a level above its natural capacity. The cuff tubing is then connected by a temporary plastic connector to the pressure-regulating balloon tubing and the pressure between the balloon and the cuff is allowed to equilibrate. The tubing to the cuff and the tubing to the balloon are each clamped with an atraumatic Silastic-shod mosquito clamp. The two tubes are disconnected and the amount of fluid remaining in the

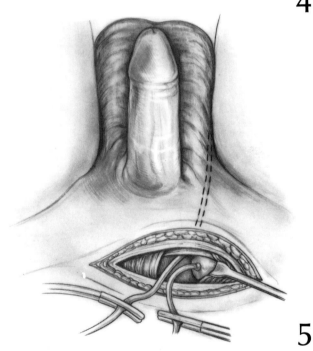

5

cuff is then measured by extracting it with a syringe connected to the tubing. This volume is carefully documented and returned into the cuff. The remaining fluid in the pressure-regulating balloon is then removed from the balloon and 40 ml is reintroduced into the balloon. The manoeuvre establishes the ideal amount of fluid within the system.

Control pump placement

6 The control pump is then placed in an accessible location for the patient. In men, a subcutaneous tunnel leading from the abdominal wound into the scrotum is established by distal blunt dissection as far into the scrotum as is technically feasible. In women, a similar subcutaneous tract is developed by distal blunt dissection into one of the labia majora. Once the pocket has been created, the control pump is inserted into the created space. The control pump is orientated so that the activation and deactivation button is readily palpable on the lateral or anterior surface. Its location is secured by placement of a 4/0 non-absorbable monofilament suture between the two limbs of the efferent and afferent tubing to prevent migration of the pump in a cephalad direction.

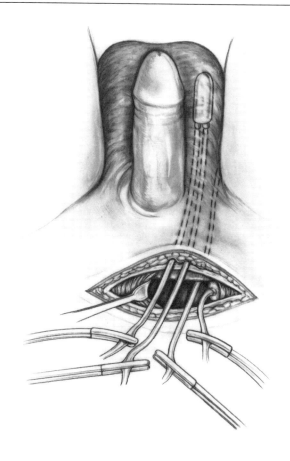

6

7 The excess portions of tubing are trimmed to an ideal length so that the appropriate connections can be made. The tubing from the cuff is connected by a special curved coupling device to the designated cuff tubing of the control pump. Similarly, the tubing from the pressure-regulating balloon is connected to the tubing-designated balloon port on the control pump by means of a straight coupling device. The shape of the coupling device (i.e. 'curved for cuff') allows ready identification should subsequent disconnection and mechanical alterations be necessary.

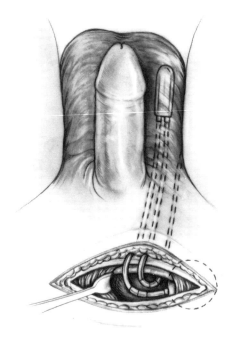

7

8 The tubing from the pressure-regulating balloon is drawn between the rectus muscles which are then reapproximated in the midline with interrupted 3/0 polyglactin (Vicryl) sutures. Similarly, the anterior rectus fascia is closed with a continuous 2/0 polyglactin running suture interrupted in the midline to allow the tubing from the pressure-regulating balloon to penetrate. All of the connections and tubings are then buried in the subcutaneous tissue with closure of Scarpa's fascia above the tubing and subsequent closure of the skin by a subcuticular 4/0 polyglactin suture.

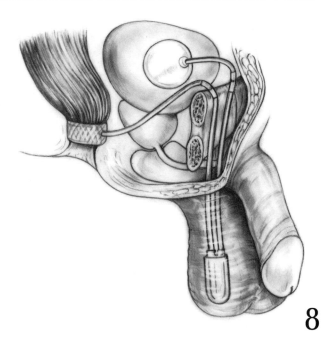

8

Postoperative care

The pressure within the anal canal is measured by manometry, both with the sphincter activated and deactivated. At the termination of the procedure, the artificial sphincter is left in the deactivated state. This is accomplished by squeezing the control pump 8–10 times until it no longer compresses. This empties fluid from the cuff into the pressure-regulating balloon. Approximately 30–40 s are allowed to pass and the control pump reservoir slowly refills. Once no further indentations in the pump can be palpated, the deactivation button is pressed. This prevents further filling of the cuff and leaves the apparatus in an inactivated state.

Antibiotic coverage is continued for 48 h with gentamicin and Unasyn (ampicillin and sulbactam). The perineal wounds are cleaned and bacitracin ointment applied twice daily. The device is left deactivated for 6 weeks, at which time the patient is seen in the anorectal physiology laboratory for device activation. Repeat anal manometry both in the resting and activated state is performed. The patient is instructed regarding mechanics of activation, deactivation and cuff emptying, and is instructed initially to activate the cuff for only 2 h each day. Activation time is gradually increased until continuous throughout the day but the cuff is left deflated at night. Once the patient is comfortable with the process, the colostomy can be taken down and bowel continuity restored. In the early period after colostomy, the cuff is left deactivated, and only when bowel function has become re-established is the cuff inflated.

Complications

The two most common complications of this procedure are infection and mechanical failure. To date, the mobidity rate in our experience with the artificial anal sphincter has been relatively low. Two of 11 patients developed an infection; one required removal and subsequent reimplantation of the device and one responded to antibiotics and delayed wound closure.

Both patients eventually achieved successful implants. The patient requiring explantation of the system did not have a stoma established. Since then, we have routinely used a colostomy (at the time of device implantation) to minimize potential infection. Mechanical failure has occurred twice in our series (two of 11, 18%). When this is recognized, exploration of the system is necessary to localize the leak or malfunctioning component. In such instances, in addition to the leaking part, the control pump should always be changed because the body fluid which enters the system after a leak may interfere with the control mechanism.

Outcome

Satisfactory continence has been achieved in 80% of patients. Eight of ten patients who have had their stomas closed report excellent continence to gas, liquid and solid stool (mean follow-up 15 months). The remaining two patients have achieved only partial continence. One was continent for over a year and then began to have deteriorating function. The other, although partially improved with respect to continence, requested re-establishment of his stoma for unrelated reasons.

Further reading

Christensen J, Sparso BO. Treatment of anal incontinence by an implantable prosthetic anal sphincter. *Ann Surg* 1992; 215: 383–6.

Wong WD, Rothenberger DA. Surgical approaches to anal incontinence. In: Bock G, Whelan J, eds. *Neurobiology of Incontinence.* Chichester: John Wiley, 1990: 246–59.

Wong WD, Rothenberger DA, Bartolo DC. An artificial anal sphincter. *Dis Colon Rectum* 1993 (in press).

Anorectal conditions: introductory comment

James P. S. Thomson DM, MS, FRCS
Consultant Surgeon and Clinical Director, St Mark's Hospital for Diseases of the Rectum and Colon, London, Honorary Consultant Surgeon, St Mary's Hospital, London, Honorary Lecturer in Surgery, The Medical College of St Bartholomew's Hospital, London, Civil Consultant in Surgery, Royal Air Force and Civilian Consultant in Colorectal Surgery, Royal Navy

In the practice of coloproctology, many patients who require treatment will have one of the troublesome anal conditions described in this section of the volume. Although surgery is often indicated, it is essential to be certain that a patient requires operative treatment because even the simplest procedure may result in complications and conservative measures are often effective. A critical review of symptoms, particularly in regard to type, location and severity, and an assessment of whether these symptoms 'match' the physical findings, is of paramount importance.

It is important that anorectal operations are not undertaken by those inexperienced in the field because there is a need for a high level of specialist training to prevent complications and to achieve the best results. In addition, adequate training will allow more procedures to be performed on a short stay or even on an outpatient basis.

Before embarking on planning the treatment of the anal disorder itself it is, of course, mandatory to exclude disease in the more proximal rectum and colon. Sometimes this has a bearing on the planning of the management of the anal problem, e.g. Crohn's disease; sometimes the symptoms may be similar, e.g. anorectal bleeding and a serious diagnosis may be potentially overlooked, and sometimes a separate asymptomatic pathology may be detected.

Although most operations will be performed under general anaesthesia, it is possible to use regional techniques (spinal or caudal blocks) or local infiltrative anaesthesia. The instruments required for anorectal surgery are generally unsophisticated, although specifically designed anal retractors are very helpful. A laser may be used to replace a scalpel or scissors, but the evidence does not suggest that this technique confers any particular advantage and it involves a large capital investment.

Haemorrhoids

Haemorrhoids may present with a variety of symptoms of which bleeding and prolapse are the most common. Discomfort and pain may also occur as the result of simple engorgement of the external plexus at defaecation or when complications such as thrombosis or fissure occur. Other symptoms include mucous discharge and its derived pruritus.

The majority of patients who present with symptomatic haemorrhoids (bleeding, pain, prolapse) will have normal bowel function, but a few may have severe constipation leading to straining at defaecation. These patients will need advice about bowel regulation and in severe cases will need to be investigated by colonic transit time, pelvic floor and anal canal studies. For the 'common' type of symptoms, dietary advice, bulking agents, injection sclerotherapy or infrared coagulation or banding are adequate treatment. However, those symptoms related to an external haemorrhoidal component will almost certainly not respond to these measures and will require operative treatment, as will those patients who have failed to respond to first-line 'office procedures'. Whether an open or closed operative technique is adopted depends on training and surgeon preference. Both methods when well done give excellent results. However, it is essential to remember two important details: secondary haemorrhoids require attention if symptomatic recurrence is to be avoided, and all the fibres of the internal sphincter must be identified and preserved to avoid postoperative problems with continence.

In the rare patient in whom there are long-standing circumferential haemorrhoids or prolapse, circumferential anoplasty (modified Whitehead haemorrhoidectomy) is regaining some popularity but care must be exercised to avoid any loss of the epithelium distal to the line of the anal valves. This anoderm must be relocated back up into the anal canal so that mucosa does not present at the anus which would result in mucous leakage ('wet anus'). The same caution must be observed for the Délorme procedure for the treatment of mucosal prolapse.

Complications of haemorrhoids such as acutely presenting haemorrhoidal thrombosis are usually managed non-operatively, although a more aggressive approach for immediate surgery has its advocates. A 'perianal haematoma' may be simply evacuated but postoperative haemorrhage may occur if the lesion is inadequately dressed with gauze and recurrence is common. An increasing number of surgeons therefore advocate immediate local resection for perianal haematomata.

Sepsis

Some of the most difficult problems for surgical treatment in the anorectum are those caused by local sepsis. The fundamental principle of operative treatment is to eradicate the sepsis while preserving full anal function. However, these two objectives are sometimes in conflict when a fistula tract crosses the sphincter mechanism and this dichotomy helps to explain the variety of techniques employed to classify and to treat fistulous disease.

While it can be presumed that most patients who have anorectal sepsis have non-specific infection (probably arising in the anal intermuscular glands), other associated pathology must be sought and excluded (e.g. Crohn's disease, intrapelvic sepsis, and occasionally pilonidal disease, infected dermoid cyst, hidradenitis suppurativa and, more recently, a resurgence of tuberculosis). Initially an abscess should be managed by simple drainage. The pus should be cultured because the presence of gut organisms is strongly indicative of an underlying fistula, but the growth of staphylococci eliminates this aetiology. Once the sepsis with its associated hyperaemia and swelling has settled a second assessment, preferably under anaesthesia, is carried out to seek possible associated pathology as described.

Although this plan provides a very general framework for management, fistula surgery has been bedevilled by difficulties with terminology. The seminal account by Parks et al.[1] has been of great value in helping us to change our emphasis for the definition of a 'low' and 'high' fistula from a simple anatomical statement of the site of the internal fistula opening in the anorectum to the use of terms to describe the functional relationship of the fistulous tract to the puborectalis component of the external anal sphincter (high fistulae being above the puborectalis and low fistulae being through or below the puborectalis muscle or superficial to the external sphincter). Most fistulae (perhaps 85%) are quite simple to treat because the fistulous tract is either subcutaneous (a bridged fissure) or intersphincteric (lying between the internal and external sphincters involving only the lower part of the external sphincter muscle itself). It should be noted that the internal opening of subcutaneous (submucous) fistula might lie at an anatomically 'high' level in the anal canal above the anorectal ring. However, because all the fistulous tract (sepsis) lies on the luminal side of the external sphincter mechanism, the lesion can be laid open without any loss of anal function. By contrast, the fistulae which traverse the sphincter mechanism (transsphincteric) can be substantially more difficult to treat and test the surgeon's skills. The 'low' variety are trans-sphincteric and pass through or below the puborectalis sling; the rare 'high' suprasphincteric variety have an internal opening above the puborectalis sling. In these fistulae it is therefore the course of the tract rather than the anatomical site of the internal opening which determines the nomenclature and this accounts for the alternative treatments which are well described in this section of the book.

Postoperative care of the wounds in these patients cannot be overvalued; pocketing, exuberant granulation tissue, mucosal bridging and the ingrowth of hair must be avoided by regular wound examination and hair shaving. If, despite these measures, there is a failure of wound closure and consolidation, other undiagnosed disorders should again be sought.

Pilonidal disease

Both pilonidal cysts and sinuses can be difficult to eradicate and a simple approach is recommended: laying open the sepsis, leaving the base in situ, and allowing it to heal with great attention to shaving local hair until the wound has healed and consolidated, which may take several months.

Rectovaginal fistula

Perhaps more accurately termed 'anovulval' or 'anovaginal' in most instances, it is often the result of childbirth injury rather than sepsis and is frequently associated with sphincter damage. Preoperative assessment of sphincter function by physiological testing and endoanal ultrasonography may therefore be of value. The excellent descriptions for operative treatment which follow should lead to successful management.

Ulceration

Anal fissure is the second most common condition seen in a rectal clinic and is by far the most common cause of anal ulceration. Other aetiologies include Crohn's disease, primary chancre, herpetic ulceration (often associated with HIV infection) and anal tumours. Many patients with the common 'idiopathic' variety of fissure are well treated by dietary change and stool bulking agents, although for recurrent or persistent fissures lateral sphincterotomy is undoubtedly the operative treatment of choice. In addition, it is usually advisable to excise a sentinal skin tag, hypertrophied anal papilla (anal polyp) and any overhanging tissue edges around the fissure.

Anal dilatation is advanced as an alternative to lateral sphincterotomy but there is no need to 'stretch' the whole of the internal sphincter, external sphincter and puborectalis sling which may result in compromised anal function. Even with lateral sphincterotomy, soiling may occur after defaecation as a result of the creation of a 'funnel-shaped' anal canal. Simple wiping with a damp cotton wool pledget to remove residual mucus and faeces will effectively help this problem and the accompanying pruritus ani.

Anal stenosis

This condition is quite uncommon and may have an inflammatory or structural aetiology. Local fungal and sometimes bacteriological infection may be difficult to treat and a dermatological opinion may be helpful. Anal stenosis because of structural damage following inappropriate surgery may be treated conservatively with a well lubricated anal dilator but may also require re-epithelialization procedures.

Condylomata acuminata

Anal and perianal warts caused by human papilloma virus, frequently associated with homosexuality, are a reminder that sexually transmitted disorders affect the anal region and may coexist with the more usual anal disorders. Inappropriate surgical treatment of anal warts may lead to excessive pain, scarring, and even anal stenosis. Although the treatment described is simple, effective and safe, careful postoperative follow-up is needed because further wart formation may occur.

Anal cancer

Malignant tumours of the anal canal are of many different histological types and are now managed by a multidisciplinary team of a surgeon, oncologist and radiotherapist. Nevertheless, surgery is important for localized disease and in the early diagnosis of these lesions.

The chapters which follow in this section of the book cover the field of anal canal disorders and will guide the surgeon well to perform careful and effective surgery.

References

1. Parks AG, Gordon PH, Hardcastle JD. A classification of fistula-in-ano. *Br J Surg* 1976; 63: 1–12.

Illustrations by Angela Christie

Evacuation and excision of perianal haematoma

T. G. Allen-Mersh MD, FRCS
Consultant Surgeon, Westminster Hospital, London, UK

C. V. Mann MA, MCh, FRCS
Consulting Surgeon, The Royal London Hospital and St Mark's Hospital for Diseases of the Rectum and Colon, London, UK

Principles and justification

A perianal haematoma usually develops suddenly as a result of occlusion and swelling of one of the haemorrhoidal veins at the anal verge. The distended vein produces a tender swelling in which thrombosis rapidly develops. The natural history of the condition is of an acutely painful swelling which persists for several days and then slowly subsides as the clot is organized leaving an external anal skin tag. Occasionally, the haematoma causes pressure necrosis of the overlying skin, and the thrombus is extruded spontaneously. Although the lesion is usually solitary, occasionally multiple thromboses occur.

Indications

The usual course for the condition is spontaneous resolution, therefore there are no absolute indications for surgical intervention. The later the patient presents, the stronger the case for conservative management.

The principal advantage of surgical intervention is that it provides immediate relief of pain because the lesion is eliminated. Therefore, if the patient is seen early (within 48h of onset), operative treatment is usually advised. Surgery is also indicated if an abscess develops to prevent the development of a subcutaneous fistula. The size of the thrombosed vein may also indicate the need for surgery, because a very large haematoma will subside to leave a large skin tag which may then be a source of pruritus and perianal soiling. Multiple lesions usually require surgical intervention.

Contraindications

The main hazard is an acute thrombosed haemorrhoid as a complication of a blood dyscrasia in acute leukaemia or polycythaemia.

Preoperative

No special preparation is required.

Anaesthesia

The operation is performed under local anaesthesia (lignocaine hydrochloride 1% with adrenaline 1:200 000). In the more nervous patient, however, where there is no contraindication, general anaesthesia may be preferred.

Operation

Position of patient

The left lateral (Sims) position with the pelvis raised on a sandbag is ideal. In an obese patient, the upper buttock may need to be strapped or held back by an assistant.

Under general anaesthesia the lithotomy or prone jack-knife position can be used.

Injection of local anaesthetic

1 The skin is gently cleansed with aqueous chlorhexidine gluconate 1:2000 solution. The finest needle should be used for the local anaesthetic injection, and the infiltration should include the skin around the area. Infiltration into the thrombus is usually not helpful and may result in premature leakage or bursting of the thrombosed area.

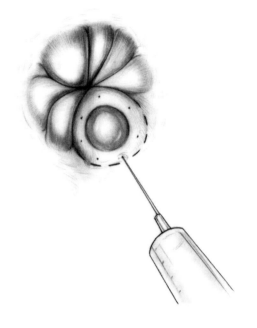

1

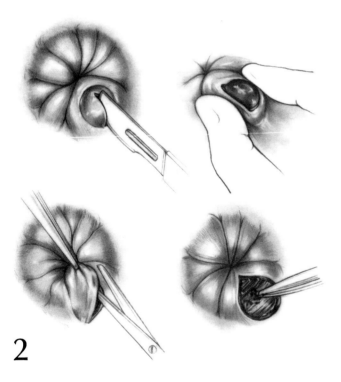

2

Evacuation of the haematoma

2 A short incision 1–2 cm long is made on the surface of the thrombosed haemorrhoid. The clot can then be removed with forceps as it is usually fairly solid. The redundant skin forming the sac around the clot is excised with fine scissors or a small scalpel.

3 After the lesion has been removed the cavity should be gently curetted to ensure that all clot has been removed. The raw area between the anal mucosa and perianal skin is left open to drain, but as the edges tend to fall together naturally, it closes spontaneously within a few days. Excision of surplus skin and mucosa at the time of removal of the thrombus reduces the likelihood of anal tag formation.

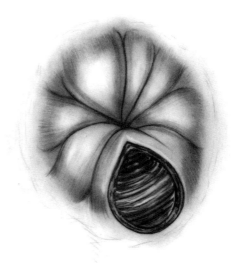

3

Postoperative care

The wound is dressed with an absorbable cellulose mesh dressing, which is simply tucked over the raw area and covered with an external pad. A stool bulking and softening agent (sterculia granules 10 ml twice daily) is prescribed for 2 weeks to ensure the passage of a soft stool while the perianal area is tender. The patient is advised to take frequent warm (sitz) baths to soothe and cleanse the operation site. It is particularly helpful if this is done after each defaecation to ensure that the anal area is kept as clean as possible.

Healing of the wound takes 5–7 days. The patient will usually be relieved by excision of the tender thrombosed area, but should be warned that some pain will return once the local anaesthetic applied for the operation has worn off. It is advisable to prescribe an oral analgesic for 2–3 days.

Complications

Infection and abscess formation

If the clot is incompletely evacuated, the wound may become infected, producing cellulitis and persisting pain. In this event, attention should be given to ensuring that adequate drainage of the wound has been achieved by further trimming of the wound edges if necessary or evacuation of any retained clot. If this is required, it is usually better done under general anaesthesia when optimal conditions are more easily achieved. Antibiotics are not usually necessary.

If an abscess develops, it should be treated in the same way as a perianal abscess by incision or deroofing under general anaesthesia. The pus should be cultured, and if *Escherichia coli* is detected, the patient should be examined to exclude the possibility of an anal fistula.

Skin tag

This will only form if evacuation, as opposed to excision, of the thrombosed haemorrhoid has been performed. If a large skin tag does form either after conservative management or inadequate excision, it can be excised under local anaesthesia.

Fistula

If large loose folds of skin remain after evacuation of the haematoma, superficial cross-healing of the wound edges can occur, leaving a subcutaneous fistula track. If this should happen, the fistula track should be laid open and the edges trimmed back so that proper healing of the wound from the base can occur.

Further reading

Bailey H. *Bailey and Love's Short Practice of Surgery*. 18th edn. London: HK Lewis, 1981: 1093 pp.

Goligher JC. *Surgery of the Anus, Rectum and Colon*. 5th edn. London: Baillière Tindall, 1984: 143 pp.

Management of uncomplicated internal haemorrhoids

Hak-Su Goh BSc, FRCS
Senior Consultant and Head, Department of Colorectal Surgery, Singapore General Hospital, Singapore

Principles and justification

Uncomplicated internal haemorrhoids do not bear pain-sensitive mucosa from or below the dentate line. They are enlarged and displaced anal cushions, which are first-degree, second-degree and small third-degree haemorrhoids and present with bleeding, perianal pruritus, or prolapse. They can be readily treated on an outpatient basis, by injection, banding, infrared coagulation, or a combination of these methods. Injection acts by stimulating submucosal fibrosis, which shrinks and anchors the anal cushions to their normal positions. Banding removes excessive internal haemorrhoidal tissues by strangulation. Infrared coagulation causes thrombosis of feeding vessels and induces haemorrhoidal involution. These techniques are all effective in treating internal haemorrhoids, but each has advantages in specific circumstances.

Management of haemorrhoids should include careful proctosigmoidoscopy to exclude inflammatory bowel disease, polyps, or carcinoma of the rectum. It is also important to alleviate factors that could aggravate or cause recurrence of haemorrhoids, such as prolonged and excessive straining at stool and chronic constipation. Apart from advice on a healthy diet of fresh fruits and vegetables, management should include a course of bulk laxative.

Infrared coagulation is a new method of treating internal haemorrhoids that is gaining widespread use. It acts by the generation of infrared light that penetrates tissue and instantly converts to heat to coagulate the tissue. When applied to the base of a haemorrhoid, the mucosa and blood vessels in the submucosa are coagulated and sealed to the muscularis. This reduces blood flow to the haemorrhoid, causing it to involute.

Indications

Injection is effective in controlling bleeding, particularly when the haemorrhoids are not bulky (first-degree and small second-degree haemorrhoids). It is useful in recurrent bleeding following haemorrhoidectomy and can be used to supplement banding. Smaller primary, as well as accessory, haemorrhoids can be injected after the larger ones have been banded. Sometimes this method is helpful for pruritus, but it is usually ineffective for bulky or prolapsing haemorrhoids.

Banding serves as the 'gold-standard' for the treatment of uncomplicated internal haemorrhoids. It is particularly effective for bulky and prolapsing haemorrhoids (second-degree and third-degree haemorrhoids).

Infrared coagulation is effective in bleeding haemorrhoids. It is useful in hepatitis B or human immunodeficiency virus (HIV)-positive patients, as it does not cause bleeding or tissue sloughing. It is particularly useful in patients who are receiving anticoagulants, who are immunocompromised, or who are pregnant. Like injection, it is not very effective for prolapse.

Contraindications

Injection should not be used in the presence of thrombosis or sepsis, active inflammatory bowel disease, or in bleeding associated with immunodeficiency disorders, such as acute leukaemia. While injection can be repeated, the interval should not be within 3 weeks because of the risk of causing injection ulcers which can bleed profusely. Injection is best avoided during pregnancy.

Banding should not be used for external haemorrhoids. All contraindications for injection also apply to banding.

Preoperative

No special preparation or anaesthesia is needed for injection of haemorrhoids. Occasionally, a simple enema (Fleet) can be administered when the rectum is loaded with soft faeces.

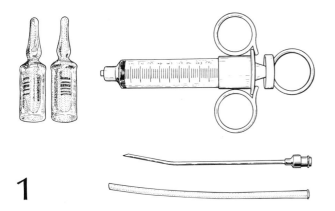

1

Operations

Position of patient

For injection, banding, or infrared coagulation of haemorrhoids, patients can be placed in either the left lateral (Sims) position or the semi-inverted (jack-knife) position on a proctological table.

INJECTION OF HAEMORRHOIDS

Instruments

1 With increasing awareness of hepatitis B and HIV infections, a 10-ml disposable plastic syringe with a three-finger grip and a long angulated needle has replaced the traditional Gabriel glass syringe. The sclerosant used is 5% phenol in vegetable oil (almond). A wide-bore plastic 'straw' facilitates drawing of the oily sclerosant into the syringe. A pair of long forceps and small pieces of gauze should be kept handy for wiping mucosal surfaces or for applying pressure if there is bleeding during injection. A lighted proctoscope provides a steady, bright illumination.

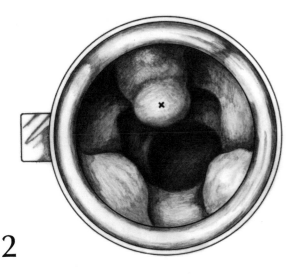

2

Injection

2 Injection is at the base of the haemorrhoids and into the submucosal plane. All the haemorrhoids can be injected in one session, and 3 ml of sclerosant is used for each site. It is best to start with the lowest haemorrhoid, so that if bleeding or leakage occurs, the remainder will not be completely obscured.

Precautions

3 Injection should be painless. If there is pain, the needle has been placed too near the dentate line and should be withdrawn and placed higher up the anal canal. If there is resistance, the injection is in the wrong plane, particularly if there is blanching of the mucosa. It indicates that the injection is in the mucosa and can cause ulceration with the risk of bleeding. The needle should be advanced into a deeper plane. When bleeding occurs on withdrawal of the needle, it is easily stopped by pressure. If bleeding does not stop with pressure, the area should be ligated with a rubber band.

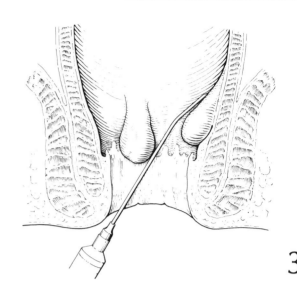

3

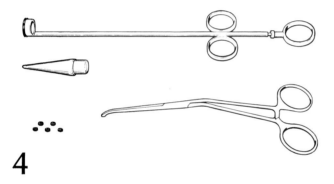

4

BANDING OF HAEMORRHOIDS

Instruments

4 Many versions of haemorrhoid ligators are available. They all have the same basic design, with a drum to trap haemorrhoidal tissue and a triggering mechanism to fire rubber bands. The instrument with the simplest design is often the most reliable. Two rubber bands are loaded onto the drum. Haemorrhoids can either be grasped with a long angulated forceps or a suction device. Grasping forceps are simple and reliable and are more widely used. A lighted proctoscope is preferred, and an assistant is needed to hold the proctoscope in place for the operator to grasp and fire at the same time.

Banding

5 With the proctoscope in place and the haemorrhoid to be banded clearly visualized, the haemorrhoid is grasped with the forceps and drawn through the drum of the ligator. The patient should not feel any pain when the haemorrhoid is grasped. The ligator is then pushed to the base of the haemorrhoid and fired. Again, there should be no pain, although the patient may feel an urge to defaecate. Banding should start with the biggest haemorrhoid, and all of them may be banded in one session provided there is no discomfort. Otherwise, one or two haemorrhoids are banded first and the remainder 4–6 weeks later.

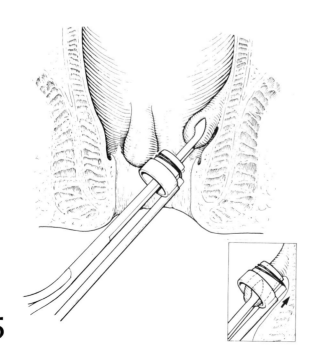

5

Precautions

6 Bands should not be placed too near the dentate line because they can catch sensitive mucosa or induce thrombosis of overlying external haemorrhoid and cause severe swelling and pain. When banding small haemorrhoids, a small volume of sclerosant or 0.5% bupivacaine hydrochloride with 1:100 000 adrenaline can be injected into the ligated mass to make it more tense and encourage sloughing.

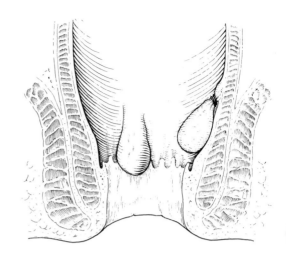

6

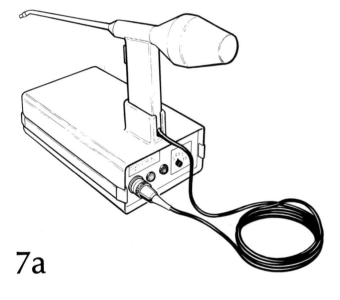

7a

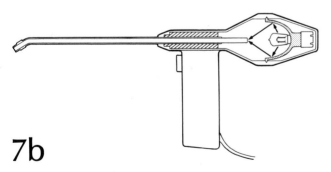

7b

INFRARED COAGULATION

Instruments

7a, b The infrared coagulator has a 15-V tungsten–halogen lamp as the infrared energy source. The light is reflected by a 24-carat gold-plated surface and carried through a quartz glass light-guide to a sapphire contact tip. The temperature at the tip reaches 100°C. The heat generated causes tissue coagulation, and the depth of coagulation is determined by the time of exposure. The automatic timer range is from 0.5 to 3.0 s, giving a coagulation depth range of 0.5–2.5 mm. The working setting is between 1.0 and 1.5 s to give a depth of 1 mm.

Coagulation

8a, b The instrument is switched on and the timer set at 1.0–1.5 s. With the haemorrhoids clearly visualized through a proctoscope, the tip of the coagulator is placed in firm contact with the base of the haemorrhoid using light pressure. The tip should not be embedded in the tissue. The instrument is then fired to the end of each automatically timed setting. A circular whitish eschar will appear on the mucosa after each exposure; three to five exposures are made in a semicircle around the base of the haemorrhoid, allowing a gap of a few millimetres between each. The tip of the coagulator should be wiped with damp gauze, after each exposure if necessary, to remove debris which may smoulder and carbonize, thereby damaging the tip.

Precautions

As each infrared exposure is so easy to execute, it is important to place the tip of the instrument accurately to avoid misfiring, thereby causing pain.

Postoperative care

No specific care is required following injection, but constipation should be treated. Patients can resume normal activities after injection. Some patients may feel faint and light-headed immediately after injection, but this is transient, lasting only 5–10 min. A short rest is all that is required.

Complications

Too much sclerosant or injection into the mucosa can cause injection ulcers, which may bleed profusely. An emergency under-running suture of the bleeding vessels may be required to stop the bleeding.

Extrarectal injection can give rise to pain and fever, or haematuria and prostatitis, if it is into the prostate. These complications may require intravenous antibiotics.

Mild tenesmoid discomfort is often felt following banding, and this is relieved with a non-steroidal anti-inflammatory drug, such as ketoprofen. A bulk laxative should be given to treat constipation and minimize the risk of prolapse due to straining.

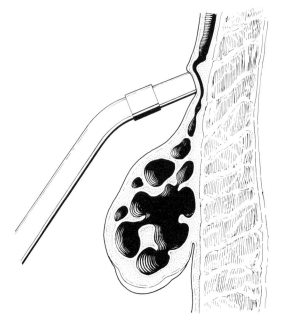

8a

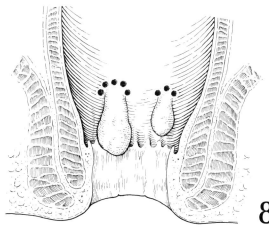

8b

When bands are placed too low or when they induce oedema and thrombosis, severe pain results. This is first treated conservatively with strong analgesics and sitz baths. If pain persists, the rubber bands should be removed under general anaesthesia.

At 7–10 days after banding the haemorrhoids slough off. In 1–2% of cases secondary haemorrhage, severe enough to require hospital admission, requires an under-running suture to control the bleeding. This is best carried out under general anaesthesia.

Very occasionally, banding of haemorrhoids can give rise to severe systemic sepsis, particularly in immunocompromised patients. Immediate intravenous antibiotics and desloughing are required to control the sepsis.

Though not common, bleeding and pain can occur within 24 h of infrared coagulation. The bleeding is mild and stops spontaneously, while pain is easily controlled with simple analgesics.

Open haemorrhoidectomy (St Mark's ligation/excision method)

T. G. Allen-Mersh MD, FRCS
Consultant Surgeon, Westminster Hospital, London, UK

C. V. Mann MA, MCh, FRCS
Consulting Surgeon, The Royal London Hospital and St Mark's Hospital for Diseases of the Rectum and Colon, London, UK

Principles and justification

Indications

Surgical treatment offers the best chance of permanent cure of haemorrhoids because no other method approaches the precision and certainty of an expertly performed operative haemorrhoidectomy. The principal indication for operative haemorrhoidectomy is large, third-degree haemorrhoids. However, second-degree haemorrhoids associated with skin tags are frequently best treated by this method as it ensures that skin tags are removed. Where other treatments, such as banding or phenol injection, have failed to relieve symptoms of haemorrhoids, operation can still cure the patient.

Occasionally, persistent bleeding from haemorrhoids can result in severe anaemia. Where bleeding from another site in the gastrointestinal tract has been excluded, operative treatment results in more rapid control than treatment by non-operative methods.

The open method combines removal of the haemorrhoidal cushions and adjacent skin tags with excellent drainage of the contaminated wound. Complications are rare and symptom relief is achieved in most cases. The main drawback of operative haemorrhoidectomy is pain during the first postoperative week; this will be discussed later.

Contraindications

All operations on the anal area are best avoided in patients with inflammatory bowel diseases such as Crohn's disease or ulcerative colitis. Patients with active pulmonary or intestinal tuberculosis should not undergo operation since tuberculous infection of the anal wounds may occur.

Patients with asymptomatic HIV disease may undergo haemorrhoidectomy, but in the more advanced stages of HIV disease (CDC group 4) wound healing is impaired and elective anal surgery should be kept to an absolute minimum. These patients may have symptoms from inflamed and ulcerated anal mucosa associated with enlarged haemorrhoids. The temptation to 'tidy' the anus by surgical excision of haemorrhoids should be resisted.

If possible, gross obesity should be reduced and skin sepsis, e.g. fungal infection, should be treated before surgery. Haemorrhoids frequently become troublesome during pregnancy and operative haemorrhoidectomy is best avoided until after delivery. Future pregnancies may cause new haemorrhoids to develop and patients should be warned of this.

Rarely, patients with portal hypertension may develop large haemorrhoids associated with portosystemic shunting. Haemorrhoidectomy in this situation can result in considerable bleeding and is probably better avoided.

Acute prolapse and thrombosis of haemorrhoids (strangulated piles) can be operated on if the patient is seen early after the onset of the complication at a time when generalized anal oedema has not yet developed. In addition to excision of the thrombosed haemorrhoid, other non-thrombosed haemorrhoids can be excised provided adequate skin bridges are preserved. Once there is obvious cellulitis of the anal margin or if there is so much oedema that adequate skin bridges cannot be preserved, it is safer not to embark on open haemorrhoidectomy.

Old age is not a contraindication to surgical treatment providing that a safe anaesthetic can be given, e.g. by a caudal method. However, an irregular bowel habit, especially constipation, should be corrected before surgery because the patient who fails to pass a regular formed stool after operation or who uses purgatives to liquefy the motions may develop faecal impaction or anal stenosis.

Haemorrhoids, however painful or disabling, are harmless. Treatment should never introduce a significant element of risk to the patient.

Preoperative

All patients who complain of bleeding from the anus should undergo rectoscopy at least to the rectosigmoid junction (20 cm from the anal verge) to confirm that a rectal source of bleeding, such as a carcinoma, is not present. Where there is darker bleeding or any suggestion of a change in bowel habit, the patient should undergo barium enema or colonoscopy. Haemorrhoidectomy should not be performed until any concurrent disease in the colon or rectum has been treated.

Other than the usual preparation to ensure that the patient is fit for anaesthetic, very little specific anorectal preparation is required for haemorrhoidectomy. The patient is admitted on the evening before or early on the morning of operation and is given a disposable phosphate enema to clear the left colon and the rectum of stool. The enema must be given at least 2 h before surgery, otherwise the enema fluid may remain within the rectum and will flow into the anal canal at the time of surgery.

Anaesthesia

Most patients are very nervous at the prospect of a haemorrhoidectomy and premedication is important in preparation for the anaesthetic.

General anaesthesia is supplemented by local anaesthetic administered by the surgeon (1% solution of lignocaine with adrenaline 1:200 000).

In elderly or unfit patients, a caudal block can be used; some surgeons employ the caudal or epidural method routinely to supplement general anaesthetic to provide excellent analgesia and relaxation of the anal sphincter. However, in the hands of the less experienced operator, the total relaxation of the internal sphincter which results from caudal anaesthesia makes internal sphincter identification more difficult, with an increased risk of internal sphincter injury.

Operation

Position of patient

The patient is placed in the full lithotomy position with the buttocks lifted over the edge of the table. Some surgeons prefer to carry out the procedure with the patient prone and the table split in a jack-knife position. Both positions are satisfactory and the choice depends on the surgeon's preference. In the conscious patient, who is being operated on under local anaesthesia, the left lateral position can be less embarrassing and uncomfortable. In these circumstances the left lateral Sims position with the buttocks raised on a sandbag offers reasonable exposure, especially if the upper buttock is firmly retracted by strapping. If the patient has cardiac or respiratory insufficiency, this position is better tolerated than full lithotomy because there is neither embarrassment of diaphragmatic action nor gross postural effects on venous return to the heart, so that the cardiac output remains stable.

Once the patient has been positioned, perianal hair can be shaved using a scalpel blade before the skin is prepared and towels applied.

Injection of local anaesthesia

1 When the patient has been anaesthetized and is in the lithotomy position, the perianal skin is prepared with a mild antiseptic solution (cetrimide 1% or aqueous chlorhexidine gluconate 1:2000). The anal canal is carefully cleaned with cotton wool pledgets soaked in cetrimide until all faecal particles have been removed.

Local anaesthetic solution is then injected subcutaneously into each haemorrhoidal mass. An injection of 2–3 ml at each site is sufficient to ensure a dry field; excessive injection distorts the operative field, making it more difficult to estimate what is to be removed and the size of the skin bridges which are to remain. Infiltration should extend beneath the mucocutaneous junction and the lining of the lower part of the anal canal, but need not include the upper half of the anal cushion.

Further local anaesthetic solution (3–5 ml) is injected into each ischiorectal fossa just to the medial side of the ischial tuberosity to block the inferior haemorrhoidal branches of the pudendal nerve. A 5-cm no. 20 needle can be passed from a central posterior puncture forwards and laterally until it strikes the periosteum of the ischial tuberosity 2.5 cm above its lowest point. The needle is then withdrawn 1–2 mm and the infiltration carried out, having ensured by aspiration that a vein has not been entered. This partial pudendal nerve block relaxes the external anal sphincter and provides useful postoperative analgesia.

It is advisable to wait for 3–5 min after local infiltration to allow the full haemostatic and anaesthetic effects to develop.

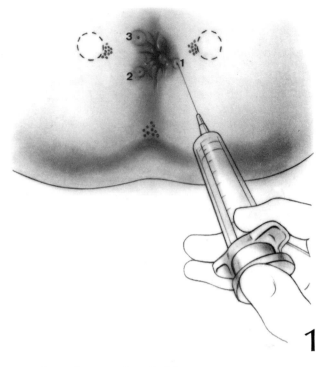

1

Display of operative field

If anal sphincter tone is increased, a gentle two-finger dilatation of the sphincter is performed to allow the anal canal to be opened. If the sphincter is of normal tone or atonic as a result of the nerve block, this step is unnecessary and may be damaging. Elderly patients should never have the sphincter dilated.

2 Dunhill forceps are placed on the perianal skin just outside the mucocutaneous junction opposite each primary haemorrhoidal cushion (left lateral, right anterior and right posterior; 3, 7 and 11 o'clock). Skin tags should be included in the area of perianal skin to be removed. Gentle traction on the forceps then brings each haemorrhoidal mass into view.

At this stage a careful note is made of the areas of skin and mucosa (skin bridges) which should remain between each area from which the haemorrhoidal cushions are to be dissected. It is usual to leave a skin bridge between each excised haemorrhoidal cushion and these should be greater than 1 cm wide to avoid a significant risk of postoperative anal stenosis.

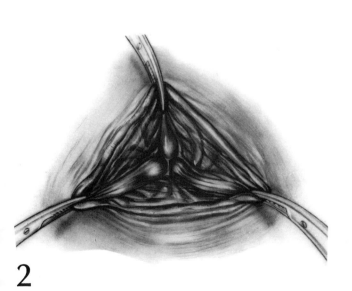

2

Triangle of exposure

3 As the internal haemorrhoids are pulled down, a second pair of Dunhill forceps is placed on the main bulk of each haemorrhoidal mass; further traction exposes the pedicles of the haemorrhoids and produces the so-called 'triangle of exposure' which is caused by the stretching of pink columnar cell mucosa between the apices of each taut pedicle. When the second pair of Dunhill forceps is clipped to each haemorrhoid, care must be taken not to include the internal sphincter muscle by taking too deep a bite. Intervening small haemorrhoids may be taken with separate forceps and approximated to the nearest primary forceps so that they are included with the main haemorrhoid in the subsequent section.

Once the triangle of exposure has been achieved the haemorrhoids are ready to be dissected and removed. It is a mistake to carry the pedicle dissection higher than this exposure allows because there is a risk of narrowing the upper anal canal if too much mucosa is gathered at the anorectal junction, and the excision of large amounts of anal epithelium will result in reduced anal sensation.

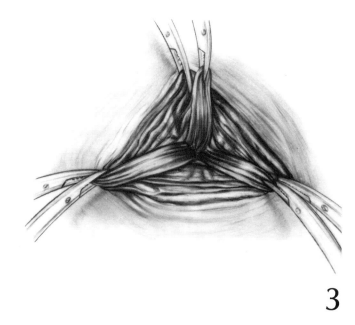

3

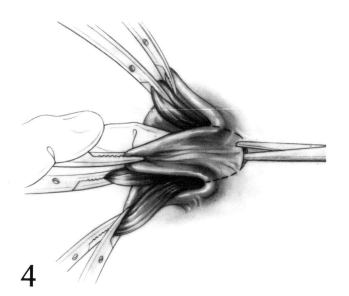

4

Start of dissection

4 The haemorrhoids are dissected in turn. For a right-handed surgeon it is convenient to start with the left lateral haemorrhoid, the others being temporarily held out of the way with slight traction by the assistant. The two forceps are held in linear fashion in the palm of the left hand, with the left forefinger in the anal canal on the pedicle of the haemorrhoid pressing lightly outwards to stretch the pedicle gently over the pulp of the finger. The blades of a pair of blunt-nosed scissors are placed alternately at each edge of the base, as seen from its cutaneous aspect, and the tissues divided towards the median plane until the incisions meet. The subcutaneous space superficial to the lowest (white) fibres of the internal sphincter and deep to the external (red) sphincter muscle is then exposed and can be opened up.

Further dissection

5   Dissection is continued in a coronal plane superficially at first, but almost at once this is changed to medial to the internal sphincter muscle and is directed towards the pedicle of the haemorrhoids in the submucosal plane. The borders of the dissection taper towards the base of the haemorrhoids and upward mobilization is not continued more than is necessary to allow easy control of the pedicle as previously defined by the triangle of exposure.

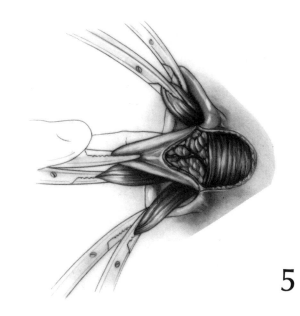

5

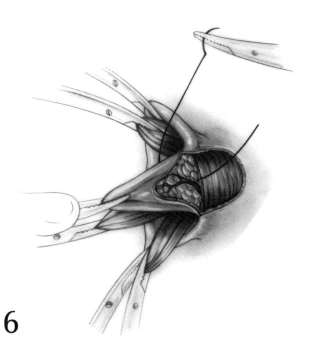

6

Ligation of pedicle

6   As the pedicle is exposed by dissection, traction on the haemorrhoid should be eased. Once the haemorrhoid has been defined, the pedicle is suture-ligated with a slow dissolving suture material (e.g. 2/0 Vicryl) with the knots tied on the luminal aspect. It is not necessary to use very strong material for the pedicle ligation; a large knot of non-absorbable material can excite a foreign body reaction and even cause a fistula.

Once the pedicle has been secured and traction on the pedicle released to check that vessels have been safely controlled by the ligature, the pedicle is cut through, leaving a good cuff. The ends of the ligatures are left long so that the pedicle can easily be identified and recovered to control persistent oozing. The pedicle is then allowed to retract to its normal position in the upper anal canal.

Procedure for remaining haemorrhoids

7 The other haemorrhoids are removed in a similar fashion. The right anterior haemorrhoid is usually the smallest and easiest to deal with, and is frequently left until last because, when the patient is in the lithotomy position, bleeding from the front of the anal canal may obscure subsequent dissection posteriorly. If the patient is prone, the sequence should be reversed. Intact bridges between perianal skin and anal mucosa must be preserved between each dissection site, and should be not less than 1 cm wide.

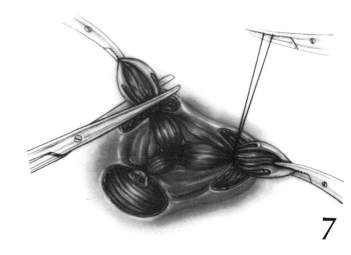

7

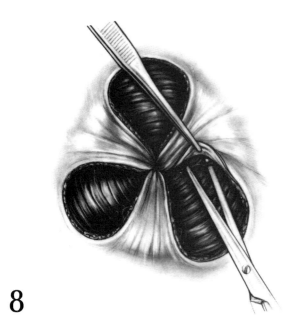

8

'Filleting' of skin bridges

8, 9 If large external veins are seen beneath the residual bridges, they can be removed by dissection beneath the margins of the bridges from each side ('filleting') or by dividing the bridges, removing the underlying veins, and then sewing the bridges back in place with fine catgut. When the divided skin bridges are being reconstituted, the rectal mucosa must not be dragged down to the anal verge, because mucus seepage from the anus would result. It may be necessary to remove a short segment of the rectal mucosa which forms the upper part of the skin bridge so that when the cut edges are sewn together the squamous epithelium is taken up into the anal canal.

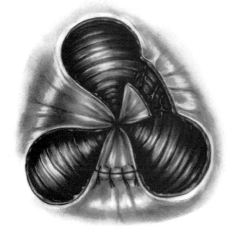

9

Trimming of wounds

10 After all the pedicles have retracted into the upper anal canal, the mucosal defects are critically inspected for persistent bleeding and for redundant flaps of mucosa or perianal skin. Any redundant tags of skin are removed, and puckering of the skin bridges can be reduced by anchoring sutures of slowly dissolving 3/0 suture material. Haemostasis of any small bleeding points, either from the mucosal edges or from the raw area of the mucosal wounds, is controlled by light application of diathermy or by ligation with 3/0 Vicryl sutures. Occasionally, in the presence of diffuse bleeding, the application of a swab soaked in adrenaline solution (1:1000) is preferred to excessive diathermy.

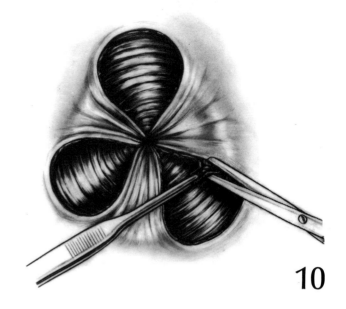

10

11

Final appearance and dressing

11 · The final appearance of the operated area should resemble a clover leaf and the wounds should be completely dry before a dressing is applied. Dressings are a matter of personal choice, except that greasy or oily materials should be avoided as they prevent proper drainage of serosanguineous exudate from the raw anal mucosal defects. Dressings such as cellulose mesh which dissolve spontaneously can be lightly tucked in over each raw area. Bulky anal packs should be avoided because they are uncomfortable. The wound should be dry at the end of the procedure and there should be no need for anal tamponade. In occasional cases, where packing is thought to be justified because of difficulty with haemostasis, the use of gelatin sponge is useful because it provides some initial tamponade and haemostasis but decomposes quite quickly. This avoids the risk of hurting the patient which occurs when a non-absorbable pack is removed from the anal canal.

A thick pad of cotton wool is then laid over the perineum and held in place by either a T bandage or Tenafix pants.

Postoperative care and complications

The dressings remain undisturbed for 24 h. They are then removed and the patient is allowed to soak the area in a warm bath. A clean pad is applied and held in place with the T bandage or Tenafix pants. The patient is started on a combination of magnesium hydroxide and liquid paraffin (Mil-Par) and Normacol (fibre) granules, both 10 ml twice daily. On this regimen, the majority of patients will have a bowel action by the third postoperative day. The patient should be encouraged to have a bath after each bowel action and clean external dressings are then reapplied. Once the patient has had a satisfactory bowel action, Mil-Par can be discontinued, but Normacol granules are continued for the first 6 weeks to ensure a soft bulky stool while the anal canal is healing.

There is some controversy about routine digital examination after haemorrhoidectomy. However, there is a risk of faecal impaction and a gentle digital examination of the anal canal and lower rectum on the fifth postoperative day is recommended. If impaction is present, a disposable sodium dihydrogen phosphate enema is given. If an impaction is not identified until a later stage, when there may be complete blockage with liquid overflow, it may even require disimpaction under anaesthesia.

Pain control may be difficult after haemorrhoidectomy, being most severe on about the third postoperative day when the first bowel action occurs. Initial pain control can be achieved with routine postoperative analgesia and a caudal block at the time of operation. Strong oral or intramuscular analgesics, including opiates, are often necessary, with a sedative (e.g. diazepam) helping to overcome the anxiety of defaecation. Other methods, such as internal sphincterotomy at the time of haemorrhoidectomy and the application of topical anaesthetic cream have been tried but do not provide any significant reduction in pain. The use of diathermy or a laser beam for haemorrhoid dissection has been claimed to reduce postoperative pain.

However, in these authors' experience, while there may be slight differences in postoperative pain using these methods, the problem of pain-induced inhibition of defaecation is not overcome. Epidural anaesthesia provides good pain control, but this approach cannot be justified because of the complications and practical difficulties of the technique.

While there are no definite contraindications to day-case haemorrhoidectomy, this can only be recommended where the patient has suitable home conditions and the medical service has made appropriate arrangements for home supervision.

In the first 24 h after operation bleeding may occur from small vessels which appeared not to be bleeding at operation because of spasm or because a ligature becomes loose. Bleeding can occur later because of stool disturbing a ligated pedicle, excessive straining in a nervous patient, or necrosis of the ligated pedicle. It is important to recognize that bleeding after haemorrhoidectomy can be life-threatening. The volume of blood passed is an unreliable guide to the extent of bleeding, because in the presence of a continent sphincter the majority of the blood may pass up into the colon. When a fall in blood pressure or rise in pulse rate occurs, re-examination of the anal canal and identification of the bleeding point is required.

A digital examination should be carried out 1 month after operation to ensure that an anal stenosis is not developing. At this stage the wounds should be granulating well but will not be fully healed. There may be some slight persisting serosanguineous discharge from the healing wounds which necessitates a small pad. During the second postoperative month the wounds should heal completely and a pad should be unnecessary after 2 months. Occasionally, one of the wounds can persist as an anal fissure with continuing pain and discharge. If this problem persists, an internal anal sphincterotomy is indicated.

Illustrations by Michael J. Courtney

Closed haemorrhoidectomy

Stanley M. Goldberg MD, FACS, FRACS
Clinical Professor of Surgery and Director, Division of Colon and Rectal Surgery, University of Minnesota
Medical School, Minneapolis, Minnesota, USA

History

Over 200 years ago the French anatomist Petit[1] first attempted to eradicate haemorrhoids without denuding the lower anal canal of its mucosa. The technique, modified by many surgeons and popularized in the USA by Ferguson[2] and Fansler[3] involves saving the anoderm, removing haemorrhoidal tissue, and replacing the anoderm into its normal position. The advantages over open haemorrhoidectomy are that the anal canal is covered with its own anoderm, postoperative dilatations are not required and primary healing is secured, resulting in much less discomfort for the patient. Frykman (unpublished) modified the partially closed technique of Fansler to a completely closed technique. Fansler advocated closing the wound only to the dentate line; however, Frykman extended closure to include the undercut and mobilized perianal skin. The same technique, used by the author's group of surgeons for 40 years, is described in this chapter.

Principles and justification

Indications

Since the advent of the rubber band ligature technique for bleeding internal haemorrhoids, indications in this unit for closed haemorrhoidectomy have been limited to prolapse, pain, bleeding not controlled by rubber band ligature or injection, and association with other surgical conditions of the anal canal, e.g. fissure and fistula.

The most frequent indication for haemorrhoidectomy in our practice today is rectal mucosal prolapse associated with prolapsing mixed haemorrhoids. Pain associated with haemorrhoids is always associated with thrombosis. When thrombosis is extensive, haemorrhoidectomy is indicated although the majority of painful thrombosed haemorrhoids can be handled with simple excision of the entire haemorrhoidal complex under local anaesthesia. When surgery is required for fissures or fistula associated with haemorrhoids, haemorrhoidectomy may be added at that time.

Preoperative

All patients undergoing haemorrhoidectomy undergo preoperative sigmoidoscopy at the time of their first examination; if they are older than 40 years and their symptoms suggest additional pathology, a barium enema examination or colonoscopy is indicated. Special care is always taken with any patient who has a history of soft stools or diarrhoea to rule out the possibility of undiagnosed inflammatory bowel disease, which is a specific contraindication for haemorrhoidectomy. The usual laboratory tests to rule out a bleeding diathesis are obtained.

The patient is informed that he will be in hospital for 1–2 days and that he should refrain from any heavy lifting for a period of 2 weeks after surgery. He is advised that complete healing will not occur for a period of approximately 3–4 weeks, and that his chance of returning to the operating room for a complication related to surgery is usually about 1%.

Oral preoperative preparation is not indicated for this technique. One disposable packaged enema is given the evening before surgery and another approximately 1 h before surgery. Neither laxatives nor antibiotics are used before operation or during the procedure.

Position of patient

1 Anorectal procedures have traditionally been performed in the lithotomy position or the left lateral position as favoured in certain parts of North America. However, the semiprone or jack-knife position is preferred, with soft rolls under the hips and ankles of the patient ensuring that the patient is comfortable on the table. The advantages of this position are that any bleeding that occurs will fall away from the operative field, it affords comfort for the operating surgeon and superior access to the operative field.

Skin preparation

No attempt is made to sterilize the skin other than using povidone-iodine (Betadine). The operative area is not shaved and adhesive tapes are applied to the buttocks to provide lateral traction.

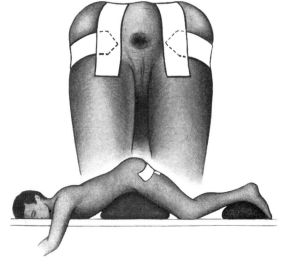

1

Anaesthesia

2 The prone position lends itself well to a combination of general and local anaesthesia. Intravenous midazolam (Versed) is used as a sedative agent, combined with 0.5% lignocaine (Xylocaine) and 1:200 000 adrenaline solution locally and 0.25% bupivacaine (Marcain). Regional anaesthesia, either spinal or caudal, can be used in this position; however, local anaesthesia is preferred as there is an inherent fear on the part of the patient of regional types of anaesthesia. With certain patients it is necessary to use an endotracheal tube in the prone position; however, in all cases local infiltration with bupivacaine and adrenaline is employed.

If local anaesthesia is used alone it is most important that infiltration be carried out correctly. A dose of 20–30 ml of a 0.5% lignocaine and 1:200 000 adrenaline solution is injected through a no. 30 needle into the skin, picking up the cutaneous nerves. After this, a direct injection of 0.25% bupivacaine with 1:200 000 adrenaline into the muscle, as illustrated, is performed to pick up the branches of the inferior rectal nerve, resulting in immediate relaxation of the sphincter muscle; neither manual dilatations nor stretching of the sphincter muscle are carried out. No specific attempt is made to inject the anoderm directly in the area of the haemorrhoids or to 'balloon up' the mucosa. The anaesthetic usually lasts for 60–180 min, more than sufficient for the operative procedure, and it also provides considerable relief in the immediate postoperative period. Elderly patients with hypertension or

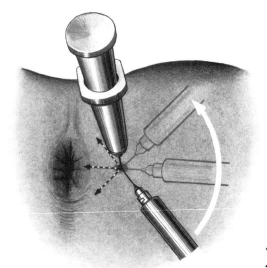

2

cardiovascular problems present no difficulty with the low concentration of adrenaline.

Another important point regarding anaesthesia is the use of minimal volumes (less than 50 ml) of intravenous solutions during surgery, a principle which has helped to keep the catheterization incidence in this unit under 3%. The author's group believes that by keeping patients dehydrated in the postoperative period their bladders are not distended, resulting in spontaneous voiding within the first 20 h.

Operation

After the introduction of local anaesthesia to relax the sphincter, the anal canal is examined digitally and then by a Pratt bivalve speculum introduced into the anal canal, examining carefully the specific haemorrhoidal areas; the operation is planned in greater detail at this point. Dilatations are not carried out with the bivalve speculum. The largest haemorrhoidal complex is removed first; the quadrants usually involved are the left lateral, right posterior and right anterior. No suction is necessary during the procedure. Small 7.5-cm² gauze sponges which fit through the operative anoscope are used as an alternative to suction. Having examined the area with the Pratt bivalve speculum, the Fansler operating anoscope is then used.

3, 4 Dissection is started on the perianal skin. No attempt is made to remove all the tissue in one motion. An elliptical incision is made with fine dissecting scissors, removing skin and haemorrhoidal tissue down to the underlying internal sphincter.

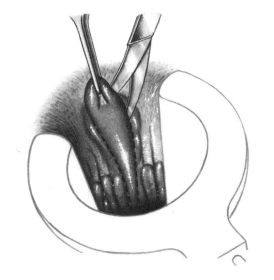

3

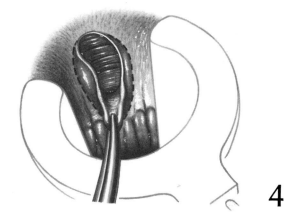

4

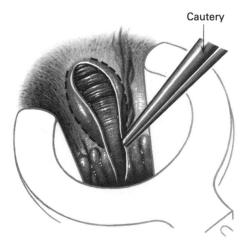

Cautery

5

5 Redundant rectal mucosa is excised high up to and sometimes even beyond the first valve of Houston to correct rectal mucosal prolapse. No crown suture is placed on the pedicle. Most of the bleeding occurs from the edges of the mucosa; individual bleeding vessels in the mucosa are coagulated using a pair of bipolar forceps. This dissection may also be performed with electrosurgical diathermy.

6 At this point the mucosa is elevated, haemorrhoidal tissue is dissected from beneath the mucosal flaps, other bleeding points are electrocoagulated, and the anodermal flaps are undercut adequately so that they can be closed without tension.

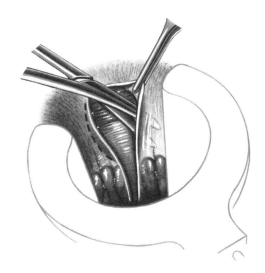

6

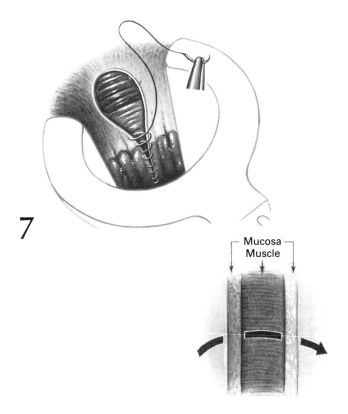

7

Mucosa Muscle

7 After dissecting the secondary haemorrhoidal vessels from beneath the anodermal skin flaps and controlling the bleeding, the wound is closed, starting at the apex using a running suture of 3/0 chromic catgut. The mucous membrane is sutured down to the underlying sphincter mechanism in an attempt to create a longitudinal scar which will prevent further prolapse. Trimming of excess skin is performed, but it is essential that the wounds be closed without tension. A loose knot is tied at the completion of the procedure. Rarely is any clamping of vessels necessary, and no pile clamps are used.

8 The procedure is carried out in three major areas and in as many additional areas as necessary. In certain cases of prolapsed thrombosed haemorrhoids, as many as six areas may be excised and primarily closed.

When the anal canal does not accept the operating anoscope easily, a partial internal sphincterotomy is carried out in the base of a wound, usually in the right posterior or left lateral quadrant. At the completion of the procedure all quadrants are examined carefully and blood clots are removed. No packing or dressing is placed in the anal canal or perianal area. The average operating time is 35 min.

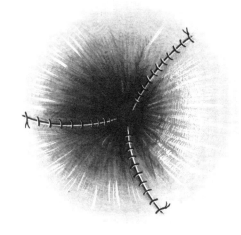

8

Postoperative care

After operation patients are encouraged to take only sips of water until such time as they void spontaneously. Since the institution of this programme of dehydration, the catheterization rate on all patients has been under 3%. Once postoperative voiding has taken place, patients are allowed fluids and food as desired. One of the advantages of the operative technique as described is that little pain is experienced. However, patients receive meperidine (pethidine) on demand for the first 3–4 days and are given an oral analgesic during their hospital stay.

Early activity is encouraged. Warm packs are applied to the perineum during the immediate postoperative period. After 24 h, patients are encouraged to take as many sitz baths as required for cleanliness and comfort. A small cotton dressing is put in the perianal area to collect whatever discharge or drainage may be present. No other local treatment is carried out. Patients are started immediately on Metamucil (ispaghula husk), one package twice daily, and Kondremul (55% liquid paraffin in Irish Moss emulsion) twice daily, the latter being stopped immediately after the first bowel movement. Because patients receive only a small (100 ml) packaged enema the evening before surgery and the morning of surgery, they usually have their first bowel action on the second or third postoperative day. If they do not, a tapwater enema is given on the third postoperative day using a soft rubber catheter.

Dilatations are not carried out in the hospital. Patients are usually discharged from the hospital on the day after surgery, with instructions not to do any lifting or straining, and to report back to the clinic in 10–14 days for examination. They are discharged with Metamucil (one package per day) and oral analgesics to use as necessary.

Complications

Skin tags may result from any operative procedure on the perianal area; however, no greater incidence of skin tag formation occurs with the closed technique. A large skin tag can be removed under local anaesthesia in the clinic; however, the author likes to have a 'pleat' so that the patient does not split the perianal skin when the anal canal opens at the time of defaecation.

Anal stenosis and stricture have been reported after the closed technique, and usually result from the removal of too much normal skin in the perianal area. With attention to detail, however, these complications have not been a problem.

Outcome

Patients return to the clinic 10–14 days after surgery and are examined very carefully, with digital and anoscopic examinations. It is apparent at this time that a percentage of the wounds have failed to remain closed; however, the majority have healed primarily. Secondary haemorrhage occurs in 0.3% of cases. Less than 1% of patients return to the operating room for a second operative procedure resulting from an unhealed wound or a persistent sinus tract. Postoperative infection has not been a problem, but in two isolated cases an attempt was made, on the part of the surgeon, to reduce postoperative pain by reinjecting the perianal tissue with local anaesthetic at the completion of the procedure, resulting in two ischiorectal abscesses. No further infections have occurred since discontinuing the reinjection technique.

Closed haemorrhoidectomy is an effective and safe alternative to open haemorrhoidectomy, resulting in rapid healing and minimal postoperative discomfort for the patient. The use of the prone position and infiltration of local anaesthetic facilitates the procedure.

References

1. Petit JL. *Traité des Maladies Chirurgicales et des Opérations qui leur Conviennent*. Volume 2. Paris: Didot, 1974: 137.

2. Ferguson JA, Mazier WP, Ganchrow MI, Friend WG. The closed technique of hemorrhoidectomy. *Surgery* 1971; 70: 480–4.

3. Fansler WA. Surgical treatment of hemorrhoids. *Minn Med* 1934; 17: 254–5.

Further reading

Bleday R, Pena J, Rothenberger DA, Goldberg SM, Buls JG. Symptomatic hemorrhoids: current incidence and complications of operative therapy. *Dis Colon Rectum* 1992; 35: 477–81.

Parks AG. Haemorrhoidectomy. *Adv Surg* 1971; 5: 1–50.

Circumferential anoplasty: modified Whitehead haemorrhoidectomy

J. C. Bonello MD
Associate Professor of Surgery and Head, Department of Surgery, University of Illinois College of Medicine at Urbana-Champaign, and Program Director, Colon and Rectal Residency Program, Carle Clinic Association, Urbana, Illinois, USA

History

In 1882, Walter Whitehead introduced a technique for the radical cure of haemorrhoids. In his paper, Whitehead stated that he invariably left strips of mucous membrane continuous with the skin, but in severe cases he removed the entire circumference of the haemorrhoidal tissue via a circumferential incision performed at the dentate line. In 1887, Whitehead himself modified his original procedure in that he presented 300 consecutive cases of haemorrhoidectomy cured exclusively by a circumferential incision. This modified procedure is known today as the Whitehead haemorrhoidectomy. Whitehead stated that it was essential that no skin be sacrificed, fearing that a contracture would result.

In the decade following his procedure, many favourable reports of Whitehead's technique appeared in the literature. The early 1900s, however, found disagreement among authors concerning the exact location of the mucocutaneous junction, generating reports with disastrous results. Afterwards, textbooks treated the procedure rather perfunctorily, citing a lack of indications. The year 1930 marked the beginning of a 30-year period during which the term 'Whitehead haemorrhoidectomy' disappeared from the literature, as various authors shunned the name Whitehead and presented their own radical procedures. Essentially all were modified Whitehead haemorrhoidectomies, using sliding skin grafts to prevent the two feared complications of the operation: mucosal ectropion and anorectal stricture.

With new anatomical studies by Goligher, Parks, Morgan and Thompson in the 1950s, coupled with the development of colonic and rectal fellowships in the USA, the 1970s saw a renaissance in colonic and rectal surgery. Trained colon and rectal surgeons, notably White, Burchell and Khubchandani, reported good to excellent results using the original or a modified Whitehead haemorrhoidectomy.

Principles and justification

A Whitehead or a modified Whitehead haemorrhoidectomy can be considered a viable alternative in a patient who has circumferential prolapsing mixed haemorrhoids. Contraindications to the Whitehead haemorrhoidectomy include: (1) minimal haemorrhoids; (2) excessive scar from previous disease or operation; (3) unusually thin, tight anoderm; (4) severe irritable bowel disease; (5) any pre-existing diseases or operations that result in chronic diarrhoea; (6) patients with incarceration, strangulation, or both, presenting 24 h or more after onset of symptoms (a relative contraindication).

Preoperative

All patients with third-degree and fourth-degree haemorrhoidal disease should undergo adequate preoperative assessment, including sigmoidoscopy and, if over 45 years of age, a barium enema. Usually only one Fleet enema is given before surgery.

Anaesthesia

Spinal, saddle or caudal anaesthesia is used in the majority of patients. Occasionally, a patient with a shallow anal canal can be operated on with local anaesthesia supplemented by intravenous sedation.

Operation

Position of patient

The prone jack-knife position is used (*see* page 49).

Incision

1 After confirmation of the diagnosis with a bivalve retractor, a 2/0 or 3/0 suture is placed deep in the proximal rectal mucosa beyond the internal haemorrhoid-bearing tissue. This serves as a marker and prevents retraction of proximal rectal mucosa once it is cut. It is usually placed posteriorly. With curved, double-pointed operating scissors, dissection is begun at the dentate line and continues along this line for one-third to one-half the circumference of the anal canal.

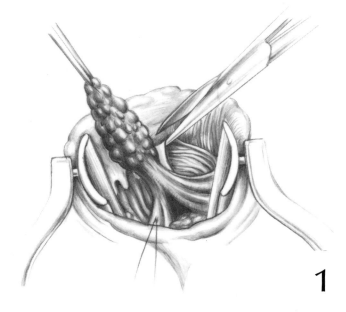

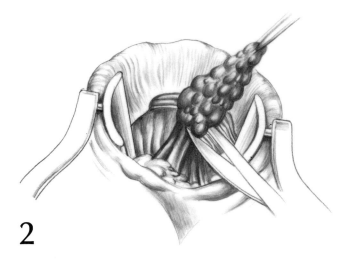

2 Using a minimum number of clamps, the cut edge of haemorrhoid-bearing rectal mucosa and associated mucosal prolapse is elevated by sharp dissection from the underlying white internal sphincter muscle throughout the length of the initial incision. The haemorrhoidal mass is then transected.

3 The distal cut edge of the anoderm is elevated and its undersurface debrided of external varices. Skin tags from previous external haemorrhoids can be removed. Over-diligence at this point can and has created flap necrosis, resulting in healing by secondary intention.

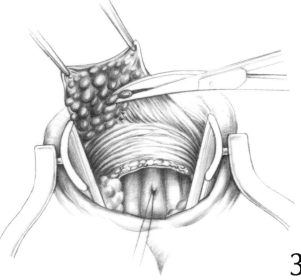

Anastomosis

4 The suture previously placed in the proximal rectal mucosa is used to approximate the cut mucosal edge to the internal sphincter 1 cm proximal to the caudal edge of the sphincter and the cut edge of anoderm. This is done from the posterior position, then to the left and to the right.

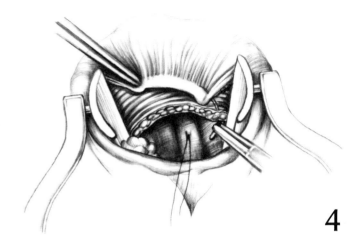

4

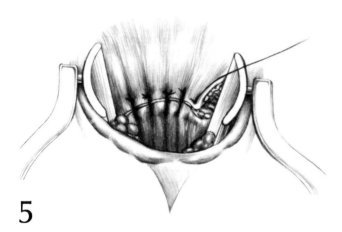

5

5 The anoderm must be pulled tightly away from the previous suture before placing the next one. Sutures are begun at the anterior position, progressing to the left anterior and the right anterior positions, again pulling the anoderm tight.

Excision of excess anoderm

6 This should create a section of redundant anoderm at the left lateral and right lateral positions.

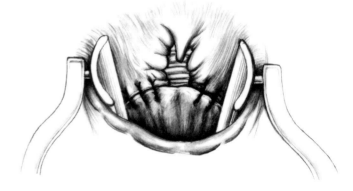

6

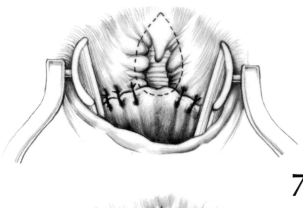

7

7, 8 The redundancy is excised in the usual closed haemorrhoidectomy fashion and closed with a running 3/0 or 4/0 Vicryl (polyglactin) suture.

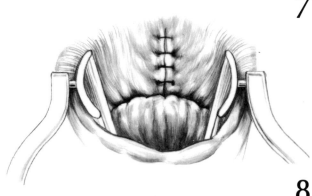

8

Wound closure

9 A roll of Gelfoam is then placed in the anal canal and a sterile dressing is applied.

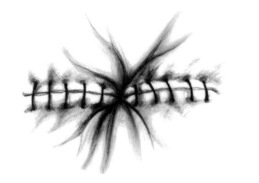

9

Postoperative care

Postoperative care is directed towards production of a soft stool, and all patients are given a bulk laxative and a stool softener. Stimulant laxatives and mineral oil are not allowed as diarrhoea must be prevented. Antiperistaltic agents or narcotic analgesics may be used to promote slight constipation in patients with loose stools. Urinary catheterization is very common after this radical procedure. Patients are usually discharged on the third or fourth day following surgery.

If a contracture occurs, a simple lateral sphincterotomy should suffice.

Outcome

Between 1 January 1970 and 1 January 1980, 356 modified Whitehead haemorrhoidectomies were performed at the Carle Foundation Hospital in Urbana, Illinois. The most common complication was urinary retention. Five patients experienced postoperative strictures. Of these, three required a second procedure and one required a third. There were no cases of faecal incontinence or rectal seepage (wet anus).

Further reading

Bonello JC. Who's afraid of the dentate line? The history of the Whitehead haemorrhoidectomy. *Am J Surg* 1988; 156: 182–6.

Management of acute anorectal sepsis

R. H. Grace FRCS
Consultant Surgeon, The Royal and New Cross Hospitals, Wolverhampton, UK

Principles and justification

Anorectal sepsis is a common minor surgical emergency; unfortunately it is often poorly managed and has a recurrence rate of 25–48% [1–3], resulting in discomfort, the need for further surgery, increased time lost from work, and damage to the anal sphincter.

Aetiology

1 Anorectal sepsis begins as an intermuscular abscess secondary to infection of an anal gland [4–8]. Extension of this downwards between the internal and external sphincters or through the lowermost fibres of the external sphincter produces a perianal abscess; extension through the external sphincter complex into the ischiorectal fossa produces an ischiorectal abscess; extension upwards or medially into the submucosal plane produces a high intermuscular or submucosal abscess. The track from the anal canal to the intermuscular abscess to the abscess cavity constitutes a fistula but not all anorectal abscesses are associated with such a fistula. Recent microbiological studies [9, 10] have shown that, although an abscess from which an intestinal organism has been cultured is likely to be associated with a fistula, those from which a skin organism is cultured (mainly *Staphylococcus aureus* or skin-derived *Bacteroides*) are not.

Indications

The diagnosis of anorectal sepsis is usually obvious: the patient complains of a painful lump by the anal canal and the severity of pain is such that the history is short. Examination reveals perianal swelling, usually associated with erythema of the overlying skin with local tenderness to palpation. There is, however, a small group of patients in whom the diagnosis may be delayed. This group complains of pain but there is no obvious swelling and no erythema; rectal examination is very uncomfortable. The unwary surgeon or general practitioner may ignore the patient's symptoms, or may consider the possibility of a fissure, but may miss the true diagnosis of submucosal sepsis. Any patient who complains of persistent anal pain of short duration in whom no fissure is visible should undergo an examination under anaesthesia as an emergency to identify the cause of the symptoms, which will frequently be found to be a submucosal abscess.

Any rationale for the initial treatment of anorectal sepsis on presentation must assume that a fistula is present because microbiology is not available; a past history of sepsis at the same site is strong evidence that a fistula is present.

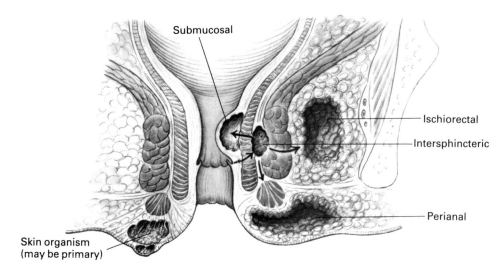

1

Surgical management

The correct management of anorectal sepsis is governed by aetiology and should relieve the immediate symptoms, prevent recurrent sepsis and minimize healing time and thereby time lost from work.

Three drainage procedures have traditionally been described: incision and drainage; saucerization; incision and drainage with primary suture.

Incision and drainage

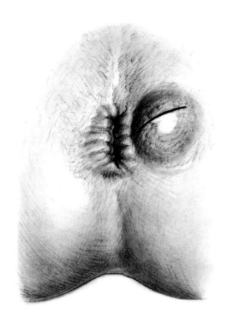

2a

2a, b Linear incision over the point of maximal tenderness or induration releases the pus; a small drain may be left *in situ*, or the wound may be lightly packed with a dilute hypochlorite dressing. This technique will relieve the immediate symptoms and minimize healing time but will do nothing to prevent recurrent sepsis if a fistula is present.

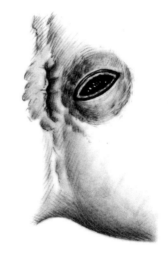

2b

Saucerization

3 A cruciate incision is made over the point of maximal tenderness or induration, followed by excision of the triangles of skin to allow 'good drainage'. If a fistula is present this technique will relieve the immediate symptoms but does not prevent recurrent sepsis and, with a large wound, is associated with a prolonged healing time.

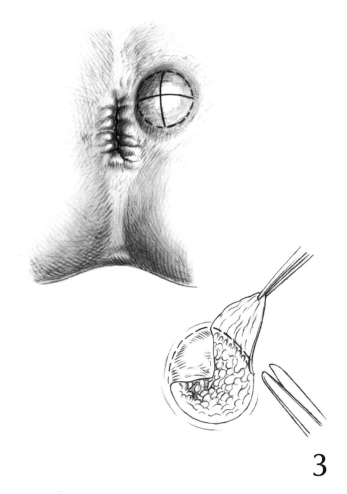

3

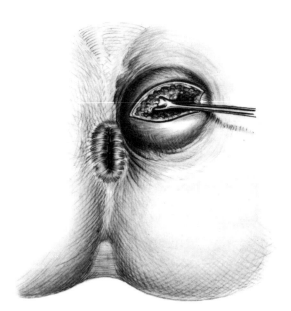

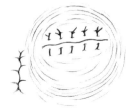

4

Incision and primary suture

4 A linear incision is made over the point of maximal tenderness or induration; the abscess cavity is curetted, and the wound sutured to obliterate this cavity. This technique, under antibiotic cover, will relieve the immediate symptoms and minimize healing time but will not prevent recurrent sepsis if an underlying fistula is present.

These three procedures all ignore the possibility of a fistula. Logical management requires the surgeon not only to drain the abscess but also to look for a fistula and treat it appropriately.

Operation

The management described in this chapter is simple, logical, and takes note of the anatomy and microbiology, recognizing that at the time of presentation no bacteriological data are available.

First examination under anaesthesia

5 The patient is examined under general anaesthesia in either the lithotomy or the jack-knife position. Visual examination and then careful palpation define the extent of induration and determine whether the abscess is perianal or ischiorectal; a large area of erythema does not necessarily indicate ischiorectal sepsis.

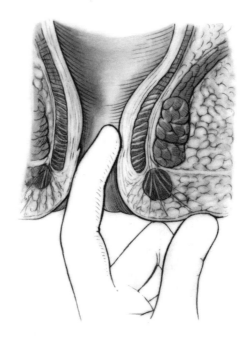

5

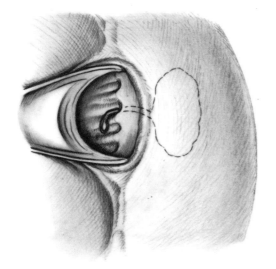

6

6 The anal canal is then inspected using a Sims or Eisenhammer speculum. The surgeon should look for pus draining into the anal canal through an internal opening at the dentate line. Gentle pressure on the abscess from the outside may help to identify the internal opening by the appearance of pus at the dentate line.

Incision and drainage

7a, b The abscess is drained through a linear incision, the cavity is curetted and the pus sent for microbiological examination. The incision may be radial (*Illustration 7a*) or circumanal (*Illustration 7b*): the radial incision may damage the underlying sphincter musculature.

The line of incision should reflect the direction of any potential fistula track: a perianal abscess will probably be associated with a low fistula track running directly towards the anal canal, which indicates a radial incision; an ischiorectal abscess may be associated with a 'high' fistula running posteriorly, or sometimes anteriorly, and a circumanal incision is preferred.

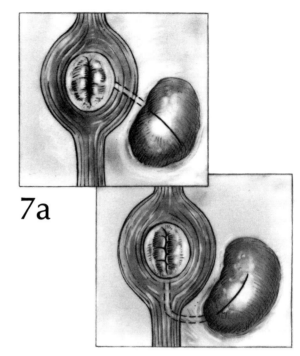

7a

7b

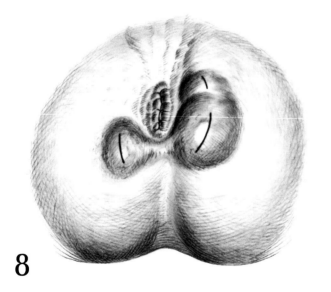

8

8 Anorectal sepsis may present with bilateral abscesses where the cavities connect in the midline and are usually associated with a fistula. Drainage of the abscess cavity will require at least one incision on either side and, depending on the extent of the sepsis, may require further incisions anteriorly or posteriorly. Most bilateral abscesses are associated with a posterior fistula.

9 In acute sepsis the relationship of the fistula track to the sphincter muscle may be difficult to establish. This is a particular problem anteriorly where the sphincter is more difficult to define because of oedema and induration. If the internal opening has been defined by the observation of pus in the anal canal it may be further defined using a hooked Lockhart-Mummery probe placed into the internal opening at the dentate line. A finger in the abscess cavity will help to identify the tip of the probe. If no pus has been observed in the anal canal, a fistula probe may be used to explore the abscess cavity and its relationship to the anal canal and the sphincter. However, all these manoeuvres should be performed with extreme caution because over-enthusiastic probing may produce a false track. When there is no obvious internal opening it is safer to await microbiology and perform a second examination under anaesthesia after the acute episode has settled.

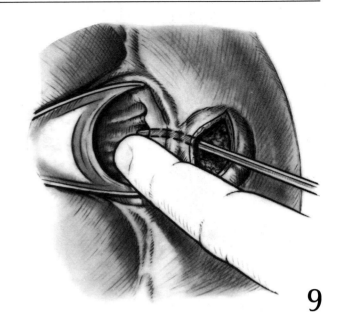

9

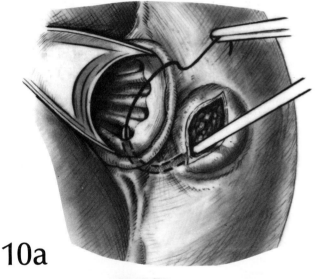

10a

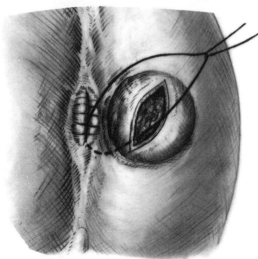

10b

10a, b If a fistula track has been defined its management depends upon the relationship of the track to the sphincter complex but oedema may make this difficult. A low fistula is easily laid open as described in the chapter on pp. 814–827. However, more complex anatomy is best managed initially by the use of a seton suture. An atraumatic 0 nylon suture on a large curved needle may be placed by guiding the needle along the groove in the Lockhart-Mummery probe; this may be done twice before tying the suture. The relationship of the seton suture to the sphincter may be further assessed at a subsequent examination under anaesthesia when the acute episode has settled.

Alternative management of the fistula is to leave its track unmarked until a second examination, when it can be treated (*see* chapter on pp. 814–827).

Microbiology

If no fistula is found at the first examination, further management depends upon the microbiology. Culture of intestinal organisms requires a second examination under anaesthesia 7–10 days later; growth of a skin organism means that no second examination under anaesthesia is required[9, 10].

Second examination under anaesthesia

If a fistula is found but not laid open at the initial examination under anaesthesia, it is defined again and then either laid open or managed with a seton suture.

If no fistula was found at the first examination, the incision is extended to give a good view of the abscess cavity which is then curetted. The fistula track will be marked by granulation tissue projecting from the fistula track into the cavity; this will remain even after the area has been curetted. The Lockhart-Mummery probe is gently passed into the track and if the fistula is low the track should be laid open and the wound edges trimmed. The management of a high fistula depends upon the extent of the external sphincter which lies below the fistula track. If a significant amount of the sphincter needs to be divided, treatment should include initial use of a seton suture. If the fistula track cannot be demonstrated, no further action should be taken.

Postoperative care

Analgesia will be required, but the patient with an abscess or abscess and fistula will rarely experience as much pain as a patient who has undergone haemorrhoidectomy.

Following first examination under anaesthesia, if no fistula is found, the abscess cavity should be packed as necessary for haemostasis with dilute hypochlorite solution in the dressing, which will be removed on the following day. The patient should be discharged home with instructions on wound management (*see* below).

Normal bowel action should be encouraged by the third or fourth postoperative day. A high-fibre diet combined with mild laxatives will ensure that there is little problem.

Wound management

The patient should bathe at least twice a day and after the bowels have been opened. The wound is irrigated with dilute hypochlorite (Milton) (1:40) solution and dressed with a flat dressing soaked in dilute hypochlorite which is tucked into the wound; the wound should not be packed and ribbon gauze should never be used. The anal dressing should be held in place with close-fitting elastic underwear which holds the dressing comfortably in place.

The passage of an anal dilator twice a day from the third postoperative day ensures that the smaller, low anal fistula wounds heal without 'bridging'. The larger, high fistula wounds do not require an anal dilator, but a further examination under anaesthesia may be required 2 weeks later to ensure that no bridging has taken place

and that the wound is healing satisfactorily. If pus is present at the later examination, there may be an unresolved problem which requires further evaluation.

Antibiotics

With adequate surgical drainage of the abscess there is no place for antibiotics in postoperative management except in cases with fulminating gangrene, tuberculosis, or in immunosuppressed patients.

Special situations

There are four special situations in which management may need to be modified.

Crohn's disease

The management of anorectal sepsis in Crohn's disease is part of the overall management of the disease and certain principles should be clearly understood:

1. Perianal sepsis is always associated with a fistula.
2. Large anal wounds do not heal well.
3. Management should be aimed primarily at relieving symptoms but with very conservative surgery.
4. There is a high incidence of recurrent sepsis if treatment does not include opening of the fistula.
5. A course of metronidazole and co-trimoxazole may be indicated.
6. Medical management may include steroids or azathioprine.

Abscess plus low fistula

Management may include laying open a fistula as the wound will be small, but simple drainage may be preferred.

Abscess with high fistula

The fistula should be laid open only with extreme caution because a large wound may be very slow to heal, or may never heal. A seton suture may be used in this situation for long-term drainage.

Abscess with multiple fistulae

The management almost certainly consists of drainage of the abscess; if sepsis continues, however, it may eventually be necessary to excise the rectum.

Tuberculous infections

This possibility should be considered in populations in whom tuberculosis is endogenous. Surgical management of the acute abscess should be on the principles already discussed because the results of bacteriological culture will not be available for at least 6 weeks. If tuberculous infection is suspected, a special request for suitable culture should be made. If it is positive, the patient will require anti-tuberculous therapy. The patient usually has evidence of tuberculosis elsewhere.

Fulminating anorectal sepsis

These infections are rare, may not be clostridial in origin[11,12] but are associated with definite mortality and considerable morbidity rates. Surgery must be radical, aiming to excise *all* the necrotic tissue until the edges are clean and bleeding; further procedures must be carried out if the first procedure is not sufficiently radical and if there is evidence of spreading cellulitis. These are the only patients with anorectal sepsis who require broad-spectrum antibiotics, taking account of microbiology when it becomes available. There may be a place for hyperbaric oxygen if there are gas-forming organisms, but the need for this has not been well defined. Control of diabetes is not usually difficult but is important.

Hydradenitis suppurativa

Hydradenitis suppurativa is a chronic low-grade sepsis of the skin which is probably associated with an abnormality of the apocrine gland system. The patient presents with multiple areas of discharge which connect by superficial subcutaneous sinus tracks. The areas most affected are the perianal skin, the perineum, the scrotum and the axillae; the nape of the neck and the face are less often involved. Men are more often affected than women. When the perineum and scrotum are involved, the condition may be very extensive and the patient may be a social outcast because of the associated offensive odour.

The microbiology of hydradenitis suppurativa has not been extensively studied but the organisms most frequently cultured are anaerobic Gram-positive cocci and the asaccharolytic group of *Bacteroides*[13].

The diagnosis is usually obvious with the classic areas of discharge with oedematous skin between external openings of the sinus tracks; the skin between these openings may be prominent and raised into thickened scarred folds. The alternating sepsis and healing causes scarring and contraction which may be a problem, particularly in the axillae with limitation of shoulder movements.

Surgical management of the perianal, perineal, and scrotal disease depends upon the extent and severity of the involvement. The oedematous folds of skin may need to be excised, but conservative surgery with preservation of skin can produce very good results. The surgical wounds in these areas heal rapidly, which is surprising in the light of the extent of the sepsis.

There is often epithelialization of some sinus tracks which should be laid open using the Lockhart-Mummery fistula probes; there is often a honeycomb of such sinuses. When they have all been laid open and curetted, the skin edges should be excised using sharp fistula scissors, preserving as much normal skin as possible.

The surgeon should accept the idea of conservative staged procedures if the involvement is extensive. The more radical procedure of wide excision of the affected skin and grafting is rarely required. There is no need for antibiotic cover.

References

1. Buchan R, Grace RH. Ano-rectal suppuration: the results of treatment and factors influencing recurrence rate. *Br J Surg* 1973; 60: 537–40.

2. Vasilevsky C, Gordon PH. The incidence of recurrent abscess or fistula-in-ano following ano-rectal suppuration. *Dis Colon Rectum* 1984; 27: 126–30.

3. Schouten WR, Van Vroonhoven TJ. Treatment of ano-rectal abscess with or without primary fistulectomy. *Dis Colon Rectum* 1991; 34: 60–3.

4. Nesselrod JP. In: Christopher F, ed. *A Textbook of Surgery.* 5th edn. Philadelphia: Saunders, 1949: 1092–114.

5. Eisenhammer S. The internal anal sphincter and the ano-rectal abscess. *Surg Gynecol Obstet* 1956; 103: 501–6.

6. Eisenhammer S. A new approach to the ano-rectal fistulous abscess based on the high intermuscular lesion. *Surg Gynecol Obstet* 1958; 106: 595–9.

7. Eisenhammer S. The ano-rectal and ano-vulval fistulous abscess. *Surg Gynecol Obstet* 1961; 113: 519–20.

8. Parks AG. Pathogenesis and treatment of fistula-in-ano. *BMJ* 1961; i: 463–9.

9. Grace RH, Harper IA, Thompson RG. Anorectal sepsis: microbiology in relation to fistula-in-ano. *Br J Surg* 1982; 69: 401–3.

10. Eykyn SJ, Grace RH. The relevance of microbiology in the management of ano-rectal sepsis. *Ann R Coll Surg Engl* 1986; 68: 237–9.

11. Ledingham IMcA, Tehrani MA. Diagnosis, clinical course and treatment of acute dermal gangrene. *Br J Surg* 1975; 62: 364–72.

12. Brightmore T. Perianal gas-producing infection of non-clostridial origin. *Br J Surg* 1972; 59: 109–16.

13. Eykyn SJ, Phillips I. Miscellaneous anaerobic infections. In: Finegold SM, George WL, eds. *Anaerobic Infections in Humans*, Volume 26. San Diego: Academic Press, 1989: 567–89.

Low anal fistula

P. R. Hawley MS, FRCS
Senior Consultant Surgeon, St Mark's Hospital for Diseases of the Rectum and Colon and Consultant Surgeon, King Edward VII Hospital, London, UK

Principles and justification

A fistula is an abnormal communication between any two epithelial-lined surfaces. An anal fistula is one in which there is an opening between the anal canal and the perianal skin. Most fistulae arise from abscesses originating in the anal glands. Anatomical studies show that there are between six and ten of these glands situated around the anal circumference, each discharging through a duct into an anal crypt, sometimes with two entering the same crypt; some crypts have no glands entering them. In at least half the cases, the glands penetrate the internal sphincter and extend into the longitudinal fibres, but not beyond them, into the external sphincter complex. Histologically, they are lined by stratified mucus-secreting columnar epithelium, but occasionally part may be lined by squamous epithelium. Cystic dilatation and infection of these glands is always situated deep to the internal sphincter muscle. Thus, the anal glands may be regarded as diverticula of the anal canal and, like diverticula in any part of the alimentary tract, are subject to stasis and secondary infection. Ducts that pass through the internal sphincter will not be able to discharge their contents so readily into the anal canal, for the muscle tone will tend to compress the lumen of the duct.

An anal fistula is virtually a sign of disease in the anal gland. This explains why there is no detectable opening into the anal canal in 30% of cases. While anal glands are distributed evenly around the circumference of the anal canal, 60% of all fistulae arise in the midline posteriorly, probably because this is the site of anal fissure, inflammation and fibrosis resulting in stasis and infection of the posterior gland. Another 20% of fistulae arise in the midline anteriorly, and the remaining 20% are distributed around the rest of the anal canal.

There are other aetiological factors. Tuberculosis, which used to be a common cause of anal fistulae, is now responsible for less than 1%. Anal fistulae are common in inflammatory bowel disease, particularly in Crohn's disease. Foreign bodies, usually from the ingestion of pieces of bone or fragments of wood, may result in a persistent fistula until these are removed. Commonly, a fistula is preceded by an abscess, and if an abscess in this region of the body is recurrent, it is almost certain that a fistula exists even if the tract cannot be identified. A neglected fistula will result in recurrent abscesses and progressive inflammation over many years. Malignancy very seldom occurs in a chronic fistula unless it is a 'congenital fistula', which is a minor degree of reduplication. Such fistulae are usually lined by rectal mucosa in their upper parts, with islands of squamous epithelium in the lower or external aspect of the fistula, and may not communicate with the anal canal. Not uncommonly malignant change occurs in these fistulae, resulting in a mucus-secreting adenocarcinoma, usually of low-grade malignancy.

A low fistula is one in which the tract can be laid open without division of the puborectalis muscle, thus preserving continence; 95% of all anorectal fistulae are low fistulae. Complex high fistulae are often iatrogenic, from injudicious probing of a low fistula with an upward extension in the intersphincteric or trans-sphincteric space. Approximately 60% of all anorectal fistulae are intersphincteric, even if their external opening is a considerable distance from the anal verge. They may cross the lower fibres of the external sphincter, but are still essentially intersphincteric. Trans-sphincteric fistulae occur in 30% of patients; a few in addition will have an upward supralevator extension that requires drainage.

Anatomy and classification of fistulae

Anatomy

1 The essential anatomy of the anal region is shown in *Illustration 1*. It should be noted that the ischiorectal fossa is a pyramidal space, the apex of which is above the anorectal ring. The anorectal ring marks the junction of rectum and anal canal and is formed by the puborectalis fibres of the levator ani muscle passing around the intestine and blending with the external sphincter. Complete incontinence results if all the anal sphincters, including the anorectal ring, are divided; section of muscle below this level may lead to some impairment of control or mucus leakage, depending on the amount of muscle divided.

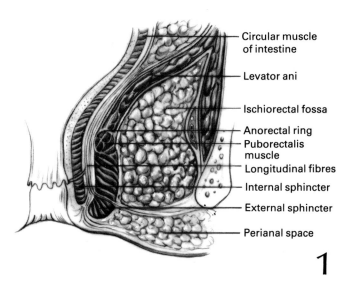

Circular muscle of intestine

Levator ani

Ischiorectal fossa

Anorectal ring
Puborectalis muscle
Longitudinal fibres
Internal sphincter
External sphincter

Perianal space

1

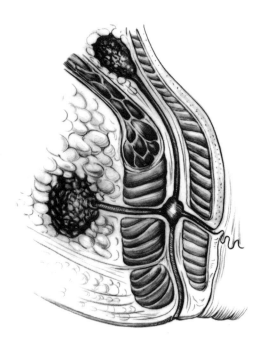

2

Classification of fistulae

2 Almost all anal fistulae result from infection of anal glands situated in the intersphincteric plane. An abscess in the anal gland leads to an abscess cavity in the intersphincteric space. From this focus infection may track laterally, medially, upwards or downwards, before or after tracking circumferentially.

[These illustrations represent the fistulae in two dimensions, but it must be remembered that in reality most are three-dimensional.]

3 About 60% of all fistulae are intersphincteric, usually passing downwards in the intersphincteric space to form a perianal abscess. When this discharges, a fistula results. The external opening is not usually close to the anus in the intersphincteric groove, but tracks laterally along the longitudinal fibres, and the external opening is 2–3 cm or more from the anal verge.

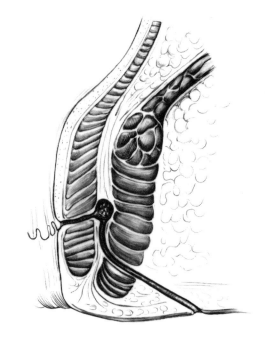

3

4 Pus may track upwards from the infected anal gland, remaining in the intersphincteric plane but pushing its way above the anorectal ring to cause a swelling and induration above the anorectal ring. This type of abscess often extends circumferentially and sometimes occurs without any downward extension, so that there is no external opening of the fistula. The abscess may break back into the anal canal by tracking medially, which gives a secondary opening, usually at a higher level than the primary opening, which is nearly always at the level of the dentate line.

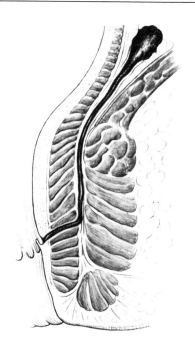

4

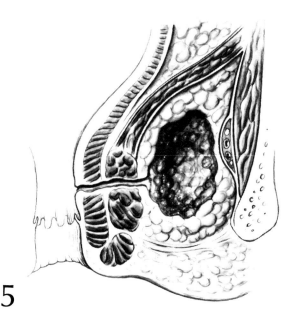

5

5 Pus from the infected anal gland may penetrate laterally through the external sphincter muscle to infect the ischiorectal fossa. This will result in an ischiorectal abscess, which will usually drain downwards through the investing fascia and the perianal fat to exit through the skin, resulting in a fistula that is termed a trans-sphincteric fistula. A difficulty arises because the site of penetration through the external sphincter muscle is often not at the same site as the tract penetrating through the internal sphincter. The fistula first tracks upwards in the intersphincteric plane and then breaks through the external sphincter at a higher level and sometimes through the puborectalis muscle. Uncommonly, the lateral extension will be above the puborectalis muscle, resulting in a true high fistula. The term 'high' trans-sphincteric fistula is the term given by some to this type of trans-sphincteric fistula, when the outward extension passes through the upper part of the external sphincter muscle. It is, however, by definition a low fistula.

6 Infection of the intersphincteric plane or ischiorectal fossa may track around circumferentially, and the fistula between the crypt and the intersphincteric plane, which usually lies in the midline posteriorly, may not be the site of penetration through the external sphincter. The trans-sphincteric part of the fistula may penetrate more laterally and also at a higher level. The ischiorectal abscesses themselves may track around circumferentially, resulting in a so-called horseshoe fistula. These trans-sphincteric fistulae and abscesses are normally limited above by the levator muscles, but may push them up on one side, suggesting a supralevator origin.

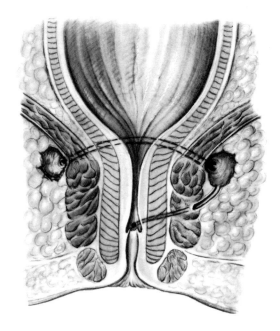

6

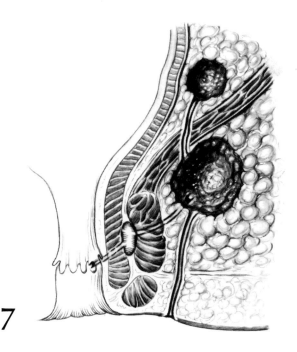

7

7 Very occasionally, the tract may spread upwards through the levator muscle and, even more uncommonly, into the rectum above the anorectal ring. Many of these high fistulae are probably iatrogenic in nature, but can occur with foreign bodies. A supralevator abscess associated with an ischiorectal abscess must be adequately drained, but if the puborectalis muscle is intact, the fistula can be dealt with as a low fistula. A supralevator hole in the rectum will need to be closed, possibly with a covering colostomy, but the primary cause must be dealt with first (as described in the chapter on pp. 828–840).

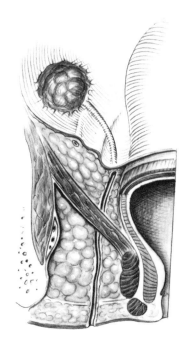

8

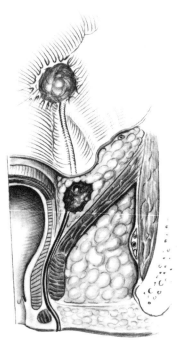

9

8, 9 Very uncommonly, a fistula arises from a supralevator origin and passes directly through the pelvic floor, either intersphincterically or through the levator, to open onto the perineal skin. These fistulae are termed extrasphincteric, and do not arise from anal gland disease. The origin is from pelvic inflammatory disease, such as diverticular disease, Crohn's disease, appendix abscess, pelvic abscess, or pyosalpinx. It may arise from a pelvic fracture penetrating the intestine. In these circumstances, the primary cause is dealt with and the fistulous tract simply curetted out, and left to heal.

Principles of operative treatment

The object of treatment of a fistula is to eradicate the septic focus and permanently eliminate the fistula tract, this being accomplished with minimal disruption to the sphincter complex. Treatment of more difficult fistulae usually results in a compromise between complete cure of the fistula and complete continence. Some surgeons take the view that it is essential to cure the septic process that causes the patient's symptoms, and that this may only be accomplished with minor degrees of sphincter impairment, such as difficulty in controlling flatus or watery stool during an attack of diarrhoea. Other surgeons will take the view that the sphincter complex must not be disrupted in any way, often resulting in a persistent fistula or even recurrent attacks of abscess formation.

There are three methods of treating a low anal fistula, depending on the preference of the surgeon. The fistula may be laid open, it may be treated with an encircling ligature known as a seton, or the sepsis may be eliminated and the origin repaired by an advancement flap. All three of these methods are used in the treatment of low anal fistulae and will be described.

The instruments that are required include a malleable probe, a set of Lockhart-Mummery probe directors and a set of lachrymal probes, as many of the tracts are narrow and fibrosed and larger probes will not pass through them. It is useful if the lachrymal probes and one of the probe directors have an eye for the passage of a seton. A pair of fistula scissors (Miltex) and an Eisenhammer retractor should be available.

Preoperative

A recurrent discharging sinus or abscess in the perineum normally indicates that a fistula is present, and this will not heal until surgery is undertaken. The patient is carefully examined including sigmoidoscopy and proctoscopy. If it is thought that the fistula may be caused by Crohn's disease, a rectal biopsy and investigations of the gastrointestinal tract should be carried out before considering whether the fistula should be treated surgically.

Preparation

The rectum should be emptied by a disposable enema or suppositories.

Anaesthesia

General anaesthesia is necessary for all except the most superficial fistulae. Full relaxation should be avoided as there should be sufficient tone in the sphincter muscles to enable the operator to palpate the external sphincter and puborectalis muscle.

Position of patient

The patient should be in the lithotomy position with the buttocks well down over the edge of the table. Alternatively, the prone jack-knife position may be used and can be helpful for the high anterior fistula.

Operative examination

The perianal region is shaved, and before starting the operation the whole area should be carefully palpated. The index finger should feel around the anus externally, identifying the intersphincteric groove and recognizing induration, whether radial or circumferential. With the index finger within the anus, the location of any induration should be identified, in which quadrants, and whether above or below the puborectalis. An internal opening may be palpable. It must be remembered that most fistulae open in the midline posteriorly, and where there is circumferential extension the opening will usually be found at this site. Most tracts can be felt as indurated ridges.

An Eisenhammer anal retractor is then inserted into the anus and the internal opening sought in the indurated quadrant. A fine malleable probe can then be inserted into the internal and external openings. An internal opening will not be obvious in about 30% of cases.

Pathological examination

Granulation tissue from the tract and any skin tag or fibrous tissue removed must be submitted for microscopic examination to exclude any specific condition, particularly Crohn's disease.

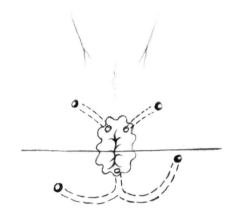

10a

Operations

SIMPLE LOW FISTULA

10a–c
The external opening and induration around the tract are palpated. Digital examination of the anal canal is then carried out to feel for an internal opening. An Eisenhammer retractor is inserted and the internal opening sought at the dentate line. Anterior tracts are often radial; posterior tracts may be horseshoe-shaped. A probe is then gently inserted into the external opening, and in a radial fistula it may pass directly through the internal opening. Even in radial fistulae, however, the tract is not always straight, and the probe must never be forced or a false passage will result. If a probe director easily passes through the fistula to exit in the anus, the tract can simply be laid open with a knife or diathermy probe.

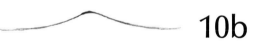

10b

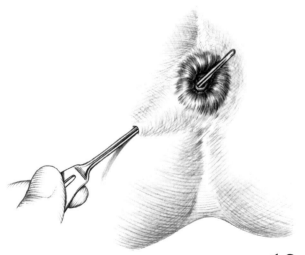

10c

11 The edges of the wound are held apart with a pair of Allis' forceps, and the granulation tissue curetted away. Careful search is made for any extensions of the fistula, particularly upwards in the intersphincteric plane, and the granulation tissue is carefully curetted away from such an extension.

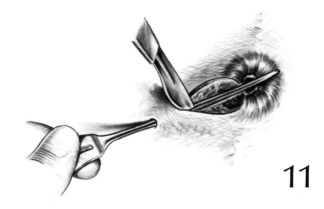

Extension of the wound

12 The wound is extended outwards for a short distance beyond the external opening, which is removed. The granulation tissue is sent for histology. When a probe cannot be passed through the fistula, or the internal opening not found, the tract is laid open from the external surface using a pair of Miltex scissors. The granulation tissue can be followed and the tract laid open until either it enters the anal canal or stops short in the intersphincteric plane. It is usually necessary in these circumstances to divide the internal sphincter to the level of the tract in order to produce a flat wound and stop pocketing.

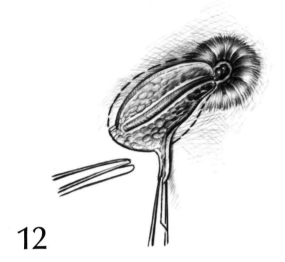

High intersphincteric fistula

13 After the lower part of the tract has been opened, it may become apparent that a higher intersphincteric tract is present because of induration in the region of the anorectal ring. A probe is then passed upwards and the tract laid open to its upper limit by dividing the internal sphincter. There may be a secondary opening which usually depicts the upper extent of the tract. It should be remembered that the tract may not run straight upwards, but may curve around.

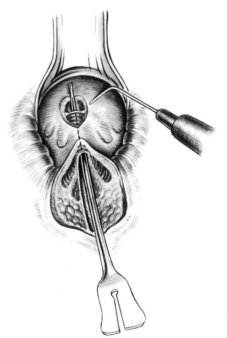

Trans-sphincteric fistula

Course of the main tract

14 The main tract of this type of fistula follows the roof of the ischiorectal fossa, i.e. it lies on the under-surface of the puborectalis and pubococcygeal muscles. The tract is horseshoe-shaped if both sides are involved, with the anterior extension on each side passing deep to the transverse perineal muscles. The communication with the anal canal is most commonly in the midline posteriorly, but not invariably so. The tract leading to the external opening on the skin is usually vertical and may descend from any part of the main circumferential tract, or multiple tracts may be present. The communication with the lumen is usually angled upwards and is often missed for this reason. If a probe is passed into the external opening, it will enter deeply parallel to the anal canal, and its tip may be palpated through the rectal wall at a level apparently above the anorectal ring. It must never be forced through at this level, or opened into the rectum, as this will result in a high fistula. The real internal opening is almost always below the anorectal ring, most commonly at the level of the dentate line.

In an extensive fistula, the internal opening may be quite small and only take a lachrymal probe angled upwards. By palpation over the fistula, the internal opening may be apparent by the appearance of a bead of pus. Injection of dyes via a small cannula placed in an external opening is not helpful in determining the extent of the tract.

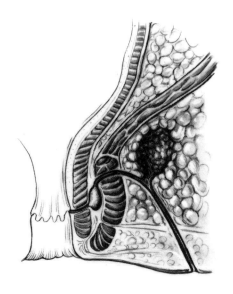

14

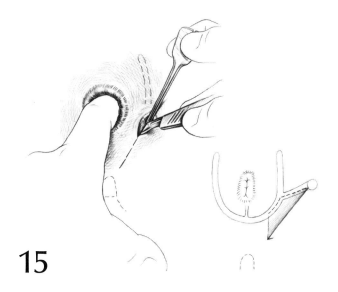

15

15 The external part of the tract is always opened first, either with a scalpel slid along a grooved director or with fistula scissors. The tract is followed by the pyogenic granulation tissue, which is curetted from the tract. It is followed backwards towards the midline and is usually extrasphincteric, but being essentially circumferential it does not cut muscle.

16 The edges of the wound are held open with a pair of Allis' forceps and the whole extent of the fistula is laid open, with any upward extensions curetted out. It is possible to leave part of the skin intact if the tract is curetted out beneath, but it is usually preferable to lay open the whole of the tract.

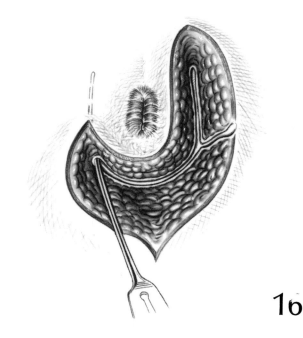

17 The tract may extend to the opposite ischiorectal fossa, but there is usually an abscess cavity full of chronic granulation tissue lying posteriorly, which may extend upwards in the precoccygeal space, occasionally extending through Waldeyer's fascia. When this posterior abscess has been laid open, the tract into the anal canal will become apparent and can be laid open if it is certain that the internal opening is below the anorectal ring. If there is any doubt, the superficial muscles only are divided, and a seton is placed around the deep part of the muscle. Muscles should always be divided at right angles to their fibres if possible, and not obliquely.

18 The wound is trimmed by bevelling the skin edges and removing part of the underlying fibrous tissue from the fistula to produce a saucer-shaped wound which will heal readily. All granulation tissue is meticulously curetted away, and a careful search should ensure that no section of the tract has been overlooked.

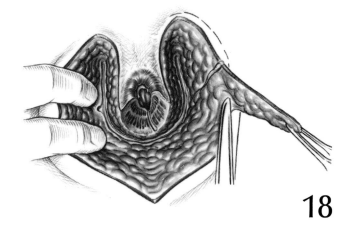

USE OF THE SETON

A seton or ligature around part of the sphincter may be used in three ways. The first is to mark the fistula if the surgeon is uncertain of the height of the tract in relation to the puborectalis muscle and does not wish to proceed with the operation. This will allow the tract to be evaluated when the patient is awake and allow definitive surgery to be carried out later.

19 The second use of the seton is to tie it loosely around the muscles after laying open the external part of the tract and draining any upward ischiorectal abscess. The internal opening is curetted out and as much granulation tissue removed as possible. The seton is then placed around the undivided muscle of the external and internal sphincter to allow drainage and healing. If this method is adopted, repeated examination under anaesthesia will be required, with further curetting of the tract, often over many months. About 50% of fistulae may heal by this method, but the other 50% will eventually require laying open before healing is obtained. It is difficult to achieve adequate drainage of high intersphincteric or trans-sphincteric extensions by this method. Its only certain place is in the treatment of fistulae associated with Crohn's disease, when a ligature of silk or Ethibond can be left in place for many months or indeed indefinitely.

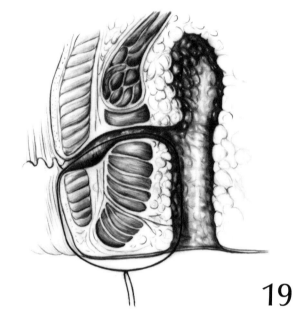

19

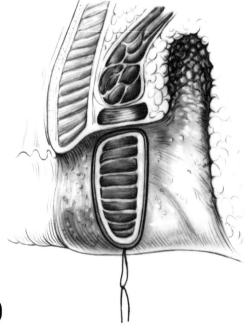

20

20 When the fistula involves the whole of the external sphincter or a substantial part of it, the surgeon may elect to use the seton as a cutting ligature. The external part of the fistula is laid open to drain it completely, and the internal sphincter laid open to the level of the primary tract, or above, until the level of the penetration of the external sphincter. The skin and mucosa are removed as if the fistula was to be laid open, but the external sphincter is preserved. A ligature of 1 silk or Ethibond is then placed around this muscle and tied tightly with a loop externally, and the ends left long.

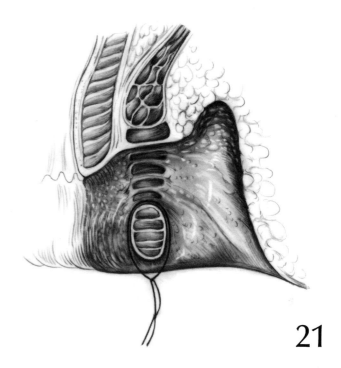

21, 22 After 2 weeks, the ligature will have cut through approximately half of the external sphincter and will be quite loose. The wound is curetted and a further seton inserted in the same tract by threading the end of the ligature through the loop tied in the previous suture and then cutting one end of the ligature and pulling the new suture through the remaining muscle. In this way, a false passage is not made. The ligature is again tied tightly, and this ligature or a successive one will cut through the muscle completely, but without allowing the ends to retract. The wound will heal and continence be achieved.

21

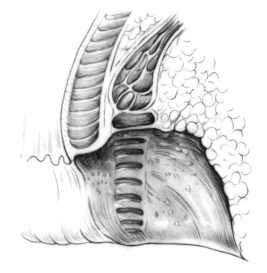

22

RECTAL ADVANCEMENT FLAP

The third method of treatment is the rectal advancement flap. This has a place in treating certain high trans-sphincteric fistulae, but is often used unnecessarily in low intersphincteric fistulae when the only piece of muscle to be divided is the internal sphincter to the dentate line, as is commonly done in any anal internal sphincterotomy.

23 With an Eisenhammer retractor in place, a rectal muscle flap of the whole rectal wall is fashioned with a broad base and elevated in the anal canal from the underlying internal sphincter muscle, exposing the perirectal fat above the anal canal.

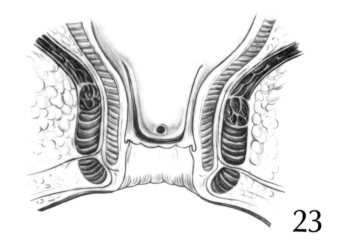

24–26 The internal opening is then excised with the base of the flap and the granulation tissue curetted out where the tract pierces the internal sphincter and the intersphincteric abscess. The external opening of the fistula is laid open and all the granulation tissue is curetted out. The defect in the internal sphincter is sutured with interrupted 2/0 polyglactin sutures or alternatively the internal sphincter can be double-breasted longitudinally and sutured. The flap is then sutured around its margins with interrupted 2/0 polyglactin sutures.

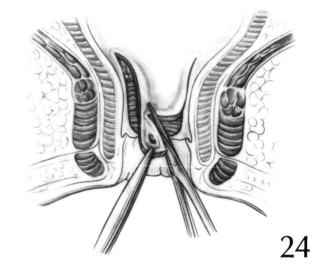

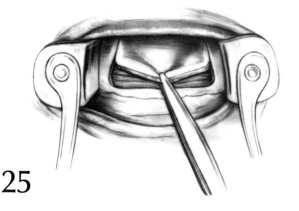

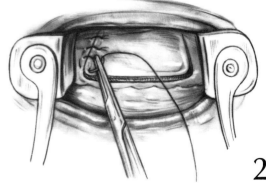

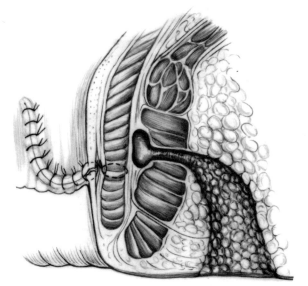

27

27, 28 The trans-sphincteric or intersphincteric part of the wound is left open to drain. It is not surprising that breakdown of these wounds commonly occurs, as they are akin to anastomoses made in an infected field. With a low intersphincteric fistula, a good result will be obtained even if the flap breaks down, but with a high trans-sphincteric or suprasphincteric fistula, breakdown of the flap will result in a further fistula, often larger than the original.

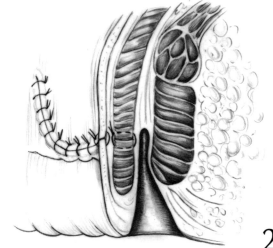

28

Postoperative care

Skin excision should be kept to a minimum, and scars should be fashioned circumferentially away from the ischial tuberosities. These are infected wounds, and cleansing and granulation tissue is stimulated with the use of 1:40 sodium hyperchlorite solution applied to flat gauze dressings. If there is significant bleeding, gauze wrung out in 1:1000 topical adrenaline solution should be inserted into the wound.

The wound heals slowly, the final scar being much smaller than the initial wound, and the anal appearance may not be grossly altered. Sphincter function is usually adequate, even when a considerable amount of the external sphincter has been divided. If necessary, the wound should be reviewed under anaesthesia, particularly if there is a persistent discharge of true pus.

High anal fistula

Philip H. Gordon MD, FRCSC, FACS
Professor of Surgery, McGill University and Director, Colon and Rectal Surgery, Sir Mortimer B. Davis Jewish General Hospital, Montreal, Quebec, Canada

It is understandable, and perhaps beneficial to the patient, that a surgeon be intimidated when a patient presents with an anal fistula associated with a *high* internal opening. Yet not all patients who have a high internal opening have problems that are necessarily difficult to manage. The reputations of some surgeons have been jeopardized because of the outcome of operations for anal fistula, and it becomes incumbent upon the surgeon to make every effort to assess the relationship of the fistulous track(s) to the sphincter mechanism. The concern, of course, is the potential double jeopardy of recurrence of the fistula and/or impairment of anal continence. Complicated fistulae challenge the ingenuity, knowledge and technical skill of the surgeon.

Before embarking upon operation for an anal fistula, it is essential that the surgeon develops an understanding of the anatomy of the pelvic floor as well as the pathogenesis of the fistula, to appreciate the origin and ramifications of the fistula. Current evidence suggests that infection of the anal glands is probably the most common cause of a fistulous abscess[1]. Obstruction of these ducts, whether secondary to faecal material, foreign bodies or trauma, will result in stasis and secondary infection. Once established, the most common course for a fistula is from the mid-anal canal downward in the intersphincteric plane to the anal verge. Infection may overcome the barrier of the external sphincter muscle, thereby penetrating the ischioanal fossa, or may extend upward in the intersphincteric plane. In addition to upward and downward tracking, pus may pass circumferentially in one of three tissue planes, the commonest being the ischioanal fossa. A horseshoe abscess may also occur in the intersphincteric plane or in the supralevator plane. It is necessary for the surgeon to make every effort to determine the relationship of these extensions to the sphincter mechanism because the operative treatment recommended will depend on the course of the fistulous track.

Many classifications of fistulae in and around the anorectal region have been described. The classification described by the late Sir Alan Parks, although very detailed, gives an accurate description of the anatomical course of the fistulous tracks[1]. This knowledge then acts as a guide to the operative treatment and has been of value to the author.

Principles and justification

The objectives of fistula surgery are simple: to cure the fistula with the lowest possible recurrence rate; to minimize any alteration of continence; and to achieve a good result in the shortest period of time. To obtain this outcome, a number of principles should be observed: the primary opening of the track must be identified; the relationship of the track to the puborectalis muscle must be established; and the least amount of muscle should be divided to cure the fistula[2]. Unfortunately, idealism and reality do not always coincide.

Indications

The presence of a discharging opening in the perineum which is either persistent or recurrent is an indication for operation. It is rare for an anal fistula to heal spontaneously. If left untreated, repeated abscesses with associated morbidity may ensue. Although non-operative methods of treatment have been attempted through the ages, it is generally accepted that the only form of treatment that affords any reliable prospective cure is surgery.

Contraindications

Surgery should be recommended unless there are specific medical contraindications to anaesthesia. Patients with established compromised anal continence present a relative contraindication because the further division of muscle required to treat the fistula might render the patient totally incontinent. Anal fistulae may be associated with active pulmonary tuberculosis, in which case the pulmonary disease should be controlled before repair of a tuberculous fistula. The presence of a 'purplish hue' discoloration of the skin and oedema around the opening should raise the suspicion that the fistula is associated with Crohn's disease. Patients with bowel symptoms suggestive of Crohn's disease should undergo gastrointestinal tract investigation by radiography or endoscopy. Control of active Crohn's disease should precede repair of an associated anal fistula. It is usually wise to avoid extensive operations for the fistula under these circumstances.

Selection of a particular operation

Controversy exists as to whether fistulotomy or fistulectomy is the more appropriate operative treatment for anal fistulae. However, there are a number of reasons for strong recommendation of fistulotomy. First, fistulectomy means the removal of the complete track and adjacent scar tissue which results in appreciably larger wounds; and second, there is a larger separation of the ends of the sphincter which results in a greater chance of incontinence and a longer healing time.

When a fistula crosses the sphincter muscle at a high level, e.g. high trans-sphincteric or suprasphincteric, there is always concern that division of the muscle *below* the track will result in impaired continence. Under these circumstances the advancement rectal flap technique is appealing[2,3]. The principles of repair include: excision of the internal opening in the anal canal; excision or curettage of the main tracks; advancement of a flap of mucosa and submucosa of rectum beyond the original internal opening; and suture of the flap to the anal canal distal to the original opening[2]. Differences in opinion exist concerning the thickness of the rectal wall to be used, use of a drain, level of advancement distally, and the need for temporary faecal diversion. The attractive features of this repair are that less sphincter requires division, contour defects are avoided, there is less pain because there is no perineal wound, and there is more rapid healing.

Preoperative assessment and preparation

Evaluation

A history should be taken and sigmoidoscopy should be performed to rule out the presence of inflammatory bowel disease, as well as to identify unusual internal openings. Should any suspicious symptoms be present, a barium enema and/or an upper gastrointestinal and small bowel barium follow-through may be indicated. For the most part, fistulography is not necessary, although in a patient with recurrent disease or if the history is suspicious of an intra-abdominal or pelvic source of sepsis, a fistulogram may prove valuable.

Patient preparation

A simple cleansing enema is all that is necessary; perianal shaving is not required. It is wise to explain to the patient the nature of the problem and its possible complications, since muscle will require division with the ever present potential for alteration of continence.

Anaesthesia

For patients with a high fistula, it is useful to perform the operation under a general or at least a regional anaesthetic. It is not uncommon to detect unexpected side branches of a fistula and these are best assessed under adequate anaesthesia.

Operation

Position of patient

Operations for anal fistula have been successfully performed with the patient in the lithotomy, left lateral and prone jack-knife positions. The author's strong preference is the prone jack-knife position.

Intraoperative assessment

Several guidelines should be kept in mind. According to Goodsall's rule, if there is an opening posterior to the coronal plane, the fistula probably originates from the dorsal midline, but if anterior, probably runs directly to the nearest crypt. Openings seen on both sides of the anal canal are likely to arise from the midline posterior crypt with a horseshoe fistula. An external opening immediately adjacent to the anal canal may suggest an intersphincteric track, while a more laterally located opening would suggest a trans-sphincteric, suprasphincteric or an extrasphincteric fistula. The further the distance of the external opening from the anal margin, the greater the probability of a complicated upward extension. When the track is low in the sphincter mechanism, palpation of the skin between the secondary opening and the anal canal will often reveal a 'cord like' structure of the fistula track. Within the anal canal it may be possible to palpate a pit indicative of an internal opening. If traction is placed on the external opening, the crypt of origin may retract into a funnel, thus identifying its location.

Introduction of an anoscope or sigmoidoscope may reveal the presence of pus exuding from an internal opening. After introduction of a probe into the track (which must always be carried out gently to avoid iatrogenic tracks and holes!), the angle the probe makes with the anal canal is helpful in determining the type of fistula. A low fistula will pass towards the anus at an angle of approximately 30° to the skin. Passage of a probe at an angle of 80° to the skin, i.e. almost parallel to the anal canal, indicates the presence of a high extension[1].

Pathological examination

Granulation tissue or any other tissue removed should be submitted for microscopic examination.

Operative technique

The different varieties of fistulae in the Parks' classification of the 'high type' will be described individually, with appropriate treatment recommendations.

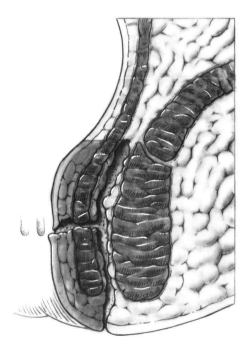

1

Intersphincteric fistula with high blind track

1   This type of fistula arises because of upward extension of the septic process in the intersphincteric plane. Treatment consists of division of the overlying internal sphincter, anoderm and mucosa as high as the blind track ascends. This procedure will unroof the infected anal gland as well as the blind extension. Little disturbance of continence will ensue because the edges of the sphincter are held together by the fibrosis of the fistulous track. Granulation tissue is curetted from the track and the edges marsupialized with an absorbable suture such as 3/0 chromic catgut. Failure to recognize the upward extension may be a cause for persistence or recurrence.

Intersphincteric fistula with high track and rectal opening

2 This type of fistula is an extension of the previous variety in which the fistula breaks back into the lower rectum. It must not be mistaken for a track that passes outside the external sphincter. If a probe passes upwards in the track parallel to the anal canal close to the lumen, the intersphincteric position of the fistula will be noted. This type of fistula is treated in an identical manner to the previous one. When incising the overlying tissue, it will be noted that the cut tissue is thin, and after the mucosa and submucosa only the pearly-white fibres of the internal sphincter are divided. No red fibres of the external sphincter will be encountered.

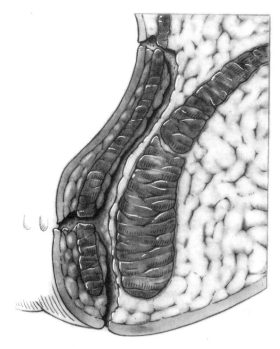

2

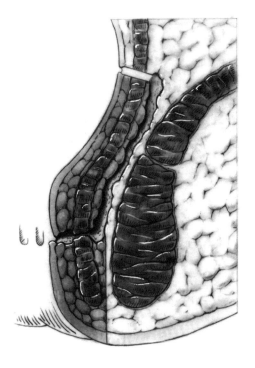

3

Intersphincteric fistula with high track without perineal opening

3 With this type of fistula, the septic process ascends in the intersphincteric plane and terminates as a blind track or may re-enter the rectum through a high secondary opening. There is no external evidence of a fistula. This variety may present in the acute phase as an intersphincteric abscess. Treatment consists of laying open the track from the distal end of the internal sphincter to as high as the blind track ascends or as high as the secondary opening. Other treatment principles are described above.

Intersphincteric fistula with extrarectal extension

4 In this variety, sepsis ascends in the intersphincteric plane and breaks out of the rectal wall into the supralevator space. It is usually encountered in the acute phase and treatment consists of drainage into the rectum, including division of the lower half of the internal sphincter to eliminate the origin of the sepsis. Thus, correct treatment is drainage into the rectum. Drainage of such an abscess through the ischioanal fossa may result in a suprasphincteric fistula which is difficult to manage.

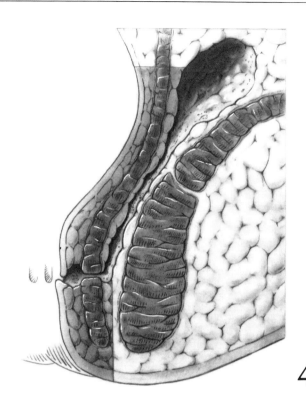

4

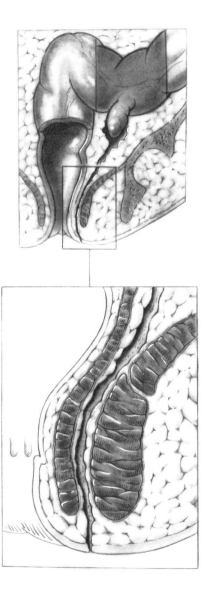

5

Intersphincteric fistula secondary to pelvic disease

5 The last type of intersphincteric fistula is not a true anal fistula, but rather originates in the pelvis. Processes such as a perforated diverticulitis or Crohn's disease might be the cause. Treatment consists of elimination of the abdominal source. No local treatment other than curettage of the track is necessary. Division of muscle is unnecessary.

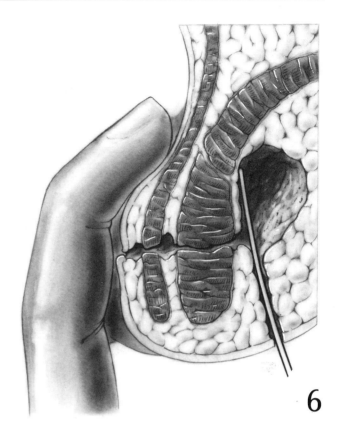

6

Trans-sphincteric fistula with high blind track

6, 7 The ease or difficulty in treating this type of fistula depends upon the level at which the track crosses the external sphincter: after so doing, the track divides into an upper and lower arm. The upper arm may reach the apex of the ischioanal fossa or even pass through the levator muscles into the supralevator space, and may cause induration above the anorectal ring which might be felt digitally through the rectum. If a probe is passed into the external opening it will go into the upper arm of the fistula and the originating track from the anal canal will not be demonstrated. A great danger is that the tip of the probe may pass through the rectal wall, thus creating an iatrogenic, suprasphincteric fistula.

The actual height and extent of the secondary track is not of paramount importance provided that it does not rupture into the rectum. Treatment consists of division of the *lower half* of the internal and external sphincter and creation of adequate drainage for the high extension.

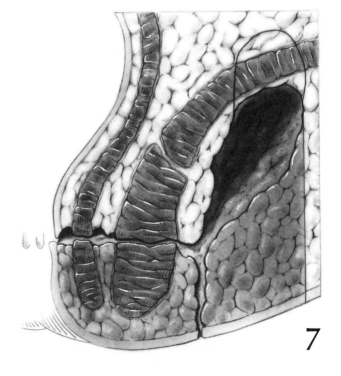

7

Trans-sphincteric fistula with high blind track treated with seton

8 When the track crosses the external sphincter at a high level, it may be deemed safer not to divide all the muscle beneath the track. Only a portion of the muscle is cut and a seton is inserted. The rationale for this manoeuvre is threefold: First, to stimulate fibrosis adjacent to the sphincter muscle so that when division of the seton-contained muscle is performed at the second stage the sphincter will not retract; second, the seton allows the surgeon to delineate the amount of muscle beneath the fistulous track better when the patient is in the unanaesthetized state; and third, the seton acts as a drain.

The internal sphincter should be divided from the level of the dentate line distally, and the overlying anoderm and a portion of the external sphincter is similarly divided. Many suture materials have been used as a seton but the author has used a heavy silk suture. Insertion of the seton is a simple matter. It is loosely tied with many knots to create a handle for manipulation.

Once inserted, the seton may be managed in several ways. Repeated handling during cleansing may eventually result in the seton 'sawing' through the muscle. More often, the seton-contained muscle requires division at a second stage 6–8 weeks later. If healing around the seton progresses rapidly, consideration can be given to removal of the seton without division of the contained muscle. The latter technique results in improved continence, but undoubtedly gives a higher incidence of fistula recurrence. The seton may also be tightened on several occasions until it eventually cuts through the contained muscle.

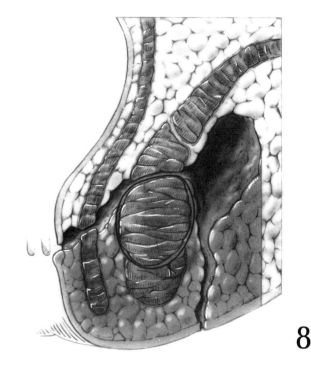

8

Clinical situations in which a seton may be considered include high level fistulae, anterior fistulae in women, patients with coexistent inflammatory bowel disease, especially Crohn's disease, elderly individuals with a weakened sphincter, individuals who have had previous operations and in whom extensive scarring is present, uncertainty of the height of the fistulous track or the amount of muscle previously cut, and the presence of multiple fistulae.

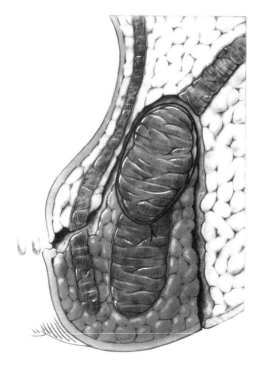

9

Suprasphincteric fistula

9 This track ascends in the intersphincteric plane above the puborectalis muscle and descends through the ischioanal fossa to the perineum. Treatment by the classic 'lay-open' procedure would result in division of the external sphincter and puborectalis muscles, rendering the patient incontinent. It is better to divide the muscle in successive stages as described for a high trans-sphincteric fistula.

Suprasphincteric fistula with high blind track

10 This extremely rare variant has an extension into the supralevator space. Once established, there is a tendency for this fistula to spread in a horseshoe fashion in the supralevator space. Because of the deposition of fibrous tissue, division of the muscle below the track may not necessarily render the patient incontinent, but it is nevertheless wise to divide the muscle in stages with the insertion of a seton. Adequate drainage of the supralevator space must be established. Should there be a horseshoe extension, bilateral drainage may be required.

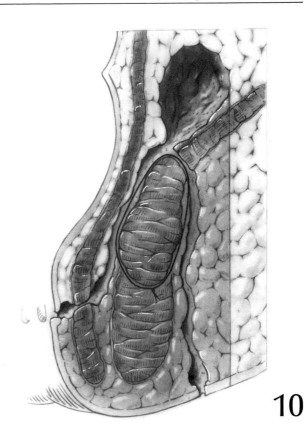

10

Advancement rectal flap

11 The course of a high trans-sphincteric fistula with the outline of the proposed flap is illustrated.

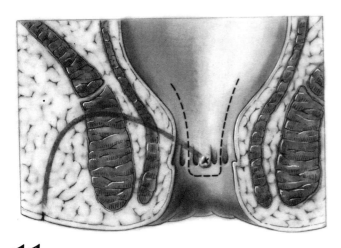

11

12 The track is cored out with a probe in the track as a guide.

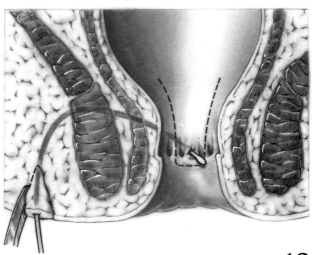

12

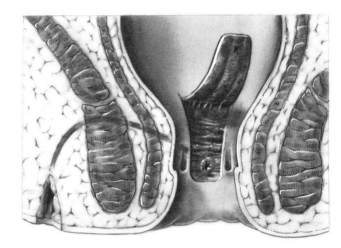

13 Excision of the track is completed with elevation of the flap, which consists of mucosa, submucosa and circular muscle fibres. The width of the proximal portion of the flap is broader than the distal end. This caution should provide good blood supply to the flap.

13

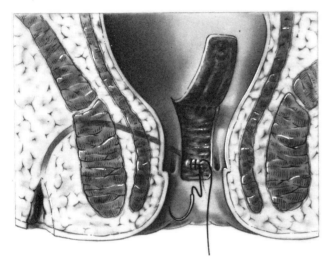

14

14 The internal opening is closed with interrupted sutures.

15 The scarred distal end of the flap is excised.

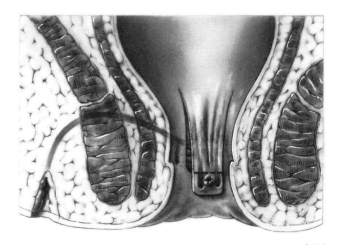

15

16 The flap is placed in position and absorbable sutures are inserted.

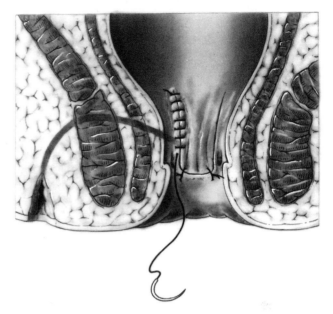

16

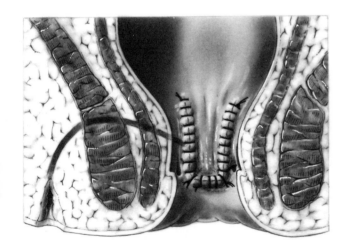

17

17 The flap is completed and the secondary fistula is left open to drain.

Extrasphincteric fistula

By definition, extrasphincteric fistulae pass outside all muscles relating to continence, and consequently division of muscle beneath the fistula will render the patient incontinent. Depending upon the cause of the extrasphincteric fistula, recommendations for treatment will differ.

Fistula secondary to anal fistula

18 A trans-sphincteric fistula with a high extension may spontaneously burst into the rectum, although this is exceedingly rare. More commonly, the secondary opening above the puborectalis muscle is iatrogenic, caused by the over-energetic probing of the surgeon during treatment of the trans-sphincteric fistula. Once established, this fistula is perpetuated by two factors: first, the focus of disease in the anal canal; and second, the continued presence of intraluminal pressure which drives debris through the track. Both factors must be eliminated for the fistula to heal.

The primary source is eradicated by division of the lower half of the internal sphincter with the adjacent external sphincter. The opening in the rectal wall is closed with non-absorbable or slowly absorbable sutures. Adequate drainage of the fistulous track must be performed, with special attention paid to elimination of

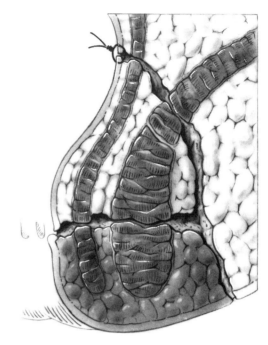

18

pocketing at the apex of the ischioanal fossa or the supralevator extension.

Before the operation the patient is given a mechanical bowel preparation, and is afterwards fed an elemental diet that effectively creates a 'medical colostomy'. It may be necessary to perform a temporary defunctioning colostomy if healing fails.

Traumatic fistula

19 A traumatic fistula may be caused in two ways: a foreign body may penetrate the perineum and enter the rectum, or a swallowed foreign body may reach the rectum and straddle the sphincter mechanism. Treatment consists of removal of the foreign body, establishment of adequate drainage, and formation of a temporary colostomy.

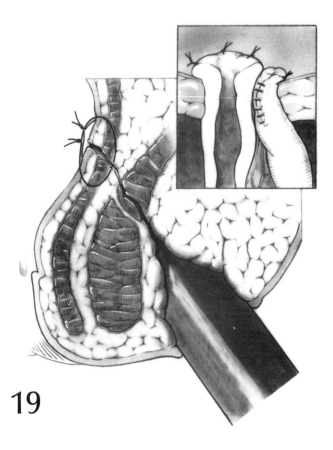

19

Fistula secondary to other anorectal disease

20 Entities such as Crohn's disease and carcinoma may result in bizarre fistulization. They are not usually amenable to local treatment and require proctectomy.

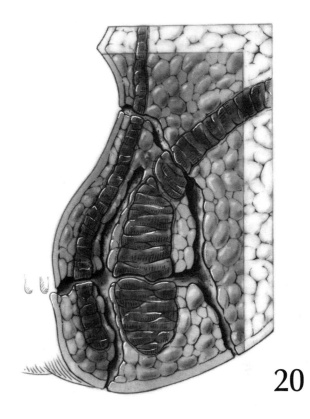

20

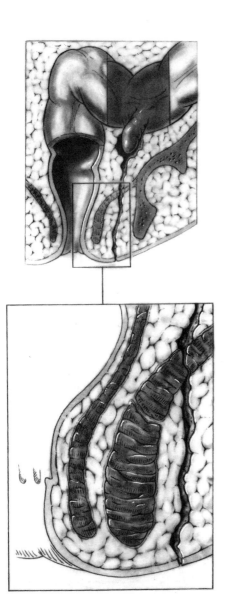

21

Fistula secondary to pelvic disease

21 Pericolic abscess caused by diverticulitis or Crohn's disease may spread through the levator muscles and discharge into the perineum through the ischioanal fossa. Once again, muscle division is not required and treatment consists of eradication of the pelvic disease.

Postoperative care

Postoperative care of the wound may be as important as the operative procedure itself. The goal is to obtain sound healing from the depths of the wound and prevent contact and premature healing of opposing skin edges. Patients are placed on an unrestricted diet and analgesics are administered as necessary. Warm baths are suggested three times a day to obtain perineal toilet. Stool softeners are prescribed to eliminate straining. Initially, weekly follow-up office visits are performed to ensure that healing is progressing satisfactorily. Packing with gauze is unnecessary. Healing times vary with the complexity of the fistula. Because some division of muscle is mandatory, patients may experience varying degrees of leakage, especially if the stools are liquid, but such symptoms generally resolve spontaneously.

In cases where fistulae are complicated by high upward extensions to the apex of the ischioanal fossa or supralevator fossa, the surgeon should examine the patient 7–10 days after the initial operation. If, during the postoperative course, there is a significant accumulation of pus, the patient should undergo re-examination under anaesthesia. If pocketing has occurred, this can be corrected; if further side tracks are discovered, they can be opened. Thus, careful follow-up of complicated fistulae may help to prevent recurrence.

Outcome

The results of fistula operations vary considerably from surgeon to surgeon. Clearly, results will depend upon the complexity of the fistula treated. In a review of the literature, rates of recurrence have ranged from 0% to 17%[4]. The author's personal experience in 160 patients revealed a recurrence rate of 6.3%. Disturbance of continence is reported in 0–39% of cases[4]. In the author's study, there was a 6% incidence of disturbance of continence but in many the problem was only temporary[5]. The dilemma facing surgeons is how to obtain adequate treatment of the fistula without causing disturbance of sphincter function. Division of too much muscle may cause incontinence. When there is doubt regarding the competence of the sphincter, it is wise to divide it in stages at successive operations. Careful assessment should be made between each stage with the patient conscious. It must be accepted, however, that cure in many complex fistulae may be associated with some loss of function, but the aim is to minimize the problem. The renewed interest in the rectal advancement flap technique may further help to decrease the incidence of alteration of continence. Similarly, the concept of seton removal without division of seton-contained muscle might decrease the incidence of alteration in continence, but will increase the incidence of fistula recurrence[6].

References

1. Parks AG, Gordon PH, Hardcastle JD. A classification of fistula-in-ano. *Br J Surg* 1976; 63: 1–12.

2. Fazio VW. Complex anal fistulae. *Gastroenterol Clin North Am* 1987; 16: 93–114.

3. Aguilar PS, Plaisencia G, Hardy TG, Hartmann RF, Stewart, WRC. Mucosal advancement in the treatment of anal fistula. *Dis Colon Rectum* 1985; 28: 496–501.

4. Gordon PH. Anorectal abscess and fistula-in-ano. In: Gordon PH, Nivatvongs S, eds. *Principles and Practice of Surgery for the Colon, Rectum and Anus*. St Louis: Quality Medical Publishing, 1992.

5. Vasilevsky CA, Gordon PH, Results of treatment of fistula-in-ano. *Dis Colon Rectum* 1985; 28: 225–31.

6. Thomson JPS, Ross AHM. Can the external sphincter be preserved in the treatment of transsphincteric fistula-in-ano? *Int J Colorect Dis* 1989; 4: 247–50.

Rectovaginal fistula: endorectal advancement flap

D. A. Rothenberger MD
Clinical Professor of Surgery and Chief, Division of Colon and Rectal Surgery, University of Minnesota Medical School, Minneapolis, Minnesota, USA

S. M. Goldberg MD, FACS, FRACS
Clinical Professor of Surgery and Director, Division of Colon and Rectal Surgery, University of Minnesota Medical School, Minneapolis, Minnesota, USA

History

A rectovaginal fistula is a congenital or acquired communication between the two epithelial-lined surfaces of the rectum and vagina located proximal to the dentate line. A fistula between the anal canal distal to the dentate line and vagina is an anovaginal fistula. Rectovaginal fistulae account for fewer than 5% of all anorectal fistulae. Numerous operative approaches and techniques have been described for repair of rectovaginal fistulae: local repairs; sliding flap advancements; sphincter-preserving transabdominal repairs; and a variety of other methods used for specific types of rectovaginal fistulae.

Principles and justification

Rectovaginal fistulae can be classified into two categories: simple and complex. Simple rectovaginal fistulae are in the low or mid-septal location, are smaller than 2.5 cm in diameter and are of traumatic or infectious aetiology. Complex fistulae are those high fistulae, larger than 2.5 cm in diameter, which are related to inflammatory bowel disease, pelvic irradiation, neoplasm, congenital abnormalities or are associated with other organ involvement (as in concomitant bladder or small bowel fistulae). One must determine whether the anal sphincter is disrupted or functioning normally. Patients with a significant rectovaginal fistula will be incontinent of stool because of the presence of the fistula, and it is sometimes hard to be absolutely certain that the anal sphincter is intact. In these cases anal manometry is used to determine competency of the sphincter muscles.

Preoperative

Examination is essential to: (1) confirm the presence of a rectovaginal fistula; (2) determine accurately the size and location of the fistula; (3) assess the state of the anal sphincter; (4) exclude fistulae involving other organs; (5) search for signs of an underlying disease state (such as an acute infection, Crohn's disease, irradiation injury or a neoplastic process); and (6) determine the presence or absence of associated proximal or distal strictures.

Rectovaginal fistula repair need not be delayed until childbearing has been completed. No operative repair should be undertaken until local inflammatory reaction has completely subsided, which is often 3–6 months after initial injury. For most simple rectovaginal fistulae, the authors prefer an endorectal advancement flap repair. A diverting colostomy is not used but an outpatient mechanical and antibiotic colonic preparation is performed.

Anaesthesia

General or regional anaesthesia is induced, a urinary catheter is inserted, and the patient is then placed in the prone jack-knife position (*see* chapter on pp. 47–50). Proctoscopic examination is carried out to ensure that the rectosigmoid is mechanically clean. A routine perianal and vaginal preparation and draping is performed. In addition to the perianal field block, submucosal and intramuscular injections of 0.25% bupivacaine with 1:200 000 adrenaline (epinephrine) solution are made along the planned routes of dissection. A headlight is invaluable to achieve good illumination of the operative field.

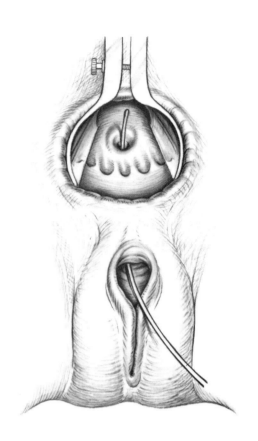

Operation

1 Exposure is gained with a bivalve anoscope and the rectovaginal fistula is identified by passing the probe through the vagina into the rectum with the patient in the jack-knife position.

1

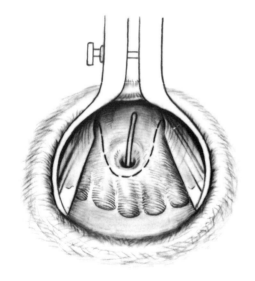

2

2 An endorectal flap which will consist of mucosa, submucosa and a portion of circular muscle is outlined around the fistula, extending approximately 7 cm proximally into the rectum. It is important to base this flap at least 4 cm cephalad to the fistula. The base should be approximately twice the width of the apex of the flap to ensure adequate blood supply.

3 The flap is raised from the apex to the base, thus exposing the attenuated septum and perineal body. Often, there is so much scar tissue near the fistula itself that it is easier to begin this dissection along the lateral portions of the endorectal flap and work distally towards the fistula.

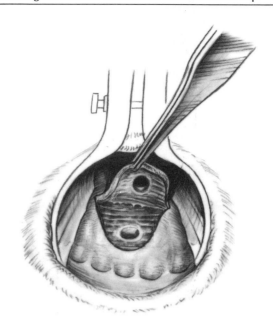

3

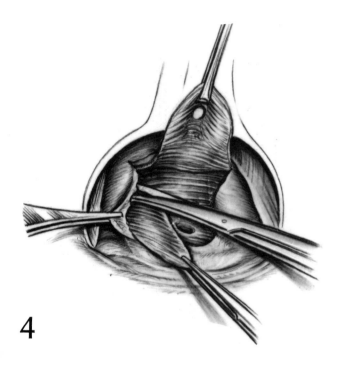

4

4 The rectal mucosa is elevated laterally from the underlying submucosa and internal sphincter muscle. This mobilization must be carried far enough laterally so that the internal sphincter and submucosa can be approximated in the midline without tension.

5 The cut edges of the internal sphincter and submucosa are next approximated in the midline without tension using 2/0 polyglycolic acid sutures in an interrupted technique.

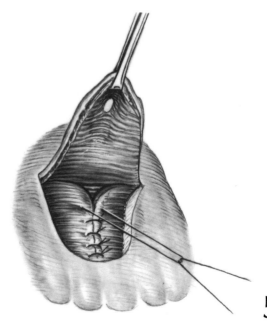

5

6 The endorectal flap of mucosa, submucosa and circular muscle is now advanced over the repaired area. Excess flap distally, including the site of the fistula, is excised.

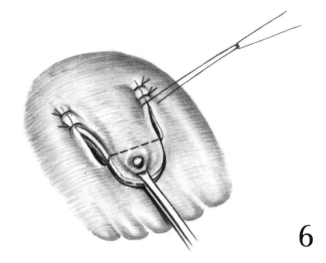

6

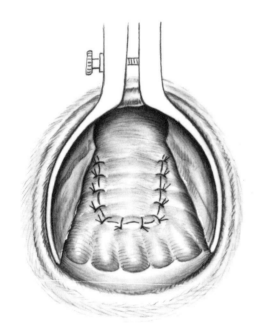

7

7 The flap is sutured in place with 3/0 polyglycolic acid sutures along each side and at the apex. Only small bites of the flap should be included in each suture.

8 The vaginal mucosa is left open for drainage.

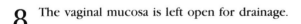

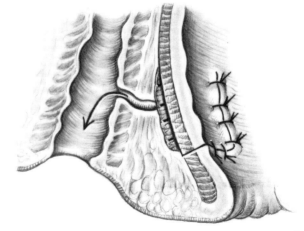

8

MODIFICATIONS OF ENDORECTAL ADVANCEMENT FLAP

Associated anal sphincter advancement flap

9 In women with an associated disruption of the anterior sphincter mechanism, the rectovaginal fistula repair is incorporated into an overlapping sphincteroplasty (*see* chapter on pp. 885–890). This procedure is begun by making a curvilinear incision which parallels the outer edge of the external sphincter muscle and which extends for at least 200–240°. An endorectal flap of mucosa and submucosa is mobilized over a 180° arc internally. Next, the external sphincter muscle is widely dissected free from its bed in the ischiorectal fat. Care is taken to preserve the branches of the pudendal nerves as they enter into the muscle posterolaterally.

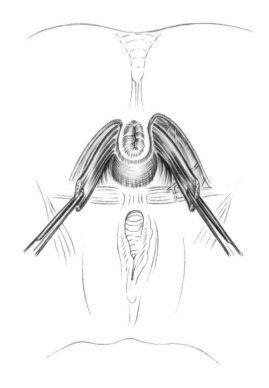

9

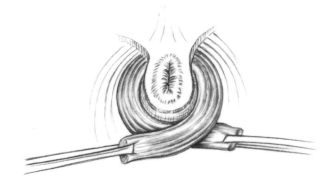

10

10 If the sphincter injury was to the distal sphincter only and the ends of muscle were completely divided or embedded only in the thin bed of scar tissue, an overlapping sphincteroplasty is accomplished. The scar is divided through the rectovaginal fistula site and the two ends of muscle overlapped to provide a snug plication around the fifth digit. Scar tissue is preserved on the severed ends of the muscle because it holds the sutures more securely than soft muscle.

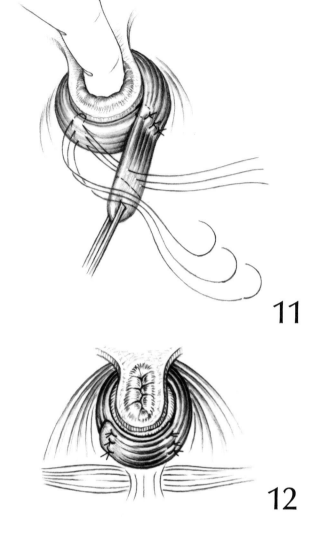

11, 12 Between four and eight horizontal mattress sutures of 2/0 polyglycolic acid are placed and then serially tied to achieve the desired degree of snugness. Tailoring sutures of 3/0 polyglycolic acid are placed as needed. Sutures should be tied securely but not so tight as to cause muscle ischaemia. This type of overlapping repair completely covers the site of the rectovaginal fistula associated with the anal sphincter disruption.

11

12

13 If the injury was more severe and the entire sphincter mechanism was disrupted, a plication of the exposed levator muscles, including the puborectalis sling, is performed before the overlapping sphincteroplasty.

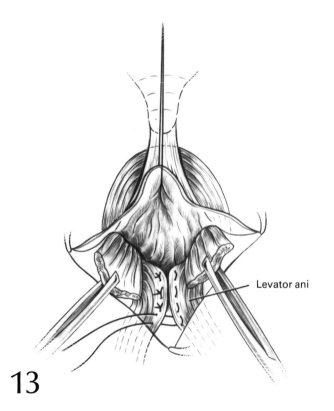

Levator ani

13

Simple rectovaginal fistula at dentate line

A small benign fistula located at or within 1 cm of the dentate line poses a special problem for the surgeon. An endorectal advancement flap technique as described above risks the possibility of creating a wet anus as the flap is advanced distal to the dentate line. For this type of very distal rectovaginal fistula, the authors prefer a modification of the flap technique described by Hoexter et al.[1].

14 A transverse elliptical incision is made around the fistula through the rectovaginal septum, thus excising the entire fistulous track.

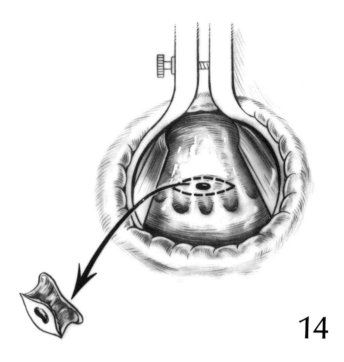

14

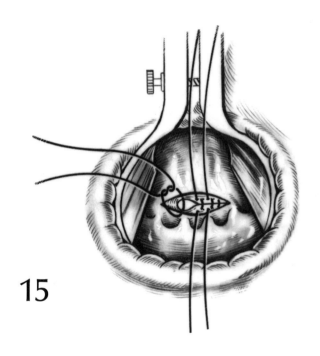

15

15 A two-layer closure of the defect in the rectovaginal septum is performed.

16 The rectal mucosa is advanced distal to the deeper portion of the repair and reapproximated. The vaginal mucosa is left open for drainage.

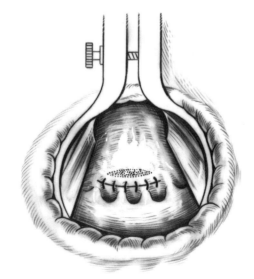

16

Complex rectovaginal fistulae

Some other approaches may be considered for complex fistula repair using the transfer of vascularized tissues. These approaches include: bulbocavernosus repair, gracilis muscle transfer, or simply an overlapping sphincteroplasty which, in effect, is a method of transferring viable muscle into an area where the complex (recurrent) fistula has occurred. In certain instances, if the recurrence of the fistula has been caused by persistent infection, a temporary colostomy might be considered at the time of repair.

Postoperative care

None of the repairs for simple rectovaginal fistula require a diverting colostomy, and this greatly simplifies postoperative care. Most patients are discharged within 24–48 h of surgery. Analgesics and warm baths are used as needed to control the pain and spasm. Perioperative antibiotics are usually discontinued after one or two doses. Regular diets with bulk agents to avoid constipation are prescribed unless a concomitant overlapping sphincteroplasty has been performed. For the latter, patients are usually kept on a low residue diet and enemas or laxatives for the first 1–2 weeks after operation, before being allowed to advance to a normal diet supplemented with bulk agents. Intercourse and vaginal tampons are proscribed for 6 weeks after repair.

Outcome

Complications are relatively few and are usually quite easily treated. A total of 81 patients ranging in age from 18 to 76 years (mean 34 years) have been treated in our unit in recent years for such simple rectovaginal fistulae. Ten patients (12%) developed complications: these were urinary retention (two), urinary tract infection (two), postoperative fever (two), bleeding that did not require re-exploration (two), and headache after spinal anaesthesia (two). These patients had had the rectovaginal fistula from 0 to 20 years before repair (mean 3.2 years). Twenty-five patients (31%) had associated anal sphincter disruption and underwent a concomitant overlapping sphincteroplasty. Postoperative follow-up ranged from 4 months to 10 years (mean 25 months). The overall success rate was 83%. The number of previous attempts at repair correlates with the failure rate[2].

References

1. Hoexter B, Labow SB, Moseson MD. Transanal rectovaginal fistula repair. *Dis Colon Rectum* 1985; 28: 572–5.

2. Lowry AC, Thorson AG, Rothenberger DA *et al*. Repair of simple rectovaginal fistula. Influence of previous repairs. *Dis Colon Rectum* 1988; 31: 676–8.

Rectovaginal fistula: vaginal repair

C. N. Hudson MChir, FRCS, FRCOG, FRACOG
Director, Clinical Academic Department of Obstetrics and Gynaecology, Medical College of St Bartholomew's Hospital, London, UK

Principles and justification

Traumatic fistulae may occur after surgery or obstetric trauma. High obstetric fistulae are almost always associated with tissue loss due to sloughing; occasionally circumferential loss of the bowel wall is present.

Inflammatory fistulae are principally caused by diverticular disease with colonic fistulae, Crohn's disease with ileal or rectal fistulae, and ulcerative colitis with rectal fistulae. Very occasionally, lymphopathia venereum, tuberculosis and actinomycosis may fistulate.

Irradiation fistulae affect the terminal ileum and colon rather more commonly than the rectum. The use of intracavitary sources for the treatment of carcinoma of the cervix may be one factor, but more fistulae arise from external beam therapy given after procedures in which a hysterectomy has been carried out and in which loops of intestine lose their mobility by adhesion within the pelvis.

Malignant disease in the alimentary canal or genital tract occasionally presents with faecal fistula. More commonly, it is seen as a preterminal complication, but malignant tissue may be involved in fistulae that are primarily traumatic or radiotherapeutic in origin. Despite the presence of tumour in a fistula, they are sometimes suitable for surgical treatment[1].

The principles of repair of rectovaginal fistulae do not differ greatly from those of repair of urogenital fistulae. Successful treatment depends on accurate diagnosis, choice of the correct operation and meticulous surgical technique.

The diagnostic problems to be resolved are:

1. The condition of the tissues and the presence or absence of associated abscess cavities.
2. The underlying pathology.
3. Accurate determination of the involved intestinal loop and the exact anatomy of the fistula.
4. The presence or absence of associated or distal stenosis of the intestine or vagina.
5. The detection of any likely subsequent impairment of anal continence.
6. The condition of associated systems: genital tract (e.g. prolapse, haematometra), urinary tract (e.g. ureteric obstruction and impending or actual urinary fistula formation).

The principles of surgical repair include excision of all unhealthy tissue, particularly where blood supply is impaired, avoidance of all tension on suture lines, both within and between individual sutures, and meticulous haemostasis to avoid haematoma formation.

Types of operation

Conservative repair operations

These are usually appropriate for simple traumatic fistulae including those of obstetric origin, in which there may have been considerable tissue loss due to pressure necrosis, but to only a selected few inflammatory fistulae in which the disorder remains entirely localized and quiescent.

Radical repair operations

By contrast to the above, these operations consist of intestinal resection with or without hysterectomy. They are suitable for ileal fistulae, fistulae involving the uterus, most colovaginal fistulae and a proportion of high rectovaginal fistulae. They will certainly be required for fistulae associated with localized inflammatory disease of the large intestine, and a proportion of fistulae due to pelvic malignant disease, particularly when the primary tumour is in the large intestine. They may occasionally be appropriate for irradiation fistulae, but should not be undertaken lightly in these cases unless there is good evidence that healthy intestine can be reached on either side of the irradiated zone. It is highly desirable to bring down vascularized tissue from outside the irradiation field in the form of a pedicle of greater omentum. If this is difficult, liberation of the omentum from the colon is required with division of one gastroepiploic artery, leaving the other to supply the pedicle.

This type of operation may also be appropriate for some high obstetric rectal fistulae, when there has been complete circumferential loss of a segment of rectum due to pressure necrosis[2]. In all the above circumstances, the success of the operation will depend on the availability of an adequate length of healthy distal intestine for anastomosis. If anastomosis is not feasible, the alternative is rectal excision and colostomy. The anal canal may then be preserved (Hartmann's operation) or removed by combined excision.

In sexually active women inflammatory perianal disease often causes severe dyspareunia, and anal preservation should not be seen as an overriding objective.

Colpocleisis

Removal of the epithelium and obliteration of the vaginal space is a surgical procedure that has a role in the management of certain difficult fistulae. It is inappropriate unless the distal vagina is healthy, and it carries the risk of the creation of an additional urinary fistula where none existed before. It will inevitably fail if there is distal intestinal stenosis below the fistula unless, perhaps, an additional procedure such as rectal fenestration is carried out.

The operation has its major place in the management of fistulae caused by irradiation; the presence of active malignant disease under these circumstances need not necessarily be a contraindication where the addition of a pedicle graft from outside the irradiated field will increase the chance of success – either the gracilis muscle or a vulval fat pad may be used.

Permanent colostomy alone

This should be reserved for patients with a fistula due to completely untreatable genital malignancy usually of cervical origin, patients too frail for definitive surgery and patients with an inactive benign condition in which the anal sphincter mechanism has been destroyed. It is emphasized that before resorting to permanent colostomy, careful evaluation of the possibility of colpocleisis should be made, because a colostomy that has not been made obligatory through rectal excision may cause great distress to the aged and infirm.

Choice of route

The abdominal route for simple closures is preferred for colonic fistulae, including those which communicate with the uterus. It is also appropriate for some high obstetric rectal fistulae particularly where access through the vagina is difficult and where this will be hindered by previous closure of the vesicovaginal fistula. It will be required if tissue loss has caused considerable adhesion to the sacrum. For irradiation fistulae, the abdominal route is only advisable when the greater omentum is to be used as a pedicle graft.

The vaginal approach is favoured for the majority of operations. Four operative vaginal techniques will be described.

The peranal route may be preferred by rectal surgeons, and the temporary paralysis of the anal sphincter following stretching by the Parks' speculum can be an advantage in preventing subsequent disruption of the suture line by flatus. The techniques employed are identical to those used through the vagina.

The transcoccygeal and transperineal approaches are probably only of historic interest but York Mason's trans-sphincteric approach, although devised as an approach to the rectoprostatic fistula of the male, has an occasional place in the management of fistulae into the female genital tract.

The number of potential surgical approaches indicates that difficult fistulae are a major surgical problem. There is a premium on successful closure at the first attempt, and the experienced surgeon achieves significantly better results than those with little direct experience.

Careful assessment and diagnosis are essential, and a better result may often be achieved by colpocleisis even by way of palliation, than mere dismissal with a colostomy.

Special contraindication

Breakdown of a surgical repair is almost always associated with peri-intestinal inflammation. This should have subsided before a subsequent attempt is made and may take up to 3 months. Rather longer may be necessary in a patient who has previously been irradiated. The decision must be based on the quality of the tissues in which it will be necessary to place sutures. Normally, no repair should be carried out simultaneously with or prior to repair of a vesical fistula, and any associated abscess cavity must have been laid open and drained so that inflammation has subsided before elective surgery.

Preoperative

Diagnosis

Although the presence of a faecal fistula is usually only too obvious, occasionally even the basic diagnosis can be very elusive. In nearly all cases, an examination under anaesthesia should be carried out. After proctoscopy and sigmoidoscopy, a probe inserted through the vaginal aperture of the fistula may be palpated on digital rectal examination or may be visible through the sigmoidoscope. If, however, the fistula is in the colon at the apex of the sigmoid loop, the intestine is almost always tethered to the pouch of Douglas, and an ordinary sigmoidoscope may be inadequate to visualize the intestinal orifice of the fistula.

Fistulography

A small Foley catheter or ureteric catheter should be inserted so that radiography can be carried out under a viewing screen. It is necessary to inject the medium even as the catheter is being withdrawn, as it is very important to determine whether a fistula is merely a simple communication between intestine and vagina or whether there is an associated abscess cavity with communications to the intestine and to the genital tract. This is particularly important when a fistula follows surgery for a primary intestinal disorder such as diverticular disease. If there is an old pericolic abscess cavity or a complicated track, it is unlikely that a vaginal operation alone will close the fistula permanently.

Endoscopic and radiographic examination of the intestine are particularly important to establish whether there is any associated or underlying intestinal disease. Even with a definite history of trauma, the persistence of a fistula can be an indication of underlying asymptomatic and hitherto unsuspected inflammatory disease of the intestine, such as Crohn's disease. If there is doubt, biopsy of the rectum and the fistula wall should be carried out. These investigations will also determine whether there is stenosis at or below the fistula site.

Preparation

The general preoperative care of all these patients is most important. High obstetric fistulae are almost always associated with a urinary fistula. The urinary fistula should always be treated first and the results of treatment will be improved if faeces are diverted from the vagina before an attempt to close the urinary fistula is made. A transverse colostomy should always be used because it will not embarrass access should a subsequent abdominal approach prove to be necessary to deal with the high rectal fistula. Preliminary colostomy is not generally regarded as essential before the preliminary repair of a straightforward rectovaginal fistula.

Apart from associated urinary fistula, there may be other sequelae to obstructed labour which require attention such as pelvic inflammatory disease, haematometra, obstructive uropathy and nerve palsies. The patient's morale may be extremely low and this aspect should not be neglected. During an extended preoperative period, anaemia, malnutrition and all infections and infestations should be treated.

Once the general condition of the patient is satisfactory, preoperative preparation in hospital should be directed more to mechanical emptying of the intestine than pursuit of bacterial sterility. After preliminary colostomy, it may be difficult to empty the distal loop by wash-out, particularly if there is any stricture formation, but this is to be regarded as very important. Leak-back through the fistula may be stemmed by packing the vagina beforehand.

With the exception of the administration of tinidazole, preoperative antibiotic therapy is better avoided. Intraoperative and postoperative administration of an antibiotic, usually cephaloridine or an aminoglycoside, may be used, but even this may not be necessary in a properly mechanically prepared intestine following transverse colostomy. If faeces have not been previously diverted, the vagina may be packed overnight before operation using noxythiolin or povidone-iodine. In a postmenopausal patient, oral oestrogen therapy may improve the quality of the vaginal epithelium.

Operations

CONSERVATIVE REPAIR OPERATIONS

Conversion to third-degree tear

1 Many small low rectovaginal fistulae represent incompletely healed complete (third-degree) perineal lacerations. The best procedure is to divide the bridge of skin and scar tissue and repair the defect as a classical third-degree laceration.

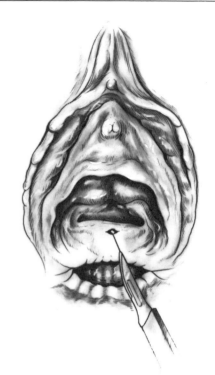

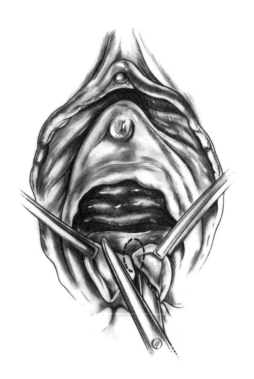

1

2 Similar considerations apply to complete destruction of the perineal body and losses of septal tissue which may extend even to the pouch of Douglas.

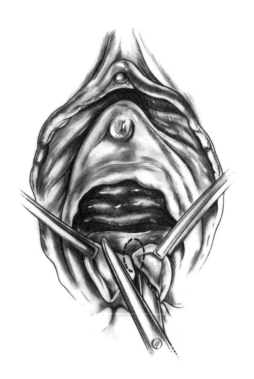

2

3 The edges and fistula track must be excised until healthy tissue has been reached. The vaginal wall must be dissected off the remnants of the perineal body until they can be exposed. In high lesions, it may be necessary to open the pouch of Douglas.

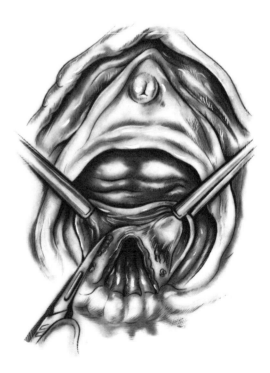

3

4 The mucous membrane of the rectum and the lining of anal canal are repaired with fine polymer sutures (polyglactin and polyglycolic acid) or extra fine chromic catgut 2/0. Traditionally, the knots are made to lie within the lumen of the intestine.

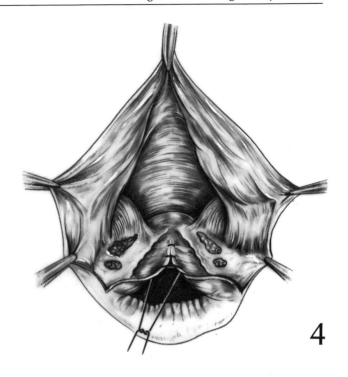

4

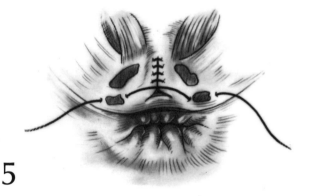

5

5 The rectal muscle and internal sphincter may be reconstructed with a series of Lembert polymer sutures (coated polyglycolic acid or polyglactin).

6 The external anal sphincter is freed where it has retracted into its tunnel on either side of the anus and reunited in front. If this is particularly tight, thus producing anal stenosis, a subcutaneous sphincterotomy may be carried out posterolaterally without subsequent impairment of function.

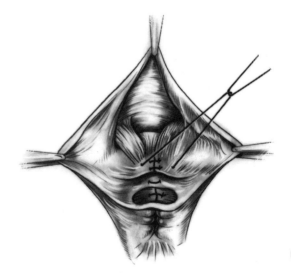

6

7–9 The remnants of the perineal body must be reunited in front of the anal canal with interrupted sutures. Attention to symmetry is important, and this may be obtained if each bite of the suture is inserted from within outwards. Closure of the vaginal epithelium is desirable in simple cases using interrupted fine catgut or polymer sutures.

Where there has been major tissue loss in the posterior wall, vaginal closure may be impossible. Peritoneum of the rectum may safely be left in this area, but it is preferable to close the pouch of Douglas with a purse-string above. Tight constricting bands in the vagina may be divided by relaxing incisions, but these should be used with caution as the blood supply may be impaired. At the lower end, it is wise to leave the navicular fossa unsutured, as a small gap allows any collection of blood and serum to discharge, thus avoiding haematoma formation. The skin over the perineum is closed with interrupted or subcuticular sutures. In major septal defects, there may be considerable reduction in rectal lumen, and such cases may need cover by a transverse colostomy.

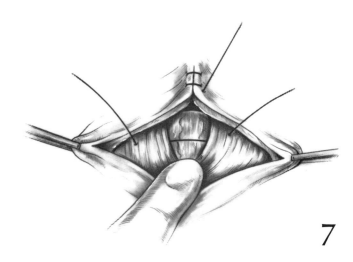

7

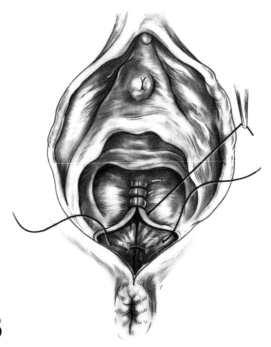

8

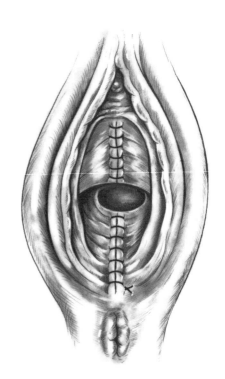

9

Purse-string and inversion

10 If the perineal body is reasonably intact, a small fistula may be treated by circumcision and inversion through a purse-string suture using a straight aneurysm needle.

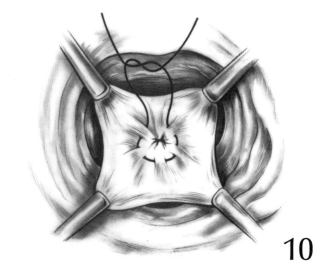

10

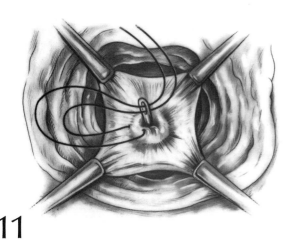

11

11 Such a fistula is best displayed by the surgeon or his assistant with an index finger in the rectum pressing the fistula area forward. When the tract has been dissected free, a purse-string suture is inserted around the base of the fistulous tract and a stay suture through the neck of the fistula is then threaded through the aneurysm needle and withdrawn.

12 Traction on this stay suture inverts the fistula tract into the anal canal through the purse-string, which can then be closed. Two or three interrupted sutures provide a second layer of muscle stitches in front of the repair. This will also serve to obliterate dead space. The vaginal epithelium is finally closed with interrupted absorbable sutures.

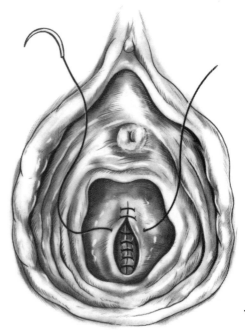

12

Flap repair

This method is suitable for moderately high fistulae. If there is reasonable access, this procedure is in fact suitable for the repair of surgical fistulae arising after hysterectomy. In such cases, the elevation of vaginal flaps denudes a small area of upper vagina which is closed off (upper partial colpocleisis).

The technique of flap repair is virtually identical to that of repair of bladder fistulae, and a Schuchardt incision may similarly be necessary. The surgeon should beware of extending this incision into the fistula, as it may interfere with vaginal closure at the end of the procedure. Exposure of the fistula may be achieved by the use of traction sutures or digital elevation via the rectum.

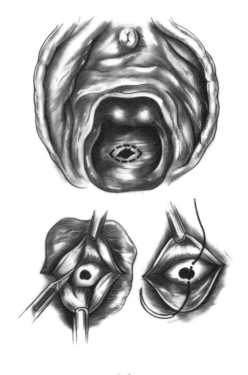

13

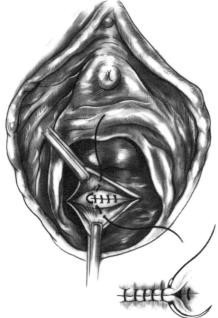

14

13, 14 A knife is used to elevate flaps around the fistula. The hole in the rectum should be repaired by interrupted sutures.

It is important that the mucous membrane should be excluded from the depths of the wound, and therefore it is probably better to avoid including it in the sutures. The direction of the suture line should be determined by the ease in which the walls of the defect can be brought together. There is very little risk of producing rectal stenosis from the repair of fistulae of this sort.

Major high fistula repair

15–17 When there has been a major injury of the posterior vaginal wall due to obstetric pressure necrosis, it may not be possible to produce sufficient mobility by ordinary flap dissection. In such cases it is desirable to open the pouch of Douglas and bring down the anterior rectal wall with its serous coat. This allows the rectal defect to be closed without tension.

There is insufficient vaginal epithelium to close the defect; therefore, it is tacked to the peritoneal covering of the anterior rectal wall, which may also be fixed to the back of the cervical stump.

Sometimes the entire vaginal wall is lost (third-degree septal loss)[3]. *Illustration 17* shows why such a lesion can only be closed with a vertical suture line. There may be considerable reduction in the lumen of the rectum, and in such cases it is advisable to cover the repair by preliminary transverse colostomy.

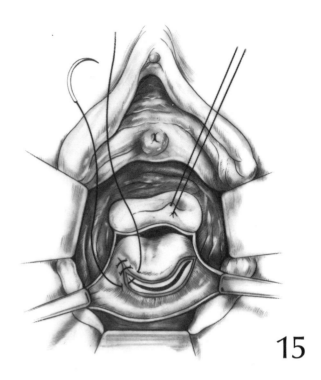

15

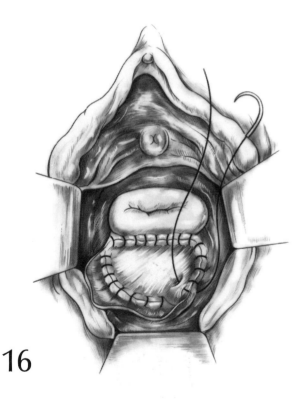

16

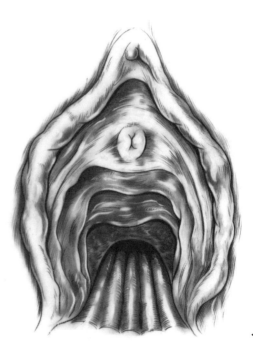

17

Transanal repair

18 This repair is best carried out with the patient in the jack-knife position. The anal canal dilated by a Parks' speculum gives a good exposure of the fistula.

The technique is identical to that used for repair through the vagina, except that sutures made of stainless steel wire may be used to close the anorectal defect.

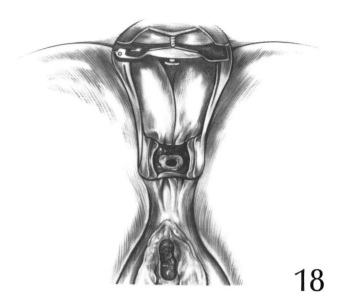

18

Trans-sphincteric repair

19, 20 The patient should be placed in the jack-knife position. An incision is made through the skin radially from the posterior aspect of the anal orifice. As this is deepened, muscle layers are identified and marked with silk sutures to aid recon-struction at the end of the procedure. When the anal canal and rectum have been fully opened, an excellent exposure of the anterior rectal wall is obtained. Closure of the incision of access should be carried out in layers with polyglycolic acid.

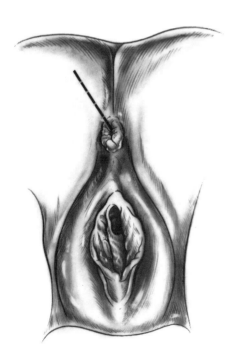

19

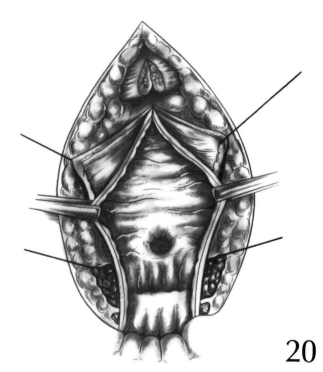

20

Colpocleisis

Upper partial colpocleisis (*see* 'Flap repair', page 856).

Lower partial colpocleisis

In this procedure the upper vagina is closed off as a 'diverticulum'. This is required for certain high vesicovaginal fistulae and is only appropriate for rectal fistulae when combined with the former. The end result is a vesicorectal fistula, and if the direction of the communication between the two viscera is oblique, this is usually a satisfactory solution to the problem of double incontinence.

Total colpocleisis

This is complete denudation of the vaginal epithelium with obliteration of the remaining space.

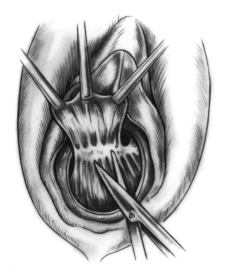

21

21 A circular incision is made around the lower vagina. The level should be somewhat oblique, preserving the maximum amount of the anterior vaginal wall in order to avoid damage to the function or integrity of the urinary tract. The upper vagina is dissected off as a full-thickness sleeve up to the margins of the fistula.

In most cases the patient will have previously undergone hysterectomy or the cervix will have been obliterated by intracavitary radiotherapy. Great care should be taken to avoid injury to the urinary tract. The fistula may be closed as previously described.

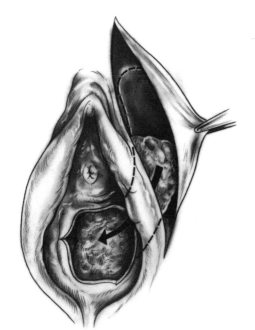

22

22 Ideally, the dead space should be obliterated by one or two tiers of sutures, but rigidity often renders this impossible. The resultant dead space may be filled by a pedicle graft of labial fat based posteriorly[4].

23 Alternatively, the gracilis muscle may be swung up, based on the proximal neurovascular bundle supplying it from the deep femoral artery. The position of this perforating vascular bundle is approximately one-third of the distance between the origin and insertion of the muscle. The muscle is diverted into the vaginal 'dead space' through a subcutaneous tunnel[5].

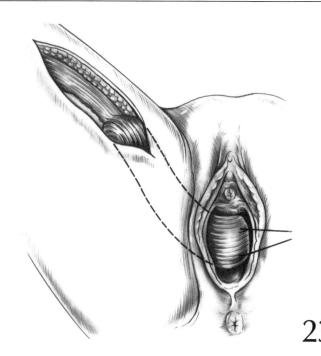

23

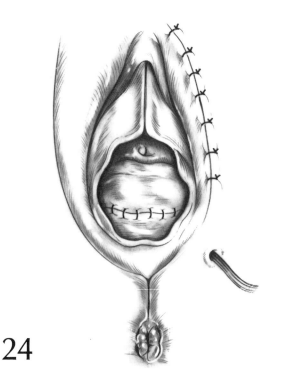

24

24 The residual sleeve of vagina needs to be elevated sufficiently by undercutting to allow transverse closure flush with the introitus. A suction drain may be brought out through a stab incision in the buttock.

Lower partial colpocleisis combined with rectal fenestration

25 This procedure may be used for palliation as an alternative to colostomy for colovaginal fistula. The upper vaginal cuff is mobilized as in total colpocleisis short of the vaginal vault. An elliptical incision is then made in the anterior rectal wall which has been denuded by the vaginal mobilization. The upper vaginal cuff is then anastomosed end-to-side to the rectum to allow the faeculent matter from the vaginal fistula to be evacuated through the rectum. The lower partial colpocleisis is closed off as above.

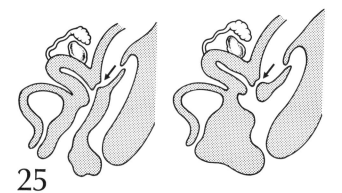

25

ABDOMINAL OPERATIONS

In some instances a preliminary right transverse colostomy will have been made. The operation is most conveniently performed in the Trendelenburg position using stirrups.

Simple repair

26 The abdomen should be opened through a left paramedian incision to allow full mobilization of the left colon if required.

The fistulous loop should be freed all round by dissection from the posterior fornix or uterus and the fistula tract divided.

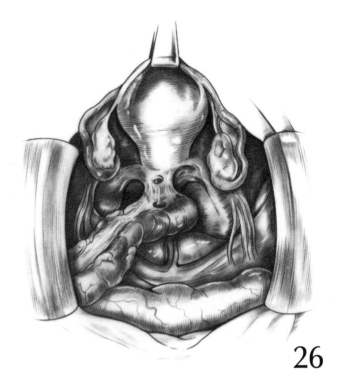

26

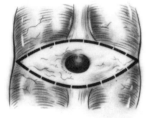

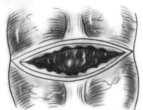

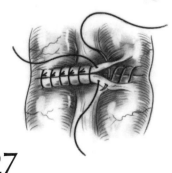

27

27 The opening in the rectosigmoid colon should be excised as a transverse ellipse so that all granulations and unhealthy tissue are removed.

The defect is repaired in two layers using a standard technique for anastomosis. This suture line should preferably lie separated from the vaginal aperture, which need not then be closed.

Any raw area in the pelvis should be covered with absorbable gauze, which also helps to keep the affected loop away from the vagina. If necessary, the greater omentum can be used for interposition.

The abdomen should be closed in routine fashion with a stab drain through the left flank down to the site of the suture line. If there is troublesome oozing from the pelvis, a suction drain may be passed out through the vaginal fistula. After the operation the anus should be dilated to admit four fingers.

Hysterectomy and repair

It has long been recognized that hysterectomy may facilitate abdominal repair of a high rectal fistula by improving access to the inferior margin of the fistula. In obstetric cases where there has been gross pelvic infection associated with slough injuries, the pouch of Douglas is often obliterated and the pelvic floor rock hard with scar tissue. The uterus is commonly fixed and adherent in the hollow of the sacrum, and this is the cause of the difficulty of access from below.

Subtotal hysterectomy with conservation of the ovaries should be carried out. The cervical stump remnant is firmly fixed in the scar tissue and the anatomy on either side is grossly distorted[6].

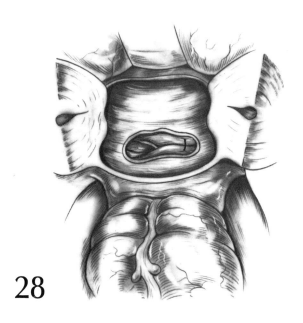

28

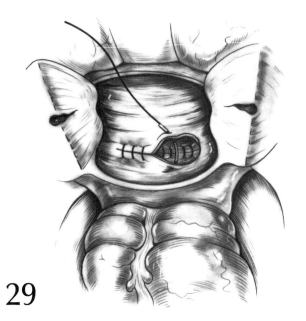

29

28, 29 A midline sagittal split of the cervical stump allows access to the fistula in the posterior fornix when the two halves of the cervix are separated.

The inferior aspect of the fistula may be freed by sharp dissection in the ordinary way. This manoeuvre avoids inadvertent inferior extension of the fistula.

Following conventional repair of the rectal aperture, the vaginal opening may also be closed and the cervical stump reunited in front as additional protection. Suction drainage is indicated.

Retrorectal mobilization and repair

30 When the uterus and vagina are not firmly adherent in the posterior part of the pelvis, dissection behind the rectum may be used to approach a high obstetric fistula. The rectosigmoid colon is first mobilized by incision of the white line and reflection of the sigmoid mesentery.

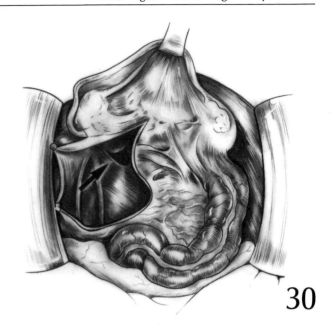

30

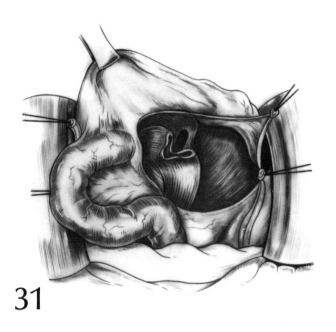

31

31 Access to the retrorectal space allows the adherent vagina and rectum to be freed from the hollow of the sacrum, and a tissue plane may be developed below the fistula between the posterior vaginal wall and rectum by blunt dissection. The fistula track may then be opened, trimmed and closed as described. Drainage is recommended.

If there has been circumferential intestinal loss due to tissue ischaemia, coloanal anastomosis comparable to the correction of a Hartmann's operation is required as described in the chapter on pp. 488–496. The EEA stapler may be particularly advantageous.

Resection and anastomosis

A resection and anastomosis for diverticular disease or carcinoma using the techniques described in the chapters on pp. 369–386 and pp. 292–306 should be used. This approach has been used for irradiation fistulae provided that intestine above the irradiated area can be brought down for a low anastomosis[7].

32 Such an operation should be covered by a pedicled omental graft, which should preferably stretch right across the pelvis and be tacked into the opened vagina[8]. The abdominal approach is likely to be more difficult and more hazardous than a vaginal operation and should not be contemplated unless it is absolutely certain that there is no reactivation of the original malignant disease.

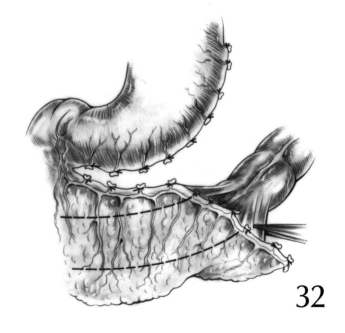

32

Postoperative care

Conservative repair operations

Dissection of a rectovaginal fistula may on occasions provoke brisk arterial haemorrhage. The question of a vaginal pack following repair has thus to be considered on its merits. In general, if a pack is necessary to achieve haemostasis, the risk of haematoma formation and breakdown of repair is high. Suction drainage through a perineal stab incision should be considered if there is any significant dead space.

The traditional management of such patients by confining the bowels for 5 days is outmoded. Nothing can be worse for a delicate stitch line at its weakest moment than for it to be stretched by a mass of descending faecal concretions. Early resort to oral laxatives is indicated, avoiding those containing liquid paraffin.

The surgeon should insist that no digital rectal examination or insertion of suppositories or enemas be performed by anyone other than himself. Failure to give this instruction may involve the administration of routine anal medication with disastrous results.

Abdominal operations

Routine postoperative care of patients who have had intestinal surgery is instituted. An infected pelvic haematoma will almost certainly cause failure, and there should be no hesitation in prescribing antibiotics. The stab drain through the flank should be left in place for 5 days or until the bowels move, whichever is later. The administration of laxatives should be encouraged as soon as ileus has subsided, but this, of course, is not important if a preliminary colostomy has been carried out. Successful closure of the fistula should be confirmed by the instillation of a large volume of blue dye down the distal loop of the colostomy before its closure is contemplated, normally about 3 weeks after operation. Rectal stenosis is not usually a problem provided there is sufficient lumen to admit a fingertip.

References

1. Hudson CN. Acquired fistulae between the intestine and the vagina. *Ann R Coll Surg Engl* 1970; 46: 20–40.

2. Bentley RJ. Abdominal repair of high rectovaginal fistula. *J Obstet Gynaecol Br Commonw* 1973; 80: 364–7.

3. Lawson JB. Injuries of the urinary tract. In: Lawson JB, Stewart DB, eds. *Obstetrics and Gynaecology in the Tropics and Developing Countries*. London: Arnold, 1967: 481–522.

4. Martius, H. Fettlappenplastik auf dem Bulbukavernosusgebiet als Fistelinahtschutzoperation. *Geburtshilfe Frauenheilk* 1940; 2: 453–9.

5. Hamlin RHJ, Nicholson EC. Reconstruction of urethra totally destroyed in labour. *BMJ* 1969; ii: 147–50.

6. Lawson JB. Rectovaginal fistulae following difficult labour. *Proc R Soc Med* 1972; 65: 283–6.

7. Moon A, Wilson E. Post-irradiation recto-vaginal fistula: cure following restorative resection of the rectum. *J Obstet Gynaecol Br Commonw* 1961; 68: 1014–18.

8. Turner-Warwick R. The use of pedicle grafts in the repair of urinary tract fistulae. *Br J Urol* 1972; 44: 644–56.

Anal cancer

J. M. A. Northover MS, FRCS
Consultant Surgeon, Director, Imperial Cancer Research Fund Colorectal Cancer Unit, St Mark's Hospital for Diseases of the Rectum and Colon, London, UK

Anal cancer is rare in developed Western countries, there being 100 cases of colorectal cancer for each new case of anal cancer. Anal cancer is relatively more common, however, in other locations, such as northern Brazil and certain parts of India. Most cases are of epidermoid origin (including squamous cell, basaloid and mucoepidermoid subtypes) while malignant melanoma and other primary types are extremely rare, and respond poorly to surgery and other forms of treatment.

Because these tumours spread mainly within the pelvis, with very few cases having overt distant spread at presentation, the treatment of anal cancer during the past half century has been surgical: radical abdominoperineal excision for anal canal tumours, while anal margin tumours have usually been removed by local excision. Results have not been satisfactory for an apparently locoregional disease. Most series published in the 1980s reported only 50–60% 5-year survival rates for both margin and canal cancers. During the past 20 years, radiation therapy or combined radiation and chemotherapy (combined modality therapy) has become the treatment of choice. Survival figures are at least as good as surgical results, but with the advantage of avoiding a colostomy.

Principles and justification

Despite the move away from surgery, the surgeon still has several important roles:

1. Initial diagnosis and assessment after treatment.
2. Excision of small tumours at the anal margin.
3. Treatment of complications resulting from non-surgical therapy or disease relapse.
4. Treatment of inguinal metastases.

Initial diagnosis and assessment after treatment

Patients with anal tumours are usually referred to a surgeon initially for confirmation of diagnosis and for staging, which requires examination under anaesthesia. The medical and the radiation oncologists should be present to make their assessment before treatment.

The full effect of radiation therapy or combined modality therapy develops about 6–8 weeks after therapy is finished. The surgeon may be asked to examine the patient at that time: if the original site of the primary tumour is soft and flat, no biopsy is required; if there is suspicion of residual disease, however, an examination under anaesthesia and biopsy should be performed.

Primary management of small margin lesions

Small lesions (TNM stage T_1, <2 cm in diameter) at the anal margin may be treated effectively by local excision alone, thus avoiding protracted non-surgical therapy. Any evidence at surgery or histological examination that the lesion is larger or more invasive than thought initially indicates a need for additional therapy.

Surgery of complications after primary treatment or disease relapse

Three situations may require surgery after primary non-surgical therapy. (1) residual tumour; (2) complications of therapy; (3) subsequent tumour recurrence.

Residual tumour

A minority of patients (10–40%) respond incompletely to radical radiation or combined modality therapy. This group will require 'salvage' surgery, but histological proof of residual disease is mandatory before such radical surgery is undertaken. The appearance of the primary tumour site can be misleading after radiation therapy; in most patients complete remission is obvious.

In some, however, a lump may remain, occasionally looking and feeling like an unchanged primary tumour. Only a generous biopsy will reveal whether the residual lump contains tumour or merely consists of inflammatory tissue. If residual disease is confirmed, previous radiation therapy does not increase the morbidity rate of radical surgery.

Complications of therapy

Some patients develop complications after radical radiation or combined modality therapy. Severe anal pain caused by radionecrosis may necessitate surgery – either colostomy (in the hope that the lesion may heal after faecal diversion) or radical anorectal excision. Occasionally, a tumour is so extensive within the sphincters or in the rectovaginal septum that incontinence or a rectovaginal fistula may develop as a direct consequence of primary tumour shrinkage. Although some rectovaginal fistulae may be amenable to repair, sphincter damage in these circumstances is unlikely to be improved by local surgery, thus necessitating abdominoperineal excision of the anorectum.

Tumour recurrence

If clinical evidence of recurrent disease is found after initial resolution, biopsy confirmation is mandatory before surgical intervention. If high-dose radiation therapy was used for primary treatment, further non-surgical therapy for recurrence is contraindicated, therefore mandating radical surgical removal. Additional conservative surgery *may* be sufficient for recurrence of anal margin tumours initially managed by local excision; radiation therapy or combined modality therapy can be considered before radical surgery is contemplated.

Treatment of inguinal metastases

Inguinal lymph nodes are enlarged in 10–40% of patients with anal cancer. Although synchronous inguinal lymph node involvement may be treated by inclusion in the radiation field of the primary lesion, some argue that it should be treated surgically. Histological confirmation of metastasis is advisable before resorting to radical groin dissection because up to 50% of cases with inguinal lymph node enlargement are caused by inflammation alone. Metachronous inguinal lymphadenopathy is most likely caused by recurrent tumour. Radical groin dissection is indicated in this situation, and may be associated with a 50% 5-year survival rate, though others have reported less favourable results. Papillon noted that the outlook following surgery and postoperative radiation therapy was better for metachronous than for synchronous groin metastases.

Preoperative

Male homosexual activity may predispose to anal cancer, probably through human papillomavirus infection. When taking a history, therefore, it is important to enquire about sexual activity to assess the likelihood of infection with human immunodeficiency virus.

Before therapy can be planned, histological type and tumour extent should be ascertained. General physical examination should include a search for inguinal lymph node involvement which is present in about one-third of cases. Digital examination of the anal canal may be difficult because of stenosis and pain. If it is possible, however, the depth of spread should be assessed, together with measurement of cephalad spread. Ultrasonography of the anal canal is a useful measure of depth of spread into the sphincters and prostate gland.

Examination under anaesthesia is an important step (particularly when initial clinical examination is difficult) with the radiotherapist present. Tissue is taken for histological examination and the tumour is staged, preferably using the TNM system for canal lesions or Papillon's system for margin tumours[1, 2]. If radiation therapy or combined modality therapy are contemplated, the risk of complications during therapy should be considered. In particular, tumours involving the rectovaginal septum may 'melt' during radiation therapy, causing a fistula. If the tumour is extensive within the vagina, a fistula is particularly likely, and this outcome should perhaps be pre-empted by constructing an initial defunctioning colostomy. In general, however, a stoma is not required before radiation therapy or combined modality therapy.

Operations

Local procedures

Local procedures can be performed in the lithotomy or in the prone jack-knife positions (*see* chapter on pp. 47–50). The author prefers the lithotomy position.

Biopsy

This may be required either for initial histological assessment for confirmation of tumour ablation following primary non-surgical therapy or to confirm recurrence. A small sliver of tissue, no more than a few millimetres in diameter and depth, is taken using a size 15 scalpel blade. It may be necessary to take a deeper biopsy specimen if there is any suggestion of subdermal residual disease.

If there is suspicion of residual or recurrent disease in the ischiorectal fossae or within the pelvis above the levator plate, a Tru-Cut needle biopsy is required. This may be performed either through the skin of the buttock or through the intestinal wall via an anal retractor, whichever is more appropriate.

Local excision

1a—c To minimize bleeding and to provide an optimal view, the area beneath the tumour is infiltrated with 1:200 000 adrenaline solution. The operative area is exposed using a Parks' anal retractor. An incision is made around the tumour, approximately 2 cm from its edge. This is extended vertically through the subdermal tissues to the outer surface of the sphincters and perianal fat, and the disc of tissue is removed by dissecting under the tumour in this plane. Before fixation the operative specimen should be pinned out on a piece of cork to ensure proper orientation for the pathologist.

The skin defect produced by local excision can be dealt with in several ways. It can be left alone, to heal by secondary intent, or the edge can be advanced circumferentially and sutured to the internal sphincter and fat of the perianal region, to minimize the skin defect. Alternatively, the skin and subcutaneous fat of an appropriate area of the buttock can be mobilized as a wedge to be advanced to the anal verge and lower canal to provide primary skin closure. The author usually employs the first option, because the wound usually contracts and heals rapidly.

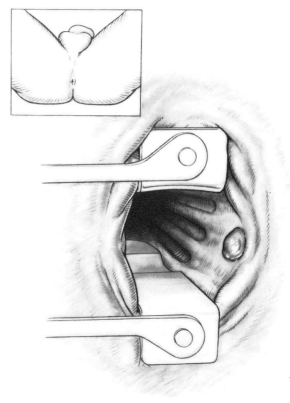

1a

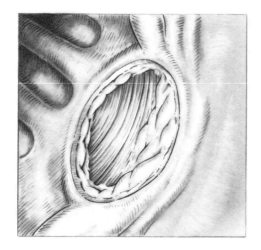

1b

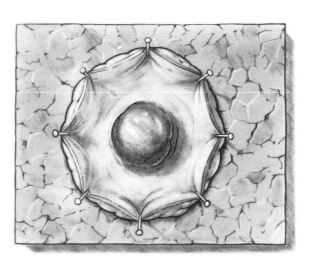

1c

ABDOMINOPERINEAL EXCISION OF THE ANUS AND RECTUM

This procedure does not differ from the operation used for low rectal cancer but some important points deserve special mention.

Perineal incision and ischiorectal dissection

Care must be taken to ensure adequate clearance of the lateral margins of the tumour. The skin incision should be at least 2 cm lateral to the tumour if its edge extends onto the perianal skin. Because the tumour may have spread to a variable extent into the ischiorectal fat, care must be taken to be radical within the infralevator compartment, taking all the ischiorectal fat and detaching the levator muscles from the bony pelvic side walls.

Perineal closure

In those patients in whom this procedure is performed after radical radiation therapy either for initial failure to control the tumour, for treatment of radionecrosis, or for later tumour recurrence, primary wound healing is less predictable than normal. If the wound edges do not come together easily, or if the tissues look unhealthy (oedematous or fibrotic due to radiation therapy), it is better to dress the wound and leave it open. If it fails subsequently to show signs of healing satisfactorily, it may be necessary to perform a skin/muscle flap transposition (a rectus abdominis flap, preferably) as a secondary procedure to expedite healing.

Postoperative care

Little specific care is needed after local excision. A bulk laxative should be prescribed to ensure easy bowel evacuation. The patient should be encouraged to bathe after each bowel movement, and apply a small damp dressing soaked in a mild antiseptic solution.

Postoperative care following abdominoperineal excision is as described in the chapter on pp. 472–487.

Complications

After local excision, early complications are uncommon; mild sepsis may require additional local toilet and dressing. The only important later complication is anal stenosis, which may result if a significant proportion of the anal margin has been removed without grafting.

Stenosis usually responds to initial dilatation under general anaesthesia, followed by regular self-dilatation by the patient.

The complications of abdominoperineal excision are discussed in the chapter on pp. 472–487.

Outcome

Anal margin cancers

Surgical series published in the past decade have reported local excision for most cancers at the anal margin. The rationale for this non-radical approach was based on the perception that margin lesions seldom metastasize, although this has not always been confirmed by long-term follow-up studies.

The largest reported series is from St Mark's Hospital, where 83 margin lesions were treated between 1948 and 1984[3]. These tumours tended to present at a somewhat earlier pathological stage than anal canal lesions. Two-thirds of patients were treated by local excision, of whom 65% survived for 5 years. All 11 patients managed by radical anorectal excision were treated with curative intent, but only four survived for 5 years. Overall the 5-year survival rate was 65% for T_1 and T_2 lesions, while patients with T_3 and T_4 cancers fared significantly worse, with only 33% surviving for 5 years.

The series reported from Copenhagen comprised 76 cases, 58 of whom were treated with curative intent, most by surgery[4]. Of the 24 (41%) who developed recurrent disease, in all but one this was local or regional. This series was followed up for longer than others, and highlighted the persisting risk of recurrence, the longest interval being 9 years after primary surgery. Of 32 patients treated by local excision only, 20 developed recurrent disease.

In contrast to these results, Greenall et al. in New York reported a corrected 88% 5-year survival following local excision, although many of their patients exhibited locoregional relapse which often responded well to further local therapy[5].

Anal canal cancers

The most extensive reported surgical experience of radical abdominoperineal excision of the rectum and anus is that of the Mayo Clinic[6], with 188 patients treated between 1950 and 1976. Thirteen (7%) of the tumours in this series were superficial lesions 2 cm or less, and were treated by local excision with excellent results. Among the 118 who underwent radical surgery, four died postoperatively, 46 developed recurrent disease, while 81 (69%) survived for 5 years. Others had less favourable results, with 5-year survival rates ranging from 20% to more than 50%.

Radiation therapy and chemotherapy

Radiation therapy

Technical advances in the 1950s have led to increased use of external beam and interstitial radiation therapy, which has produced good results[7]. Five-year survival rates are as good as with surgery, and have the advantage of avoiding the need for a stoma in the majority of cases.

Combined modality therapy

Combined modality therapy using 5-fluorouracil, mitomycin C and 3 Gy of radiation produces 'cures' in most cases including some that are too advanced for any hope of surgical cure[8]. With wider experience, it is now clear that higher doses of radiation therapy (45–60 Gy) should be used (usually divided into two courses to minimize morbidity), with intravenous 5-fluorouracil at the beginning and end of the first radiation therapy course, and a single bolus of mitomycin C given on the first day of therapy. Modifications of chemotherapy dose regimen are necessary for elderly patients and those with extensive ulcerated tumours. Prophylactic antibiotics should be prescribed in frail patients, the elderly and those with extensively ulcerated or necrotic tumours. It has yet to be determined whether similar levels of local tumour control and survival can be achieved without chemotherapy, which might avoid some morbidity.

References

1. UICC. In: *TNM Classification of Malignant Tumours.* Geneva: UICC, 1982.

2. Papillon J, Montbarbon J. Epidermoid carcinoma of the anal canal. *Dis Colon Rectum* 1987; 30: 324–33.

3. Pinna Pintor M, Northover JMA, Nicholls RJ. Squamous cell carcinoma of the anus at one hospital from 1948 to 1984. *Br J Surg* 1989; 76: 806–10.

4. Jensen SL, Hagen K, Harling H, Shokouh-Amiri MH, Nielsen OV. Long term prognosis after radical treatment for squamous-cell carcinoma of the anal canal and anal margin. *Dis Colon Rectum* 1988; 31: 273–8.

5. Greenall M, Quan S, Stearns M *et al.* Epidermoid cancer of the anal margin. Pathologic features, treatment and clinical results. *Am J Surg* 1985; 149: 95–101.

6. Boman B, Moertel C, O'Connell M *et al.* Carcinoma of the anal canal. A clinical and pathologic study of 188 cases. *Cancer* 1984; 54: 114–25.

7. Papillon J, Mayer M, Montbarbon J, Gerard J, Bailly C. A new approach to the management of epidermoid carcinoma of the anal canal. *Cancer* 1983; 51: 1830–7.

8. Nigro ND. An evaluation of combined therapy for squamous cell cancer of the anal canal. *Dis Colon Rectum* 1984; 27: 763–6.

Illustrations by Gillian Oliver

Lateral subcutaneous internal anal sphincterotomy for anal fissure

M. J. Notaras FRCS, FRCSEd, FACS
Consultant Surgeon, Barnet General Hospital and Honorary Senior Lecturer and Consultant Surgeon, University College Hospital, London, UK

Principles and justification

Examination of the lower half of the anal canal by separation of the buttocks to open up the perianal region will reveal the presence of any simple anal fissure, as they are located below the dentate line and are always confined to the anoderm in the mid-posterior position (90%) or the mid-anterior position (10%). The anoderm is that part of the anal skin that lies between the dentate line and the anal verge and is the squamous lining of the anal canal.

1 An acute fissure is a superficial splitting of the anoderm and may heal with conservative management. Once the fissure is recurrent or chronic, operation is required for a permanent cure. A chronic fissure is recognized by the presence of transverse fibres of the internal sphincter in its floor. A late stage in the development of a chronic fissure is the formation of a large fibrous polyp from the anal papilla on the dentate line at the upper end of the fissure. Infection of the sentinel pile that develops at the lower end of the fissure at the anal verge may lead to the formation of a superficial fistula.

Fissures that are multiple or extend above the dentate line should be viewed with suspicion as a simple anal fissure never extends above the dentate line. These complex fissures are usually signs of more serious diseases, such as ulcerative colitis, Crohn's disease, tuberculosis, or syphilis. When associated with large rubbery inguinal lymph nodes, they may indicate a primary syphilitic infection, and smears from the anal canal should be taken for dark-ground illumination before digital or endoscopic examination contaminates the field with lubricant.

It must be remembered that anal sexual intercourse is necessary for the transmission of anal syphilis, so this infection must be considered in patients suspected of, or known to engage in, this form of sexual activity. Serological tests must be performed, and the possibility of acquired immune deficiency syndrome considered.

Human immunodeficiency virus (HIV)-positive patients with anal conditions should be identified, as it is important to distinguish fissures from ulcers. Biopsies should be taken from any suspicious fissure or ulcer, and in HIV-positive patients viral culture of part of the biopsy specimen is essential. Sphincterotomy performed for an HIV-positive homosexual patient infected with cytomegalovirus or herpetic ulcer may result in faecal incontinence combined with slow healing of the wound.

An intersphincteric sinus or abscess may be mistaken for a chronic anal fissure unless excluded by careful examination. A subcutaneous fistula may also be present in a sentinel haemorrhoid (*see Illustration 1*).

Treatment of anal fissure

Lateral subcutaneous internal anal sphincterotomy has been shown to have many advantages over other forms of treatment, such as anal dilatation and mid-posterior internal sphincterotomy performed through the floor of the fissure. It has rapidly gained acceptance as it may be performed as an outpatient procedure under local or general anaesthesia. Its main advantages are that it avoids an open intra-anal wound, the divided internal sphincter is bridged by skin, there is minimal anal wound care, postoperative anal dilatation is unnecessary and relief from symptoms is almost immediate, with the fissure becoming painless and healing within 3 weeks.

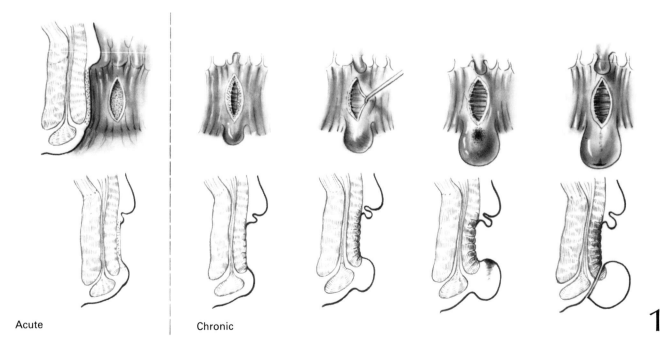

Acute   Chronic

1

Preoperative

The author prefers no bowel preparation so that the urge to defaecate after the operation is not delayed. The patient may be placed in the lithotomy, lateral or jack-knife position according to the preference of the surgeon. Sigmoidoscopy should be performed on all patients.

Anaesthesia

The procedure may be performed under general or local anaesthesia or a combination of methods. The author supplements general anaesthesia with local anaesthesia, which permits a lighter general anaesthetic to be used. A local anaesthetic combined with dilute adrenaline solution helps to reduce bleeding and immediate postoperative pain.

Approximately 10 ml of local anaesthetic agent (0.5%

lignocaine hydrochloride with 1:200 000 adrenaline) is infiltrated subcutaneously into the perianal area on each side of the anus. The inferior haemorrhoidal nerves are blocked on each side by injection of 5–7 ml into each ischiorectal space along the medial aspect of each ischial tuberosity. A further 5 ml is injected directly into the external sphincter muscle on each side of the anus.

When local anaesthesia is used alone, it should be supplemented by diazepam, 10–20 mg intravenously (according to age and weight), and sometimes also pethidine hydrochloride, 50–100 mg intravenously. This technique sedates patients adequately, and although conscious throughout the procedure, they usually have no memory of the event. After the operation patients will need to rest for 1–2 h until the effects of local anaesthesia have subsided and the sphincters have recovered.

Operations

CLOSED TECHNIQUE

The lithotomy position is used.

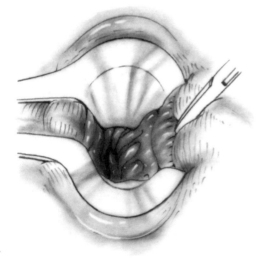

2a

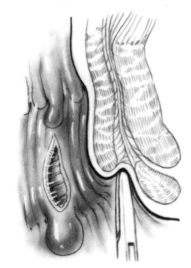

2b

$2a, b$ A bivalved anal speculum (Parks', Eisenhammer or Goligher) is introduced into the anal canal and opened sufficiently to stretch the anus slightly. The internal sphincter is then felt as a tight band around the blades of the speculum. Its lower border is easily palpated and can be demonstrated by gently pressing a pair of forceps into the intersphincteric groove. The floor of the fissure should be probed for a sinus or fistula.

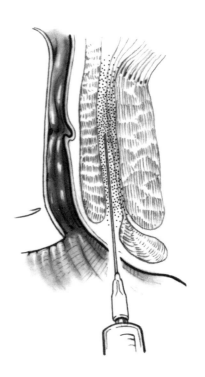

3a

3a, b Local anaesthetic agent, 2–3 ml, is introduced under the mucosa and anoderm. The anal lining is lifted away from the internal sphincter by the infiltration of local anaesthetic, thus reducing bleeding and the risk of perforation by the scalpel blade in the closed technique. It also facilitates dissection if the open technique is used.

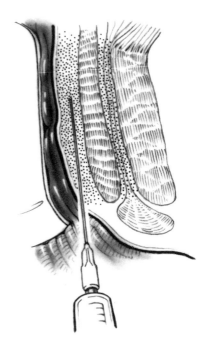

3b

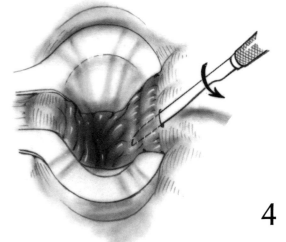

4

4, 5 After the internal sphincter has been identified, a narrow-bladed scalpel (52L 'Beaver' cataract knife) is introduced through the perianal skin at the mid-lateral aspect of the anus (3 o'clock). It is pushed cephalad with the flat of the blade sandwiched between the internal sphincter and the anoderm until its point is just above the dentate line.

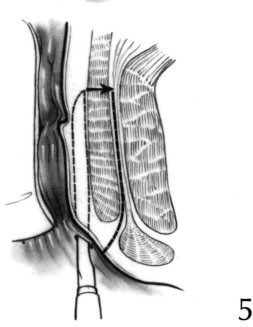

5

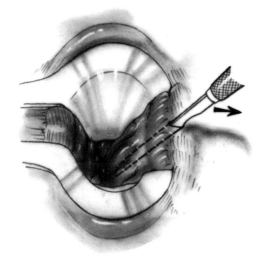

6

6 The sharp edge of the blade is then turned towards the internal sphincter, and by incising outwards and laterally the internal sphincterotomy is performed. As the scalpel blade cuts through the internal sphincter there is a characteristic 'gritty' sensation, and with completion of the division there is a sudden 'give', indicating that the blade has reached the outer surrounding ring of external sphincter muscles.

7   Another variation of the technique is to introduce the blade between the external and internal sphincter muscles via the intersphincteric groove, and then to perform the sphincterotomy by cutting inwards towards the mucocutaneous lining.

Whichever technique is used, the aim is to preserve the skin bridge over the divided internal sphincter.

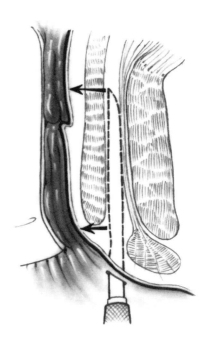

7

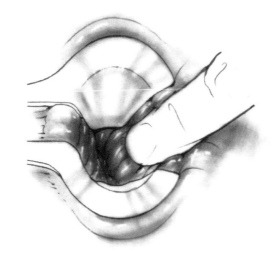

8

8   After division of the internal sphincter the completeness of the sphincterotomy may be assessed after withdrawal of the knife by pressure of the finger tip over the site. This will rupture any residual internal sphincter fibres.

Usually, there is a slight ooze of blood from the small external wound, but this is soon arrested by tamponade as the external sphincters recover and contract around the internal sphincter. The external wound is left open to allow drainage.

9 If there is a large sentinel tag, it is removed with sharp-pointed scissors without damaging the sphincters and with minimal excision of the perianal skin. All overhang is removed. Fibrous polyps are excised if present.

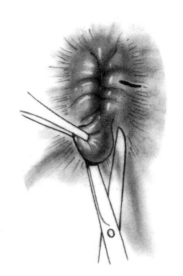

9

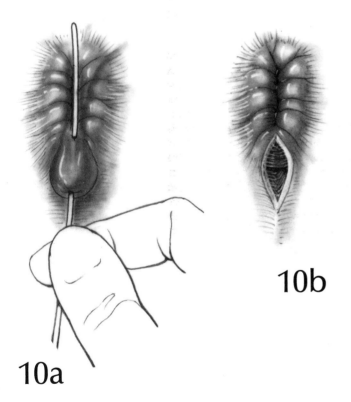

10a

10b

10a, b A fistula in a sentinel tag (when present) should be laid open. The tract passes through some of the superficial fibres of the lower border of the internal sphincter. It is tempting also to perform a complete internal anal sphincterotomy through the fissure and the rest of the sphincter above the sentinel tag, but results are better if the surgeon confines himself merely to laying open the fistula and then performing a lateral subcutaneous sphincterotomy. This avoids the development of a 'key-hole' deformity in the mid-posterior position, which may lead to perianal soiling (as described in the chapter on pp. 885–890).

A dressing is laid on the anal area. Intra-anal dressings are contraindicated as they cause postoperative pain. Once bleeding has ceased no dressings are required. The patient is encouraged to have a bowel action as soon as the inclination develops.

OPEN TECHNIQUE

If the surgeon is not happy with the closed technique because of fear of damage to the external sphincter muscle, the open method is equally applicable. The author originally practised this technique, but with experience found the closed technique simpler and more expeditious.

11a, b
A bivalved anal speculum is inserted into the anus to stretch the internal sphincter slightly to assist its identification, as described in the closed method.

A local anaesthetic with adrenaline is injected into the subcutaneous area selected for the procedure. A radial incision is made into the perianal skin just below the inferior border of the internal sphincter. This incision is preferred to the circumferential type, as the wound is left unsutured and open for drainage and the edges of the wound will approximate naturally.

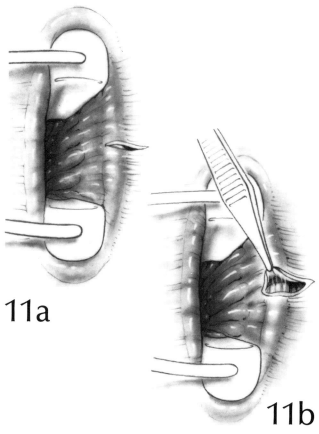

11a

11b

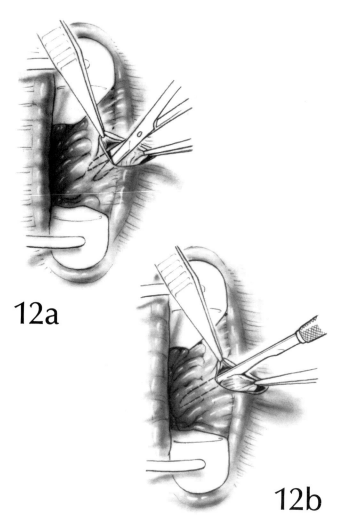

12a

12b

12a, b
The upper end of the incision is grasped with a pair of forceps and dissection with narrow-bladed scissors is carried out to separate the anoderm from the internal sphincter. The latter is recognized by its white fibres. To facilitate dissection and the sphincterotomy, its lower border may be grasped with forceps.

The exposed internal sphincter is then divided by a narrow scalpel blade or scissors.

13 The wound is left open to allow free drainage. A 'lay-on' dressing of gauze is placed over the anus. Intra-anal dressings should not be used, as they cause postoperative pain.

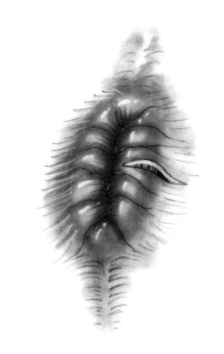

13

ANAL STENOSIS

14a–c Patients may have marked anal stenosis caused by chronic and repeated ulceration. It may also follow a previous haemorrhoidectomy or the prolonged use of mineral oils ('paraffin anus').

In those cases where there has been no previous anal surgery, bilateral subcutaneous lateral sphincterotomy may be of value. The sphincterotomy is performed on one lateral side, and if considerable tension remains in the internal sphincter on the opposite side, a second lateral subcutaneous sphincterotomy is indicated.

When there has been a previous haemorrhoidectomy, it is usual for scarring of the anoderm to extend beyond the dentate line to the rectal mucosa. There is usually fibrosis in the internal sphincter deep to these areas. In such cases, the author selects a site for the sphincterotomy in the healthiest tissue between the areas of scarring. It may also be necessary to make release incisions in the scarred mucosal areas but these are made superficially. Patients are advised to use an anal dilator for up to 2 months after the procedure.

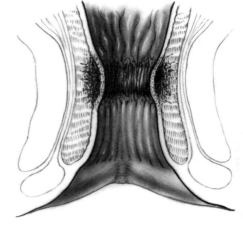

14a

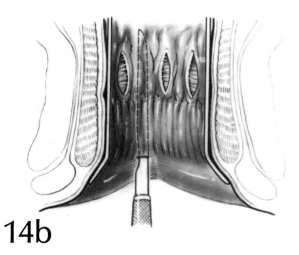

14b

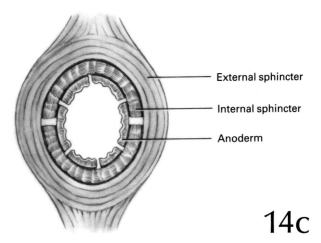

External sphincter

Internal sphincter

Anoderm

14c

Mucosal prolapse

Andrew McLeish MD, FRACS
Senior Colorectal Surgeon, Austin Hospital, Heidelberg, Victoria, Australia

The majority of patients with rectal mucosal prolapse do not require surgery, which is reserved for those with either extensive or continuing prolapse after treatment with sclerosant or rubber bands. Most patients are elderly women and there is frequently an element of external anal sphincter weakness.

Principles and justification

Excision of redundant mucosa

There is usually an excess of anorectal mucosa, which is excised, but care must be taken not to excise too much to prevent subsequent anal stenosis.

Tethering of remaining mucosa

The aim is to tether the remaining prolapsing mucosa within the anal canal to the internal anal sphincter by scar tissue throughout the length of the anal canal and the distal 1–2 cm of rectum.

Differences from haemorrhoidectomy

In contrast to haemorrhoidectomy, it is unusual to excise associated skin tags or redundant perianal skin with anal mucosectomy. Furthermore, the extent of dissection up into the rectum is less than that of haemorrhoidectomy. The basic principles of surgery, however, are similar for both haemorrhoidectomy and mucosal prolapse excision.

Circumferential mucosectomy

This operation is to be avoided because of the high incidence of subsequent anal stenosis and the risk of advancing mucus-secreting mucosa from the upper anal canal or rectum down to the anal verge, resulting in persistent anal leakage and moisture. Rarely, circumferential mucosectomy is indicated for severe anorectal mucosal prolapse with marked redundancy of mucosal folds; it is then important to excise only the distal rectal mucosa so that the circumferential suture line sits at the level of the anorectal junction.

Non-operative management

Most patients with minor prolapse, particularly segmental prolapse, can be treated with an injection of 5% phenol in almond oil applied to the mucosa in the upper anal canal. Moderate prolapse is treated with rubber band ligatures which should also be applied to the mucosa of the upper anal canal and not the externally prolapsed mucosa. Both procedures can be repeated several times if necessary.

Preoperative

Assessment

The diagnosis of anal mucosal prolapse is usually obvious on direct inspection of the anus with the patient in the left lateral position, and asking the patient to strain. Where there is difficulty in distinguishing between mucosal prolapse and haemorrhoids, the patient is treated as having haemorrhoids.

If any doubt exists as to whether the patient might have a full-thickness rectal prolapse, then examination under anaesthesia is indicated and, if the anterior rectal wall can be readily prolapsed with grasping forceps, the diagnosis is confirmed. Full-thickness prolapse should not be treated by anal mucosectomy.

Endoscopic examination of the rectum is important to exclude pathologies such as prolapsing villous tumour, rectal carcinoma or solitary rectal ulcer.

There is no place for anorectal physiology studies unless there is weakness of the anal sphincter which might be suitable for surgical repair. Mucosal prolapse is often associated with weakness of the external anal sphincter, which is usually unsuitable for repair. However, if surgical repair of the sphincter is to be undertaken, any mucosal excision should be performed as a subsequent procedure.

Segmental mucosal prolapse may occur where previous anorectal damage has occurred, e.g. after anal fistulectomy. Care should be taken not to excise too much of the visible mucosa as the latter may be contributing to continence.

Preparation

Although day case surgery is occasionally suitable, most patients require hospitalization for several days. Medically fit patients can be admitted on the day of surgery. Apart from anaesthetic assessment, the only preparation is the use of two rectal laxative suppositories several hours before operation to ensure an empty rectum. Shaving is seldom required and should only be done in the operating room.

Anaesthesia

Because the patient is placed in the prone jack-knife position for the operation, relaxant anaesthesia is used, with or without premedication. Although administration of anaesthesia is easier when the patient is in the lithotomy position, any benefit is far outweighed by the superior surgical access afforded by the jack-knife position.

Local anaesthetic is infiltrated in the plane between the anal mucosa and internal anal sphincter, using a total of 20 ml 1% prilocaine with 1:200 000 adrenaline. The injected solution facilitates dissection in the correct plane and reduces perioperative bleeding.

At the completion of the procedure, a caudal injection of 10 ml 0.5% bupivacaine with 1:200 000 adrenaline provides excellent postoperative analgesia for several hours.

Occasionally, a low spinal anaesthetic is used in place of general anaesthesia.

Operation

Position of patient

The patient is placed in the prone jack-knife position with the pelvis supported on several pillows and flexed to 90°, with the abdomen free to allow respiration, the buttocks strapped apart, and a slight head-down position of the table (*see Illustration 4* on page 49).

Infiltration

1 The submucosa is infiltrated in four quadrants with 20 ml of anaesthetic solution, starting with the right posterior quadrant from the anal verge to just above the anorectal junction. The left index finger is inserted into the anus to guide the position of the infiltrating needle.

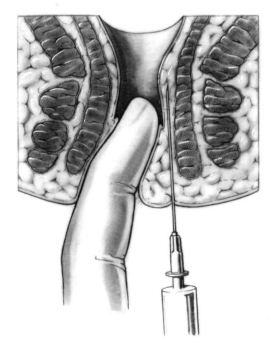

1

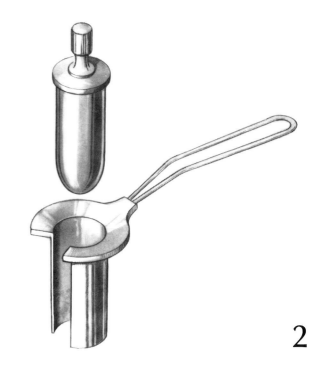

2

Retraction

$2, 3$ A lubricated Fansler operating anoscope is
inserted, pushing the prolapsed mucosa back
into its correct position. This particular retractor affords
excellent exposure, allows easy suturing because the
circumferential curve is similar to the passage curve of a
26-mm tapered needle, and the surgical assistant can
easily alter the angle of the anal canal by manipulating
the handle. Unlike operating with the patient in the
lithotomy position, the entire operating team can see
every detail of the operation.

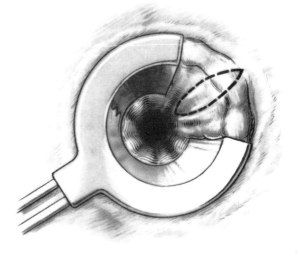

3

Mucosal excision

4–6 Starting at the anal verge in the right posterior quadrant, the anal mucosa is tented up by fine-toothed dissecting forceps and excised in a strip as far up as 1–2 cm above the anorectal junction. The underlying internal anal sphincter is bared, but it must not be divided. If skin tags are present they are excised in continuity with the mucosa.

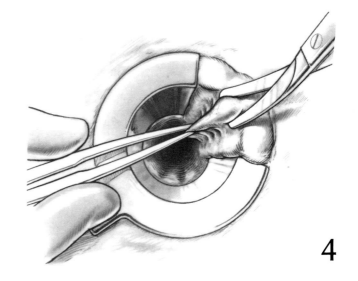

4

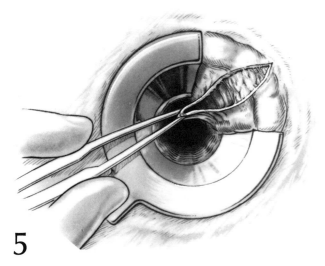

5

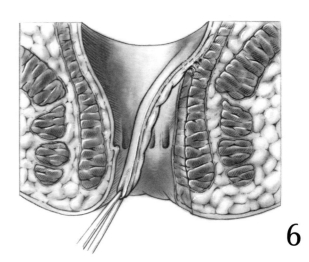

6

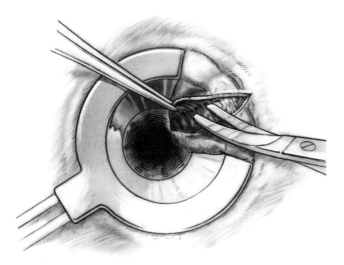

7

Haemostasis

Haemostasis is secured with diathermy forceps. The vessels are small and occur mainly at the upper apex of the dissection in the submucosa. Occasionally, they perforate the internal anal sphincter.

Remaining mucosa

7 The edges of the residual mucosa are dissected from the underlying internal anal sphincter to allow tension-free closure of the mucosal defect.

Closure of defect

8 Closure of the defect is started at the upper apex with an absorbable suture such as 2/0 chromic catgut on a 26-mm tapered needle, with inclusion of the internal anal sphincter with each bite. The suture must not be under tension or the mucosa will tear, and the knot at the anal verge should be tied loosely to avoid undue postoperative discomfort and formation of skin tags secondary to oedema.

Care must be taken with anterior wound closure in a woman with an attenuated rectovaginal septum, as sutures placed too deeply can result in a rectovaginal fistula.

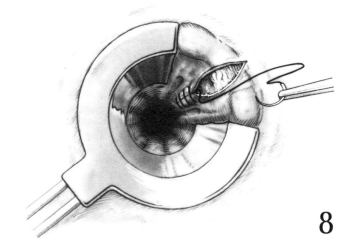

8

Remaining quadrants

9 The procedure is repeated in the other three quadrants. Provided that all suture lines are completed with the Fansler anoscope in place, the possibility of a subsequent anal stenosis is remote.

The previous suture lines are inspected to ensure that no bleeding is present, and a dry gauze dressing is placed on the perianal skin. No internal anal dressing is used.

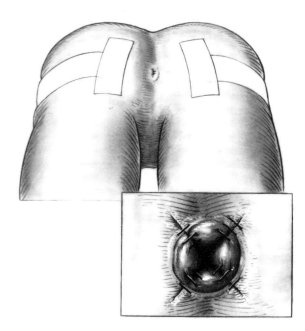

9

Postoperative care

The perianal dressings are changed as required; they can be discontinued after 48 h. Warm salt baths promote anal comfort and ambulation plus daily aperients encourage early bowel movement. Initially, pain is controlled with narcotic analgesia, but after 24–48 h a non-codeine oral analgesic is recommended. Anal mucosectomy is not as painful as haemorrhoidectomy because there is usually less removal of perianal skin.

Complications

Bleeding occurring within the first 24 h is caused by inadequate haemostasis during operation. Secondary haemorrhage at 7–10 days usually stops spontaneously, but occasionally requires direct suturing under anaesthesia. The incidence of secondary haemorrhage is approximately 1%. Disruption of a suture line is not an unusual event and the wound is allowed to heal by secondary intention. Urinary retention can occur and may require short-term catheterization.

Outcome

Small amounts of residual mucosal prolapse can usually be treated satisfactorily by sclerosant injection or rubber banding. Persistent straining at stool may result in minor recurrences of prolapse, particularly if there is weakness of the anal sphincter mechanism. The overall results of anal mucosectomy are most satisfactory.

Illustrations by Angela Christie

Anoplasty

Gregory C. Oliver MD
Associate Clinical Professor of Surgery, Robert Wood Johnson School of Medicine, Piscataway, New Jersey
and Muhlenberg Hospital, Plainfield, New Jersey, USA

Robert J. Rubin MD
Clinical Professor of Surgery, Robert Wood Johnson School of Medicine, Piscataway, New Jersey and
Muhlenberg Hospital, Plainfield, New Jersey, USA

Principles and justification

Anoplasty is a surgical procedure employed to reconstruct an anal defect utilizing local perianal tissues. The common conditions for which this technique is used are anal stenosis, mucosal ectropion and intractable recurrent anal fissures unresponsive to lateral internal sphincterotomy in a patient without a diarrhoeal disorder.

Two techniques are employed for anal stenosis depending on the severity of the underlying condition. Multiple anotomies may be performed for the more limited mucocutaneous scarring that may follow an amputative haemorrhoidectomy, while island flap advancement is selected for the major anal reconstructive procedures where there is significant loss of anoderm. A full-thickness island is preferred to a rotational flap in most cases, because it is simple to perform, surgical time is short, and it is readily accomplished under local anaesthesia with a very high success rate[1,2]. The standard V–Y skin advancement flap was attractive in the past because of its simplicity, but too often it is complicated by skin loss due to the precarious blood supply to the tip of the graft. This V–Y concept can be modified to an island flap with subsequent improvement in flap viability. The shape of the island flap is of importance only insofar as the flap configuration fills the anal canal defect without tension on the suture line.

An island flap is constructed by designing a suitably shaped piece of perianal skin which will comfortably fill the anal defect. A complementary partial internal lateral sphincterotomy may be performed beneath the anal incision to establish adequate luminal size before flap advancement. Most often the flap is diamond-shaped to replace loss of anoderm in patients with stenosis or triangular in the case of mucosal ectropion.

The advantage of the operation is that, in addition to the pliable full-thickness skin, adequate subcutaneous tissue is included with the flap. This easily allows the supple vascularized skin pedicle to be advanced into the anal defect. The inclusion of the subcutaneous tissue provides vascularity for the entire island flap, which improves graft viability and wound healing.

Preoperative

A sodium acid phosphate/sodium biphosphate enema is administered the evening before and the morning of the surgical procedure. Parenteral antibiotics should be considered perioperatively, as the wounds will soon be contaminated with the passage of faeces.

Anaesthesia

The procedure is routinely performed under local anaesthesia with bupivacaine hydrochloride 0.25% with adrenaline 1:200 000, adding hyaluronidase, 150 units, to each 30 ml of local anaesthetic solution used, complemented by intravenous sedation.

Operations

Position of patient

The operations are performed in the prone jack-knife position. The buttocks are taped laterally to the table for initial anal exposure, but these tapes should be released before suturing the flap in place to relieve wound closure tension.

ISLAND FLAP ADVANCEMENT FOR ANAL STENOSIS

Incision

1 The stenosis is viewed in the prone jack-knife position.

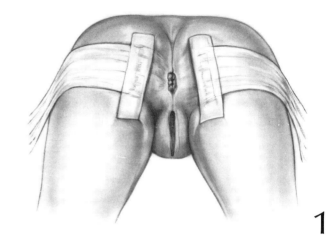

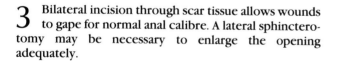

2 A lateral linear incision is made through the stenotic area. A lateral partial internal sphincterotomy may be needed. In the case of mucosal ectropion, a defect is created by excising the ectropion, and a triangular flap is advanced.

3 Bilateral incision through scar tissue allows wounds to gape for normal anal calibre. A lateral sphincterotomy may be necessary to enlarge the opening adequately.

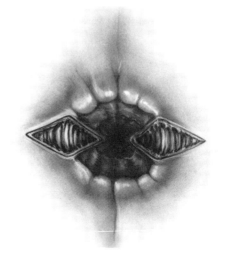

4 Island flaps are constructed so that perianal skin and attached subcutaneous and vascular elements will fill the defect created as described above. For mucosal ectropion correction, the flap is designed to fill the excisional defect. The diamond flap is usually twice as long as it is wide; it is really two isosceles triangles.

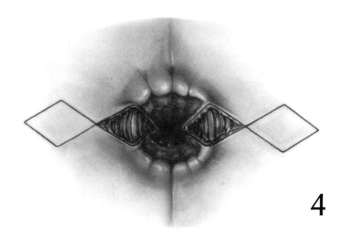

4

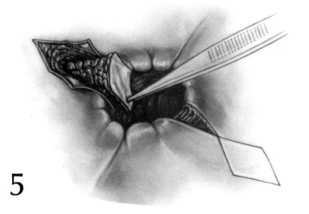

5

5 Full-thickness skin and subcutaneous tissue are incised deeply and circumferentially so that a tension-free island of tissue can slide into the stenotic defect. It is sutured in place with absorbable polyglycolic acid suture. Great care is taken not to undermine the flap, as this will disrupt its blood supply. This flap cannot be created over an area of scarring because its success depends on a supple, vascularized subcutaneous base.

6 The harvest sites are best closed primarily. This helps to hold the advanced island flap in place without tension.

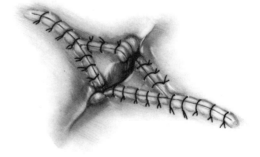

6

ISLAND FLAP ADVANCEMENT FOR NON-HEALING ANAL CANAL WOUNDS

7 Non-healing anal canal wounds are excised circumferentially, and the newly configured island flap is advanced into the proposed defect.

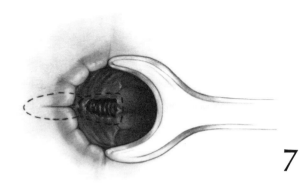

7

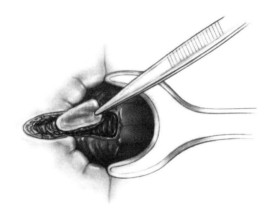

8

8 The fully mobilized island flap with its continuous vascular pedicle is advanced in a tension-free fashion to fill the previously excised defect.

9 The island flap is sutured in place to fill the excision site of the unhealed wound, and the donor site is closed.

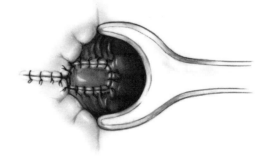

9

MULTIPLE ANOTOMIES FOR MILD TO MODERATE ANAL STENOSIS

10 The stenotic area is placed under tension. A Ferguson–Hill retractor is selected that will fit the anal canal without causing tearing.

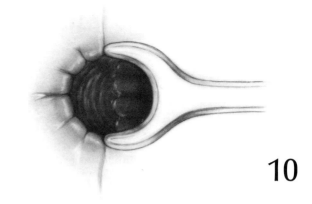

10

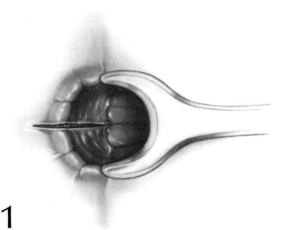

11

11 An incision is made through the stenotic tissue, thus locally releasing the stenosis and allowing the wound to gape.

12 The next larger size of Ferguson–Hill retractor is inserted when the anotomies are sufficient to permit it.

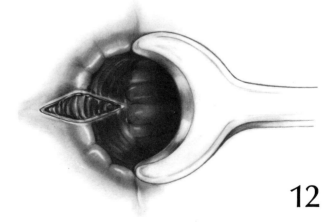

12

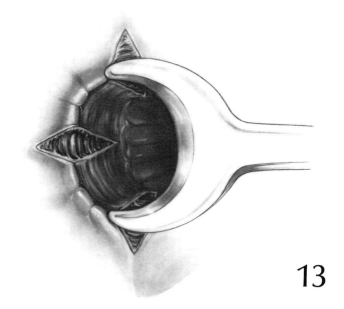

13 Enough anotomies (up to four quadrants) are made until the 3.5-cm diameter Ferguson–Hill retractor can be easily inserted. A partial lateral internal sphincterotomy may be performed with either the closed or open technique during the performance of anotomies to allow sufficient anal canal expansion. All wounds are left open to heal by secondary intent.

13

Postoperative care

When island flap advancements are selected as a technique to correct severe anal stenosis, the authors maintain intravenous antibiotic cover for perioperative prophylaxis (one preoperative and two postoperative doses). Additionally, a limited bowel-confining regimen, consisting of a clear liquid diet, oral codeine phosphate and diphenoxylate hydrochloride with atropine sulphate (Lomotil) is prescribed. This regimen is continued for 48 h.

Local wound care consists of painting the wounds with povidone-iodine solution twice daily and instituting sitz baths once bowel function has resumed. If a seroma or haematoma is noted beneath the flap, local evacuation is carried out.

When multiple anotomies are selected as a technique to correct mild to moderate stenosis, the authors do not use intravenous antibiotics nor a bowel-confining regimen. These patients can generally return home on the day of the operation.

Weekly clinic examinations are necessary until healing is complete, to ensure that restenosis does not occur. Digital dilatation of the healing anal canal may be necessary during follow-up.

References

1. Caplin DA, Kodner IJ. Repair of anal stricture and mucosal ectropion by simple flap procedures. *Dis Colon Rectum* 1986; 29: 92–4.

2. Pearl RK, Hooks VH, Abcarian H, Orsay CP, Nelson RL. Island flap anoplasty and mucosal ectropion for the treatment of anal stricture. *Dis Colon Rectum* 1990; 33: 581–3.

Illustrations by Angela Christie and the late Robert Lane

Perianal and anal condylomata acuminata

James P. S. Thomson DM, MS, FRCS
Consultant Surgeon and Clinical Director, St Mark's Hospital for Diseases of the Rectum and Colon, London, Honorary Consultant Surgeon, St Mary's Hospital, London, Honorary Lecturer in Surgery, The Medical College of St Bartholomew's Hospital, London, Civil Consultant in Surgery, Royal Air Force and Civilian Consultant in Colorectal Surgery, Royal Navy, UK

R. H. Grace FRCS
Consultant Surgeon, The Royal and New Cross Hospitals, Wolverhampton, UK

Principles and justification

Condylomata acuminata are caused by infection of stratified squamous epithelium with human papilloma virus (HPV); HPV types 6, 11, 16 and 18 are those usually recovered. A significant proportion of affected patients are homosexual.

This disease has an interesting natural history, because although most patients require treatment, spontaneous regression does occur. The presence of purple or black lesions among the more usual pink warts indicates that spontaneous regression might occur. Malignant change has been reported, but in the majority of patients the disease follows an entirely benign course with varying numbers of warts.

The condition known as 'giant condylomata', however, is a different and rare lesion. This is a very well differentiated squamous cell carcinoma, which usually extensively involves the anal canal and perianal skin and requires radical treatment.

Assessment

The diagnosis of perianal condylomata acuminata is usually obvious, but it is important to determine accurately the extent of the disease, because warts may also be present within the anal canal or lower rectum and on the external genitalia. In women (approximately one-fifth of affected patients), the vulva, vagina and cervix must be assessed. For all patients, recurrence is likely if not all the lesions are treated.

Differential diagnosis of perianal warts is condylomata lata, a secondary manifestation of syphilis. Condylomata acuminata are commonly transmitted by sexual contact, and other forms of sexually transmitted disease should be excluded. The cooperation of a physician who specializes in these diseases should be sought in the management of patients, not only to diagnose but also to screen for other sexually transmitted disorders, and contacts should be traced.

Principles of treatment

Small numbers of warts confined to the perianal skin may be treated by the repeated application of 25% podophyllum resin in compound benzoin tincture. Surgical treatment, however, will be required if: (1) there is no response to podophyllum, (2) there is extensive involvement of the perianal skin, and (3) if there is involvement of the anal canal and lower rectum.

The traditional method of removing condylomata acuminata used diathermy or electrocautery. Although this technique satisfactorily removed the lesions, it resulted in damage to the surrounding normal skin and to the base of the small wounds created after removal of the warts. Treatment of adjacent lesions resulted in a confluent area of tissue destruction with considerable discomfort in the postoperative period. Healing was slow, and scarring occasionally resulted in stenosis of the anal canal.

Scissor excision avoids the use of diathermy or cautery except in controlling the occasional persistent bleeding point. A solution of adrenaline 1:300 000 in physiological saline is injected subcutaneously and submucosally. This separates the warts from each other, because even large lesions have an area of normal skin between them. This allows the maximum amount of healthy skin and mucosa to be preserved when individual warts are removed by sharp-pointed scissors. The resulting small wounds heal rapidly with minimal discomfort to the patient. Usually, it is possible to remove all the warts on one occasion, but if there is a large number, removal may best be done in two stages with an interval of approximately 1 month.

Occasionally confluent lesions in the upper anal canal cannot be removed individually. Total circumferential submucosal excision is feasible, and as the extent is seldom more than 2 cm, the wound can be closed by inserting interrupted catgut sutures to approximate the lower rectal mucosa at the dentate line.

Laser equipment may be used, and an operating microscope may be of value, particularly for intra-anal lesions, which may be rendered white by applying acetic acid.

Preoperative

The rectum should be empty; a disposable enema the evening before operation usually provides adequate preparation.

Anaesthesia

This operation is best performed under general anaesthesia, but caudal anaesthesia provides adequate relaxation of the anal canal.

Small scattered lesions involving only the perianal skin can be excised after infiltration of local anaesthetic, but many patients find this difficult to endure.

Operation

1 Adrenaline 1:300000 in physiological saline is injected subcutaneously. Approximately 50–75 ml solution is injected into each perianal area. This is best done in quadrants so that the solution is injected in a particular area immediately before excision is begun; if all the solution is injected initially, absorption occurs and the benefit of the 'ballooning' effect is lost. While the injection is being given, the needle of the syringe should be moving so that an intravenous injection is avoided.

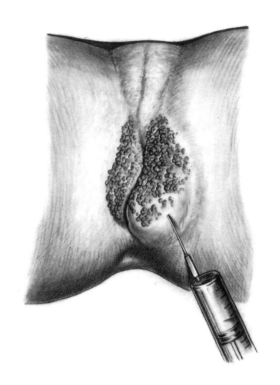

Excision of warts

2,3 Warts are individually removed, preserving as much normal skin as possible using a pair of fine-toothed forceps and scissors. There is usually little haemorrhage, but a persistent bleeding point may be controlled by diathermy.

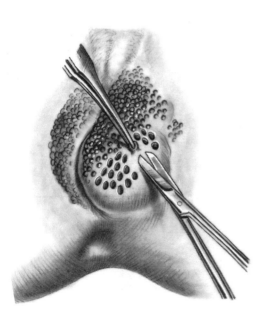

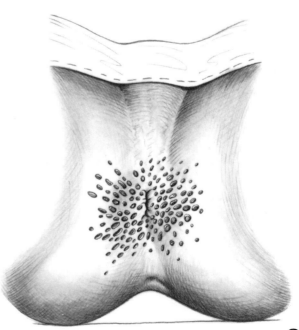

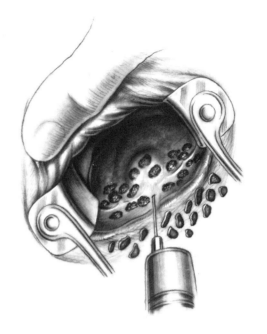

4

Removal of warts from within the anal canal

4, 5 With the aid of an anal retractor, such as the Parks' retractor, adrenaline is injected submucosally. The warts are again removed individually, preserving the mucosa between them. A large mucosal defect may be sutured with 3/0 chromic catgut to approximate the mucosa of the lower rectum to the dentate line.

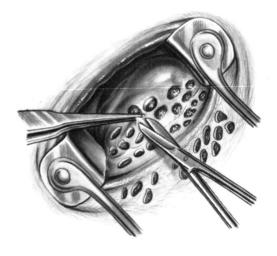

5

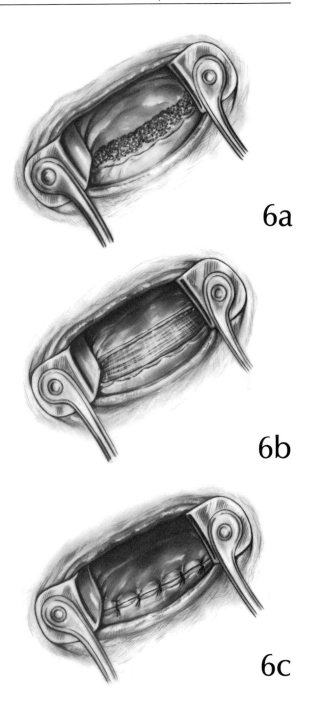

6a

6b

6c

Circumferential lesions

6a–c Circumferential lesions may be removed in the same way. The defect, which is seldom more than 2 cm in length, is closed by approximating the distal rectal mucosa to the line of the anal valves with about 12 fine catgut sutures.

Wound dressing

When all the warts have been removed, a gauze dressing soaked in physiological saline and enclosed within a sheet of Surgicel is inserted into the anal canal and used to cover the perianal area. A pressure dressing is then applied with the aid of a T bandage or with a pair of close-fitting elastic pants. The Surgicel acts as a haemostatic agent and also makes a very satisfactory non-stick dressing, because after 24 h it becomes very slippery, thus facilitating its removal.

Postoperative care

Little discomfort is experienced after this procedure, and the patient requires minimal analgesia. A normal diet should be started immediately after the operation, and the passage of a satisfactory stool is ensured by prescribing a bulk laxative. If extensive warts are removed from the anal canal, an anal dilator (No. 1 St Mark's dilator) should be passed twice a day with the aid of 1% lignocaine gel.

The warts can recur, and patients should be warned about this possiblity. If warts continue to recur after repeated operations, a chemotherapeutic ointment (5-fluorouracil) may be used. The role of this agent, however, in the treatment of condylomata acuminata requires further study.

Further reading

Prasad ML, Abcarian H. Malignant potential of perianal condyloma acuminatum. *Dis Colon Rectum* 1980; 23: 191–7.

Simmons P, Thomson JPS. Sexually transmitted diseases (and warts). In: Decosse JJ, Todd IP, eds. *Anorectal Surgery*. Edinburgh: Churchill Livingstone, 1988: 132–48.

Thomson JPS, Grace RH. The treatment of perianal and anal condylomata acuminata: a new operative technique. *J R Soc Med* 1978; 71: 180–5.

Procedures for pilonidal disease

John U. Bascom MD, PhD, FACS
Consulting and Attending Surgeon, Sacred Heart General Hospital, Eugene, Oregon, USA

History

Surgeons pursuing inappropriate goals may create pilonidal problems. The result can be great disability, long hospitalization and persistent open wounds, but the fault may not lie with the surgeon who only follows published but out-of-date recommendations. Both simple primary treatments that avoid complications and a curative operation for the complications of ill-advised surgery will be described.

Pilonidal disease was first described 150 years ago. It seemed a simple condition, but resulted in unexpected healing problems and unexplained recurrences. Some indolent wounds defied all treatment, although wide excision seemed to offer a solution. The use of wide excision increased during World War II until nearly 80 000 men had been hospitalized by 1945 for an average of 55 days each, in a vain attempt to cure the disease. Immobilization of these needed troops led the Surgeon General in the USA to issue an edict prohibiting wide *en bloc* excision and mandating simple linear incision.

In the past, the surgical approach has been to treat the secondary abscess rather than the two aetiological issues: the nearly invisible midline cutaneous 'pits', and the potent but invisible forces across the natal cleft.

In pilonidal disease, less treatment is better than more. The condition is often self-limiting and non-operative methods can cure[1]. Most pilonidal lesions create only a mild nuisance, and they are rare in patients older than 40 years. By contrast, most substantial problems associated with pilonidal disease are iatrogenic and therefore the surgeon must understand and confront the factors that create the disease to prevent these complications.

Principles and justification

Pilonidal cysts are not embryonic in origin and the disease is not congenital but acquired. Occasionally, congenital dimples will appear over the distal sacrum, but they do not give rise to pilonidal disease. Dimples are easily distinguished from pilonidal pores and are seldom a source of symptoms. Unusual midline epidermal cysts may develop over the lower spinal cord and communicate with the skin, but they are easily distinguished from pilonidal disease.

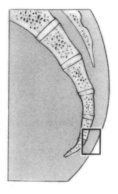
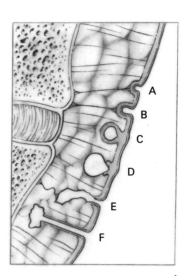

1

1 Pilonidal disease is a condition of the epidermis that begins with forces that stretch the normal hair follicle (A) in the natal cleft[2]. This results in a small hole in the skin called a 'pit' (B), which represents an enlarged hair follicle. Histological sections taken near a pilonidal pit show various sizes of enlarged hair follicles in otherwise normal skin. Each follicle holds a single hair surrounded by rings of keratin, and under these influences it becomes inflamed. When the mouth of the follicle becomes closed by inflammation (C), the combination of a 'vacuum' beneath the follicle and the pressure within the follicle drives keratin into the subcutaneous fat creating an acute abscess (D) with its associated pain caused by pus under pressure. A chronic abscess (E), the most common form of the disease, appears and persists after spontaneous or surgical drainage. Thus, by definition, this pilonidal lesion is an abscess and not a cyst because it has no epithelial lining.

In long-standing lesions, however, a tube of epithelium (F) may develop by slow growth down the wall of a chronic abscess. This lining develops no rete pegs and no skin structures or hair follicles. Tubes develop in approximately 10% of patients and are usually only 2–5 mm in length, but occasionally they may extend to 2 cm or more. Epithelial tubes must be removed or marsupialized to prevent the development of epithelial inclusion cysts.

The reduced subcutaneous pressure in the natal cleft, which is one of the factors that causes keratin to be drawn down through the thin base of the hair follicle, was identified and measured by Brearley[3]. The negative pressure develops because of the tension between the skin attachment to the midline skeleton and the weight of the hanging buttocks when a patient is in the erect position. Measurements show that most pilonidal pits develop precisely over the angle of the sacrum where the maximum negative pressure leads to follicle stretching and rupture.

Although hair shafts may play a role in the origin of the disease, hair appears in only half of these abscesses. Hair is often a secondary invader, however, gathered into the natal cleft and then sucked into the abscess cavity by the negative pressure already discussed and propelled by rubbing of tissue against the scales of shed hairs.

The natal cleft itself is of great aetiological importance. Pilonidal lesions occur only in skin clefts, most commonly the natal cleft, and never on convex surfaces. In severe disease, a surgeon's attempt to preserve the natal cleft may not only allow the condition to persist, but complex wounds sometimes develop because of the creation of a deep residual cleft, and the tension that pulls the skin away from the sacrum. Wounds under such tension do not heal, and the moist conditions in the cleft encourage the growth of anaerobic bacteria[4], which also interfere with healing. Thus, in severe disease, treatments to obliterate the cleft are always useful, while in primary disease, treatments to obliterate the cleft are only occasionally helpful.

Operations

ACUTE PILONIDAL ABSCESS

Indications and contraindications

All patients with acute pilonidal abscesses seek treatment for a hot, red, exquisitely tender bulge deep in the natal cleft; aspiration or open drainage provides relief of symptoms, with antibiotics being necessary after aspiration but not after open drainage.

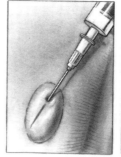
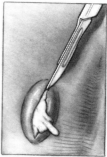
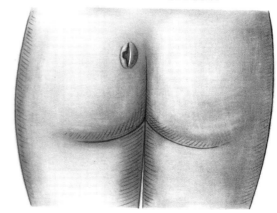

Anaesthesia

2 Patients appreciate the comfort of oral oxycodone before anaesthesia, but it is prompt drainage that relieves the pain. The effects of local anaesthesia are blunted in inflamed tissue, thus extensive infiltration is impractical and can be very painful. Slow superficial injection of the local anaesthetic mixture into the area of the incision is sufficient (bupivacaine hydrochloride, 0.5%, with adrenaline, 1:200000, and buffered 1:10 with sodium bicarbonate solution, 50 mmol/l).

Incision

The abscess can be aspirated, but this author prefers to incise it laterally. If an incision is used, the surgery to be performed on the abscess in its chronic form 1 week later can be anticipated by incising 2.5 cm from the midline. The knife blade is advanced through the fat towards the midline. When pus appears, advancement of the knife is stopped. The pus does not need to be cultured and the abscess cavity should not be packed. A 1-cm button of skin is cut away from the lateral edge of the incision, which prevents premature resealing and is less painful than packing. Daily showers should be encouraged, and a mini-pad to protect clothing from drainage is useful.

Outcome

Patients with an acute pilonidal abscess treated in this fashion will obtain comfort within hours of aspiration or open drainage. Although this treatment is incomplete, the abscess seldom requires redrainage within 7 days, by which time the midline pits become visible and can be excised (see method for chronic pilonidal abscess described below).

CHRONIC PILONIDAL ABSCESS

Indications and contraindications

A chronic abscess is the most common form of pilonidal disease and is best treated by abscess drainage and pit excision, but other options are also discussed below. Patients with a midline pit who complain of a discharge or natal cleft pain and those with recent acute drainage (even if they are currently asymptomatic) should be treated surgically, because a pocket of granulations is usually present.

Midline wounds larger than 1 cm, congenital midline dimples, pilonidal pits without symptoms and the chronic abscess of many years' duration which has multiple deep tracts (such tracts may extend in several layers down toward the sacrum and are better laid open and allowed to heal by second intention) are not suitable for this treatment. Care must be taken to identify the patient who complains of pain on sitting and has no natal cleft pit, but has a sharp spur on the coccyx. Removal of the spur through a laterally placed incision gives relief.

Drainage and pit excision

This procedure attacks the source of the disease but does not create a large unhealing wound. It is simple enough for office or outpatient use and patients can return to work the following day.

Preoperative

Preoperative aspirin users are best deferred for 3 weeks without aspirin to allow for platelet recovery. One hour before surgery, oxycodone is given for comfort during injection of local anaesthetic agent. Oral cephalexin, 250 mg, and metronidazole, 400 mg, are given orally at the same time. Before taping the buttocks apart, the separated buttocks are pulled in all directions to help identify all the pits; magnification and good lighting are of value.

Anaesthesia
Bupivacaine hydrochloride, 0.5%, with adrenaline, 1:200 000 (for less bleeding), provides prolonged local anaesthesia. Patients appreciate warmed solutions being applied to the skin and slow infiltration through a fine (number 30) needle is advocated. The addition of 1 ml of sodium bicarbonate solution (50 mmol/l) to each 10 ml of anaesthetic solution neutralizes the irritating effect of the local anaesthetic. Except for exceedingly sensitive patients, general anaesthesia is unnecessary.

Incision

Incisions in the midline should be avoided whenever possible. The forces and conditions that created the pilonidal problem will tend to disrupt a suture line. Thus, when entering the abscess cavity, one or more incisions should be placed laterally away from the midline.

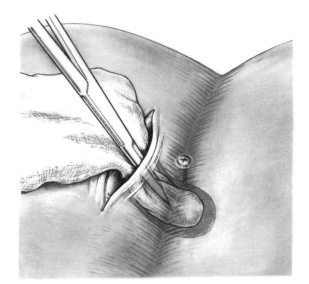

3 An incision is made 2.5 cm to one or both sides of the midline. The fat is left *in situ* on the overlying skin. The incision is made long enough to be able to see inside the entire cavity quite clearly. Incision length adds nothing to disability and does not delay healing. Scrubbing with gauze removes granulations, hair and debris. This scrubbing reveals a fibrous wall. Branch cavities must be carefully sought, and these need to be opened and scrubbed. In 10% of patients it is necessary to excise a small segment of fibrous abscess wall when infiltrated with hair.

3

4   The point of the haemostat is thrust into the cavity, directing it against the underside of the midline skin, and rubbed firmly. This identifies the follicle that started the trouble and other enlarged follicles that require removal.

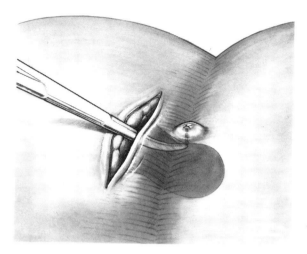

4

5   All enlarged pits are cut out, cleaned out and removed. The tip of a number 11 blade is used to excise the pit by taking a piece of tissue the size of a grain of rice. Multiple pits are excised individually as far as is feasible. The deep end of the removed specimen is inspected. A complete excision shows either soft, ill-defined, red-brown granulations or fibrous tissue. A tiny, clean, and 'macaroni-like' end, which is seen in about 5% of cases, indicates that a deeper part of an epithelial tube remains. This must be excised or inclusion cyst formation is likely.

Skin punches or curettes used vigorously is an alternative method of pit excision. The resulting small defects may be sutured with a subcuticular removable monofilament or allowed to heal secondarily.

The large lateral wound is left open to allow drainage. The lateral wound should not be packed because packing causes pain and serves no purpose.

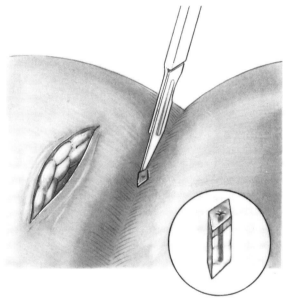

5

Postoperative care

Antibiotic coverage is continued for three doses. The patient should be encouraged to wash the wound with soap and water during a twice-daily shower. An immediate return to normal sitting and other activity should also be suggested. A dressing to protect clothing is useful. After 2 days a mini-pad inside the underwear suffices.

Sutures are removed on the seventh day. The patient is examined each week until certain of solid midline healing. Most patients need only one or two postoperative visits.

Complications
The most common complication is a slowly healing midline wound, which occurs in about 10% of patients. Most respond to careful local hygiene and shaving, but occasionally a wound will require a small pack, silver nitrate, or minimal marsupialization. The rare non-healing wound will yield to a smaller repeat of pit excision or to a Karydakis procedure. On rare occasions, patients have increasing pain and watery drainage in the postoperative period and this indicates superficial cellulitis which should be vigorously treated with appropriate antibiotics.

Outcome

The technique described above for lateral drainage of the abscess and excision of pits has been used in over 430 patients. Follow-up of 92% of 200 patients showed no large unhealed wounds. Treatment approached the ideal of no disability because half the patients returned to school or work the day following treatment. Mean healing time was 3 weeks and recurrent abscess or epithelial inclusion cysts appeared in only 5% of patients, with all recurrences being smaller than the original presenting problem.

Other treatment options

Non-operative management

6 The picking out of invading hairs, a few weekly local hair shavings, and emphatic instruction on cleanliness have healed many lesions, but the approach requires diligence. Results are not as prompt as those associated with pit excision, but the freedom from complications is unequalled.

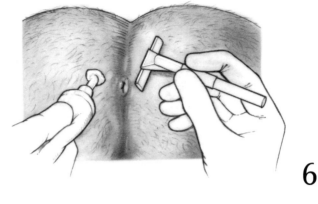

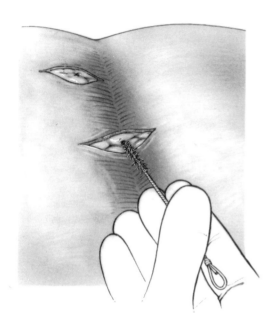

Pit excision and cavity brushing

7 This limited surgery is worth considering[5]. A transverse excision of the pit gives access to the cavity which can then be thoroughly cleaned. Unlike a vertical incision, the tissue tension associated with transverse incisions will tend to pull the wound closed rather than open.

Midline incision

8 A midline incision is acceptable if it lays open the cavity through all openings, but it is not recommended as initial treatment. Trimming back the skin edges prevents early closure. Deep tissues should not be removed. Marsupialization (suturing down the edges of the wound) may speed healing but may increase wound tension. The two disadvantages of midline vertical incision are the need for packing and the occasional resistant wound which does not heal. Such wounds, formerly disastrous, now fortunately respond to secondary repair described below. Primary closure should never be used after a midline incision because it is very often followed by recurrent sepsis and local skin breakdown.

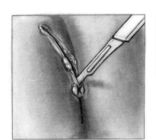

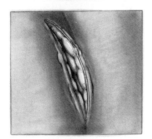

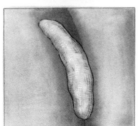

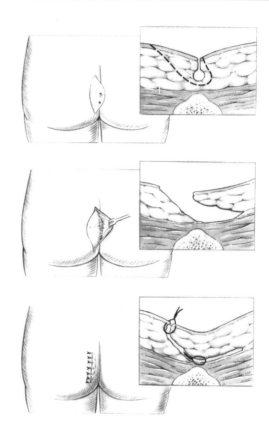

Karydakis operation[6]

9 An eccentrically placed skin excision is used followed by a limited excision of subcutaneous tissue. This method offers the advantages of incision closure, fresh skin is brought into the midline, and the natal cleft is flattened. The main disadvantages of the operation are the removal of substantial amounts of tissue and the mobilization of fat, which may risk postoperative abscess formation under the skin flap.

Procedures not recommended

There is no place in the treatment of chronic pilonidal abscess or any other pilonidal problem for wide midline excisional surgery. *En bloc* excisions down to the sacrum should never be used. This procedure attacks the wrong target. Such wounds suffer from slow healing or non-healing. Thus, the use of retention sutures or pressure packs have no place in current treatment of pilonidal disease.

9

COMPLEX PILONIDAL WOUNDS

Cleft closure

Indications and contraindications

Excessive and inappropriate pilonidal surgery may give rise to considerable patient morbidity with weeks in hospital, wounds packed open for years, or a succession of failed operative procedures. The cleft closure operation can resolve these problems and is indicated for any wound that remains unhealed at 3 months, for primary treatment of large or complex defects, and for any major secondary surgery. This operation should not be used, however, for most primary treatments nor for a small recurrent abscess with only a pinhole midline opening, which should be treated as a primary chronic abscess.

The four advantages of the operation are prompt and secure healing in even the largest wounds, stability in the presence of complications, suitability for outpatient surgery, and a low rate of recurrence. Furthermore, the operation moves the suture line away from the midline natal cleft. It heals without functional defect or significant cosmetic changes.

Preoperative

The patient should be assessed while he is standing, by marking the outer line of contact of the buttocks with a felt pen. A tentative repair is sketched on the patient's skin and then a gloved finger is used to explore the natal cleft with the patient sitting, bending and standing until the geometry of the closure is familiar.

Anaesthesia
General anaesthesia is required. Local anaesthetic suffices for smaller versions of this procedure. At the start of the operation, intravenous cefapirin sodium, 1 g, and metronidazole, 1 g, are given to protect against common pathogens including anaerobes.

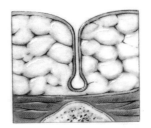

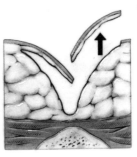

General principle

10 The general principle of the procedure is shown in the illustration. It accomplishes a skin transfer by lifting a flap of extra skin from the donor buttock and drawing it across the midline onto the recipient buttock.

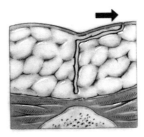

10

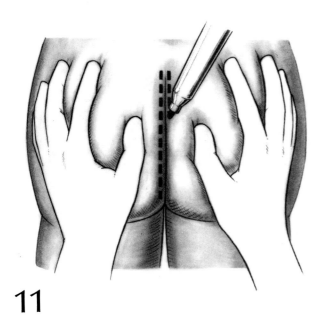

11

Incision

11 The patient is re-examined in the jack-knife position for rectal fistulae, a potent source of failure. The buttocks are pushed together and the outer line of their contact is marked with a felt pen.

12 The buttocks are taped apart and before skin preparation, bupivacaine hydrochloride and adrenaline are infiltrated to limit blood loss and give prolonged postoperative comfort. The incision for the donor flap should be sketched, with a view to raising the flap from the least damaged side of the natal cleft, full thickness and fat free.

The incision is commenced on the recipient side, off the midline and above the top of the natal cleft. The knife should slant down and across the midline at an acute angle just above the unhealed wound. Inferiorly, the incision turns sharply to cross the midline at right angles cephalad of the anus, and then it should turn again so that the lower end of the incision points towards the anus.

The skin from the midline incision is elevated to the surface of the donor buttock at the line of natural contact. Cephalad to the anus the perianal skin is weak. Therefore, the surgeon should leave some extra subcutaneous tissue attached. It may be necessary with low-lying wounds to extend undermining of the anal

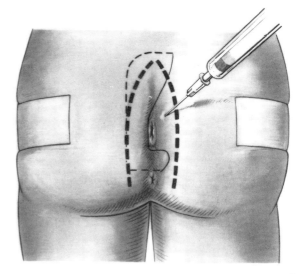

12

flap into the subcutaneous sphincter fibres. Rotation of this anal flap will relieve tension at the anal end of the closure and prevent skin necrosis. At the upper end of the incision, undermining continues above the top of the natal cleft, because leaving the upper cleft attached to the sacrum invites recurrence.

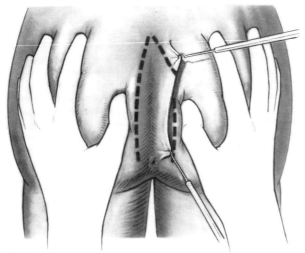

13

13 The recipient side is measured. The donor flap itself is used as a template. The tapes are released and the buttocks are pushed together. The donor flap is gently pulled across the midline. Any skin overlapped by the donor flap is marked for removal. A loose donor flap, which would fold down between the fat layers, should be avoided. Below the level of the end of the sacrum, the skin is marked for removal to the natural line of contact, but not beyond. The removal of more skin risks postoperative discomfort from skin tension while the patient is in the sitting position.

14 Skin to be discarded is elevated out to the marked limit of removal. This prepares a bed to receive the donor flap. It also unroofs the unhealed wound.

From the bed of the unhealed wound, granulations and debris are scrubbed away with gauze. The 2–3-mm sheet of scar that forms the base of the wound is excised. The scar will heal if left in place, but removal often relieves tissue tension to a surprising extent. To further free tissues, a knife is pulled across strands of scar in the fat between sacrum and buttock skin on each side. Fat or muscle should not be mobilized. As much fat as possible is saved to provide padding. Bleeders should be carefully cauterized.

Exposed fat over so vast an area gives alarm, but with release of the retracting tapes, the fat falls to the sacrum. Most of the raw surface disappears as fat from right meets fat from left. The donor flap covers the remainder. After a final check 'fit', skin from the recipient side is excised.

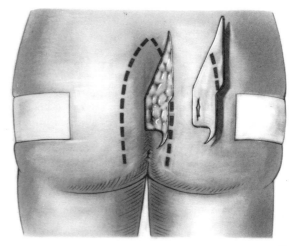

14

Wound closure

15 To finish cleft closure, a suction drain is pulled through a stab wound. The Blake drain gives the least pain on removal. The drain is sewn and taped securely because accidental removal delays healing. Fat is approximated with small bites of 4/0 polydioxanone suture to position the skin for closure. Closure is started by tacking the rotated anal flap roughly into position. The skin edges should now lie together without tension. Deep bites in fat for wound strength are unnecessary. The skin incision is closed with a subcuticular pull-out using 3/0 polypropylene and bringing a cross-stitch to the surface at intervals to simplify later removal. Sutures are reinforced with skin tapes. The wound is covered with a light dressing.

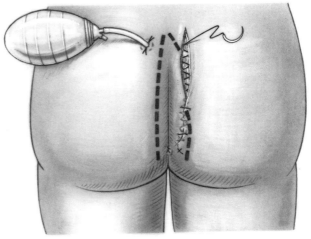

15

Postoperative care

The patient may be discharged after recovery from anaesthesia and may sit in the car on the way home. Written instructions should be given for daily showers, twice daily iodophore swabbing, changes of absorbent cotton near the anus four times daily, and 4 days of oral cephalexin and metronidazole at 250 mg each four times daily. The drain is removed at 4 days and the pull-out suture at 1 week. Examination should be performed weekly until healing is complete. Most patients resume activities on the fourth postoperative day.

Complications

Complications of cleft closure are uncommon. Infection responds quickly to opening the inferior 2 cm of the wound and administering antibiotics. Small patches of skin necrosis heal and do not affect the result. Haematomas respond best to evacuation under anaesthesia and reclosure over a drain. Postoperative discomfort on sitting is rare and largely avoidable. Irritated areas quickly respond to careful cleansing. Small recurrences respond to local revision and flattening.

Outcome

Thirty-five referred patients underwent cleft closure. They had sought help for recurrent disease after one to five operations, or for surgical incisions unhealed after periods of 6 months to 20 years. Most patients left the outpatient facility the day of cleft closure. Most wounds healed primarily, a few with minor intermittent discomfort. All wounds were healed within 3 months, and at 6 months to 7 years all wounds remain healed. Three chronic unhealed perineal wounds after total colectomy for Crohn's disease responded similarly.

Alternative procedures for complex wounds

Local care

Repeated local shaving and meticulous hygiene may help some complex wounds. Holding the buttocks apart with tape to allow the cleft to dry may occasionally help. This form of treatment, however, should not be prolonged because the likelihood of a good outcome is small.

Skin grafts

Split-thickness skin grafts to a granulating surface are seldom successful, and if on occasion a preliminary healing is achieved, the skin surface remains vulnerable. Therefore, split-thickness skin grafts are not recommended.

Z-plasty

16 Full thickness Z-plasty requires mobilization of fat and carries a suture line across the risk-prone midline natal cleft. The distal end of the Z is placed beside the cleft and not within it. In the author's experience, the cleft closure procedure is to be preferred.

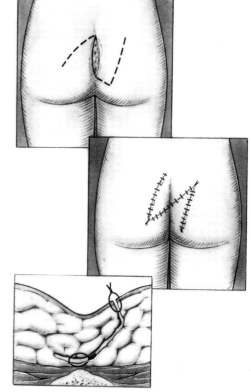

References

1. Allen-Mersh TG. Pilonidal sinus: finding the right track for treatment. *Br J Surg* 1990; 77: 123–32.

2. Bascom JU. Pilonidal disease: long-term results of follicle removal. *Dis Colon Rectum* 1983; 26: 800–7.

3. Brearley R. Pilonidal sinus: a new theory of origin. *Br J Surg* 1955; 43: 62–8.

4. Marks J, Harding KG, Hughes LE. Staphylococcal infection of open granulating wounds. *Br J Surg* 1987; 74: 95–7.

5. Lord PH, Millar DM. Pilonidal sinus: a simple treatment. *Br J Surg* 1965; 52: 298–300.

6. Karydakis GE. Easy and successful treatment of pilonidal sinus after explanation of its causative process. *Aust NZ J Surg* 1992; 62: 385–9.

16

List of products

Allen stirrups, Allen Medical Systems, Ohio, USA
Allis' clamps, Codman, Massachusetts, USA
Asepto syringe, Bectin-Dickensen, Franklin Lakes, New Jersey, USA

Babcock clamps, Codman, Massachusetts, USA

Cameron electrode, Cameron-Miller Inc, Chicago, Illinois, USA
CEEA stapler, US Surgical Corporation, Connecticut, USA/AutoSuture,
    Ascot, UK
CEEA premium stapler, US Surgical Corporation, Connecticut,
    USA/AutoSuture, Ascot, UK
Coloshield, Deknatel Inc, USA
Colyte, Reed and Carnrick, Pitscataway, New Jersey, USA

Dacron, Du Pont, Wilmington, Delaware, USA
Debakey forceps, Codman, Massachusetts, USA
Dennis clamp, Codman, Massachusetts, USA
Dexon, Davis & Geck, Gosport, UK
DHC stapler, Ethicon, Edinburgh, UK/Johnson & Johnson, Texas, USA

Eisenhammer retractor, Seward Medical, London, UK
Endo-Babcock, US Surgical Corporation, Connecticut, USA
Endo dissector, US Surgical Corporation, Connecticut, USA
Endo-Gauge, US Surgical Corporation, Connecticut, USA
Endo-GIA stapler, US Surgical Corporation, Connecticut, USA
Endo-Grasp, US Surgical Corporation, Connecticut, USA
Ethibond, Ethicon, Edinburgh, UK
Ethilon, Ethicon, Edinburgh, UK

Fansler anoscope, Baxter-Muller, Chicago, Illinois, USA

Gastrografin, Schering Health Care, UK
Gelfoam (gelatin sponge), Upjohn, Kalamazoo, Michigan, USA
Gelpi retractors, Aesculap, San Francisco, California, USA
GIA stapler, Autosuture, Ascot, UK/US Surgical Corporation,
    Connecticut, USA
Glassman clamp, Codman, Massachusetts, USA
GoLytely, Braintree Laboratories, Maryland, USA
Gore-tex, W L Gore & Associates, Flagstaff, Arizona, USA

Ivalon sponge implant (polyvinyl alcohol sponge), Unipoint
    Industries, North Carolina, USA

Karaya, Bullen, Liverpool, UK
Keith needle, Codman, Massachusetts, USA

Lang Stevenson's clamps, Codman, Massachusetts, USA
Lipiodol, May & Baker, Dagenham, UK
Lomotil, Searle, High Wycombe, UK
Lone Star retractor, Lone Star Medical Products, Houston, Texas, USA

Marlex, C P Bard, Massachusetts, USA
Maryland dissector, Solos, Georgia, USA
Maxon, Davis & Geck, Gosport, UK
Metzenbaum scissors, Codman, Massachusetts, USA
Mil-Par, Sterling Health, UK
Miltex scissors, Seward Medical, London, UK

Nelaton catheter, Indoplas, Sydney, Australia
NICE device, Neuromed, Florida, USA
Normacol, Norgine, Oxford, UK
NuLytely, Braintree Laboratories, Maryland, USA

PDS, Ethicon, Edinburgh, UK
Pennington forceps, Pilling, Philadelphia, USA
Picolax, Ferring, Middlesex, UK
Pratt bivalve speculum, Baxter Hospital, Illinois, USA
Prolene, Ethicon, Edinburgh, UK

Redivac, Biomet, Bridgend, UK
RL 60, Ethicon, Edinburgh, UK/Johnson & Johnson, Texas, USA
Roticulator 55, US Surgical Corporation, Connecticut, USA/
    AutoSuture, Ascot, UK

Salvati protoscope, Electro Surgical Instrument Co., Rochester, New
    York, USA
Satinsky clamp, Codman, Massachusetts, USA
Shoemaker's clamps, Codman, Massachusetts, USA
Silastic, Dow Corning, Reading, UK
Steridrape, Johnson & Johnson, Texas, USA
Steristrips, Johnson & Johnson, Texas, USA
Stomahesive, Johnson & Johnson, Texas, USA
Surgicel, Johnson & Johnson, Texas, USA
Surgilon, Johnson & Johnson, Texas, USA
Surgities, Johnson & Johnson, Texas, USA
Surgiwhips, US Surgical Corporation, Connecticut, USA

TA 55 stapler, AutoSuture, Ascot, UK/US Surgical Corporation,
    Connecticut, USA
TA premium stapler, AutoSuture, Ascot, UK/US Surgical Corporation,
    Connecticut, USA
Teflon, Du Pont, Wilmington, Delaware, USA
Ti-Cron, Ethicon, Edinburgh, UK
Tribiotic, 3M Health Care, Loughborough, UK
Tru-Cut, Travenol Laboratories, Thetford, UK/Deerfield, Illinois, USA

Unasyn, Roerig, New York, USA

Valley Lab diathermy, Valley Laboratory, Colorado, USA
Valtrac, Davis & Geck, New Jersey, USA
Ventrol drain, Mallinckrodt, Athlone, Eire
Vicryl, Ethicon, Edinburgh, UK

Index